Cardiac Electrophysiology Methods and Models

Daniel C. Sigg · Paul A. Iaizzo
Yong-Fu Xiao · Bin He
Editors

Cardiac Electrophysiology Methods and Models

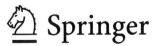 Springer

Editors
Daniel C. Sigg
Department of Integrative Biology
and Physiology
University of Minnesota Medical School
Minneapolis, MN
USA
siggx001@umn.edu

Yong-Fu Xiao
Cardiac Rhythm Disease Management
(CRDM)
Medtronic, Inc.,
Mounds View, MN
USA
yong-fu.xiao@medtronic.com

Paul A. Iaizzo
Department of Surgery
University of Minnesota
Minneapolis, MN
USA
iaizz001@umn.edu

Bin He
Department of Biomedical Engineering
University of Minnesota
Minneapolis, MN
USA
binhe@umn.edu

ISBN 978-1-4419-6657-5   e-ISBN 978-1-4419-6658-2
DOI 10.1007/978-1-4419-6658-2
Springer New York Dordrecht Heidelberg London

Library of Congress Control Number: 2010934635

Springer is part of Springer Science+Business Media (www.springer.com)

Preface

Cardiovascular disease is the major cause of morbidity and mortality worldwide. While significant progress has been made in treating some major subcategories of cardiac disease, such as arrhythmias and ischemic heart disease, significant unmet needs remain. This, in turn, implies a great need for future basic, applied, and clinical research and, ultimately, therapeutic developments.

Even with major medical advances, every day in the USA alone, thousands of patients die due to the underlying arrhythmias. In this disease category, atrial fibrillation is the most common arrhythmia, affecting millions of patients around the world at any given time. To understand its complex causes in varied populations, the underlying mechanisms, and/or optimal therapies, the scientific and medical communities face tremendous challenges, and this requires great effort and cooperation. In other words, there is currently a major public need to continue to develop new and better therapies for treating or preventing arrhythmias. Accordingly – and fortunately – an ever-increasing number of biomedical, pharmaceutical, and medical personnel are interested in studying various aspects of arrhythmias at basic, translational, and applied levels. Not only has our overall understanding of the molecular basis of disease dramatically increased, but we are also seeing a growing number of available and emerging molecular, pharmacological, and device treatment-based therapies.

We recognize that there is a need, albeit one that poses a great challenge, to provide guidance for researchers in this field in the form of a practical, state-of-the-art handbook dedicated to cardiac electrophysiology models and methods. As such, one of our primary goals was to showcase the various authors' expertise on key research methods and protocols, pinpointing their advantages and pitfalls, and provide readers with a single resource with a focus on practical implementation and collaborative cross-functional research. Further, it was our vision to create this book, which is very much focused on practical methods and implementation, and yet provide enough theory so that the principles can be clearly understood and easily applied. Finally, it should be noted that this textbook has been primarily written by scientists and clinicians from various leading academic and industrial research institutions from across the globe, whose work has had a major impact on arrhythmia research.

We hope that this textbook will be a helpful reference for those teaching and/or studying cardiac electrophysiology. We are grateful to all the authors for their excellent contributions, to Monica Mahre for her outstanding administrative support, and to Springer publishers for making this book a reality.

Twin Cities of Saint Paul and Minneapolis,   Daniel Sigg, MD, PhD
Minnesota, USA,   Yong-Fu Xiao, MD, PhD
October 28, 2009   Bin He, PhD
                                                                   Paul A. Iaizzo, PhD

Contents

Part III   Putting It All Together

Contributors

David G. Benditt, MD, FACC, FHRS, FRCPC
Department of Medicine, University of Minnesota, Minneapolis, MN, USA

Rudolf Billeter, PhD
School of Biomedical Sciences, Queens Medical Centre, University of Nottingham
Medical School, Nottingham, UK

Mark R. Boyett, PhD
Cardiovascular Medicine, School of Medicine, University of Manchester,
Manchester, UK

Jacques M.T. de Bakker, PhD
Department of Experimental Cardiology, Academic Medical Center,
Amsterdam, The Netherlands

Halina Dobrzynski, PhD
Cardiovascular Medicine, School of Medicine, University of Manchester,
Manchester, UK

J. Kevin Donahue, MD
Heart and Vascular Research Center, Case Western Reserve University
School of Medicine, Cleveland, OH, USA

David Donaldson, MD
Heart Center, Massachusetts General Hospital, Boston, MA, USA

Michael D. Eggen, PhD
Departments of Surgery and Biomedical Engineering, University of Minnesota,
Minneapolis, MN, USA

Michael Fauler
Institute of Applied Physiology, Ulm University, Ulm, Germany

MaryAnn Goldstein, MD
Pediatric Emergency Medicine, Minneapolis, MN, USA

Ian D. Greener, PhD
Heart and Vascular Research Center, Case Western Reserve University
School of Medicine, Cleveland, OH, USA

Bin He, PhD
Department of Biomedical Engineering, University of Minnesota, Minneapolis,
MN, USA

Alexander J. Hill, PhD
Department of Surgery, University of Minnesota and Medtronic, Inc.,
Mounds View, MN, USA

Boris Holzherr
Institute of Applied Physiology, Ulm University, Ulm, Germany

Peter J. Hunter, PhD
Auckland Bioengineering Institute, The University of Auckland,
New Zealand

Paul A. Iaizzo, PhD
Department of Surgery, University of Minnesota, Minneapolis, MN, USA

Deborah A. Jaye, MS
Cardiac Rhythm Disease Management, Medtronic, Inc., Mounds View, MN, USA

Karin Jurkat-Rott, MD
Institute of Applied Physiology, Ulm University, Ulm, Germany

Rodolphe P. Katra, PhD
Department of Biomedical Engineering, College of Engineering, University of
Alabama at Birmingham, Birmingham, AL, USA

Pipin Kojodjojo, MRCP, PhD
Department of Cardiology, St. Mary's Hospital and Imperial College Healthcare
NHS Trust, London, UK

Timothy G. Laske, PhD
Department of Surgery, University of Minnesota, Medtronic, Inc., Minneapolis,
MN, USA

Jong-Kook Lee, MD, PhD
Department of Cardiovascular Research, Research Institute of Environmental
Medicine, Nagoya University, Nagoya, Japan

Frank Lehmann-Horn, MD
Institute of Applied Physiology, Ulm University, Ulm, Germany

Xiaohuan Li, MD
Department of Medicine, Cardiovascular Division, University of Minnesota,
Minneapolis, MN, USA

Chenguang Liu, MS
Department of Biomedical Engineering, University of Minnesota, Minneapolis, MN, USA

Fei Lü, MD, PhD, FACC, FHR
Department of Medicine, Cardiovascular Division, University of Minnesota, Minneapolis, MN, USA

Louisa Malcolme-Lawes, MRCP, BSc
Department of Cardiology, St. Mary's Hospital and Imperial College Healthcare NHS Trust, London, UK

Abdul Mansoor, MD, PhD
Department of Medicine, University of Minnesota, Minneapolis, MN, USA

Moussa Mansour, MD
Heart Center, Massachusetts General Hospital, Boston, MA, USA

Gwilym M. Morris, MRCP, MA, BmBCh
Cardiovascular Medicine, School of Medicine, University of Manchester, Manchester, UK

John T. Nguyen, MD, MP
Department of Medicine, Cardiovascular Division, University of Minnesota, Minneapolis, MN, USA

David P. Nickerson, PhD
Auckland Bioengineering Institute, The University of Auckland, New Zealand

Alena Nikolskaya, PhD
Medtronic, Inc., Minneapolis, MN, USA

Mohammad Nurulqadr Jameel, MD
Department of Medicine, University of Minnesota, Minneapolis, MN, USA

James C. Perry, MD, FACC, FHRS
Department of Pediatrics, Cardiology Division, University of California San Diego/Rady children's Hospital, San Diego, CA, USA

Nicholas S. Peters, MRCP, FRCP, MD
Department of Cardiology, St. Mary's Hospital and Imperial College Healthcare NHS Trust, London, UK

Jason L. Quill, PhD
Departments of Surgery and Biomedical Engineering, University of Minnesota, Minneapolis, MN, USA

Eric S. Richardson, PhD
Departments of Surgery and Biomedical Engineering, University of Minnesota, Minneapolis, MN, USA

Scott Sakaguchi, MD, FACC, FHRS
Cardiovascular Division, Department of Medicine, University of Minnesota,
Minneapolis, MN, USA

Tushar V. Salukhe, MRCP, MD
Department of Cardiology, St. Mary's Hospital and Imperial College Healthcare
NHS Trust, London, UK

Vinod Sharma, PhD
Cardiac Rhythm Disease Management, Medtronic, Inc., Minneapolis, MN, USA

Daniel C. Sigg, MD, PhD
Department of Integrative Biology and Physiology, University of Minnesota,
Minneapolis, MN, USA

Nicholas D. Skadsberg, PhD
Medtronic, Inc., Mounds View, MN, USA

Bruce H. Smaill, PhD
Auckland Bioengineering Institute and Department of Physiology,
University of Auckland, Auckland, New Zealand

Maria Strom, MS
Heart and Vascular Research Center, Case Western Reserve University
School of Medicine, Cleveland, OH, USA

Richard Sutton, DScMed, FRCP, FACC, FHRS, FESC
Europace, St. Mary's Hospital and Imperial College, London, UK

Yukiomi Tsuji, MD, PhD
Department of Cardiovascular Research, Research Institute of Environmental
Medicine, Nagoya University, Nagoya, Japan

Harold V.M. van Rijen, PhD
Department of Medical Physiology, University Medical Center Utrecht,
Utrecht, The Netherlands

Yong-Fu Xiao, MD, PhD
Cardiac Rhythm Disease Management, Medtronic, Inc., Mounds View, MN, USA

Joseph Yanni
School of Medicine, University of Manchester, Manchester, UK

Chapter 1
Clinical Cardiac Electrophysiology: An Overview of Its Evolution

David G. Benditt, Scott Sakaguchi, MaryAnn Goldstein, and Richard Sutton

Abstract Clinical cardiac electrophysiology represents a convergence of five key medical sciences, each with a unique (albeit occasionally overlapping) evolutionary history. Without any one of the following five elements, the modern clinical cardiac electrophysiologist would be less well equipped to address many common problems as effectively as currently expected: (1) electrocardiographic assessment; (2) device therapy including pacing, defibrillation, and monitoring; (3) intracardiac recordings, stimulation, and/or autonomic assessments; (4) mapping (both epicardial and endocardial) with associated imaging and/or navigation; and (5) pharmacologic therapies such as antiarrhythmic and anticoagulation drugs.

This chapter is designed to provide readers with a brief overview of the evolution of each of these aspects of modern clinical cardiac electrophysiology practice, and also to illustrate how they interact to facilitate our understanding and treatment of common clinical conditions. Inevitably, space and time preclude a comprehensive review of each subject. Such a review would span more than 100 years, encompass contributions from throughout the world, and emanate from the effort and insight of scientists, engineers, clinicians, and often volunteers and patients too numerous to mention. Furthermore, in many cases the origin of seminal work remains controversial. As a result, some readers may differ with our interpretation of some of the cited events. Nevertheless, our primary goal is to provide an appropriate perspective that will enhance appreciation of the more detailed and focused chapters to follow.

1.1 Electrocardiography

Electrocardiography (ECG) is perhaps the most fundamental of all the sciences that make up modern clinical electrophysiology. Without these essential body surface recordings of the heart's electrical action and the amazingly insightful interpretations

D.G. Benditt (✉)
Department of Medicine, University of Minnesota, Minneapolis, MN, USA
e-mail: bendi001@umn.edu

D.C. Sigg et al. (eds.), *Cardiac Electrophysiology Methods and Models*,
DOI 10.1007/978-1-4419-6658-2_1, © Springer Science+Business Media, LLC 2010

received from clinicians long before an electrode catheter was ever inserted into the human heart, the development of modern clinical cardiac electrophysiology may not have materialized. It was the need to better understand ECG findings that primarily led to studies of the cardiac conduction system and the underlying mechanisms of elicited arrhythmias; only then was it possible to develop current approaches to treatment, including pharmacologic, interventional, and/or surgical therapies.

The study of heart rhythm, and occasionally rhythm disturbances, dates back many centuries. Descriptions of pulse examination are found dating from the sixteenth-century BC in Egypt, the eighth-century BC in China, and the third-century BC in Greece (including notable observations on irregular pulses by Galen in the second-century AD).[1] However, it was not until the second half of the nineteenth century that recordings of the heart's electrical activity from the body surface set the stage for the modern era of heart rhythm analysis and treatment.

Augustus Waller is credited with recording the first cardiac body surface ECG tracing.[2] Waller was born in Paris in 1856, but ultimately became a professor of physiology at the University of London, and made his landmark recordings at St Mary's Hospital in London in 1887. Interestingly, St Mary's Hospital remains a busy medical facility today (Fig. 1.1), and continues to be notable for contributions to heart rhythm study and care. Waller is also credited with popularizing the term

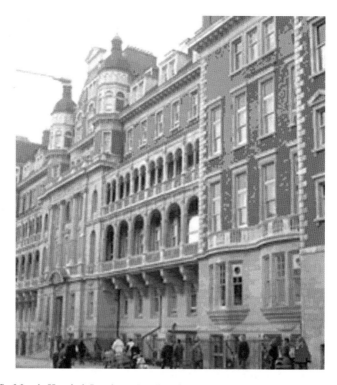

Fig. 1.1 St. Mary's Hospital, London, UK. Site of Waller's first ECG recordings

electrocardiogram for English usage (Willem Einthoven used the term as early as 1905, but in Dutch[3]) when he used it in the title of a 1917 paper presented before the Physiological Society of London ("A Survey of 2000 Electrocardiograms"). In any case, despite Waller's important contributions, the birth of modern electrocardiography is most often credited to Einthoven, working in The Netherlands.[3,4] Einthoven began to work on ECG recording in the mid-1890s using methods similar to those used by Waller, but it was his subsequent development of the string galvanometer and his publication of these methods in 1903 that ultimately placed ECG recording in the realm of worldwide accessibility. Additionally, Einthoven importantly innovated the lettering code still used for ECG description (P, Q, R, S, T), and described the use of the bipolar limb leads and the so-called Einthoven triangle, a concept that continues to be used by modern electrocardiographers to describe ECG features. Rightly so, Einthoven received a Nobel Prize for this work in 1924.

Perhaps the single most important contributor to ECG and arrhythmia analysis in the first half of the twentieth century (and still considered one of the most important arrhythmologists of all time) was Sir Thomas Lewis. Working in London in the 1920s and 1930s, Sir Thomas was both an experimentalist as well as a clinician; his analysis of virtually every recorded cardiac arrhythmia set the standard for future workers. He published numerous scientific papers related to heart rhythm analysis along with several books, each of which is considered a classic. In particular, his landmark book "The Mechanism and Graphic Registration of the Heart Beat" remains not only a collector's item (Fig. 1.2) but, more importantly, is an exceedingly insightful teaching tool for even the modern interventional electrophysiologist.[5] For example, the concept of the *ladder diagram* to analyze cardiac conduction and arrhythmias is derived from Sir Thomas' approach to the evaluation of cardiac arrhythmias.

In terms of American electrocardiography, Paul Dudley White is reputed to have established the first ECG laboratory in the United States, in 1914, after spending a year in London under the tutelage of Sir Thomas. However, while widely regarded as one of America's most important cardiologists from the 1920s until his death in 1973, his most evident contribution to arrhythmology was the 1930 publication (along with Louis Wolff of Boston and the eminent English cardiologist John Parkinson) of the manuscript describing Wolff–Parkinson–White (WPW) syndrome (Fig. 1.3).[6] This condition ultimately became the *Rosetta Stone* for cardiac electrophysiologists attempting to understand reentry as a basis for clinical tachyarrhythmias in the human heart. It should be noted that, at approximately the same time as the publication of the description of WPW syndrome, Frank N. Wilson, working at the University of Michigan, introduced unipolar chest leads using the *Wilson terminal* as the ground for each electrode. Importantly, this concept remains in use today in all ECG laboratories.[7]

During the 1930s and through the period of World War II, the study of cardiac arrhythmias using the ECG gradually migrated from Europe to the United States. Primarily, it was the exodus of scientists from Europe during this time period that facilitated the subsequent prominence of the United States in the field of arrhythmology. Relative to this period, many important names could be listed as having

THE MECHANISM

AND

GRAPHIC REGISTRATION

OF

THE HEART BEAT

BY

SIR THOMAS LEWIS, M.D., F.R.S., F.R.C.P., D.Sc., C.B.E.,

Honorary Consulting Physician, Ministry of Pensions;
Late Consulting Physician in Diseases of the Heart (Eastern Command);
Physician of the Staff of the Medical Research Council;
Physician and Lecturer in Cardiac Pathology, University College Hospital, London;
Fellow of University College, London.

3rd Edition.

LONDON :
SHAW & SONS Ltd., FETTER LANE, FLEET STREET, E.C.4.
Printers and Publishers.

Fig. 1.2 Front page of Sir Thomas Lewis' "The Mechanism and Graphic Registration of the Heart Beat, 3rd edition"[5]

made relevant contributions, but perhaps the most notable were Alfred Pick and Richard Langendorf (interestingly backed by Louis N. Katz, one of the most influential cardiologists of his day). Both Pick and Langendorf were alumni of the University of Prague (studying under the noted electrocardiographer and arrhythmologist Max Winternitz) and worked there together prior to World War II. Langendorf escaped to the USA in 1939. Pick fortunately survived the war in Europe, and subsequently arrived in the USA in the late 1940s, joining Langendorf and Katz in Chicago. Not surprisingly, numerous interesting and notable anecdotes are ascribed to these individuals. Often such stories began with those related to Langendorf's efforts to "recruit" Pick out of war-torn Europe. The more recent

The American Heart Journal

| VOL. V | AUGUST, 1930 | No. 6 |

Original Communications

BUNDLE-BRANCH BLOCK WITH SHORT P-R INTERVAL
IN HEALTHY YOUNG PEOPLE PRONE TO
PAROXYSMAL TACHYCARDIA

LOUIS WOLFF, M.D., BOSTON, MASS., JOHN PARKINSON, M.D., LONDON,
ENG., AND PAUL D. WHITE, M.D., BOSTON, MASS.

Fig. 1.3 Title from manuscript describing Wolff–Parkinson–White syndrome[6]

vignettes, dating from the 1960s and 1970s, relate to the general understanding that, at major scientific meetings after an arrhythmia abstract presentation, nobody stood to ask a question until Dr. Pick had had an opportunity to do so; as such, everyone in the room waited patiently, except for the speaker. Additionally, many of the current most senior clinical cardiac electrophysiologists will clearly recall their personal stories surrounding the trepidation associated with being called to the front of the room to analyze "unknown" ECGs (with very thick noisy baselines characteristic of older ECG recorder systems) during the annual Pick–Langendorf "Interpretation of Cardiac Arrhythmias" course held at Chicago's Michael Reese Medical Center (usually in the depth of winter). This was *the* original interactive teaching course and ran for approximately 25 years (ending in 1980); it can reasonably be considered the precursor of today's well-known (and comparably anxiety provoking) teaching course led twice each year by Mark Josephson and Hein Wellens.

It should be emphasized that Pick and Langendorf's insightful analyses of complex arrhythmias using only the surface ECG were remarkable. Among the many novel concepts derived from their studies of complex arrhythmias were *concealed conduction* (now recognized daily in clinical electrophysiology practice), the presence of nonconducted His bundle extrasystoles (a rare event, but usually good for one question on clinical electrophysiology board examinations), and the presence of *mother* and *daughter* waves in atrial fibrillation. In regard to the latter point, the concept of mother and daughter waves remains a topic central to the world of atrial fibrillation ablation. "In fibrillation, the mother circus ring is still supposed to be present, but its diameter is shorter, and the pattern of both its path and that of its daughter impulses is variable" (p. 406).[8]

It is important to note that, in subsequent investigations employing advanced intracardiac recordings, modern electrophysiologists have substantiated most of Langendorf's and Pick's insights, providing evidence of their brilliance. Their work is summarized in a 1956 classic textbook "Clinical Electrocardiography" by Professors Katz and Pick, which is an extension of an earlier 1941 volume by Katz; the 1956 book is difficult to find, but very much worth the effort (Fig. 1.4).[8]

Clinical
Electrocardiography

Part I

THE ARRHYTHMIAS

WITH AN ATLAS
OF ELECTROCARDIOGRAMS

By

LOUIS N. KATZ, A.B., M.A., M.D., F.A.C.P.

DIRECTOR, CARDIOVASCULAR DEPARTMENT, MICHAEL REESE HOSPITAL,
CHICAGO, ILLINOIS; PROFESSORIAL LECTURER IN PHYSIOLOGY,
UNIVERSITY OF CHICAGO, CHICAGO, ILLINOIS

AND

ALFRED PICK, M.D.

PHYSICIAN-IN-CHARGE OF HEART STATION AND RESEARCH ASSOCIATE,
CARDIOVASCULAR DEPARTMENT, MICHAEL REESE HOSPITAL,
CHICAGO, ILLINOIS

Illustrated With 415 Engravings

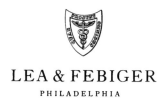

LEA & FEBIGER
PHILADELPHIA

Fig. 1.4 Front page from Katz and Pick's classic arrhythmia book[8]

The 1950s and 1960s represented an era in which the spread of ECG technology inevitably resulted in a widening of academic study of the ECG, and in-depth analyses of atrioventricular (AV) conduction disturbances (including bundle branch block) and various tachyarrhythmias. Further, interest in the prognostic implications of ECG findings fueled the novel incorporation of ECG records (never officially used before, even in the selection of aircrew during World War II) into major epidemiological enterprises exemplified by the Framingham study and the University of Manitoba Heart follow-up study. During this same period, Mauricio Rosenbaum, working in Buenos Aires, contributed the concept of *hemiblocks* (also termed fascicular blocks, 1967)[9]; Francois Desertenne in France introduced the term *torsade de pointes* (1966) for a unique form of ventricular tachycardia[10]; and Leo Schamroth, a Belgian by birth who spent all of his productive work career in South Africa, published perhaps the most comprehensive treatises on the ECG evaluations of cardiac arrhythmias.[11] Of interest, these latter works are not well known to current generation cardiologists and electrophysiologists in the United States, most of whom are much more familiar with the teachings of Henry Marriott, Schamroth's Bermuda-born English-trained American competitor.[12]

From the mid-1980s until today, one additional ECG challenge remained to be explored, namely the use of ECG recordings in one form or another to provide sudden cardiac death risk stratification.[13–15] To this end, ECG recording techniques provided insight on (1) signal-averaged ECG; (2) heart rate variability; (3) microvolt T-wave alternans; and more recently (4) heart rate turbulence. Unfortunately to date, none of these methods has met expectations in terms of positive predictive value for identifying high-risk individuals.

By the mid-1980s, excluding the risk stratification aspect just mentioned, a new era of ECG analysis began to emerge, one that is associated with the development of intracardiac and intraoperative electrogram recordings and initial forays into cardiac activation mapping. However, before proceeding with that aspect of clinical electrophysiology, we should alter course somewhat in our historic review to discuss the temporally parallel efforts in the 1950s–1970s that resulted in the birth of device-based therapies for treatment of cardiac rhythm disturbances.

1.2   Device Therapy: Pacing, Defibrillation, and Monitoring

It is considered reasonable to identify the historical origins of *implantable device therapy* to when there was a totally implantable system capable of reliably stimulating a heart that, left on its own, had an inadequate intrinsic rate. This point in time is best assigned to1958, when the first totally implanted pacing system was placed in a patient by a team led by surgeon Ake Senning and engineer designer Rune Elmqvist in Sweden.[16–18] Although this first implant was effective only for a few hours, it was a landmark achievement. In fact, this patient had subsequent implants and survived for over 40 years, becoming a well-known personality in medical circles (e.g., he was a frequent guest at events sponsored by many of the most well-known pacemaker companies, whose devices he ultimately utilized).

Subsequent to the initial application of the most basic fixed-rate, nonprogrammable, asynchronous short-lived implantable pacemakers, the evolution of implantable devices progressed rapidly to provide (1) increasingly more physiologic pacemaker capabilities with longevities exceeding a decade; (2) the ability to terminate tachycardias by rapid stimulation methods, cardioversion, and/or defibrillation capabilities;

(3) long-term diagnostic monitoring; and most recently (4) hemodynamic support. The history of this evolution is complex and thus will only be briefly summarized here.

1.2.1 Early Development

Solitary reports exist regarding early twentieth-century experiences with electrical cardiac stimulation at various sites from Europe to Australia. Nevertheless, credit for the earliest practicable electrical cardiac stimulator is generally accorded to Alfred Hyman who, working in New York in the early 1930s, developed a portable electrical clock-generator that successfully stimulated hearts in an experimental setting by means of a transthoracic needle. Hyman also seems to have been the first to coin the term *artificial pacemaker*, and also reported its use in a patient.[16,18–20] The stimuli were applied to the right atrium via a transthoracic needle. The device was intended for use during resuscitation but its use aroused considerable adverse criticism and the experiments were abandoned. During this period, clinical use remained sporadic and scientific clinical studies were never initiated, in part due to the intervention of World War II.

The late 1940s witnessed increased interest in cardiac stimulation during surgery. Among the more prominent contributions at the time was the work of Bigelow, Callaghan, and Hopps from Toronto, who stimulated the right atrium by a transvenous approach during open-heart surgery using a device powered from a wall plug.[16,18] The electrode was bipolar and proved to be the forerunner of today's stimulation leads. Unfortunately, at this time they had not thought to stimulate the heart from the ventricles.

In the early 1950s, Zoll succeeded in pacing the heart by using two external skin-mounted chest electrodes connected to an external pacemaker.[16,21] Interestingly, this concept remains available today as part of a comprehensive external cardioverter-defibrillator system in which the cutaneous electrodes offer backup pacing capability. However, because of discomfort due to this type of pacing, this approach is not widely used except in the most dire bradycardic emergencies. More specifically, transcutaneous pacing tends to activate skeletal muscles and pain fibers as well as initiate skin inflammation, thereby having the potential for causing considerable morbidity. Fortunately, the need for widespread use of transcutaneous pacing was short-lived. In August 1958, Seymour Furman, then a surgical resident at Montefiore Hospital, Bronx, New York (and later one of the founding members of the North American Society of Pacing and Electrophysiology, now the Heart Rhythm Society) introduced a transvenous electrode into the right ventricle and succeeded in stimulating the heart for 96 days[22]; once again, this pacemaker required power from an external source. Meanwhile, in the same year and, in part, triggered by the need to maintain pacing despite power outages, Lillehei and Bakken at the University of Minnesota, used a battery-powered transistorized external pacemaker for the first time (Fig. 1.5).[16,18–23] As noted previously, it was also the same year that Senning and Elmqvist performed the first pacemaker implantation using an epicardial lead.

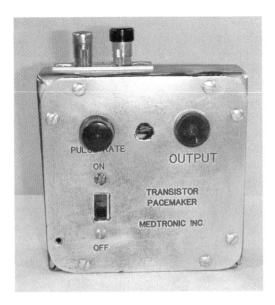

Fig. 1.5 Photograph of first transistorized wearable external pacemaker; the approximate dimensions were 10 × 10 × 3 cm. This was designed by Earl Bakken in 1957

1.2.2 Initial Evolution of Implantable Pulse Generators

Early developments in cardiac pacing substantially improved the prognoses for patients with surgically induced complete *heart block* and ultimately for other individuals with life-threatening bradycardias. However, the first implantable devices offered only asynchronous fixed-rate pacing, meaning that they were incapable of sensing any intrinsic cardiac electrical activity, and they also had very limited longevities (often measured in months). It is important to note that throughout the early development of cardiac pacemakers, battery longevity was a major limitation. The 1958 pacemaker designed by Elmqvist (see above) had an inductive recharging circuit for noninvasive recharging of nickel–cadmium batteries.[16-18] While rechargeable devices were conceptually interesting (e.g., the Pacesetter Inc. rechargeable device of the early 1970s), battery technology at the time provided insufficient device longevity. In addition, the idea that elderly and infirm patients should be responsible for frequently recharging their potentially life-saving pacemakers was probably neither prudent nor welcomed by the patients; apart from the obvious inconvenience, the weekly (or even more frequent) recharging process reminded patients of their dependence on technology and their inevitable mortality. Indeed, even today with modern advances in rechargeable batteries, this concept remains essentially untested. Meanwhile, Chardack and Greatbatch were adopting mercury–zinc batteries, routinely used by watch-makers, for use in pacemakers.[18,24] At the time, mercury–zinc technology offered about a 1-year longevity (later increased to approximately 2 years) without the need for recharging.

These batteries were primarily mounted in epoxy cast pacemakers that had enough porosity to permit dissipation of the hydrogen gas that they produced. Unfortunately at the same time, the employed epoxy allowed body fluids to access circuitry causing precipitous pacemaker system failures.

In 1970, a nuclear-powered implantable pacemaker with a 20-year or longer expected longevity was introduced.[25] However, this concept caused the following problems: (1) potential release of radioactivity; (2) ultimate issues with device disposal; and (3) potential inconvenience for travel by pacemaker wearers. Moreover, batteries with a lifetime in excess of 20 years prevented patients from taking advantage of the progress in circuit technology. Consequently, following the introduction in 1972 of lithium–iodine battery technology,[26] which offered the potential for service lifetime greater than a decade and with reliable and predictable battery depletion patterns, all former power sources became obsolete. Note that lithium–iodine cells remain the principal energy source for modern pacing devices.

Interestingly, the introduction of pacemakers that could sense and thereby pace only when needed (so-called *demand* pacemakers) had been the subject of study as early as the mid-1950s (e.g., an external demand system was used by Leatham and colleagues),[27] but did not become available for implantation until the early 1960s. Despite the earlier work of others, the demand pacemaker is attributed to Barouh V. Berkovits (another Prague émigré) who pioneered the application of this feature in implantable devices.[28–29] This *demand* innovation not only reduced power consumption, but also diminished the possibility (albeit very small) of a pacing stimulus falling on the so-called *cardiac vulnerable period* (more or less the peak of the T-wave) and triggering a tachyarrhythmia. Berkovits also pioneered the first dual-chamber pacemaker which he called the *bifocal* at the time (Fig. 1.6).[29]

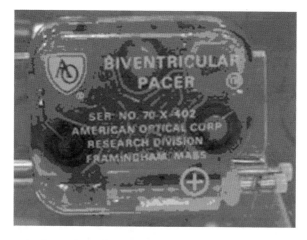

Fig. 1.6 Photograph of an early version of the *bifocal* pacemaker designed by Barouh Berkovits

1.2.3 Pacing Lead Development

Despite innovations in achieving transvenous access and endocardial stimulation, the transvenous approach for cardiac pacing was limited by instability of the leads and their tendency to fracture. On the other hand, the favored epicardial technique had its own problems, particularly the tendency for pacing threshold to rise over time requiring implantation of high-output larger devices. Additionally, early epicardial lead longevity was a major problem particularly due to conductor failure.

Ultimately, endocardial leads incorporated multifilar coiled wire designs that yielded more robust conductors, capable of withstanding many years of repetitive flexing. Further, by the mid-1970s tined-tip leads (innovated by Paul Citron, Medtronic, Inc.), providing a means to engage the trabeculae lining of the right ventricle, became commercially available.[30] In combination, these innovations increased average lead longevity to roughly parallel or exceed that of the lithium–iodine power source, and further reduced acute endocardial lead dislodgement rates from approximately 10 to 1%.[30] Consequently, the endocardial approach for permanent pacing became the dominant technique. Compared to epicardial pacing, endocardial pacing offered a less invasive approach, providing the following advantages: (1) the possibility of therapy without general anesthesia; (2) the ability to be performed in centers without cardiac surgery services; and (3) improved pacing thresholds and lead longevity.

Initially, endocardial leads were implanted via cut-down over the cephalic vein in the delto-pectoral groove. This method is still used by some surgeons, but has the limitation of being difficult to place more than one lead. Consequently, the percu-taneous puncture of the subclavian vein gradually became predominant in the late 1980s and early 1990s. This method made the implantation procedure quicker and easier, yet presented a new set of problems including the potential complications of (1) inducing a pneumothorax; and/or (2) causing a subclavian crush of the lead, i.e., insulation and conductor damage where the lead(s) passed through the tough sub-clavian ligament/subclavius muscle and was thereby the fulcrum for vigorous flexion. Direct puncture of the axillary vein over the first rib, pioneered at the University of Minnesota by Jean E. Magney and colleagues, has largely obviated these problems associated with subclavian vein access.

In addition to changes in vascular access, at about the same time bipolar pacing leads became increasingly popular. The move away from unipolar pac-ing permitted detection of spontaneous cardiac signals with less risk of inap-propriate detection of noncardiac signals (particularly, skeletal myopotentials that were notorious for causing inappropriate pacing stimulus inhibition).[31,32] The value of bipolar sensing was instrumental for facilitating safer sensing in the atrium, where spontaneous signals tend to be of low amplitude (compared to the ventricles) and the amplifier sensitivity setting must often be greater than that used for the ventricle (i.e., increasing risk of sensing undesirable extrane-ous signals).

1.2.4 Later Pacing System Advances

Important technical developments during the 1970s substantially improved pulse generator reliability, longevity, and safety. Most notable among these innovations were hermetic sealing, lower power hybrid circuit technology, and improved component protection.[16,33] Providing appropriate credit for these advances is difficult to assign; scores of engineers and scientists working in many countries and together with all the device manufacturers contributed hundreds of refinements. Altogether, these contributions made the promise of increasingly reliable and more widely available implantable devices a clinical reality. For example, hermetic sealing protected circuitry from disruption by seepage of biological fluids that had been a major problem associated with earlier pulse generator systems. Hybrid technology, as opposed to use of discrete components, was especially critical in terms of simplifying manufacturing, reducing power consumption, and thereby substantially increasing the number of potential pacemaker functions without compromising service life or increasing size. Further, protection was incorporated to diminish adverse impact on device operation of strong external electric fields (e.g., defibrillator shocks, surgical cautery) and to prevent pacing at excessively high rates (so-called *run away*), a condition occasionally encountered with certain component failures. In sum, reliability improved, sizes were reduced, longevity increased, and the base of potential implanting physicians was broadened as devices became more readily implanted in the pre-pectoral region with leads passed via punctures of the subclavian veins.

Throughout the late 1970s and 1980s, many additional pacemaker features were added as electronic designs and manufacturing became more efficient. Of these, the development of transcutaneous telemetry communication was seen as invaluable. This advance allowed for both testing and programming of the pacemaker to better understand and often overcome pacing problems, and also allow for more effective device follow-up care. It is important to note that difficulties with sensing or high pacing thresholds could often be overcome by reprogramming alone. With all the other innovations that were incorporated into devices, it now became possible to deal with the complex problems of providing more physiological pacing modes. Thus, despite earlier work with atrial sensing and ventricular pacing by Folkman in the late 1950s and Nathan in the early 1960s,[33] it was only as a result of the technical advances in the mid-1970s that implantable rate adaptable devices (initially VDD mode) appeared. Thereafter, the even more advanced DDD pacing mode became feasible, a concept introduced in 1977 by Funke (he termed it the *Universal pacemaker*).[34] The first implants of commercially available DDD systems in humans took place in Europe in the late 1970s.

As pacing systems evolved, so did the types of conditions for which they were prescribed. Whereas the earliest devices focused on treatment of excessive bradycardia in patients with complete heart block, the physician community gradually recognized the important benefits of pacing in other conditions, particularly sinus node dysfunction (initially termed *sick sinus syndrome*). In fact, by the mid-1980s, sinus node disease surpassed AV block as the largest single pacemaker indication. In that setting, it soon became evident that *atrial tracking* (i.e., triggering the pacemaker rate based on the native sinus rate) was not always the optimum method for providing heart rate response, as many patients exhibited severe chronotropic incompetence. Consequently, the concept of sensor-based rate-adaptive pacing emerged with the objective of providing a more reliable heart rate response.

In 1981, Anthony (Tony) F. Rickards[35] conceived the idea that pacing rate could be controlled by detection of the duration of the stimulus-T interval, which is analogous to the QT interval and reflects the prevailing catecholamine drive to the heart. However, while a pacemaker based on Rickards' concept was offered commercially, a competitive piezoelectric sensor system introduced in 1983, and based on the work of Anderson and colleagues,[36] was simpler and more effective, and thus became more widely adopted. In essence, pacing rates were adjusted based on the degree of vibration induced in the sensor by relative body movement (i.e., activity). While this method has many limitations, the relative advantages were readily understood by pacing physicians and these devices became highly successful in the marketplace. Some years later, in the early 1990s, the vibration concept was modified into an accelerometer configuration. The accelerometer sensor remains the most widely used today (although occasionally partnered with other sensors, particularly a minute ventilation sensor). Other sensor technologies, apart from the stimulus-T method discussed above, were also introduced in the mid-1980s, but none of these achieved levels of success comparable to that of the piezoelectric *activity* sensor. These additional sensor technologies included (1) temperature-based pacing; (2) a respiratory rate or tidal volume sensor; (3) an oxygen sensor; and/or (4) a ventricular pressure (dP/dt) system.[37] Currently, sensors for rate-adaptive pacing remain the norm in modern pulse generators.

As pulse generators became smaller and the use of multiple pacing leads (primarily one atrial and one ventricular) became routine, there was need for lower profile leads with slippery surfaces that permitted pacing leads to more readily pass over each other. It was noted that silicone rubber, the material of choice up to that time, did not have sufficient slipperiness and had relatively low tear strengths (i.e., was easily damaged; the tougher silicone rubber now in use was not available at the time).[38] In addition, manufacturers of silicone were contemplating stopping production, in part due to fallout from the silicone breast implant litigations prevalent in the early 1980s. Consequently, in this setting, the employment of polyurethane insulation seemed optimal.[38] Polyurethane (particularly those known as 80A and 55D) offered both toughness and slipperiness. Additionally, it allowed for the possibility of reducing coating thickness, thus allowing for smaller overall lead cross-sectional diameters. The 80A form proved more flexible than the 55D, and was initially the most widely used for leads; unfortunately, the biostability of 80A was later found to be an issue resulting in insulation defects and loss of pacing function. Later forms of polyurethane along with tougher silicones have largely resolved these issues.

Optimizing the electrode–myocardial interface has always been a challenge for pacing lead manufacturers.[39] Throughout the early years of endocardial pacing, the stability of pacing leads became a growing concern. As many as one in ten lead implants needed to be redone as a result of acute dislodgements. As alluded to earlier, in order to address this problem in the mid-1970s, tines were added at the end of conventional endocardial leads to enhance passive fixation.[30] The use of tines proved to be very effective in the ventricle, but even more secure methods were sought for atrial applications. Exposed and *sugar-coated* screws (helixes) were available, but many physicians were reluctant to use them; consequently, a retractable screw system was sought. In approximately 1977, Bisping introduced a sheathed screw electrode that superseded the previously available fixed unsheathed screws for fixation.[40] Over the next decade, the retractable screw technology evolved and now this type of *active* lead fixation remains very popular (all manufacturers offer a version of it). Active fixation permitted placement of leads effectively anywhere in the right heart (e.g., right ventricular septal site pacing), but in particular it facilitated stable atrial sensing and pacing (previously only the right atrial appendage offered stable pacing). In 1983, steroid eluting leads were introduced in order to limit endocardial inflammation and consequent rise in pacing threshold associated with newly placed pacing leads.[39] This innovation essentially eliminated early and late threshold rises, and was particularly important for pediatric patients, in whom exit block at the electrode–myocardium interface had been a common clinical problem. Finally, the tip electrode surface received considerable attention in the 1980s.[39] Specialized coatings enabled small electrode tips to have, in effect, much larger active surface areas. The results were lower stimulation thresholds (less energy/battery drain) as well as better sensing.[41]

1.2.5   More Recent Pacing System Advances

Among the important developments in pacing in the early 1990s was the introduction of a standard lead connector and header configuration (IS-1 standard). Obtaining industry-wide agreement among vigorous competitors to develop such a standard must be considered, in itself, an impressive achievement; the result permitted interchangeability of leads and generators among manufacturers. This agreed upon standard was an in-line bipolar system that also allowed for reduction in the size of the header, and thus the overall pulse generator profile.

Later in the 1990s and in the first years of this century, devices became increasingly capable of monitoring internal and external operations. Thus, it is now routine to be able to assess information on the frequency of atrial and ventricular pacing, battery longevity, lead impedance, frequency of detected tachyarrhythmias, and most recently, assessment of transpulmonary electrical impedances as markers of evolving volume overload (usually the result of worsening heart failure).[42,43] Further, advances in transcutaneous telemetry allow device interrogation and reprogramming to be performed from out of the operative field, and also allow complete transtelephonic evaluation of the pacing system from home, thereby reducing the number of patient trips to the follow-up clinic.

Apart from technological advances, the current decade of cardiac pacing has been characterized by numerous developments of clinical guidelines from the major professional societies, i.e., based on results of large multicenter clinical trials aimed at establishing an evidence base for appropriate device indications and mode selection.[44,45] For example, among the many important clinical observations, these trials revealed that *over-pacing* of the right ventricle should be avoided in order to preserve ventricular function over the long term.[46] In addition, findings supported the value of left ventricular-based pacing for improving cardiac function in patients with systolic heart failure (so-called cardiac resynchronization therapy or CRT).[47–53]

The concept that biventricular pacing may ultimately improve cardiac performance began to be studied long before the first clinical publications of the 1990s. The earliest studies date from the beginning of the 1970s and were led by Tyers,[54,55] then working in Philadelphia, Derek Gibson and colleagues in London,[56] and researchers under the direction of DeTeresa in Madrid.[57] However, at that time, technology limited the ease with which left ventricular leads could be placed and kept stable. In 1994, Serge Cazeau and associates from Paris provided the first clinical report of CRT.[47] Thereafter, the technique rapidly gained momentum. Specifically, Jean-Jacques Blanc and Claude Daubert in France and Angelo Auricchio in Germany were among the early contributors to a substantial wave of literature combining this new cardiac pacing modality (subsequently termed cardiac resynchronization therapy or CRT) with the assessment of cardiac hemodynamics. Subsequently, a series of large randomized controlled trials confirmed the value of CRT. In general, the outcomes of MUSTIC, MIRACLE, PATH-CHF, COMPANION, and CARE-HF[49–53] convinced not only the pacing community but also many heart failure specialists that CRT was a valuable adjunct to overall heart failure patient management.

1.2.6 Emergence of Implantable Defibrillators

Studies regarding the use of electrical shock to terminate arrhythmias have a long history. However, the origins of clinical defibrillation therapy may be best timed to the observations of Claude Beck in Cleveland in 1947[58] who defibrillated a 14-year-old patient in the operating room (Fig. 1.7). Later, the work of Zacouto and Bouvrain[59] and Lown[60] in the early 1960s provided further foundation for its therapeutic benefits; it was not until the 1960s that transthoracic defibrillation became an accepted therapy.

The ultimate development of implantable clinical devices for internal defibrillation (ICDs) is attributable to the persistence of Mirowski and Mower, yet it should be noted that their first proposals met with considerable scepticism and resistance.[61] The initial device (so-called AID®, Intec Corp., Pittsburgh, PA) had limited functionality, was very large, and required an open-chest procedure to place the epicardial electrodes. The pulse generator resided in the abdomen, as it was much too

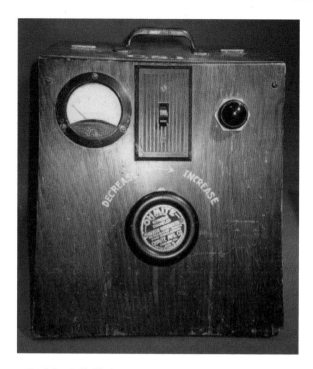

Fig. 1.7 Photograph of the defibrillation generator used by Claude Beck in 1947

large to fit anywhere else. These initial ICD implantations, beginning in 1980, required that the patient had to have survived two cardiac arrests (the chances of that were remote indeed). By the mid-1980s, the indications had broadened and transvenous leads became available (although device size still demanded an abdominal implant site). An alternative approach to the prevention of cardiac arrest was the use of a lower energy implantable cardioverter as proposed by Zipes and colleagues.[62] The cardioverter concept was based upon the view that early intervention (when the tachyarrhythmia was still presumably reasonably organized) would require less energy, be delivered more rapidly (i.e., shorter charge time), and thus would require a smaller device; however, physicians did not feel comfortable with this approach and the notion lapsed. High-energy (≥ 30 J) delivery ICD devices decisively won the day.

Transvenous pre-pectoral ICD implantation gradually evolved through the 1990s, as size was reduced in successive device generations. Further, the number of ICDs implanted has rapidly grown annually, as clinical studies such as AVID, CASH, CIDS, MUSTT, MADIT, MADIT2, and SCD-Heft have all provided incontrovertible evidence that ICD therapy was more effective for preventing sudden death in high-risk populations (principally individuals with low ejection fractions) than was achievable with any other available treatments (Fig. 1.8).[63–70] Other developments in the 1990s included adoption of biphasic shocks, inclusion of the generator's case in

1st UM Implant 1986
Surgical-Abdominal site

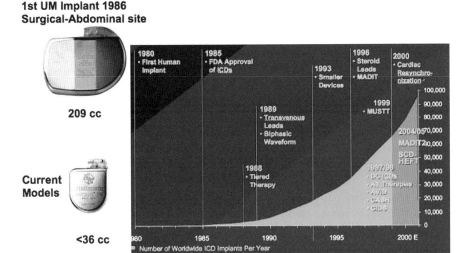

Fig. 1.8 Photographs of early and later implantable cardiac defibrillators (ICDs; *left*) and graph illustrating growth of ICD use since their introduction in the early 1980s (*right*). Images courtesy of Medtronic, Inc., Minneapolis, MN

the defibrillation circuit (so-called *active can* innovated by Gust Bardy of Seattle), and dual coil leads.[71] Taken together, these advances made ICD treatment more readily available to more patients and, at the same time, easier to deliver. As a result, more centers could then offer this treatment that was previously confined to a few sites. Current ICDs offer all of the functionality of modern pacemakers (including CRT capability when indicated), and are able to be fully interrogated by long-distance communication.

1.2.7   Ambulatory Monitoring

Ambulatory ECG (AECG) monitoring has rapidly become accepted as essential for optimizing arrhythmia diagnoses. The first developed AECG device was attributed to Norman Holter in the late 1940s, but practical application of this technology did not occur until almost 20 years later.[72] Progressively smaller and more user friendly iterations of the so-called *Holter* monitor developed over time; these set the standard for AECG monitoring well into the 1990s. Furthermore, Holter-type monitors are still used and are capable of providing full disclosure rhythm recordings for 24- or 48-h periods. In addition, in the 1970s and 1980s, so-called *event* recorders became available. These offered the patient the opportunity to trigger the device when symptoms occurred and were often prescribed for months at a time; in fact, they are still used in this manner. However, the problems of short recording durations of Holter devices, and the need for patients to respond to occasionally serious symptoms with event recorders were obvious limitations. To overcome the first problem, Krahn, Klein, and colleagues innovated the concept of insertable (implantable) loop recorders (ILRs).[73] The ILR initially offered almost 2 years of monitoring capability; newer models have even greater longevity. To deal with the second problem, that is the need for the patient to trigger the event recorder when symptoms occur (something that is often not possible if the patient is stressed or otherwise incapacitated), automatic wireless data transmission from mobile cardiac outpatient telemetry (MCOT) devices to a 24/7 monitoring center were developed.[74] Most recently, the MCOT concept has been incorporated into an ILR configuration, i.e., an implanted monitor that is capable of communicating data via wireless telemetry to a central monitoring facility.

While the ILR is a well-established tool in clinical electrophysiology, the potential value of long-term patient hemodynamic monitoring for both diagnostic and treatment assessment is increasingly being recognized as useful. The first iteration of such technology was the implantable device that directly or indirectly measured left atrial pressure.[75] These instruments permitted the detection of hemodynamic changes in heart failure patients before emergency room or hospital care becomes necessary (thereby saving considerable healthcare expenses). The potential for similar systems to facilitate care of other chronic disease states is only now beginning to be explored.

In summary, the past 50 years have been marked by impressive developments in device therapies associated with both cardiac arrhythmia and cardiac arrest. In particular, the cost and size of implantable devices has progressively been reduced, while availability, functionality, and reliability have substantially increased. Nevertheless, it should be noted that, like any developing technology, inevitably failures have occurred. Fortunately, these have been uncommon and, given the intense clinical monitoring (including home monitoring and national registries) that has become the current standard, are quickly recognized.

The evolution of device therapy was certainly critically dependent on the understanding of cardiac arrhythmias introduced by the electrocardiographers discussed earlier; however, of perhaps even greater importance was the development of cardiac arrhythmia initiation and termination by electrical stimulation techniques that derived from observations in operating rooms and in the newly evolving clinical electrophysiology laboratories of the late 1960s and 1970s.

1.3 Intracardiac Recording, Stimulation, and Autonomic Assessment

In principle, modern interventional cardiac electrophysiology requires development of three primary skills: (1) the ability to record and interpret intracardiac electrograms; (2) insights into the initiation and termination of arrhythmias by intracardiac electrical stimulations; and (3) the innovation of transcatheter ablation methodologies.

1.3.1   Early Studies Using Transcatheter Recordings

The study of the cardiac conduction system has a long history in basic science laboratories of the last decades of the nineteenth century and the first half of the twentieth century. The anatomic findings of His, Purkinje, and Bachmann are now permanently attached to the cardiac structures they first described. Other major contributors in the same era include Keith and Flack (sinus node), Tawara (AV node), and Mahaim (controversial bypass tracts), Sir Thomas Lewis, Brian Hoffman, Gordon Moe, Paul Cranefield, Michael Rosen, and Maurits Allessie (see Chap. 4 for more details on this history).

In the clinical arena, intracardiac electrophysiologic recording began in Staten Island, New York in the late 1960s. The key innovation was the ability to record electrograms from the His bundle. It was Paul Puech who, in 1957, reported that he made such a recording during a heart catheterization procedure.[76] Yet, it is Benjamin Scherlag (then at the Staten Island Public Health Hospital under the direction of Anthony Damato, and now in Oklahoma City) and colleagues who are accorded credit for developing the technique to record His bundle electrograms in humans using transvenous catheters in 1969.[77] It is this transvenous catheter approach that permitted direct assessment of clinical cardiac conduction system disturbances, and led to the development of a better understanding of their pathophysiology and prognoses. Of historical interest, Damato's laboratory in that era was the source of many first-generation US clinical cardiac electrophysiologists, including John J. Gallagher (who became the program leader at Duke University), Mark Josephson (who established electrophysiology at the University of Pennsylvania), Ken Rosen (founder of the extensive University of Illinois electrophysiology group in Chicago), and Masood Akhtar (who remains director of the impressive electrophysiology program in Milwaukee).

1.3.2   Premature Electrical Stimulation and Entrainment

As important as intracardiac conduction system recordings have become, it was the insights of Durrer and Wellens in the early 1970s that led to (1) a better understanding of the electrical activation of the human heart (among the earliest applications of epicardial mapping); (2) the value of using intracardiac recording in conjunction with cardiac electrical stimulation for the triggering and mapping of tachycardia circuits; and (3) the use of pacing as an antitachycardia tool within implanted devices (Fig. 1.9).[78–82] In fact, Wellens' concise treatise on the subject published in 1971 remains a classic in the field.[81]

The landmark work from Dirk Durrer and Hein Wellens contributed a clear understanding of the clinical utility of employing programmed electrical stimulation (PES) of the heart to initiate and terminate many tachyarrhythmias, a technique now used daily in electrophysiology laboratories. These observations set the stage for

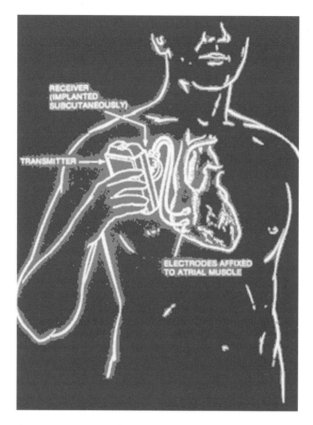

Fig. 1.9 Illustration depicting use of a manually activated antitachycardia pacing system. This device was triggered by an external box and signals were then transmitted to an implanted antenna-pacemaker system. Therapy was directed at pace-terminable supraventricular tachycardias. Image courtesy of Medtronic, Inc., Minneapolis, MN, USA

intraoperative and later catheter-based mapping for the subsequent treatment of complex arrhythmias. Notably, PES was employed by Gallagher and colleagues at Duke to study preexcitation,[83] Albert L. Waldo (then at University of Alabama in Birmingham, now in Cleveland) to study postoperative atrial tachyarrhythmias (including classic studies of atrial fibrillation and flutter),[84-86] Akhtar and Denker to study properties of the conduction system, and Josephson and colleagues in studies of ventricular tachycardia.[87-89] More specifically, Gallagher's work in the mid-1970s comprised innovations in epicardial mapping of accessory AV connections, and incorporated the many surgical innovations devised by Will Sealy for dividing such connections. At the same time, Josephson's contributions included intraoperative endocardial mapping of ventricular tachycardias that led to Alden Harken Jr.'s innovative ablative surgery. The Josephson–Harken endocardial surgical procedure focused on the newly discovered arrhythmogenic regions along border zones of infarct-related scars; this innovative, a curative approach, not only captured a great deal of medical attention but also public interest. Interestingly, a report in a prominent weekly US newsmagazine at the time popularized the term *Pennsylvania Peel* for this surgical technique.

Fundamental understanding of mechanisms of many common tachycardias remained controversial well into the 1970s. Even in the simplest case, that of WPW syndrome, the concept of longitudinal dissociation of the conduction system as a basis for preexcitation lived on in the literature. However, when Howard Burchell (then working at the Mayo Clinic) induced temporary block in an accessory pathway during surgery (Fig. 1.10),[90] and Anderson and Becker[91] provided anatomic descriptions of such connections, the evidence favoring accessory AV connections being the basis of WPW syndrome became incontrovertible. The first successful surgical ablation of an accessory pathway was performed at Duke University in the early 1970s. Thereafter, the Duke group led by John Gallagher and Will Sealy not only perfected the diagnostic electrophysiological laboratory evaluation of preexcitation syndromes, but also developed the methods for surgical ablation of accessory connections.[83,92] Shortly thereafter, the London, Ontario group led by George Klein (a Gallagher protégé) and Gerard Guiraudon importantly contributed to advancing surgical techniques for preexcitation with introduction of the closed heart epicardial approach. Incidentally, James Cox, who later became known as the innovator of the surgical approach for atrial fibrillation (i.e., the MAZE procedure) began his career in this fertile Duke environment before making his mark at Washington University in St Louis.

In the 1980s, bradyarrhythmias received less attention than tachyarrhythmias, as most of the insights into clinical conduction disease had already been made. Specifically, the productive electrophysiology group at the University of Illinois led

Atrioventricular and Ventriculoatrial Excitation in Wolff-Parkinson-White Syndrome (Type B)

Temporary Ablation at Surgery

By Howard B. Burchell, M.D., Robert L. Frye, M.D., Milton W. Anderson, M.D., and Dwight C. McGoon, M.D.

SUMMARY

A patient with an atrial septal defect, paroxysmal tachycardia, and the Wolff-Parkinson-White syndrome (type B) had epicardial exploration to determine the nature of the excitation anomaly. Right bundle-branch block in association with the WPW syndrome (type B) was evidenced by the late activation (0.12 sec) of the epicardium over the outflow tract of the right ventricle. Early activation of the base of the right ventricle (near the atrioventricular groove at the right border of the heart) was interpreted as indicating an actively conducting atrioventricular muscle bridge (bundle of Kent) in this region. During paroxysms of tachycardia, the ventricular area excited much later than when sinus mechanism was present, and the adjacent right atrium was excited in sequence. This sequence supported the concept of a circus movement, that is, movement from atrium to ventricle via atrioventricular bundle (His) and ventricle to atrium via a muscle bridge (Kent). Injection of procaine into the base of the right ventricle abolished the pre-excitation of the ventricle.

Fig. 1.10 Title and abstract from the first description of temporary ablation of an accessory pathway in Wolff–Parkinson–White syndrome[90]

by Kenneth Rosen had already examined the electrophysiologic features of most aspects of clinical conduction disease. Similarly, Maurice Lev (also working in Chicago), Jean Lenegre (in Paris), and Thomas James (in Birmingham, Alabama) all provided careful pathologic insights into these cardiac conduction disturbances. Nevertheless, Ahktar and Denker (in Milwaukee) continued to provide complex and fascinating insights into the physiology of infranodal conduction.[93–95] These latter observations are often overlooked today, but nonetheless they are classical examples of the use of PES to better understand both cardiac conduction physiology and disease. At about the same time, in the mid to late 1970s and early 1980s, Harold Strauss (at Duke) and William Mandel and colleagues (in Los Angeles), and Onkar Narula (in Florida), basing their work on the clinical observations of Irene Ferrer and the laboratory observations of J. T. "Tom" Bigger Jr. at Columbia University in New York,[96–100] devised clinical electrophysiological laboratory studies to assess sinus node dysfunction. Strauss is best known for the development of the sinoatrial conduction time test, whereas Mandel popularized overdrive suppression as a test of sinus node function [sinus node recovery time (SNRT)]. Additionally, Mandel and Jordan also brought to light key aspects of the effects of autonomic tone and drugs on sinoatrial function.[100]

One of the most important contributions to clinical electrophysiology in the 1980s was Al Waldo's observations on *entrainment*[24,85,101,102] a concept that evolved from his postoperative arrhythmia studies in Birmingham. Entrainment provided not only an intellectual foundation for understanding clinical macro-reentry tachycardias, but also has become a tool used daily in electrophysiology laboratories to establish the presence of a reentry mechanism and to assess the location of tissues critical to the maintenance (and successful ablation) of these same arrhythmias. While originally proven using the accessory AV connection (i.e., so-called AV reentry) model of macro-reentry, most current generation clinical electrophysiologists first become familiar with entrainment in assessment of atrial flutter.[101] In this regard, much of our understanding of the macro-reentry nature of atrial flutter (both typical counter-clockwise and less common clockwise forms) is based on the work of Francisco (Paco) Cosio in Madrid (a self-trained electrophysiologist who did his initial cardiology training in Minneapolis, Minnesota).[103] Cosio confirmed the inferior vena cava-tricuspid annulus isthmus-dependent nature of this macro-reentry right atrial tachycardia. Now, it is standard practice for electrophysiologists to *entrain* the tachycardia from that isthmus, thereby confirming its key role in the circuit in each patient before proceeding to permanently eliminate the circuit by transisthmus ablation (usually by radiofrequency energy applications).

Finally, in terms of current interest in treatment of atrial fibrillation, Maurits Allessie's work in the experimental laboratory was particularly insightful and contributed two currently very important concepts: (1) atrial fibrillation begets atrial fibrillation; and (2) remodeling of the atria occurs during prolonged periods of atrial fibrillation, making reversion to stable sinus rhythm increasingly more difficult.[104] Of course, with regard to the latter notion, the reverse was also observed. If atrial fibrillation is terminated and sinus rhythm restored for a prolonged period, *reverse remodeling* can occur in many cases, thereby enhancing the chance that sinus rhythm will be maintained.

1.3.3 Ablation

Selective transcatheter ablation of small regions of cardiac tissue critical to maintenance of cardiac arrhythmias, such as the cavo-tricuspid isthmus in the case of atrial flutter, derives in part from both the surgical experience alluded to briefly earlier as well as experimental and clinical work by Melvin Scheinman at the University of California-San Francisco and John Gallagher at Duke University.[105,106] In the mid-1970s, both studied the use of DC shock delivered from a conventional external defibrillator using modified connectors, with the energy (200–300 J) directed through conventional electrode catheters to the target tissues. The initial target organ of primary interest was the AV junction, and the goal was to induce permanent AV block in patients with atrial fibrillation and excessively rapid ventricular rates. Shortly thereafter, the same DC shock method was used (despite considerable anxiety among practitioners) with remarkable safety and effectiveness to treat posteroseptal accessory pathways, drug-resistant left ventricular tachycardia, or even tachycardias arising in the right ventricular outflow tract. Given the rather crude activation mapping of arrhythmias at the time, the somewhat indiscriminate nature of DC shock damage proved paradoxically to be advantageous. However, it should be noted that complications did arise when this approach was applied within the more fragile coronary sinus in an attempt to address laterally positioned accessory AV connections.

   The use of DC energy as an ablative energy source was ultimately superseded by introduction of radiofrequency (RF) energy (comparable to conventional cautery) in the early 1990s. It should be noted that many individuals contributed importantly to this advance, with Warren (Sonny) Jackman in the United States and Karl Heinz Kuck in Germany being particularly notable leaders in the field.[107–109] Importantly, RF energy could be much more precisely directed and therefore was inherently safer than DC shock ablation; one result of this development was expansion of *indications* for ablation. In particular, attention was immediately focused on ablation of the so-called *fast* AV nodal pathway, and then later and more successfully (and with a much lower risk of inducing AV block) the currently preferred *slow* pathway target. Thereafter, RF energy was directed toward ablation of accessory AV connections at virtually all sites, atrial ectopic tachycardias, and ultimately atrial fibrillation.

   Subsequently, techniques for applied ablation to reduce susceptibility to atrial fibrillation were based, in part, on the prior surgical observations by Cox and colleagues[110] but, in addition, as a result of the publication in 1997 of the observed importance of pulmonary vein triggers by Michel Haissaguerre and co-workers in Bordeaux,[111,112] with important contributions being provided by John Shwartz in the United States and Shih-Ann Chen and colleagues in Taiwan among others. More specifically, ablation of apparent triggering activity from small muscle bundles within the pulmonary veins and occasionally cardiac venous structures showed considerable success in preventing paroxysmal atrial fibrillation, but pulmonary vein stenosis was a worrisome risk and atrial fibrillation recurrence rates were high. Consequently, isolation of the veins by antral ablation lines became more popular, tended to improve success rates, and diminished complications, although the previously unseen risk of esophago-atrial fistula became a rare, but frightening, concern.

Apart from RF energy, other ablation methodologies have received increasing interest. Specifically, Gallagher and Sealy at Duke, in the 1970s, were the first to assess the role of cryothermia for cardiac tissue ablation during surgical procedures for arrhythmia therapy.[113,114] They deemed this a particularly valuable technique, as it achieved a structurally solid and electrically homogenous ablation lesion. However, the applicability of catheter delivery of cryothermic lesions did not emerge for more than 15 years later.[115,116] Catheter-delivered cryothermia for ablation purposes was developed in Montreal in the 1990s and, after a slow start, is now widely used. Many electrophysiologists prefer cryothermic ablation for safety reasons, especially to prevent inadvertent injury to the cardiac conduction system when they are working around the AV node area. It should be mentioned that laser ablation has also been evaluated, but to date has not been widely applied.

1.3.4 Autonomic Disturbances and Genetically Determined Susceptibility to Arrhythmias

During the 1980s and 1990s, cardiac electrophysiologists began to take an increasing interest in the role of autonomic disturbances as a cause of cardiac arrhythmias and, in particular, syncope and other forms of what has come to be termed *autonomic dysfunction*.

Among the earliest clinical investigators to study the impact of autonomic variations on tachyarrhythmias were Phillipe Coumel in Paris[117,118] and Menashe Waxman in Toronto. Each developed new insights into neural effects in ventricular and supraventricular tachyarrhythmias. Waxman also identified the potential for isoproterenol to accentuate susceptibility to neurally mediated reflex syncope in susceptible individuals.

The relative importance of autonomic effects on ischemia-related arrhythmias became of particular interest in this era. The experimental work from Zipes' laboratory at the University of Indiana was particularly critical in revealing the asymmetry of neurological input to myocardial tissues and associated electrophysiological consequences that occur when a ventricular region has suffered myocardial infarction.[119,120]

Within a few years of the innovation of diagnostic head-up tilt testing for assessing susceptibility to vasovagal syncope by Kenny and Sutton in London in 1986, the study of neurally mediated syncope became a routine part of the electrophysiology laboratory globally.[121] Initially, prolonged head-up tilt testing (up to 1 h) was used alone, but that approach had obvious practical limitations. In 1989, Benditt's group introduced a shorter head-up protocol in which isoproterenol provocation was used if drug-free tilt was nondiagnostic.[122] Thereafter, nitroglycerin provocation was introduced by Antonio Raviele (Venice) in the mid-1990s,[123,124] and subsequently modified by Brignole and colleagues to be called the *Italian Protocol*; this protocol has become the most widely accepted and employed methodology worldwide. It is generally considered that the use of a drug challenge during tilt improved the test diagnostic utility with only a small cost in false positives.

In the late-1990s, the study of syncope was rendered easier and much more efficient by the availability of ILRs as described earlier. A number of studies supportive of the value of ILRs in this setting emanated from Italian investigators, primarily led by Michele Brignole (Lavagna).[125,126] The so-called ISSUE studies have helped to define the causes of syncope in a variety of clinical settings (i.e., *isolated* forms, syncope in the setting of known conduction system disease, etc.), and have also focused on the role of pacing in various types of neurally mediated syncope disease.

In the first decade of this century, electrophysiologists gradually began to become interested in and take responsibility for evaluating and treating patients with postural syncope and other less well-defined orthostatic intolerance syndromes (e.g., postural orthostatic tachycardia syndromes, so-called *anoxic reflex seizures*, and functional dysautonomia). It also became apparent in this period that the care of these clinical problems required a multidisciplinary approach, enlisting the help of individuals with neuroscience, geriatric, pediatric, and/or emergency department skills.

1.3.5 Channelopathies: Genetically Determined Arrhythmias

During the past 25 years, one of the most rapidly growing aspects of arrhythmia research and care has been the broader recognition of the impact that genetics has on both susceptibility to rhythm disturbances and various drug effects.[127–132] In the 1970s, pharmacogenetics focused on a few drug–genetic interactions (most often metabolic issues), but little attention was paid to proarrhythmic possibilities. The latter came to light with recognition that certain antiarrhythmic agents (particularly Vaughan–Williams Class IA and III) provoked QT interval prolongation and increased potential for torsade. This phenomenon was particularly a risk in premenopausal women. Later, the important molecular biological studies innovated by Michael Vincent and Mark Keating in Utah and Peter Schwartz in Milan began to point out various genotypic and phenotypic forms of long QT syndrome (LQTS).[127–129] Ultimately, it was suspected that drug effects and genetic susceptibility work together to increase torsade de pointes risk in many individuals without phenotypic LQTS in the baseline state. The efforts of both Peter Schwartz (Milan, Italy) and Arthur Moss (Rochester, NY, USA), who created a registry of LQTS patients and their follow-up, have substantially impacted the manner in which LQTS patients are managed, particularly with regard to exposure to antiarrhythmic drugs and many other drug classes (e.g., antibiotics, antidepressants, antianginals, gastrointestinal remedies, etc).

In addition to LQTS, a number of other syndromes predisposing individuals to often life-threatening arrhythmias have come to light. Through the efforts of the Brugada brothers, the *Brugada syndrome*, although uncommon, is now widely recognized.[130] As noted earlier, arrhythmogenic (right) ventricular dysplasia (ARVD) was first recognized by Guy Fontaine (Paris), and has been the subject of an important follow-up registry directed by Frank Marcus in Arizona.[131] In ARVD, the initial genes being identified point away from a *channelopathy* and toward an abnormality in cell–cell connections (desmosomes). Furthermore, short QT syndrome, some forms of atrial fibrillation, and idiopathic ventricular fibrillation are other recognized genetically associated conditions, and many more are likely to be identified in years to come.

Ultimately, one sought after clinical goal would be the ability to provide curative gene therapy. However, while gene *replacement* therapy is not yet a reality, *gene-directed* therapy seems possible. For example, mexiletine, an infrequently used Class 1B antiarrhythmic drug (in the same class as lidocaine), may be used effectively in patients with LQTS3 because the underlying problem is a residual sodium channel current. Potentially, other gene-directed treatments will emerge as well. For the present, in most instances, the only reliable treatment for most of these life-threatening arrhythmia syndromes is ICD implantation.

1.4   Epicardial and Endocardial Mapping, Imaging, and Navigation

The concept of mapping whole heart activation was first considered in experimental models in the early part of the twentieth century, but substantial technologic development was needed before such mapping could be applied clinically.

Perhaps the most impressive use of activation mapping in the early 1970s was the work of Durrer and colleagues in Amsterdam. The detailed activation of the human heart was obtained in reanimated specimens and the hand-drawn color images were published in *Circulation* at the insistence of Howard Burchell, who was editor at the time.[133] Interestingly, a number of the original colored images are now found in the holdings of the Bakken Museum in Minneapolis.

Initially cardiac activation mapping evolved from ECG recordings on the body surface. At Duke in the early 1970s, Madison Spach and D. Woodrow Benson Jr. developed sophisticated methods to evaluate cardiac activation using numerous body surface electrodes.[134–135] The resulting maps provided considerable insight into arrhythmia activation patterns, but were limited in applicability due to difficulty of reproducing the technology (at the time) and the complexity of interpreting the data.

The first practical intraoperative multisite activation mapping systems were developed by Fontaine, Guiraudon, and Frank (France) and by Gallagher and colleagues at Duke in the mid-1970s.[83,136,137]Gallagher's system used multielectrode

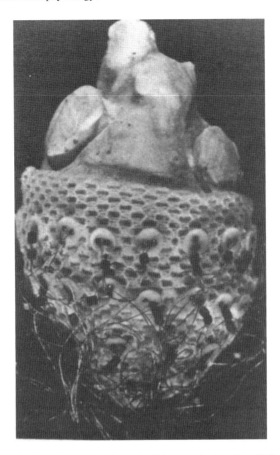

Fig. 1.11 Photograph of multiple electrode *sock* of the type designed by Gallagher in the 1970s for intraoperative mapping

epicardial sock for intraoperative arrhythmia activation mapping (Fig. 1.11). Everything from the choice of the fabric, the design of the reusable electrodes, and the development of a computer-based measurement system proved to be challenging. Ultimately, however, this was the first step in facilitating assessment of cardiac activation during arrhythmias in the surgical suite.

Subsequent to the work at Duke, epicardial mapping evolved at several sites. Perhaps one of the most substantial developments was the combined epicardial–endocardial recording systems used by Boineau, Cox, and Scheussler at Washington University in St Louis, MO.[138] The resulting studies not only improved our understanding of sinoatrial activation in the human, but set the stage for Cox's iterative development of the MAZE procedure for surgical therapy of atrial fibrillation.

More recently, as computers have become smaller and, at the same time, increasingly more powerful and directional catheter technology has become more sophisticated, 3D electro-anatomic mapping of the cardiac chambers has become an essential

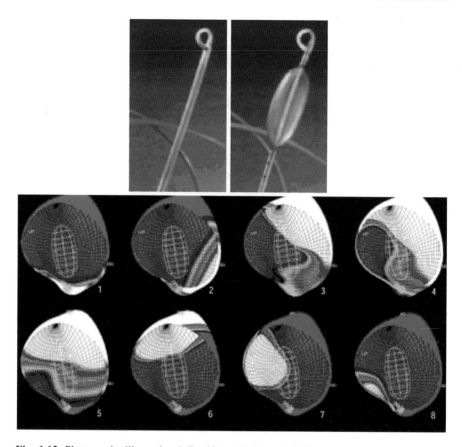

Fig. 1.12 Photographs illustrating inflatable multielectrode balloon system (*top*) and typical intracavitary activation map recording from the noncontact recording system commercialized by Graydon Beatty (*bottom*). Photos courtesy of Endocardial Solutions Inc., Division of St. Jude Medical, Inc., St. Paul, MN, USA

capability of clinical electrophysiology laboratories (CARTO®, Biosense-Webster, and IVAVX®, Endocardial Solutions, Inc.). The earliest noncontact mapping system was developed by Taccardi in Italy in the late 1980s[139] and refined by Rudy at Case Western Reserve University in Cleveland. Thereafter, Graydon Beatty and colleagues at the University of Minnesota developed a commercial mapping system in the mid-1980s.[140] A unique aspect of the system developed by Beatty is a catheter-delivered expandable multielectrode balloon to assess endocardial activation on a beat-by-beat basis and display it for the operator to examine (Fig. 1.12). The system permits conventional point-by-point intracavitary mapping as well.

The two principal 3 D mapping systems in current use utilize triangulation location methods to monitor catheter sites within the cardiac chambers and thereby construct an activation sequence picture. Both systems facilitate the development of ablation strategies for complex arrhythmias. More recently, both systems can also merge the activation maps with previously acquired Computed Tomographic (CT) images of the patient's heart. Thus, the arrhythmia activation is displayed on a cardiac image specific to the patient being evaluated.

Workers interested in mapping and ablation of ventricular tachycardia, atrial ectopic arrhythmias, and atrial fibrillation have been assisted greatly by the 3D imaging technology. These techniques are now being further advanced by use of various robotic devices (including magnetic catheter guidance in one system). It is considered that robotic technologies offer the prospect of more precise and repeatable catheter movement and positioning together with less radiation exposure for operators, nurses, and technicians.

1.5 Antiarrhythmic Drug Therapy

During approximately the first 60 years of the twentieth century, antiarrhythmic drug therapy was limited to one or two membrane-active agents and various digitalis preparations.[141,142] Quinidine was available throughout this time period, with procainamide being introduced in the early 1950s. In the 1960s, lidocaine (only for parenteral use) was introduced, and became the most important agent for urgent care of patients with ischemic ventricular tachyarrhythmias until amiodarone became available in the United States in the early 1980s.[143] Bretylium (and later an orally available analog bethanidine) was also used at that time parenterally for its reported antifibrillatory action, but its tendency to induce orthostatic hypotension and persisting uncertainty regarding its effectiveness undermined its acceptance.[144,145] Finally, given the limited options available, especially in terms of orally active drugs, phenytoin (Dilantin®, primarily known for its antiepileptic action) was often considered part of the physician's antiarrhythmic armamentarium. Yet, it should be noted that phenytoin is rarely used in this capacity today.

Various beta-adrenergic blockers and calcium-channel blockers (diltiazem and verapamil) became available in the 1970s and early 1980s. These drugs found multiple applications in the treatment of hypertension, ischemic heart disease, and/or other cardiovascular problems. Yet, in regard to antiarrhythmic use, their principal impact has been in management of supraventricular tachyarrhythmias; in this context, they essentially eliminated the use of digitalis preparations.

The late 1970s and early 1980s saw the introduction of a number of new antiarrhythmic agents, i.e., disopyramide (a Class IA drug) became available in the United States in 1977.[142,146] Initially, disopyramide appeared to be a major addition to antiarrhythmic drug therapy. However, ultimately its prominent negative inotropic effects, troublesome anticholinergic side effects (e.g., dry eyes, dry mouth, constipation), and tendency to result in marked QT interval prolongation resulted in disopyramide being relegated to, at most, a niche role. Similarly the orally absorbable lidocaine look-alikes, tocainide and mexiletine, were introduced with the anticipation that they would be as effective for ischemia-induced arrhythmias and as hemodynamically tolerable as lidocaine; unfortunately this hope did not materialize. Tocainide was eventually withdrawn due to hematologic adverse effects, and mexiletine (a drug that often causes substantial nausea) is only used sporadically.

During the early phase of the *antiarrhythmic drug era*, at least in terms of ventricular tachyarrhythmias, the prevailing hypothesis was that suppression of ventricular ectopy was desirable and would be an effective marker for a proposed treatment's ability to prevent sudden death. The concept was reinforced (albeit indirectly) by evidence that mortality in ischemic heart disease patients correlated with the severity of ambient ventricular ectopy. Thus, the utility of an antiarrhythmic drug was tested by assessing its ability to suppress premature ventricular beats (PVBs). The new Class IC drugs (principally flecainide, encainide, and propafenone) excelled in PVB suppression and became known as *PVB killers*, as did the related agent moricizine. However, when the PVB suppression theory was tested in a large multicenter randomized trial (Cardiac Arrhythmia Suppression Trial, CAST) in which mortality was assessed (i.e., comparing placebo versus flecainide, or encainide, or moricizine), the results caused considerable dismay.[147] In fact, in the CAST trial, mortality was greater in all active drug groups compared to placebo. Thus, the PVB suppression era came to an abrupt end and a new model was needed.

In the late 1970s and early to mid-1980s, about the same time as the CAST study was being undertaken, antiarrhythmic drug testing for prevention of life-threatening arrhythmias was a prominent feature in the electrophysiology laboratory. Such testing was pioneered by multiple groups including (1) Gallagher at Duke; (2) Wellens in the Netherlands; (3) Ronnie Campbell in Newcastle; (4) John Fisher in New York; (5) Mark Josephson in Philadelphia; and (6) Geoff Hartzler (who later became a major figure in the then emerging field of coronary angioplasty) and Jim Maloney at the Mayo Clinic.[148–150] In this model, various antiarrhythmic drugs and dosages were administered to hospitalized patients and, after a suitable time period, treatment efficacy was then tested using pacing and extrastimulus testing in the laboratory. The desired endpoint was demonstration that an arrhythmia that was initially inducible in the drug-free state was no longer induced in the presence of drug(s) therapy. Yet this approach to selecting treatment often proved frustrating, as the arrhythmia (albeit slowed by drugs) often remained inducible. Further, the stimulation protocols tended to vary from operator to operator, making multicenter assessment of this approach among centers almost impossible. The ESVEM trial and MUSTT study were notable exceptions in which careful protocol control was effected.[151,152] In any case, the process usually involved an in-hospital stay of many days, often required testing of several drugs, and was very expensive. In the end, by the mid-1980s, with the arrival of amiodarone in the United States (it was available years earlier in Europe), the era of electropharmacological drug testing closed. Amiodarone was simply not testable in that manner for both pharmacological (i.e., very long half-life) and clinical experiential reasons.

The most important additions to antiarrhythmic drug therapy in the 1980s and 1990s, apart from amiodarone, were sotalol and dofetilide. Specifically, sotalol was found to be very useful for control of certain supraventricular arrhythmias (particularly atrial fibrillation) and was also found to be safe in the setting of low ejection fraction patients (perhaps in part because of its beta-blocker attributes). Likewise, dofetilide was found to have a similarly neutral mortality effect in sick patients.

However, due to its complex dosing needs and QT prolongation action (and the regulatory environment at the time when it was introduced), dofetilide in the United States was limited to in-hospital treatment initiation. Nevertheless, both drugs continue to play an important role today. Dronedarone, an amiodarone analog, has recently also become available.

One of the most valuable lessons of the *antiarrhythmic drug era* was recognition that all antiarrhythmic agents had the capability to aggravate arrhythmias (so-called proarrhythmia).[153] It soon became evident that certain patient-related factors were important contributors to this risk, particularly diminished ejection fraction, ongoing ischemia, female gender and genetic susceptibility (i.e., some cases of proarrhythmia may represent polymorphisms or *subclinical* cases of channelopathies discussed earlier). As a result, with the exception of amiodarone, sotalol, and dofetilide, most available antiarrhythmic drugs were no longer considered sufficiently safe for treatment of the sickest patients.

Disappointing clinical experience with antiarrhythmic drugs in the case of life-threatening problems, the increasingly complex regulatory hurdles in the United States and Europe (stimulated, in part, by recognition of the proarrhythmic potential of these agents), extremely high development costs, and the arrival of ICD therapy have markedly undermined new antiarrhythmic drug development worldwide. Currently, in the United States, only azimilide (in development for almost 15 years) and dronedarone (an amiodarone look-alike without the iodine component) offer new therapeutic opportunities. Additionally, a few agents directed at specific membrane channels (e.g., I_f channel blockade to slow heart rate, ivabradine) are being critically assessed. Others have been put on hold, and the likelihood of being offered many clinical useful options in the foreseeable future is remote.

1.6 Conclusion

Over the past five decades, clinical cardiac electrophysiology and pacing has been characterized by rapid growth with a multifaceted nature. During this period, this specialty has expanded sufficiently to warrant the founding of several scientific organizations, in particular the Heart Rhythm Society (formerly the North American Society of Pacing and Electrophysiology, NASPE), the European Heart Rhythm Association (EHRA, a subdivision of the European Society of Cardiology), the Asian-Pacific Heart Rhythm Society (APHRS), the Chinese Society of Pacing and Electrophysiology, and the Japan Heart Rhythm Society (JHRS). These and other societies not only serve as a source of professional education, but have also been instrumental in the development of numerous invaluable clinical practice guidelines (e.g., pacing and antitachycardia therapy, atrial fibrillation, syncope, etc.) and have had an important impact on government health policies and insurance company attitudes.

This chapter has provided a brief overview of some of the key developments in this field. Inevitably, many important individuals and contributions have been omitted, for which we apologize. In any case, it should be apparent that the advances associated with developments in clinical cardiac electrophysiology and pacing cover a broad range of technologies and have benefited the treatment of a wide range of conditions, from heart block and other bradyarrhythmias to tachyarrhythmias, syncope and less well characterized autonomic disturbances of cardiovascular control, heart failure, and cardio-pulmonary resuscitation. Furthermore, this knowledge and associated technology developments are now being increasingly adapted to treatment of conditions in other body systems, including the brain, stomach, intestines, and bladder.

References

1. Luderitz B. History of the Disorders of Cardiac Rhythm. New York: Future Publishing, 1995:1–6.
2. Waller AG. A demonstration on man of electromotive changes accompanying the heart's beat. J Physiol 1887; 8:229–34.
3. Einthoven W. Ueber die Form des menschlichenElektrocardigramms. Pflugers Arch 1895; 60:101–23.
4. Einthoven W. Ein neues Galvanometer. Ann Phys 1903; 12:1059–71.
5. Lewis, T. Mechanism and Graphic Registration of the Heart Beat. London: Shaw and Sons Ltd., 1925.
6. Wolff L, Parkinson J, White PD. Bundle-branch block with short P-R interval in healthy young people prone to paroxysmal tachycardia. Am Heart J 1930; 5:685–704.
7. Wilson FN, Johnston FD, MacLeod AG, et al. Electrocardiograms that represent the potential variations of a single electrode. Am Heart J 1933; 9:447–58.
8. Katz LN, Pick A. Clinical Electrocardiography. Part 1. The Arrhythmias. Philadelphia: Lea & Febiger, 1956.
9. Rosenbaum MB, Elizari MV, Lazarri JO. Los hemibloqueous. Buenos Aires: Paidos Publisher, 1967.
10. Dessertenne F. La tachycardie ventriculaire a deux foyers opposes variables. Arch Mal Coeur Vaiss 1966; 59:263–72.
11. Schamroth L. Disorders of Cardiac Rhythm. Oxford: Blackwell Publishers, 1971.
12. Upshaw CB, Silverman ME, Henry JL Mariott: lucid teacher of electrocardiography. Clin Cardiol 2007; 30:207–8.
13. Beithardt G, Borggreffe M, Haerten K. Ventricular late potentials and inducible ventricular tachyarrhythmias as a marker for ventricular tachycardia after myocardial infarction. Eur Heart J 1986; 7:127–34.
14. Huikuri HV, Makikallio T, Airaksinen KE, et al. Measurement of heart rate variability: a clinical tool or a research toy? J Am Coll Cardiol 1999; 34:1878–83.
15. Chow T, Joshi D. Microvolt T-wave alternans testing for ventricular arrhythmia risk stratification. Expert Rev Cardiovasc Ther 2008; 6:833–42.
16. Sutton R, Fisher JD, Linde C, et al. History of electrical therapy for the heart. Eur Heart J 2007; Suppl I:13–110.
17. Elmqvist R, Senning A. An implantable pacemaker for the heart. In: Smyth CN, editor. Proceedings of the Second International Conference on Medical Electronics. London: Iliffe & Sons Ltd., 1960:253–4.
18. Schechter DC. Exploring the Origins of Electrical Cardiac Stimulation. Minneapolis, MN: Medtronic Inc., 1983.
19. Hyman AS. Resuscitation of the stopped heart by intracardial therapy. II. Experimental use of an artificial pacemaker. Arch Int Med 1932; 50:283–305.
20. Mugica J. Survol historique de la technologie de la stimulation cardiaque. ***RBM 1989; 11:221–4.

21. Zoll PM. Resuscitation of the heart in electrical standstill by external electric stimulation. N Engl J Med 1952; 247:768–72.

22. Furman S, Robinson G. Stimulation of the ventricular endocardial surface in control of complete heart block. Ann Surg 1959; 841–6.

23. Bakken EE. One Man's Full Life. Minneapolis, MN: Medtronic Inc., 1999.

24. Chardach WM. Heart block treated with an implantable pacemaker. Past experience and current developments. Prog Cardiovasc Dis 1964; 6:507–20.

25. Norman JC, Sandberg GW, Huffman FN. Implantable nuclear-powered cardiac pacemakers. N Engl J Med 1970; 283:1203–7.

26. Greatbatch W, Lee JH, Mathias W, et al. The solid-state lithium battery: a new improved chemical power source for implantable cardiac pacemakers. IEEE Trans Biomed Eng 1971; 18:317–23.

27. Cook P, Davies JG, Leatham A. External electric stimulator for treatment of ventricular standstill. Lancet 1956; 271:1185–9.

28. Berkovits BV, Castellanos A Jr, Lemberg L. Bifocal demand pacing. Circulation 1969; 40:44–9.

29. Castillo CA, Berkovits BV, Castellanos A Jr, et al. Bifocal demand pacing. Chest 1971; 59:360–4.

30. Mond H, Sloman G. The small tine pacemaker lead: absence of displacement. Pacing Clin Electrophysiol 1980; 3:171–7.

31. Fetter J, Bobeldyk GL, Engman FJ. The clinical incidence and significance of myopotential sensing with unipolar pacemakers. Pacing Clin Electrophysiol 1984; 7:871–9.

32. Levine PA, Caplan CH, Klein MD. Myopotential inhibition of unipolar lithium pacemakers. Chest 1982; 82:461–5.

33. Sutton R, Bourgeois I. The history of cardiac pacing. In: Sutton R, Bourgeois I, Ryden L, editors. The Foundations of Cardiac Pacing: An Illustrated Practical Guide to Basic Pacing, Vol. 1, Part 1. New York: Futura Publishing Co. Inc., 1991:319–24.

34. Funke HD. Die optimierte sequentielle Stimulation von Vorhof und Kammer-ein neuartiges Konzept zur Behandlung bradykarder Dysrhythmien. Herz Kreisl 1978; 10:479–83.

35. Rickards AF, Norman J. Relation between QT interval and heart rate: new design of physiologically adaptive cardiac pacemaker. Br Heart J 1981; 45:56–61.

36. Humen DP, Anderson K, Brumwell D, et al. A pacemaker which automatically increases its rate with physiological activity. In: Steinbach K et al., editors. Cardiac Pacing. Darmstadt: Steinkopff Verlag, 1983:259–65.

37. Benditt DG, Milstein S, Gornick CC, et al. Sensor-triggered rate-variable cardiac pacing: current technologies and clinical implications. Ann Int Med 1987; 107:714–24.

38. Stokes K. The biostability of polyurethane leads. In: Barold S, editor. Modern Cardiac Pacing. New York: Futura Pub. Co., 1985:173–98.

39. Stokes KB, Kriett JM, Gornick CC, et al. Low threshold cardiac pacing leads. IEEE Med Biol Soc 1983; 100–3.

40. Bisping HJ, Kreuzer J, Birkenheir H. Three-year clinical experience with a new endocardial screw-in lead with introduction protection for use in the atrium and ventricle. Pacing Clin Electrophysiol 1980; 3:424–35.

41. Stokes K, Bornzin G. The electrode-biointerface: stimulation. In: Barold S, editor. Modern Cardiac Pacing. New York: Futura Pub. Co., 1985:33–78.

42. Wang L, Fundamentals of intra-thoracic impedance monitoring in heart failure. Am J Cardiol 2007; 99:3G–10G.

43. Yu C, Wang L, Chau E, et al. Intrathoracic impedance monitoring in patients with heart failure: correlation with fluid status and feasibility of early warning preceding hospitalization. Circulation 2005; 112:841–8.

44. Gregoratos G, Abrams J, Epstein AE, et al. ACC/AHA/NASPE guidelines update for implantation of cardiac pacemakers and antiarrhythmia devices: summary article: a report of the American College of Cardiology, American Heart Association task force on practice guidelines (ACC/AHA/NASPE committee to update the 1998 pacemaker guidelines). J Am Col Cardiol 2002; 40:170–1719.

45. Vardas PE, Auricchio A, Blanc JJ, et al. Cardiac pacing and cardiac resynchronisation therapy-European Society of Cardiology Practice Guidelines. Eur Heart J 2007; 28:2256–95.
46. Wilkoff BL, Cook JR, Epstein AE, et al. Dual-chamber pacing or ventricular back-up pacing in patients with an implantable defibrillator: the dual chamber and VVI implantable defibrillator trial (DAVID) trial. JAMA 2002; 288:3115–23.
47. Cazeau S, Ritter P, Bakdach S, et al. Four chamber pacing in dilated cardiomyopathy. Pacing Clin Electrophysiol 1994; 17:1974–9.
48. Blanc JJ, Etienne Y, Gilard M, et al. Evaluation of different ventricular pacing sites in patients with severe heart failure. Results of an acute hemodynamic study. Circulation 1997; 96:3273–7.
49. Cazeau S, Leclerq C, Lavergne T, et al. Multisite stimulation in cardiomyopathies (MUSTIC) study investigators. Effects of multisite biventricular pacing in patients with heart failure and intraventricular conduction delay. N Engl J Med 2001; 344:873–80.
50. Abraham WT, Fisher WG, Smith AL, et al. The MIRACLE Study Group. Multicenter Insynch randomized clinical evaluation. Cardiac resynchronization in chronic heart failure. N Engl J Med 2002; 346:1845–53.
51. Auricchio A, Stellbrink C, Sack S, et al. Pacing therapies in congestive heart failure (PATH-CHF) study group. Long-term clinical effect of hemodynamically optimized cardiac resynchronization therapy in patients with heart failure and ventricular conduct ion delay. J Am Coll Cardiol 2002; 39:2026–33.
52. Bristow MR, Saxon LA, Boehmer J, et al. Comparison of medical therapy, pacing and defibrillation in heart failure (COMPANION) investigators. Cardiac resynchronization therapy with or without an implantable defibrillator in advanced chronic heart failure. N Engl J Med 2004; 350:2140–50.
53. Cleland JGF, Daubert J-C, Erdmann E, et al. The cardiac resynchronization-heart failure (CARE-HF) study investigators. The effect of cardiac resynchronization on morbidity and mortality in heart failure. N Engl J Med 2005; 352:1539–49.
54. Tyers GFO. Optimal electrode implantation site for asynchronous dipolar cardiac pacing. Ann Surg 1968; 167:168–79.
55. Tyers GFO. Comparison of the effect on cardiac function of single-site and simultaneous multiple-site ventricular stimulation after A-V block. J Thorac Cardiovasc Surg 1970; 59:211–7.
56. Gibson DG, Chamberlain DA, Coltart DJ, et al. Effect of changes in ventricular activation on cardiac hemodynamics in man. Comparison of right ventricular, left ventricular, and simultaneous pacing of both ventricles. Br Heart J 1971; 33;397–400.
57. De Teresa E, Rodriguez-Bailon I, Moreau J, et al. Haemodynamics of ventricular depolarization sequence during permanent cardiac pacing. In: Santini M, editor. Progress in Clinical Pacing. Milan: Springer-Verlag, 1984:888–92.
58. Beck CS, Pritchard WH, Feil HS. Ventricular fibrillation of long duration abolished by electric shock. JAMA 1947; 135:985–6.
59. Bouvrain Y, Guedon J, Zacouto F. The treatment of ventricular tachycardia by external electric shock. Arch Mal Coeur Vaiss 1962; 55:257–74.
60. Lown B, Amarasingham R, Neumann J. New method for terminating cardiac arrhythmias: use of synchronized capacitor discharge. JAMA 1962; 182:548–55.
61. Mirowski M, Reid RR, Mower MM, et al. Termination of malignant ventricular arrhythmias with an implanted automatic defibrillator in human beings. N Engl J Med 1980; 303:322–4.
62. Zipes DP, Hegger JJ, Miles WM, et al. Early experience with an implantable cardioverter. N Engl J Med 1984; 311:485–90.
63. AVID Investigators. A comparison of antiarrhythmic-drug therapy with implantable defibrillators in patients resuscitated from near-fatal ventricular arrhythmias. N Engl J Med 1997; 337:1576–83.
64. Connolly SJ, Gent M, Roberts RS, et al. Canadian implantable defibrillator study (CIDS): a randomized trial of the implantable cardioverter defibrillator against amiodarone. Circulation 2000; 101:1297–302.

65. Kuck KH, Cappato R, Siebels J, et al. Randomized comparison of antiarrhythmic drug therapy with implantable defibrillators in patients resuscitated from cardiac arrest: the cardiac arrest study Hamburg (CASH). Circulation 2000; 102:748–54.
66. Moss AJ, Hall WJ, Cannom DS, et al. Improved survival with an implanted defibrillator in patients with coronary disease at high risk for ventricular arrhythmia. Multicenter automatic defibrillator implantation trial investigators. N Engl J Med 1996; 335:1933–40.
67. Bigger JT Jr. Prophylactic use of implanted cardioverter defibrillators in patients at high risk for ventricular arrhythmia after coronary artery bypass graft (CABG) patch trial investigators. N Engl J Med 1997; 337:1569–75.
68. Buxton AE, Lee KL, Fisher JD, et al. A randomized study of the prevention of sudden death in patients with coronary artery disease. Multicenter unsustained tachycardia trial investigators. N Engl J Med 1999; 341:1882–90.
69. Moss AJ, Zareba W, Hall WJ, et al. The multicenter automatic defibrillator implantation trial II investigators. Prophylactic implantation of a defibrillator in patients with myocardial infarction and reduced ejection fraction. N Engl J Med 2002; 346:877–83.
70. Bardy GH, Lee KL, Mark DB, et al. Sudden Cardiac Death in Heart Failure (SCDHeFT) Investigators: Amiodarone or an implantable cardioverter-defibrillator for congestive heart failure. N Engl J Med 2005; 352:225–37.
71. Bardy GH, Yee R, Jung W. Multicenter experience with a pectoral unipolar implantable cardioverter-defibrillator. Active Can Investigators. J Am Coll Cardiol 1996; 28:400–10.
72. Holter NJ. New method for heart studies. Continuous electrocardiography of active subjects over long periods is now practical. Science 1961; 134:1214–20.
73. Krahn A, Klein GJ, Yee R, et al. Final results from a pilot study with an implantable loop recorder to determine the etiology of syncope in patients with negative non-invasive and invasive testing. Am J Cardiol 1998; 82:117–9.
74. Joshi AK, Kowey PR, Prystowsky EN, et al. First experience with a mobile cardiac outpatient telemetry (MCOT) system for the diagnosis and management of cardiac arrhythmia. Am J Cardiol 2005; 95:878–81.
75. Bourge RC, Abraham WT, Adamson PB, et al. Randomized controlled trial of an implantable continuous hemodynamic monitor in patients with advanced heart failure: the COMPASS-HF study. J Am Coll Cardiol 2008; 51:1073–9.
76. Puech P, Latour H, Grolleau R, et al. L'activite electrique du tissu de conduction auriculo-ventriculaire en electrocardiographie intracavitaire. Arch Mal Coeur Vaiss 1970; 63:500–20.
77. Scherlag BJ, Lau SH, Helfant RH, et al. Catheter technique for recording His bundle activity in man. Circulation 1969; 39:13–8.
78. Durrer D, Ross JP. Epicardial activation of the ventricles in a patient with Wolff-Parkinson-White syndrome (type B). Circulation 1967; 35:15–21.
79. Durrer D, Schoo L, Schuilenburg RM, et al. The role of premature beats in the initiation and the termination of supraventricular tachycardia in the Wolff-Parkinson-White syndrome. Circulation 1967; 36:644–2.
80. Wellens HJ, Schuilenberg RM, Durrer D. Electrical stimulation of the heart in patients with Wolff-Parkinson-White syndrome, type A. Circulation 1971; 43:99–114.
81. Wellens HJJ. Electrical Stimulation of the Heart in the Study and Treatment of Tachycardias. Leiden, The Netherlands: Kroese, 1971.
82. Wellens HJJ, Durrer DR, Lie K. Observations on mechanisms of ventricular tachycardia in man. Circulation 1976; 54:237–44.
83. Gallagher JJ, Pritchett ELC, Sealy WC, et al. The preexcitation syndromes. Prog Cardiovasc Dis 1978; 20:285–327.
84. Waldo AL, MacLean WA, Cooper TB, et al. Use of temporarily placed epicardial atrial wire electrodes for the diagnosis and treatment of cardiac arrhythmias following open-heart surgery. J Thorac Cardiovasc Surg 1978; 76:500–5.
85. Waldo AL, MacLean WA, Karp RB, et al. Entrainment and interruption of atrial flutter with atrial pacing: studies in man following open heart surgery. Circulation 1977; 56:737–45.

86. Waldo AL, Wells JL Jr, Cooper TB, et al. Temporary cardiac pacing: applications and techniques in the treatment of cardiac arrhythmias. Prog Cardiovasc Dis 1981; 23:451–74.
87. Josephson ME, Horowitz LN, Farshidi A. Continuous local electrical activity. A mechanism of recurrent ventricular tachycardia. Circulation 1978; 57:659–65.
88. Josephson ME, Horowitz LN, Farshidi A, et al. Recurrent sustained ventricular tachycardia. 2. Endocardial mapping. Circulation 1978; 57:440–7.
89. Josephson ME, Horowitz LN, Farshidi A, et al. Recurrent sustained ventricular tachycardia. 1. Mechanisms. Circulation 1978; 57:431–40.
90. Burchell HB, Frye RL, Anderson MW, et al. Atrioventricular and ventriculoatrial excitation in Wolff-Parkinson-White syndrome (type B). Temporary ablation at surgery. Circulation 1967; 36:663–72.
91. Becker AE, Anderson RH, Durrer D, et al. The anatomical substrates of Wolff-Parkinson-White syndrome: a clinicopathological correlation in seven patients. Circulation 1978; 57:870–9.
92. Sealy WC, Gallagher JJ, Pritchett ELC. The surgical anatomy of Kent bundles based on electrophysiological mapping and surgical exploration. J Thorac Cardiovasc Surg 1978; 76:804–15.
93. Denker S, Lehmann MH, Mahmud R, et al. Divergence between refractoriness of His-Purkinje system and ventricular muscle with abrupt changes in cycle length. Circulation 1983; 68:1212–21.
94. Denker S, Lehmann M, Mahmud R, et al. Effects of alternating cycle lengths on refractoriness of the His-Purkinje system. J Clin Invest 1984; 74:559–70.
95. Denker S, Lehmann MH, Mahmud R, et al. Facilitation of macroreentry within the His-Purkinje system with abrupt changes in cycle length. Circulation 1984; 69:26–32.
96. Strauss HC, Saroff A, Bigger JT Jr, et al. Premature atrial stimulation as a key to the understanding of sinoatrial conduction in man. Presentation of data and critical review. Circulation 1973; 47:86–93.
97. Benditt DG, Strauss HC, Scheinman MM, et al. Analysis of secondary pauses following termination of rapid atrial pacing in man. Circulation 1976; 54:436.
98. Narula OS, Samet P, Javier RP. Significance of the sinus node recovery time. Circulation 1972; 45:140–58.
99. Jordan JL, Yamaguchi I, Mandel WJ, The sick sinus syndrome. JAMA. 1977; 237:682–4.
100. Jordan JL, Yamaguchi I, Mandel WJ. Studies on the mechanism of sinus node dysfunction in the sick sinus syndrome. Circulation 1978; 57:217–23.
101. Waldo AL, MacLean WA, Karp RB, et al. Entrainment and interruption of atrial flutter with atrial pacing: studies in man following open heart surgery. Circulation 1977; 56:737–45.
102. Waldo AL, Plumb VJ, Arciniegas JG, et al. Transient entrainment and interruption of the atrioventricular bypass pathway type of paroxysmal atrial tachycardia. A model for understanding and identifying reentrant arrhythmias. Circulation 1983; 67:73–83.
103. Cosio FG, Arribas F, Barbero JM, et al. Validation of double-spike electrograms as markers of conduction delay or block in atrial flutter. Am J Cardiol 1988; 61:775–80.
104. Wijffels CEF, Kirchhof CJHJ, Dorland R, et al. Atrial fibrillation begets atrial fibrillation. A study in awake chronically instrumented goats. Circulation 1995; 92:1954–68.
105. Scheinman MM, Morady F, Hess DS, et al. Catheter-induced ablation of the atrioventricular junction to control refractory supraventricular arrhythmias. JAMA 1982; 248:851–5.
106. Gallagher JJ, Svenson RH, Kasell J, et al. Catheter technique for closed chest ablation of the atrioventricular conduction system. A therapeutic alternative for the treatment of refractory supraventricular tachycardia. N Engl J Med 1982; 306:194–200.
107. Jackman WM, Wang X, Friday KJ, et al. Catheter ablation of accessory atrioventricular pathways (Wolff-Parkinson-White syndrome) by radiofrequency current. N Engl J Med 1991; 324:1605.
108. Jackman WM, Beckman KJ, McClelland JH, et al. Treatment of supraventricular tachycardia due to atrioventricular nodal reentry by radiofrequency catheter ablation of slow pathway conduction. N Engl J Med 1992; 327:313–8.

109. Kuck KH, Schluter M, Eiger M, et al. Radiofrequency current catheter ablation of accessory atrioventricular pathways, Lancet 1991; 337:1557–61.
110. Cox JL, Boineau JP, Schuessler RB, et al. Successful surgical treatment of atrial fibrillation: review and clinical update. JAMA 1991; 266:1976.
111. Haissaguerre M, Jais P, Shah DC, et al. Spontaneous initiation of atrial fibrillation by ectopic beats originating in the pulmonary veins. N Engl J Med 1998; 339:659–66.
112. Haisaguerre M, Jais P, Shah DC, et al. Electrophysiological end point for catheter ablation of atrial fibrillation initiated from multiple pulmonary venous foci. Circulation 1999; 101:1409–17.
113. Harrison L, Gallagher JJ, Kasell J, et al. Cryosurgical ablation of the A-V node-His bundle: a new method for producing A-V block. Circulation 1977; 55:463–70.
114. Ohkawa S, Hackel DB, Mikat EM, et al. Anatomic effects of cryoablation of the atrioventricular conduction system. Circulation 1982; 65:1155–62.
115. Timmermans C, Ayers GM, Crijns HJ, et al. Randomized study comparing radiofrequency ablation with cryoablation for the treatment of atrial flutter with emphasis on pain perception. Circulation 2003; 107:1250–2.
116. Aoyama H, Nakagawa H, Pitha JV, et al. Comparison of cryothermia and radiofrequency current in safety and efficacy of catheter ablation within the canine coronary sinus close to the left circumflex coronary artery. J Cardiovasc Electrophysiol 2005; 16:1218–26.
117. Coumel Ph. Autonomic arrhythmogenic factors in paroxysmal atrial fibrillation. In: Olsson SB, Allessie MA, Campbell RWF, editors. Atrial Fibrillation: Mechanisms and Therapeutic Strategies. New York: Futura Publishing, 1994:171–85.
118. Coumel Ph. Autonomic influences in atrial tachyarrhythmias. J Cardiovasc Electrophysiol 1996; 7:999–1007.
119. Zipes DP, Rubart M. Neural modulation of cardiac arrhythmias and sudden cardiac death. Heart Rhythm 2006; 3:108–13.
120. Zipes DP. Ischemic modulation of cardiac autonomic innervation. J Am Coll Cardiol 1991; 17:1424–5.
121. Kenny RA, Bayliss J, Ingram A, et al. Head-up tilt: a useful test for investigating unexplained syncope. Lancet 1986; 1:1352–5.
122. Almquist A, Goldenberg IF, Milstein S, et al. Provocation of bradycardia and hypotension by isoproterenol and upright posture in patients with unexplained syncope. N Engl J Med 1989; 320:346–51.
123. Raviele A, Gasparini G, Di Pede F, et al. Nitroglycerin infusion during upright tilt: a new test for the diagnosis of vasovagal syncope. Am Heart J 1994; 127:103–11.
124. Raviele A, Menozzi C, Brignole M, et al. Value of head-up tilt testing potentiated with sublingual nitroglycerin to assess the origin of unexplained syncope. Am J Cardiol 1995; 76:267–72.
125. Brignole M, Menozzi C, Maggi R, et al. The usage and diagnostic yield of the implantable loop-recorder in detection of the mechanism of syncope and in guiding effective antiarrhythmic therapy in older people. Europace 2005; 7:273–9.
126. Brignole M, Sutton R, Menozzi C, et al. International Study on Syncope of Uncertain Etiology 2 (ISSUE 2) Group. Early application of an implantable loop recorder allows effective specific therapy in patients with recurrent suspected neurally mediated syncope. Eur Heart J 2006; 27:1085–92.
127. Moss AJ, Zareba W, Benhorin J, et al. ECG T-wave patterns in genetically distinct forms of the hereditary long QT syndrome. Circulation 1995; 92:2929–34.
128. Zareba W, Moss AJ, Schwartz PJ, et al. Influence of genotype on the clinical course of the long QT syndrome. International Long QT Registry Research Group. N Engl J Med 1998; 339:960–5.
129. Priori S. Long QT and Brugada syndromes. From genetics to clinical management. J Cardiovasc Electrophysiol 2000; 11:1174–80.
130. Brugada J, Brugada R, Brugada P. Right bundle-branch block and ST segment elevation in leads V1 through V3: a marker for sudden death in patients without demonstrable structural heart disease. Circulation 1998; 97:457–60.
131. Marcus Fl, Fontaine G, Guiraudon, et al. Right ventricular dysoplasia. A report of 24 cases. Circulation 1982; 65:384–95.

132. Lehnart SE, Ackerman MJ, Benson DW Jr, et al. Inherited arrhythmias: a National Heart, Lung, and Blood Institute and Office of Rare Diseases workshop consensus report about the diagnosis, phenotyping, molecular mechanisms, and therapeutic approaches for primary cardiomyopathies of gene mutations affecting ion channel function. Circulation 2007; 116:2325–45.

133. Durrer D, van Dam RT, Freud GE, et al. Total excitation of the isolated human heart. Circulation 1970; 41:899–912.

134. Benson DW Jr, Sterba R, Gallagher JJ, et al. Localization of the site of ventricular preexcitation with body surface maps in patients with Wolff-Parkinson-White syndrome. Circulation 1982; 65:1259–68.

135. Benson DW Jr, Spach MS. Evolution of QRS and ST-T-wave body surface potential distributions during the first year of life. Circulation 1982; 65:1247–58.

136. Harrison L, Ideker RE, Smith WM, et al. The sock electrode array: a tool for determining global epicardial activation during unstable arrhythmias. Pacing Clin Electrophysiol 1980; 3:531–40.

137. Gallagher JJ, Kasell JH, Cox JL, et al. Techniques of intraoperative electrophysiologic mapping. Am J Cardiol 1982; 49:221–40.

138. Boineau JP, Canavan TE, Schuessler RB, et al. Demonstration of a widely distributed atrial pacemaker complex in the human heart. Circulation 1988; 77:1221–37.

139. Taccardi B, Arisi G, Macchi E, et al. A new intracavitary probe for detecting the site of origin of ectopic ventricular beats during one cardiac cycle. Circulation 1987; 75:272–81.

140. Kadish A, Hauck J, Pederson B, et al. Mapping of atrial activation with a noncontact, multielectrode catheter in dogs. Circulation 1999; 99:1906–13.

141. Surawicz B. Brief history of cardiac arrhythmias since the end of the nineteenth century: Part I. J Cardiovasc Electrophysiol 2003; 14:1365–71.

142. Surawicz B. Brief history of cardiac arrhythmias since the end of the nineteenth century: Part II. J Cardiovasc Electrophysiol 2004; 15:101–11.

143. Singh BN, Venkatesh N, Nademanee K, et al. The historical development, cellular electrophysiology and pharmacology of amiodarone Prog Cardiovasc Dis 1989; 31:249–80.

144. Bacaner M, Benditt DG. Management of ventricular tachycardia and fibrillation with bethanidine an orally absorbable bretylium analog. Circulation 1981; 64:36–41.

145. Green AF. The discovery of bretylium and bethanidine. Br J Clin Pharmacol 1982; 13:25–34.

146. Benditt DG, Pritchett ELC, Wallace AG, et al. Recurrent ventricular tachycardia in man. Evaluation of disopyramide therapy by intracardiac electrical stimulation. Eur J Cardiol 1979; 9:255–76.

147. Anonymous. Preliminary report: effect of encainide and flecainide on mortality in a randomized trial of arrhythmia suppression after myocardial infarction. The Cardiac Arrhythmia Suppression Trial (CAST) Investigators. N Engl J Med 1989; 321:406–12.

148. Fisher JD, Cohen HL, Mehra R, et al. Cardiac pacing and pacemakers. II. Serial electrophysiologic-pharmacologic testing for control of recurrent tachyarrhythmias. Am Heart J 1977; 93:658–68.

149. Hartzler GO, Maloney JD. Programmed ventricular stimulation in management of recurrent ventricular tachycardia. Mayo Clin Proc 1977; 52:731–41.

150. Horowitz LN, Josephson ME, Farshidi A, et al. Recurrent sustained ventricular tachycardia 3. Role of the electrophysiologic study in selection of antiarrhythmic regimens. Circulation 1978; 58:986–97.

151. The ESVEM Investigators. Determinants of predicted efficacy of antiarrhythmic drugs in the Electrophysiologic Study versus Electrocardiographic Monitoring trial. Circulation 1993; 87:323–9.

152. Wyse GD, Talajic M, Haflee GE, et al. Antiarrhythmic drug therapy in the Multicenter Unsustained Tachycardia Trial: drug-testing and as-treated analysis. J Am Coll Cardiol 2001; 38:344–51.

153. Benditt DG, Bailin S, Remole S, et al. Proarrhythmia: recognition of patients at risk. J Cardiovasc Electrophysiol 1991; 2:S221–32.

Part I
Overview

Chapter 2
Basic Cardiac Electrophysiology: Excitable Membranes

Deborah A. Jaye, Yong-Fu Xiao, and Daniel C. Sigg

Abstract Cardiomyocytes are excitable cells that have the ability to contract after excitation; therefore, each heartbeat is an event of electrical–mechanical coupling. Cardiac electrical activity at different levels can be measured through variable means and modified by different drugs or medical devices. Understanding the basic mechanisms of cardiac excitation is essential not only to a physiologist, but also to a cardiologist, because cardiac arrhythmias are a major health issue in our society and clinical practice. Diagnosis and therapy of arrhythmias requires understanding the cause or origin of each arrhythmia and making decisions to control or eliminate the arrhythmia. Advances in basic research enhance our understanding of normal cell, tissue, and organ function (physiology) and also disease processes (pathophysiology), and hopefully lead to better clinical diagnosis and improved clinical therapies, either directly or indirectly. Cardiomyocytes are the main component of a heart. Their electrical activity is fundamentally a bioprocess determined by the transmembrane potential, a voltage difference between the intracellular and extracellular compartments. During a normal cardiac cycle, mechanical contraction always follows electrical excitation. This chapter provides a basic overview of membrane excitability of cardiomyocytes and other excitable cells (i.e., neuronal and skeletal).

2.1 Introduction

The most critical job of the heart is to expel blood to the whole body, and transport critical nutrients to and remove waste products from the tissues. The heart is a muscular pump with rhythmic electrical activity and muscle contraction. Cardiac electrical activity results from fluxes of sodium, potassium, calcium, and chloride ions across the cell membrane. These ion fluxes, or membrane currents, can be measured and analyzed at the level of single channel or whole cell by patch clamp, or whole body by ECG.

D.C. Sigg (✉)
Department of Integrative Biology and Physiology, University of Minnesota,
Minneapolis, MN, USA
e-mail: siggx001@umn.edu

D.C. Sigg et al. (eds.), *Cardiac Electrophysiology Methods and Models*,
DOI 10.1007/978-1-4419-6658-2_2, © Springer Science + Business Media, LLC 2010

The main mechanism of cardiac excitation and contraction is the excitability of the cell membrane, which is the term used to describe the ability of a cell to depolarize or be depolarized to initiate an action potential. Membrane excitability depends on the action of ion channels, ion pumps, and ion transporters or exchangers embedded in the lipid bilayer surrounding a cell. An external stimulus delivered to an excitable cell causes a rise in the resting membrane potential or the voltage gradient across the membrane. Once a critical level, or threshold, is reached, the membrane permeability to ions is altered, causing a depolarizing inward current and initiating an action potential.[1] This property is not unique to cardiac cells but is shared by neurons as well as skeletal and smooth muscle cells. However, non-excitable cells cannot be depolarized to induce an action potential either with or without stimulation.

Before delving into the characteristics of the cardiac action potential, one needs to understand the basic concepts of membrane structures, ion channels, and ion currents contributing to the action potential. The following sections describe how ion channels affect membrane excitability.

2.2   Cell Membrane

The cell membrane is composed of a phospholipid bilayer with its hydrophobic interior and various proteins inserted (Fig. 2.1a). The lipid bilayer itself is impermeable to ions, but embedded channel proteins in the membrane can selectively allow passage of ions.[2] The plasma membrane serves as a barrier to maintain the ionic concentrations in the intra- and extracellular compartment. Due to channel ion selectivity, the compositions of fluids inside and outside the cell are different (Table 2.1). The cell membrane has a charge across it, a transmembrane potential, and is polarized (Fig. 2.1b). The inside of excitable cells is more negative than the outside, resulting in an overall negative potential. Depolarization occurs when the negativity of the transmembrane potential is reduced, while repolarization is the restoration of the resting membrane potential.

Depolarization and repolarization are effectively modulated by a series of ion fluxes across the cell membrane in which are embedded numerous proteins. Some of them span the cell membrane to form pores or channels allowing the passive or active transport of ions. Each type of ion channel is highly selective to permit only one or more specific ions (Fig. 2.1a). Two factors affecting passive diffusion through the membrane are electric potential and ion concentration, or the electrochemical gradient. When the ion concentration is greater in one region, the tendency is for the ions to move to the area of lower concentration due to diffusion forces. Similarly, movement of ions is promoted by electrical forces. Like a capacitor, excitable membranes store energy in the form of electrochemical gradients that can be discharged to transmit electrical signals in tissues. In the electric circuit analogy, the pores form a conductive branch in parallel with the capacitive lipid bilayer (Fig. 2.1b). Ohm's law, which defines the relationship

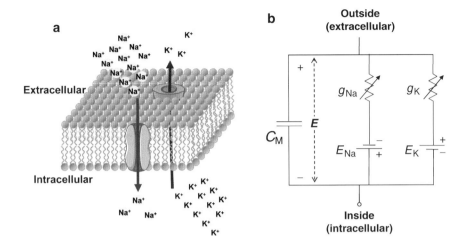

Fig. 2.1 Three-dimensional view of a representative section of a schematic plasma membrane with embedded proteins, such as Na$^+$ channel and K$^+$ channel (**a**) and an equivalent circuit (**b**). The cell membrane acts like an equivalent circuit with a capacitive branch (C_M), representative of the lipid bilayer, and with conductive branches (g_{Na} and g_K), representative of sodium – and potassium-selective pores, as well as the corresponding electromotive forces (E_{Na} and E_K), representative of the sodium and potassium equilibrium membrane potentials

Table 2.1 Major ionic components of intra- and extracellular fluids and equilibrium potentials of major ions

Ion	Intracellular concentration (mEq/L)	Extracellular concentration (mEq/L)	Equilibrium potential (mV)
Na$^+$	15	140	70
K$^+$	135	4	−94
Ca^{2+}	2×10^{-4}	4	132
Mg^{2+}	40	2	
Cl$^-$	4	120	−90
HCO$_3^-$	10	24	
HPO$_4^{2-}$	20	4	
SO$_4^{2-}$	4	1	
Proteins$^-$, Amino acids$^-$, Urea, etc.	152	1	

between current, voltage, and conductance or resistance in an electric circuit, also governs in describing the electrical properties of membranes.[3]

In addition to ion movement down the electrochemical gradient through ion channels, intracellular concentrations of sodium, potassium, and calcium are maintained by active transport via pumps spanning the cell membrane. The sodium–potassium exchange pump is electrogenic, meaning it creates an electrical potential across the cell membrane and generates a large concentration gradient for sodium and potassium. Sodium is pumped outside the cell at a ratio of 3:2 with potassium being pumped inside the cell, leaving a deficit of positive ions inside the cell. Additionally, calcium pumps and the sodium–calcium exchanger transport calcium ions out of the cytoplasm to achieve a low intracellular calcium concentration.

2.3 Membrane Electrophysiology

2.3.1 Resting Membrane Potential

The origin of resting and action potentials lies in the relative concentrations inside and outside the cell and in the permeability of the membrane to that ion. The resting potential is the transmembrane potential that exists when the electrical and chemical forces are exactly equal and there is no net movement of ions across the cell membrane. In most cardiac cells, the typical resting membrane potential is about −85 to −90 mV (Fig. 2.2). In skeletal muscle and nerve, the resting potential is −95

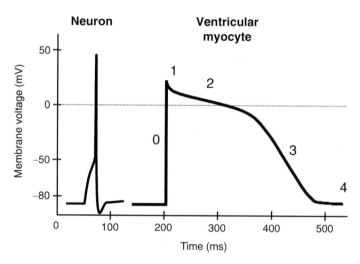

Fig. 2.2 Representative action potentials (APs) of a neuron and ventricular myocyte. Note the morphological differences between the two APs. Regular contractile myocytes have a true resting membrane potential (about −90 mV) at phase 4 in the panel that remains constant near the equilibrium potential for K^+ (E_K). When an AP is initiated, there is a rapid depolarization phase (phase 0) which is caused by activation of fast Na^+ channels. Phase 1 is an initial repolarization due to the opening of transient outward K^+ channels (I_{to}). However, because of the large increase in the inward L-type Ca^{++} currents at the same time and the transient nature of I_{to}, the repolarization is delayed with a plateau (phase 2). This plateau phase prolongs the AP duration and distinguishes the cardiac AP from the much shorter AP in neuron. Continuous repolarization activates another type of K^+ channel (I_K) and, along with the inactivation of Ca^{++} channels, leads to the rapid repolarization (phase 3)

and −90 mV, respectively, while in smooth muscle it is −50 to −60 mV.[4] The terms resting potential and action potential are reserved to describe the transmembrane potential of excitable cells. Non-excitable cells, such as fibroblasts and endothelial cells, cannot initiate and propagate an action potential and thus do not have a corresponding resting potential.

2.3.2   Equilibrium Potential and the Nernst Equation

The flow of ions across the cell membrane is determined by the ion concentration, or chemical gradient, as well as the electrical gradient. For any given ion, the concentration gradient across the cell membrane promotes diffusion of that ion. The electrical gradient across the membrane that prevents the net diffusion of the ion is called the equilibrium potential for that ion. The equilibrium potential is also known as the Nernst potential because it is calculated with the Nernst equation, which is valid for any permeant in a steady state.

$$V = -\frac{RT}{zF}\ln\frac{C_i}{C_o} = -61.5 \cdot \log\frac{C_i}{C_o}, T = 37^\circ C \tag{2.1}$$

Equation (2.1), Nernst Equation, where V is the membrane potential, R the gas constant, T the absolute temperature, z the valence of the ion, F the Faraday constant, and C_o and C_i the concentration of the ion outside and inside the cell.

When the cell membrane is permeable to multiple ions, the membrane potential that prevents the net diffusion of any of the permeant ions across the membrane is determined by the Goldman–Hodgkin–Katz equation. For a membrane permeable to sodium, potassium, and chloride, the membrane potential is defined as follows:

$$V_m = -61.5 \cdot \log\frac{P_{K^+}[K^+]_i + P_{Na^+}[Na^+]_i + P_{Cl^-}[Cl^-]_o}{P_{K^+}[K^+]_o + + P_{Na^+}[Na^+]_o + P_{Cl^-}[Cl^-]_i} \tag{2.2}$$

Equation (2.2), Goldman–Hodgkin–Katz equation for the membrane potential across a cell membrane permeable to K^+, Na^+, and Cl^-. P=membrane permeability (cm/s); V_m is in mV.

The equilibrium potentials for the common ions in cardiac muscle are shown in Table 2.1. By evaluating the equilibrium potentials of various ions, we understand where active transport processes come into play. The equilibrium potential for potassium is almost exactly equal to the resting membrane potential, which prevents the movement of potassium outside the cell. However, for sodium, both the concentration gradient and the membrane potential favor movement of sodium inside the cell. Based on the Nernst and Goldman equations, the electrochemical gradients cause diffusion of sodium into the cell, which should lead to steady-state conditions. However, the sodium–potassium exchanger offsets diffusion by continuously pumping sodium out and potassium into the cell.

2.3.3   Ion Channels and Membrane Currents

Ion channels embedded in the cell membrane are proteins that have the ability to transport ions across the membrane, but their permeability to ions is highly selective. Each type of channel only allows passage of one or more specific ions. In excitable membranes, the three major classes of cation-selective ion channels are sodium, potassium, and calcium. Permeability of the channels is controlled by gates that open and close in response to changes in voltage potential (voltage gating) or chemical binding (chemical or ligand gating). While some types of potassium channels are ligand gated, the potassium, sodium, and calcium currents contributing to the action potential in normal hearts are regulated by voltage-gated channels. At the resting membrane potential (−85 to −90 mV for most cardiomyocytes), the majority of potassium channels are in the open state, but sodium channels are closed.[5] Opening of the voltage-gated sodium channel in response to a less negative cytoplasm (threshold) causes a large amount of sodium to enter the cell and is the basis for initiation of an action potential. Table 2.2 summarizes the major electrophysiological properties of excitable membranes of nerve, cardiac myocyte, skeletal, and smooth muscle cells. Chapter 3 further details the gating properties of ion channels.

By convention, inward currents are defined as movement of positive charge, such as Na^+, into the cell or negative charge, such as Cl^-, out of the cell, whereas outward currents are generated by positive charge leaving the cell or by negative charge moving into the cell. Because the inside of the cell is negatively charged at rest, inward currents are considered depolarizing and outward currents are repolarizing. Actually, many different ions dynamically move in and out of a cell at the same time during an action potential. Therefore, the instant membrane potential at a distinct time in an action potential is determined by the sum of all ion movements across the membrane.

2.3.4   Action Potential

The most efficient signal conduction in excitable tissue is the initiation and propagation of action potentials. When an excitatory stimulus causes the membrane potential to become less negative and beyond a threshold level, the permeability of the

Table 2.2   Major electrophysiological properties of excitable membranes

Cell type	Resting membrane potential (mV)	Action potential duration (ms)	Conduction velocity (m/s)
Nerve			
Large myelinated	−80 to −90	0.2–1	100
Muscle			
Cardiac	−85 to −90	200–300	0.3–0.5
Skeletal	−80 to −90	1–5	3–5
Smooth	−50 to −60	10–50	

membrane to ions changes, the cell rapidly depolarizes, and the membrane potential reverses transiently prior to repolarization. This process describes the action potential that includes depolarization and repolarization (Fig. 2.2). Unlike skeletal muscle, cardiac muscle is electrically coupled so that the wave of depolarization propagates from one cell to the next, independent of neuronal input. A significant amount of what we know about action potentials today is based on the seminal studies by A. L. Hodgkin and A. F. Huxley in the squid giant axon in the 1950s[6] and, more recently, by Luo and Rudy[7,8] in the ventricular myocyte. In the classical experiments published by Hodgkin and Huxley, the timing and amplitude of the ionic currents contributing to the squid axon action potential were measured in voltage clamp experiments and characterized mathematically. The Luo–Rudy model was built on the Hodgkin–Huxley model and characterizes the ionic contributions to the ventricular cardiac action potential. These models are discussed further in Chapter 7 of this book.

Morphologically, cardiac action potential has its unique characteristics. Figure 2.2 compares the action potentials of a neuron and ventricular cardiomyocyte. One of the distinguishing characteristics of the cardiac action potential is the plateau and longer action potential duration. In nerve fibers, the action potential is of a short duration (0.2–1 ms), whereas the cardiac action potential is typically 200–300 ms in human cardiomyocytes. Skeletal muscle action potential is similar to the nerve action potential in shape and duration (1–5 ms). These major differences from skeletal and neuronal cells can be explained by contributions of calcium currents in the cardiac action potential. The plateau and longer action potential duration are critical for cardiomyocytes, because myocardial contraction is more dependent on extracellular Ca^{2+} to enter into cells. Table 2.3 summarizes the main ion fluxes across the cardiac plasma membrane during an action potential. In addition, the ionic contributions to the cardiac action potential are discussed in more detail in Chapter 3 of this book.

2.3.5   *Refractoriness*

The ability of the heart to respond to a stimulus depends on the time that elapsed since its last contraction.[5] There are four states of refractoriness throughout the action potential (Fig. 2.3): (1) absolute refractory period (ARP) or effective refractory period (ERP), which is the period during which an electrical stimulus, no matter how great the stimulus, will not elicit an action potential because the membrane is not sufficiently repolarized and sodium channels have not completely recovered from the inactivated state; (2) relative refractory period (RRP), which requires a larger stimulus to initiate an action potential; (3) supernormal period (SNP), during which the threshold is lower than typically required to generate an action potential; and (4) normal excitability.[5] During RRP and SNP, the cell is slower to depolarize and the amplitude and duration of the action potential are smaller than those elicited after the cell has fully repolarized. Full recovery time, or

Table 2.3 Major ion fluxes across cardiac plasma membrane during action potential

Current	Selective ion	Current direction	Phase	Effect
I_{Na}	Na^+	Inward	0	Depolarization
$I_{Ca,T}$	Ca^{2+}	Inward	0	Depolarization
I_{to}	K^+	Outward	1	Early repolarization
$I_{Ca,L}$	Ca^{2+}	Inward	2	Plateau
I_{Kr}	K^+	Outward	3	Repolarization
I_{Ks}	K^+	Outward	3	Repolarization
I_{K1}	K^+	Outward	4	Resting potential
I_f	K^+/Na^+	Inward	4	Depolarization/ pacemaking

Source: Modified from Katz[9] and Whalley[10]

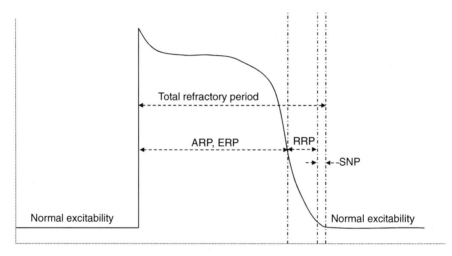

Fig. 2.3 Cardiac AP and refractory period. The total refractory period is comprised of the (1) absolute refractory period (ARP) or effective refractory period (ERP), which is the period during which an electrical stimulus will not elicit an AP because the membrane is not sufficiently repolarized and sodium channels have not completely recovered; (2) relative refractory period (RRP), which requires a larger stimulus; and (3) supernormal period (SNP), during which the threshold is lower than typically required to generate an AP. Normal excitability exists outside of the total refractory period. See Chap. 3 for a detailed discussion of cardiac action potentials

the total refractory period, encompasses the ARP, RRP, and SNP.[9] The membrane responsiveness to electrical stimulus is different in the periods of ARP, RRP, SNP and normal state (Fig. 2.4). The duration of the total refractory period varies with the time course of repolarization, which is shorter in nerve and other types of muscle cells. Duration also varies in the region of the heart with atrial being shorter than ventricular. It also decreases as heart rate increases. The activity of the autonomic system can significantly modify the duration of the cardiac refractory period.

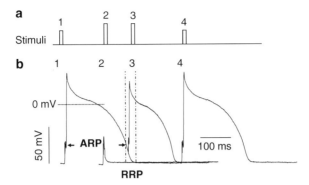

Fig. 2.4 Responsiveness of canine ventricular myocytes to electrical stimulation. (**a**) Marks of stimulation pulses delivered at different time periods (1, 2, 3, and 4) during a cardiac cycle. (**b**) APs initiated by the stimuli delivered at the times corresponding to those in panel (**a**). A pulse stimulus initiated an action potential (1). If a pulse fell in the absolute refractory period (ARP with the *arrows*) of an AP, no AP was induced even with super-threshold stimulation (2). During the relative refractory period (RRP with *dotted lines*), an AP could be generated after super-threshold stimulation (3). After full recovery, a normal AP (4) was initiated with the threshold stimulation as in (1). The notch on the upstroke of the depolarization phase of the AP was a stimulation artifact

2.3.6   Excitation–Contraction Coupling

Excitation of healthy cardiomyocytes always is followed by their mechanical contraction. Excitation–contraction coupling is a biological process in which an action potential triggers a cardiac myocyte to mechanically contract. Therefore, it is a process whereby an electrical signal (i.e., action potential) is converted to a mechanical process (i.e., myocyte contraction). While this process can be explained on a single myocyte level, in normal physiology, the process is orchestrated and coordinated at a whole organ level through the coordinated depolarization and repolarization of the entire heart, which starts with the depolarization of the sinoatrial node and ultimately leads to depolarization and subsequent contraction of the atria and ventricles. This is facilitated by the strong coupling of the cardiac myocytes and the cells of the conduction system via gap junctions. The key contractile proteins in the heart are actin and myosin, while troponins are the key regulatory proteins. Troponin I inhibits the actin binding site of myosin during diastole where cytosolic calcium concentrations are very low. Once an action potential depolarizes the cellular membrane, calcium ions enter the cell during phase 2 of the action potential through voltage-gated (L-type) calcium channels. This calcium triggers further release of calcium to the cytoplasmic compartment from the sarcoplasmic reticulum (SR) through ryanodine receptors. The free calcium then binds to troponin C. Troponin C induces a conformational change in the regulatory complex, thereby enabling troponin I to expose a site on the actin molecule. The actin molecule is then able to bind to the myosin ATPase located on the myosin head. The binding subsequently leads to hydrolysis of ATP, and a conformational change occurs in the

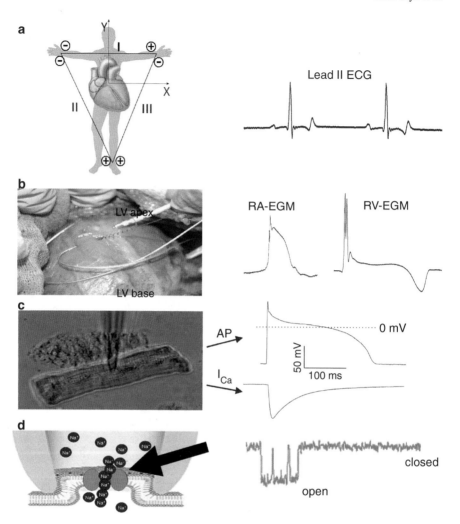

Fig. 2.5 Different levels of cardiac electrophysiological recordings. (**a**) Standard limb lead configuration forming Einthoven's triangle (*left panel*) and electrocardiogram (ECG) signal from Lead II (*right panel*) (adapted from www.cvrti.utah.edu/~macleod/bioen/be6000/labnotes/ecg/figures/limbleads.jpg. (**b**) Epicardial mapping of the canine left ventricle to record local electrograms at the tissue level (*left panel*) and endocardial electrogram recorded from the right atrium (RA-EGM) or from the right ventricle (RV-EGM) with placement of a Medtronic modified 3830 lead with 4-mm tip-to-ring spacing to a porcine heart (*right panel*). (**c**) Whole-cell patch clamp of a human ventricular myocyte (*left panel*) isolated from disposed biopsy tissue; morphology of ventricular AP and inward L-type Ca^{2+} current trace recorded by the whole-cell patch clamp method (*right panels*). (**d**) Schematic diagram of single channel recording configuration and inward single channel currents after a voltage pulse

actin–myosin complex. The result of these changes is a mechanical movement between the myosin heads and the actin, and a shortening of the sarcomere. At the end of the phase 2 of the action potential, calcium entry slows and calcium is removed from the SR via an ATP-dependent calcium pump (SERCA ATPase). This eventually lowers the cytosolic calcium concentration and removes calcium from troponin C. Calcium is also being removed from the cell by the sodium–calcium-exchanger pump (NCX). A conformational change in the troponin complex is being induced by the reduced cytosolic calcium, leading to troponin I inhibition of the actin binding site. At the end of the cycle, a new ATP binds to the myosin head, displaces ADP, restores the initial sarcomere length, and the cycle starts over.

2.4   Summary

The membrane of cardiomyocytes is excitable. Cardiac electrical activities can be measured and quantified at different levels (Fig. 2.5). The fundamental mechanism of this excitability is due to impermeability to ions of the lipid bilayer and highly selective permeability to ions of the proteins embedded in the membrane. As selective passage of ions across the plasma membrane, the components of ions are differently distributed in the intra- and extracellular compartments. Such imbalanced distribution in the resting state causes more negative than positive ions in the intracellular compartment and results in a transmembrane potential of −85 to −90 mV in most cardiomyocytes. Electrical, chemical, or mechanical stimulation can depolarize cardiomyocytes to a threshold level and initiate an action potential. In the normal heart, each electrical activity is followed by a mechanical contraction. However, abnormalities of initiation and conduction of electrical impulses in a heart can lead to arrhythmias and mechanical failure. More accurate diagnosis and proper therapy of electrical abnormalities of the heart require current knowledge of basic cardiac electrophysiology.

References

1. Hurst JW. The Heart, Arteries and Veins, sixth edition. New York: McGraw-Hill, 1985.
2. Alberts B. Molecular Biology of the Cell, third edition. New York: Garland Publishers, 1994.
3. Hille B. Ion Channels of Excitable Membranes, third edition. Sunderland, MA: Sinauer, 2001.
4. Guyton AC, Hall JE. Textbook of Medical Physiology, tenth edition. Philadelphia: Saunders, 2000.
5. Milnor WR. Cardiovascular Physiology. New York: Oxford University Press, 1990.
6. Hodgkin AL, Huxley AF. A quantitative description of membrane current and its application to conduction and excitation in nerve. J Physiol 1952; 117:500–44.
7. Luo CH, Rudy Y. A dynamic model of the cardiac ventricular action potential. I. Simulations of ionic currents and concentration changes. Circ Res 1994; 74:1071–96.
8. Luo CH, Rudy Y. A dynamic model of the cardiac ventricular action potential. II. After depolarizations, triggered activity, and potentiation. Circ Res 1994; 74:1097–113.
9. Katz AM. Physiology of the Heart, fourth edition. Philadelphia: Lippincott Williams & Wilkins, 2006.
10. Whalley DW, Wendt DJ, Grant AO. Basic concepts in cellular cardiac electrophysiology: Part I: ion channels, membrane currents, and the action potential. Pacing Clin Electrophysiol 1995; 18:1556–74.

Chapter 3
Cardiac Action Potentials, Ion Channels, and Gap Junctions

Jacques M.T. de Bakker and Harold V.M. van Rijen

Abstract Interplay between various ion channels in the membrane of cardiomyocytes is responsible for depolarization and repolarization of the heart cells, whereas cell-to-cell coupling, mediated by gap junction proteins, is involved in propagation of the action potential through the heart. In this chapter, the different phases of the action potential of heart cells are discussed and the role and characteristics of the most important ion channels that are active during these phases are conferred. Differences in the expression of the various ion and gap junction channels under normal conditions are described. Also discussed are changes in ion and gap junction channel expression and distribution that occur in cardiac disease. Finally, the role of ligand-gated and stretch-activated ion channels is addressed briefly.

3.1 Introduction

Contraction of the heart is preceded by electrical activity that spreads through the heart in a coordinated manner. Action potentials of the heart cells (cardiomyocytes) that are responsible for electrical activity are generated by interplay of various ion channels and exchangers.[1] Propagation of the action potential depends on channel proteins (gap junctions) that connect the cells electrically.[2] The heart harbors various types of cardiomyocytes that exhibit different biophysical properties caused by differences in ion channel expression. This gives the heart cells their specific electro-physiological characteristics. Cells in the sinoatrial node must orchestrate the electrical activity of the heart and therefore these cells exhibit regular, spontaneous depolarizations. From the sinoatrial node, activation spreads through the atria and initiates atrial contraction. Contraction of the ventricles must follow that of the atria after a delay to allow adequate filling of the ventricles. This implies that the electrical impulse after leaving the atrium must be delayed before entering the ventricles.

J.M.T. de Bakker (✉)
Department of Experimental Cardiology, Academic Medical Center, Amsterdam,
The Netherlands
e-mail: j.m.debakker@amc.uva.nl

D.C. Sigg et al. (eds.), *Cardiac Electrophysiology Methods and Models*,
DOI 10.1007/978-1-4419-6658-2_3, © Springer Science+Business Media, LLC 2010

For this reason, the atrioventricular (AV) node, which connects the atria and ventricles electrically, exhibits very slow conduction. In addition, some cells in the AV node demonstrate spontaneous activity, although at a much lower rate than activity of the sinoatrial node. A special combination of ion channels, gap junction channels, and myocardial architecture accounts for these unique properties of both the sinoatrial and AV node. Once the ventricle has been reached by the electrical impulse, ventricular cells must be activated rapidly to optimize pump function. The fast distribution of electrical impulse through the ventricles is mediated by the specific conduction system, consisting of the bundle of His, the bundle branches, and the Purkinje system. Cells of the specific conduction system have a special composition of ion channels to allow fast propagation (>1 m/s). Also here, special structural and functional characteristics, such as a large cell size, a peculiar distribution of gap junction channel proteins along the cell border, and a fibrous sheet around the bundle branches, are present and result in high conduction velocity. The bundle branches shade off into the Purkinje network that finally transfers the impulse to the cells of the working myocardium. Again, cells with special electrical characteristics are present to allow a safe electrical connection between the small Purkinje strands and the large working myocardium.

3.2 Phases of the Action Potential

Cardiac cells are electrically excitable and exhibit, like many other cells of vertebrates, an electrical potential across the membrane in the resting state. Depending on the cell type, the transmembrane voltage ranges from –60 to –90 mV, where the intracellular space is negative with respect to the extracellular space. The resting membrane potential is caused by differences in ion concentrations that exist between the intracellular and extracellular milieu. The difference in ion concentration between the intra- and extracellular space will give rise to diffusion of ions across the membrane, generating a potential difference that will counteract the diffusion and finally result in electrochemical equilibrium. This equilibrium potential is described by the Nernst equation.[3] Because various ions are present, conductance of the different ion channels plays a role in determining the equilibrium potential. In addition, conductivity of the ion channels is often voltage dependent. At rest, most ion channels, except for the potassium channel, are virtually closed. For this reason, the resting membrane potential is determined mainly by the potassium concentrations inside and outside the cell. See Chapter 2 for further discussion of the equilibrium potential.

A typical ventricular action potential is generated in case a depolarizing current, usually from activated neighboring cardiomyocytes, reduces the membrane potential toward about –60 mV. At this value of the membrane potential, sodium channels open and the membrane potential will move toward the sodium equilibrium value of about +20 mV. This depolarization phase is fast (within milliseconds) and is meant to activate neighboring cells, and also to open the calcium channels to initiate cardiac contraction. This initial phase of the cardiac action potential is called

Fig. 3.1 Action potential of a ventricular cardiomyocyte. Numbers indicate different phases of the action potential. In *gray* are the major currents running during the different phases

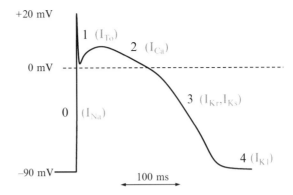

phase 0 and causes the upstroke of the action potential (Fig. 3.1). Shortly after the sodium channels open, they close (inactivate) again. In addition, a first repolarization is initiated by a particular potassium (K^+) channel that generates a transient outward current (I_{To}). This repolarizing current causes a notch in the action potential of some types of cardiomyocytes. These two processes define *phase 1* of the action potential. In contrast to action potentials generated in neurons, the cardiac action potential exhibits a plateau phase, an interval at which the membrane potential maintains a value close to the value reached at the end of phase 0. The plateau phase is maintained by calcium current (I_{Ca}) that generates a depolarizing current and is called *phase 2* of the action potential. In fact, the plateau phase is present because of a delicate balance between depolarizing (inward) and repolarizing (outward) currents. Repolarization of the action potential is caused by inactivation of the depolarizing currents and changes in the conductance of various potassium channels, which result in an increase in repolarizing current. This period of the action potential is called *phase 3*; the prevailing repolarizing currents finally bring the membrane potential back to its initial resting value of -60 to -90 mV. The resting state that follows is called *phase 4* and is maintained by another potassium current (I_{K1}).

3.3   Ion Channels

Ion channels that are responsible for the depolarizing and repolarizing currents through the membrane consist of complex proteins. These proteins form pores (channels) across the lipid bilayer that composes the cell membrane. Ion channels are not simple structures that gradually open and close. Patch clamp measurements revealed that there are, in fact, only two states for the channels – closed or open. In patch clamp recording, a microelectrode (glass pipette with a tip diameter of 1 μm) contacts the cell surface. With gentle suction a tight electrical seal is formed where the cell membrane contacts the mouth of the microelectrode. By varying the concentrations of ions in the medium on either side of the membrane patch, one can test which ion will pass the channel. With appropriate electronic circuitry and voltage across the membrane patch, the current can be measured. The current behaves in a peculiar way; even at constant conditions the currents switch abruptly on and off, as though an on/off switch were being randomly jiggled (Fig. 3.2). If conditions are changed, the random behavior continues, but with different probability. If the condition tends to open the channel, it will spend a much greater proportion of time in the open conformation, although it will not remain open continuously.[4]

Ion channels differ with respect to ion selectivity, that is the type of ions they allow to pass, and gating, the condition that influences their opening and closing. For voltage-gated channels, the probability of being open is controlled by the membrane potential. Ligand-gated channels are controlled by the binding of a molecule (ligand) to the channel protein, whereas stress-activated channel opening is controlled by a mechanical force applied to the channel. In heart muscle, all three types of channels are present. Voltage-gated ion channels play a major role in propagation of the action potential under normal conditions. They have specialized charged protein domains, called *voltage sensors*, which are sensitive to changes in the membrane potential. Changes above a certain threshold value exert sufficient electrical force on these domains to encourage the channel to close or open. The most important voltage-gated ion channels for the cardiac cell are the sodium (Na^+), calcium (Ca^{++}), and potassium (K^+) channels.

3.3.1 Voltage-Gated Channels

3.3.1.1 Sodium Channel

The sodium channel is the major voltage-gated ion channel for depolarization.[5] The mammalian genome contains at least nine sodium channel genes, of which the *SCN5A* gene is the most important one in cardiac tissue. Sodium channels consist of various subunits, but only the principal (α) subunit is required for function. The pore-forming α subunit is large (predicted molecular weight 227 kDa in rat and man) and consists of four homologous domains (I–IV), each comprising six transmembrane

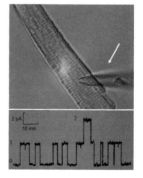

Fig. 3.2 *Upper panel*: Cardiomyocyte with patch electrode (*white arrow*) attached to the cell membrane. *Lower panel*: Ionic current recorded with the patch pipette. Note that the on/off switching occurs between zero and two discrete levels (1 and 2)

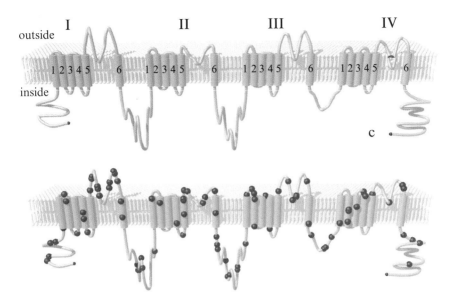

Fig. 3.3 Schematic drawing of the SCN5A sodium channel, showing the four domains (I–IV), each comprising six transmembrane segments (S1–S6). The highly conserved S4 region (*purple color*) acts as the channel's voltage sensor. *Red dots* in the *lower panel* indicate sites where mutations in the gene have been found in humans

segments (Fig. 3.3). They may co-assemble with auxiliary β subunits that are important modulators of the sodium channel function. Patch clamp studies revealed that the conductivity of these channels is 85 pS in the open state.

The time course of opening the channels occurs after a delay, which implies that a simple two-state model is not applicable. Therefore, Hodgkin and Huxley assumed the voltage-gated sodium channels to have three types of states: deactivated (closed), activated (open), and inactivated (closed) (Fig. 3.4). Channels in the deactivated state are supposed to be blocked by an *activation gate* (m), which opens in response to a stimulus. Inactivation is thought to be due to an inactivation (h) gate that blocks the channel shortly after it has been activated. Closing of the h-gate (inactivation of the channel) is slower than closing of the m-gate. Therefore, the channel remains open (activated) for a few milliseconds after depolarization. The inactivation is removed when the membrane potential of the cell repolarizes following the falling phase of the action potential. This allows the channels to be activated again during the next action potential.

The temporal behavior of sodium channels can be modeled by a Markovian scheme or by the Hodgkin–Huxley-type formalism. In the former scheme, each channel occupies a distinct state with differential equations describing transitions between states; in the latter, the channels are treated as a population affected by three independent gating variables.[6] Each of these variables can attain a value between 1 (fully permeable to ions) and 0 (fully nonpermeable), the product of these variables yielding the percentage of conducting channels.

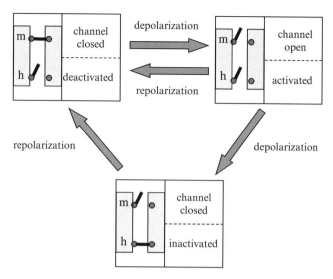

Fig. 3.4 Schematics of the three states of a sodium channel. If the membrane potential is increased to –60 mV, the m-port opens (*right box*). Closing of the h-port is also caused by depolarization, albeit at a slower rate (*lower box*). Thus, the channel only opens for a few milliseconds. If the opening of the m-port is delayed, the system will inactivate (repolarize) immediately (*repolarization arrow* between the *upper two boxes*). Finally in state three, during normal repolarization, the m-port closes and h-port opens (*left box*)

Many mutations in the *SCN5A* gene have been described and give rise to Brugada or long QT syndrome (LQT3) (Fig. 3.3). These syndromes are associated with sudden cardiac death due to ventricular fibrillation. Arrhythmias may be caused by either a loss or gain of function. Loss of function is often associated with reduced sodium current. In the heterozygous mutations (homozygous mutations are usually not compatible with life), the sodium channels generated by the mutated gene are often functionally inactive, but changes in the biophysical characteristics of the channels may occur as well.

Reduced sodium current will affect propagation of the action potential and may be arrhythmogenic. However, there is redundancy in the heart with regard to sodium current. Studies in heterozygous sodium channel knockout mice, which have only 50% of the sodium current present in wild type animals, reveal only an 18% reduction in conduction velocity[7] (Fig. 3.5). The reason that arrhythmias occur in patients with reduced sodium channel expression is therefore more complex and might be related to structural changes that also occur due to the mutation.

During the plateau phase of the action potential, the sodium current is virtually zero. Gain of function mutations in the sodium channel give rise to a persistent sodium current during the plateau phase. This persistent inward current prolongs the action potential and may disturb the delicate balance between depolarizing and repolarizing currents during the plateau phase toward depolarization. In this manner, early after-depolarizations may occur.

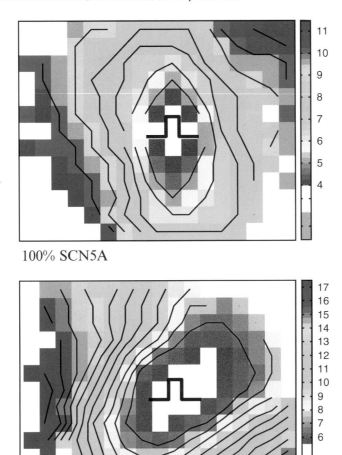

100% SCN5A

50% SCN5A

Fig. 3.5 Epicardial activation maps of the right ventricle of a wild type mouse heart (*upper panel*) and the heart of a heterozygous SCN5A mouse (50% SCN5A expression, *lower panel*). The heart was electrically stimulated at the center of the electrode (*markers*). Lines are isochronal lines at distances of 1 ms. Note that isochronal lines are more crowded in the *lower panel*, indicating conduction slowing. A 50% reduction in sodium channel expression reduces conduction velocity by approximately 18%

3.3.1.2   Calcium Channel

The calcium channel not only mediates maintenance of the plateau phase of the action potential, but is also involved in pacemaker depolarization in the sinoatrial node [the funny current I_f and the (lack of) inward rectifier current (I_{K1}) are involved in pacemaking as well] and slow conduction in the AV node. Calcium channels are very selective with permeability to calcium being 1,000-fold higher than the permeability of potassium and sodium. Two types of voltage-dependent calcium channels play a role in cardiac muscle, the L-type (long-lasting) calcium channel and the T-type (transient) calcium channel. T-type calcium channels have a conductance of less than 10 pS and the current they carry is called $I_{Ca,T}$.[8] These channels open as the fast depolarization passes (-50 mV) but, like the sodium channel, they inactivate immediately if the change in potential is low. $I_{Ca,L}$ is the current carried by the L-type calcium channel. A major difference with the T-type channel is that this *long-lasting* channel inactivates at a much lower rate, implicating that the current persists for a much longer period. Activation of the channel starts at a membrane potential of -40 mV, and conductance of the $I_{Ca,L}$ channel is 16 pS, almost double that of the fast type. Calcium antagonists that are used clinically, like nifedipine and verapamil, mainly block the L-type calcium channel and do not affect the T-type. The L-type calcium channel is important in maintaining the plateau phase, while T-type channels are important in initiating an action potential. Although T-type channels are found in ventricular cells, they probably do not contribute to the upstroke of the action potential of these cells, because their relatively small and transient current component is dominated by the coincidental and much larger sodium current. Because of their rapid kinetics, T-type channels are commonly found in cells undergoing rhythmic electrical behavior. They are found in pacemaker cells (i.e., sinoatrial node and AV node) of the heart that control the heartbeat.

L-type calcium channels consist of five subunits called α_1, α_2, δ, β, and γ, of which α_1 is the pore-forming subunit that shows remarkable homology with the pore-forming subunit of the voltage-dependent sodium channel. The associated subunits have several functions including trafficking (controlling the amount of α_1 subunit expressed at the cell membrane) and modulation of gating. The channel protein forming the α_1 subunit is more than 2,000 amino acids long and consists as the sodium channel of four internally homologous domains (I–IV). Each domain spans the membrane six times. The gating mechanism is similar to that of the sodium channel, consisting of two different opening mechanisms with varying threshold potentials and different kinetics for opening and closure.

Calcium channels are not only involved in cardiac excitability, but also play a crucial role in the mechanical properties of the cardiomyocytes. The inflow of calcium into the cell triggers release of calcium from the endoplasmatic reticulum, which activates interaction sites between the actin and myosin filaments of the sarcomeres, leading to contraction. L-type calcium channels play an important role in arrhythmogenesis, because they are capable of mediating the inward current that underlies some types of triggered arrhythmias like early after-depolarizations. Calcium channels can also support slow conduction in reentrant circuits.

3.3.1.3 Potassium Channels

More than 12 potassium channels are involved in the electrophysiology of cardiomyocytes under normal or pathologic conditions. A number of these potassium channels are involved in shaping the action potential of the cardiac cells. The configuration of cardiac action potentials varies considerably among species and different regions of the heart, which is largely attributable to the diversity in expression of the different types of time- and voltage-activated potassium channels.

The Inward Rectifier Current (I_{K1})

As illustrated before, the resting membrane potential is stabilized and maintained by a potassium current, the I_{K1}. This current is called *inward rectifying* because it passes current more easily into the cell. At membrane potentials below the reversal (Nernst) potential of the channel, the inward rectifying K$^+$ channels support the flow of positive charge into the cell, pushing the membrane potential back to the resting potential (Fig. 3.6). When the membrane potential is higher than the resting potential, the channels move charge out of the cell; however, this current is much smaller. The high conductance around the reversal potential (steep slope in Fig. 3.6) for I_{K1} helps to maintain a stable diastolic membrane potential. However, upon depolarization, the large conduction is shut down by the rectification, and other potassium channels are allowed to control the plateau phase. The functional channel is assumed to be assembled from four subunits with two transmembrane segments.[9]

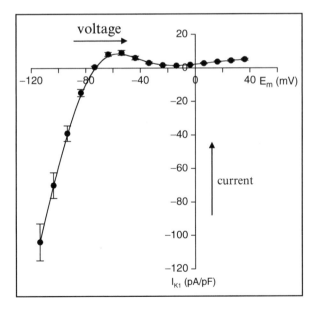

Fig. 3.6 Voltage–current relationship of the inward rectifier current (I_{K1}). The corresponding channel was expressed in HEK (human embryonic kidney) 293 cells. Inward currents (negative values) are large, whereas outward currents (positive values) are small

The Transient Outward Current (I_{To})

The I_{To} plays an important role in phase 1 of the action potential. I_{To} rapidly activates and subsequently inactivates and underlies the initial rapid repolarization phase of the action potential. This current is responsible for the notch in the early phase of the action potential. Additionally, this current is prominent in the atria, which may be the cause of the shorter action potential duration in the atrium. I_{To} may influence the balance between inward and outward ionic currents during the plateau phase and, in this way, may modulate action potential duration and refractoriness. For example, a transmural gradient of I_{To} expression in ventricular myocardium underlies the dramatic difference in phase 1 repolarization across the ventricular wall.

Two kinetic variants of cardiac I_{To} have been identified: fast I_{To}, called $I_{To,1}$ and slow I_{To}, called $I_{To,2}$. $I_{To,1}$ is formed by assembly of K(v4.2) and/or K(v4.3), alpha pore-forming voltage-gated subunits, while $I_{To,2}$ is comprised of K(v1.4) and possibly K(v1.7) subunits. Several regulatory subunits and pathways modulating the level and biophysical properties of cardiac I_{To} have been identified. An important electrophysiological change in cardiac disease is the reduction in I_{To} density with a loss of heterogeneity in I_{To} expression and an associated action potential prolongation. Transmural differences in I_{To} expression in the right ventricle have been associated with the occurrence of ST-segment elevation and cardiac arrhythmias in the Brugada syndrome.[10]

The Delayed Rectifier Currents $(I_{Kr}$ and $I_{Ks})$

Two potassium currents contribute to the repolarization of the cardiac cell in the terminating phase (phase 3) of the action potential: (1) the slow delayed rectifying current, I_{Ks}; and (2) the rapid delayed rectifying current, I_{Kr}.[9] The rapid component of the delayed rectifier has unique features in its specific block by the methanesulfonanilide class of antiarrhythmic drugs like E-4031 and dofetilide; in contrast to I_{Ks}, I_{Kr} is half-activated at −20 mV and increases as a function of membrane potential up to approximately 0 mV. During repolarization of the action potential, I_{Kr} rapidly recovers from inactivation and causes the current to peak at −40 mV. I_{Kr} channels are encoded by the *hERG* gene that can form heteromultimers with two other potassium channel proteins KCNE1 and KCNE3. The hERG potassium channel comprises four identical subunits, each containing six transmembrane domains. Abnormalities in this channel may lead to either LQT2 syndrome (loss of function mutations) or short QT syndrome (gain of function mutations).[11] Both may lead to fatal cardiac arrhythmias due to repolarization disturbances of the cardiac action potential. The *hERG* gene is the human homolog of the Ether-a-go-go gene found in the *Drosophila* fly. When flies with mutations in this gene are anesthetized with ether, their legs start to shake like a popular dance at the Whisky a Go Go nightclub in West Hollywood, California.

The slow activating delayed rectifier current I_{Ks} gradually increases during the plateau phase of the action potential because its activation is delayed and very slow. I_{Ks} plays a role in determining the rate-dependent shortening of the cardiac action potential. The channels have less time to deactivate during the shortened diastolic interval as heart rate increases and I_{Ks} channels accumulate in the open state during rapid heart rates and contribute to the faster rate of repolarization. I_{Ks} is a potassium selective current that activates at -30 mV and has a linear current–voltage relationship. Its time course for activation is extremely slow. The single-channel conductance is only 1–6 pS and its magnitude is modulated by divalent cations. Elevated Ca^{++} increases I_{Ks}. The KvLQT1 protein that forms the I_{Ks} channel is encoded by the *KCNQ1* gene. Mutations in the gene can lead to a defective protein, and several forms of inherited arrhythmias such as LQT1, short QT syndrome, and familial atrial fibrillation have been described. Co-expression of KvLQT1 with minK results in a sevenfold increase in current magnitude, marked slowing of the time course of activation, and a 20-mV depolarizing shift in the voltage dependence of activation.

The Ultra-Rapid Delayed Rectifier Current (I_{Kur})

A potassium current that is absent in the ventricles, but present in the atrium, is the ultra-rapid delayed rectifier current (I_{Kur}). This current plays an important role in human atrial repolarization. It is a potassium selective outwardly rectifying current with a single-channel conductance of 10–14 pS.[12]

3.3.2 Ligand-Gated Channels

Voltage-gated ion channels activate/inactivate depending on the voltage gradient across the plasma membrane, while ligand-gated ion channels activate/inactivate depending on binding of ligands to the channel. These channels are usually activated under abnormal conditions. The acetylcholine-activated potassium current has a similar current–voltage relation as the inward rectifier potassium current, but only carries current ($I_{K,Ach}$) if acetylcholine concentration is high ($>5 \times 10^{-8}$ M). The conductivity of the channel is larger than that of I_{K1} (50 versus 40 pS); however, the mean opening time is much shorter than that of I_{K1}.[13]

The ATP-sensitive potassium channel ($I_{K,ATP}$) is closed under normal conditions. The channel only opens as ATP concentration of the cell reduces from its normal value of 3–0.5 mmol. In its open state, conductivity of the channel is 90 pS, which is the largest one of the ion channels found in cardiomyocytes. Reduction of ATP occurs during ischemia, which triggers opening of the channel; opening of the K_{ATP} channel is considered to be the molecular basis of ST-segment changes observed during acute ischemia.

3.3.3 Stretch-Activated Channels

Mechanosensitive ion channels open under the influence of stretch or pressure, and they play a role in mechano-electrical feedback. Opening of the channels allows ions, to which they are permeable, to flow down their electrochemical gradients into or out of the cell, causing a change in membrane potential.[14]

3.3.4 Exchangers

The sodium-calcium exchanger has a crucial role in maintaining a delicate balance between calcium influx and efflux. In order to keep the appropriate concentrations of sodium and potassium, the sodium–potassium pump drives sodium out and potassium into the cell through an active process.

3.3.5 Electrophysiological Heterogeneities in Ion Channel Expression

The role of action potential duration heterogeneities as a substrate for unidirectional conduction block and reentry has been supported by simulation studies from Viswanathan and Rudy.[15] In hypertrophied and failing myocardium, the inherent differences in action potential duration may be enhanced by changes in density, distribution, or properties of the potassium currents.

Other studies have shown that, in the healthy heart, heterogeneous expression of repolarizing voltage-gated potassium channels is not limited to the left ventricle, but interventricular differences exist as well. Whole-cell voltage-clamp recordings showed that mean peak I_{To1} densities are significantly higher in cells isolated from mouse right (RV) than left ventricle (LV). In contrast, the densities of I_{To2} in murine RV, LV apex, and LV base cells are not significantly different.

Myocardial cells isolated from RV and LV midmyocardium of the canine heart revealed that I_{To1} density was significantly larger in the RV than the LV, while steady-state inactivation and rate of recovery were similar. I_{Ks} currents were considerably larger in the RV, but I_{Kr} and I_{K1} were not different. The higher values of I_{To1} and I_{Ks} may well explain the shorter action potentials in the RV compared to the LV.

Also, sodium channels seem to be distributed heterogeneously throughout the heart. Cardiomyocytes isolated from subendocardial and subepicardial layers of the rat heart show that a transmural gradient of sodium current is present in the LV. Sodium current in the LV subendocardium was significantly larger than at the sub-epicardium (-49.7 ± 2.5 pA/pF versus -32.9 ± 3.2 pA/pF). The sodium current in the RV was similar to that at the left subendocardium of the LV (-49.7 ± 3.7 pA/pF). Functional studies on the consequence of this difference have yet to be performed.

3.3.6   Changes in Ion Channel Expression by Cardiac Remodeling

Heart disease is associated with cardiac remodeling or changes in the electrical and mechanical properties of the myocardium. These changes involve alterations in ion and gap junction channels as well as structural modifications. Structural changes may include replacement fibrosis, increased cell size and interstitial collagen deposition, as well as myocyte disarray, but also loss of cardiac myocytes, depending on the underlying disease. Cardiac hypertrophy and heart failure often reveal increased collagen deposition and increased heterogeneity of connexin expression, whereas cell size is increased. Myocardial infarction is associated with loss of cardiomyocytes, which is followed by a reparative process that replaces dead cells by replacement fibrosis to maintain structural integrity of the myocardium. Fibrous tissue formation in the infarcted heart is an ongoing process that even involves noninfarcted myocardium, although to a lesser extent. It has been shown that heart failure, regardless of ischemic or nonischemic etiology, is characterized by progressive loss of cardiac myocytes, often through apoptosis mechanisms, further decreasing cardiac function.

In the infarcted heart, Connexin 43 expression is reduced in areas remote from the infarcted zone, whereas it is disrupted in the infarct border zone. In addition, sodium current has been shown to be reduced by more than 50%. These remodeled parameters will impair conduction and may give rise to ventricular arrhythmias.

Dilated cardiomyopathy (DCM) is the most common form of cardiomyopathy, but constitutes a heterogeneous group of disorders. DCM is a disease of the heart muscle in which ventricular dilation is accompanied by contractile dysfunction of the LV and/or RV. In DCM, histology is usually not specific but shows substantial myocyte hypertrophy. Mild focal and interstitial fibrosis as well as *ghost cells* (myocytes without myofibrillary elements) and apoptosis are present. Connexin 43 expression from patients with DCM is heterogeneously reduced and gene expression of the voltage-gated sodium channel has been shown to be reduced to 30–50% of controls.[16] These changes all favor the vulnerability of arrhythmias.

Hypertrophic cardiomyopathy (HCM) is a disorder that is often caused by mutations in genes encoding sarcomeric proteins. Although HCM is characterized by LV wall thickening due to hypertrophied cardiomyocytes, the major characteristic feature of HCM is myofiber disarray. Focal and widespread interstitial fibrosis is present as well. Arrhythmogenic right ventricular cardiomyopathy (ARVC) is an inherited disorder associated with mutations in desmosomal proteins, proteins that are considered important for rigidity of cells and cell signaling. ARVC is characterized by progressive replacement of the RV myocardium by fatty and fibrous tissue. However, remodeling of Connexin 43 has been observed in Naxos disease, a plakoglobin mutation causing ARVC; this form of ARVC shows a high incidence of arrhythmias and sudden cardiac death.

The expression of many other ion channels is affected by heart failure. For example, a significant reduction of I_{K1} and especially I_{To} has been reported in cardiomyocytes from patients with severe heart failure.[17] I_{To} is most markedly affected in pacing-induced heart failure in the dog heart. In human atrial fibrillation, I_{Kur} has been shown to be reduced, but many other ion channel abnormalities have been reported as well.

3.4 Gap Junctions

For propagation of the cardiac action potential, heart cells need to be coupled electrically. The coupling is mediated by gap junction proteins.[18] Next to conduction of ions, these proteins form conduits for intercellular communication allowing exchange of ions, nutrients, metabolites, and small molecules including peptides. Six connexin (Cx) units assemble into a hemi-channel (connexon), which resides in the membrane of cardiomyocytes. At sites where the membranes of neighboring cells are close together and connexons from two adjacent cells face each other, they form a channel connecting the cells across the intercellular space (Fig. 3.7). The gap junction proteins are called *connexins*, membrane proteins that have molecular weights ranging from 25 to 50 kDa.

Connexins are not only present in the heart, but control cell-to-cell communication in various other cell types. Up to 24 different connexin types have been described. In the heart, Cx40, Cx43, Cx45, and Cx30.2 are most important for propagation of the electrical impulse. The numbers refer to the molecular weight of the connexins in Dalton. Cardiac connexins exhibit distinctive unitary conductance, voltage sensitivity, and ion selectivity. Cx43 has the largest conductance, whereas the lowest occurs for Cx30.2 (9 pS). In Table 3.1, the different characteristics are shown. Next to intercellular voltages, gap junction conduction is modulated by a variety of other factors, as variations in Ca^{2+}, pH, and phosphorylation. During the course of ischemia, decreased ATP levels, increased intracellular Ca^{2+} concentrations, and acidosis determine gap junction closure through Cx43 dephosphorylation and internalization into the cytosol. Anesthetics, hormones, and neurotransmitters all affect gap junction conduction, which should be considered in experimental and clinical studies in which gap junctions play a role.

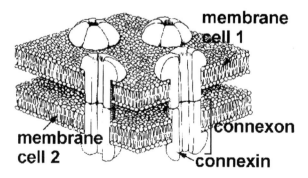

Fig. 3.7 Schematic drawing of cell-to-cell coupling by gap junction proteins

Table 3.1 Electrophysiological properties of cardiac connexins

Connexin	Conductance	Voltage sensitivity	Ionic selectivity anion/cation
Cx43	50–150	Low	0.13
Cx40	180	Moderate	0.29
Cx45	25	High	0.20
Cx30.2	9	Low	Unknown

3.4.1 Gap Junction Distribution in Cardiac Tissue

Using immunohistochemical approaches, cardiac connexin distribution has been studied. The different connexins present are not evenly distributed within the heart. Cx40 is present in the atrium, the AV node, the bundle branches, and the Purkinje system. The amount of Cx40 expression, however, highly differs between the different tissue types, being low in the AV node and high in the specific conduction system and the atrium. Cx43 is the major connexin in the ventricular working myocardium, but is also present in atrial myocardium where it co-localizes with Cx40. Cx45 is mainly found in co-localization with Cx40 in the bundle branches. Cx30.2 is predominantly localized in the conduction system of the heart, with particularly high levels in the sinoatrial and AV node; Cx43 levels are lower in sinoatrial and AV nodes compared to atrial or ventricular working myocardium.

3.4.2 Redundancy of Connexins

In the heart, there is a high redundancy in connexin expression with regard to conduction of the electrical impulse. Studies with conditional Cx43 knockout mice have shown that a 50% reduction of Cx43 expression does not affect conduction velocity in the ventricles.[19] Cx43 expression must decrease by 90% to affect conduction, but even then conduction velocity is reduced by only 20%. Similar studies with Cx40 knockout mice showed that conduction block occurred in the right bundle branch, but Cx45 was still able to maintain conduction in the left bundle branch, albeit at reduced velocity.[20] Also, the effect on conduction velocity in the atrium was marginal and, in some studies, even absent. Exchange of Cx40 by Cx45 also hardly affected conduction in the bundle branches. Interestingly, Cx30.2 was shown to decelerate impulse conduction through the AV node.[21]

Despite redundancy, reduced connexin expression will finally impair conduction velocity. In contrast to a reduction in sodium current, which can decrease conduction velocity by only threefold to about 17 cm/s in ventricular myocardium before conduction block occurs, a reduced connexin expression may decrease conduction velocity 200-fold to 0.26 cm/s before block occurs (Fig. 3.8).[22] In general, reduced connexin expression finally results in impaired conduction. Interestingly, in discontinuous cardiac tissue structures exhibiting unidirectional conduction block, such as that present at sites where myocardial bundle diameter suddenly changes, reduced

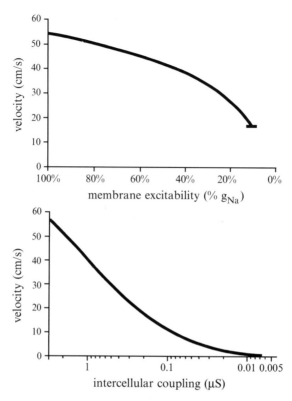

Fig. 3.8 Change in conduction velocity in simulated strands of cardiomyocytes due to reduced membrane excitability (*upper panel*) and decreased intercellular coupling (*lower panel*). Conduction block occurs at a reduction of excitability by a factor >3; conduction block occurs after a reduction of cell-to-cell coupling by a factor >300. Modified from Shaw and Rudy[22]

coupling will favor conduction. The reason is that, at such sites, the discrepancy between current supply and current demand is restored by uncoupling, mainly by reducing load.[23]

3.4.3   Gap Junction Distribution in Cardiomyocytes

In the adult heart, gap junctions are mainly located at the long ends of the cardiomyocytes where the largest intercalated disks connect neighboring cells. They exhibit a staggered arrangement of the transverse-oriented intercalated disks, and there are large areas along the cell surface that have no gap junctions (Fig. 3.9). This distribution of connexins highly differs from the gap junction as observed in neonatal cardiomyocytes. The neonatal myocyte is smaller, has a spindle shape, and the connexins are almost evenly distributed along the cell membrane. Distribution of gap junctions

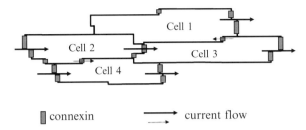

Fig. 3.9 Schematic drawing of cell-to-cell coupling. In adult cardiomyocytes under physiological conditions, connexins are present at the long ends of the cells and only sporadically side by side. Current flow in the axial direction is therefore higher (*large arrows*) in comparison to current perpendicular to the fiber direction (*small arrows*)

along the myocyte perimeter plays an important role in impulse conduction, being faster in the fiber direction as compared to propagation perpendicular to it.

3.4.4 Homomeric and Heteromeric Expression

The co-existence of different connexins in tissue indicates that channels could be assembled with more than one type of connexin. Channels formed of different connexins suggest that each one can provide channels with different gating and permeability properties. As indicated before, atrial myocytes express large amounts of Cx43 and Cx40, whereas in ventricular myocytes Cx43 and Cx45 co-localize in gap junctions and may form heteromeric/heterotypic channels.[24]

As shown before, homomeric channels formed by these connexins differ in unitary conductance, permeability, and regulation. Biochemical and electrophysiological measurements suggest that Cx43 and Cx45 extensively mix to form heteromeric channels with distinct biophysical characteristics; however, individual connexin components dominate aspects of the physiological behavior of these channels. These interactions between different connexin types may also lead to paradoxical results. For instance, it appears that deletion of Cx40 in neonatal atrial myocytes leads to an increase in electrical propagation velocity and a concomitant increase in Cx43 in atrial gap junctions.[25]

3.4.5 Remodeling of Connexin Expression

Mutations in genes that encode connexins have only rarely been identified as being a cause of human cardiac disease, but remodeling of connexin expression and gap junction organization are well documented in acquired adult heart disease, notably ischemic heart disease and heart failure.[26] Remodeling of connexins may affect the expression, distribution, and type of connexins expressed. Heterogeneous reduction

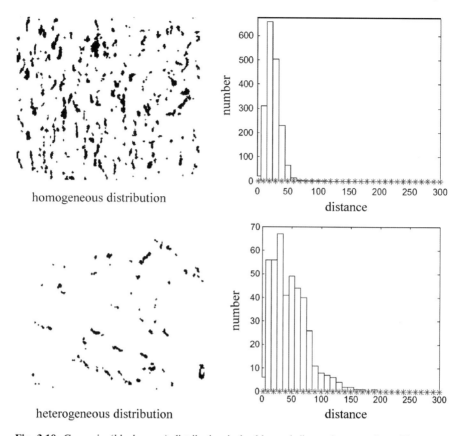

Fig. 3.10 Connexin (*black areas*) distribution in healthy and diseased myocardium. The *upper panel* shows homogeneous distribution as found in healthy myocardium. The *lower panel* shows reduced and heterogeneous distribution from a failing heart. The value of heterogeneity is determined by the standard deviation of the distances between adjacent connexin plaques (*right panels*)

in Cx43 expression occurs in various disease states like heart failure and DCM, and has been correlated with increased vulnerability for ventricular arrhythmias (Fig. 3.10). However, also in the atriums of patients with atrial fibrillation, reduced connexin (Cx40) expression and increased heterogeneity have been observed and related to the arrhythmia.

3.4.6 Transmural Differences in Connexins

Dispersion of repolarization has been reported in the hearts of a wide variety of animals and humans and has been shown to promote arrhythmias. The underlying mechanism may, at least in part, be caused by heterogeneous expression of gap junction channels. Cell-to-cell coupling through gap junctions is expected to attenuate heterogeneities between cells with different action potential durations. However, regional differences in connexin expression could counteract this equalizing process. It has been shown that Cx43 is selectively reduced in the subepicardium (by 24%) compared to deeper layers of normal canine LV.[27] The greatest dispersion of repolarization occurs within the subepicardial–midmyocardial interface, where Cx43 expression is reduced. Gap junction remodeling occurs during cardiac disease and may enlarge the electrophysiologic heterogeneities across the ventricular wall and promote dispersion of repolarization, which underlies arrhythmias. Because potassium channels are major determinants of repolarization, intrinsic heterogeneity in expression of potassium channels (transmural and apical-basal gradients) will also play a role in dispersion of repolarization.

3.5   Conclusion

In this chapter, we showed that ion channels underlie the shape of the action potential and, together with gap junction channels, highly determine propagation of the action potential. Differences in expression of the various ion channels are the cause of the varying action potentials of the different cell types. It is, however, important to realize that ion channel and gap junction channel expression may also vary in cells of the same type, even under normal conditions. These differences cause heterogeneities that are usually enlarged under pathologic conditions which may be inherited or acquired. These increased heterogeneities, together with reduced expression levels, are at the base of the occurrence of arrhythmias in the heart.

References

1. Noble D. The Initiation of the Heart Beat, second edition. Oxford: Clarendon Press, 1979.
2. Kanno S, Saffitz JE. The role of myocardial gap junctions in electrical conduction and arrhythmogenesis. Cardiovasc Pathol 2001; 10:169–77.
3. Boron WF, Boulpaep EL. Medical Physiology: A Cellular and Molecular Approach, second edition. Philadelphia: Elsevier/Saunders, 2009.
4. Hille B. Ion Channels of Excitable Membranes, third edition, Sunderland: Sinauer Associates Inc., 2001
5. Marban E, Yamagishi T, Tomaselli GF. Structure and function of voltage-gated sodium channels. J Physiol 1998; 508:647–57.
6. Bennett PB, Shin HG. Biophysics of cardiac sodium channels. In: Zipes DP, Jalife J, editors. Cardiac Electrophysiology from Cell to Bedside, third edition. Philadelphia: WB Saunders Company, 1999:67–78.
7. van Veen TA, Stein M, Royer A, et al. Impaired impulse propagation in Scn5a-knockout mice: combined contribution of excitability, connexin expression, and tissue architecture in relation to aging. Circulation 2005; 112:1927–35.
8. Balke CW, Marban E, O'Rourke B. Calcium channels: structure, function and regulation. In: Zipes DP, Jalife J, editors. Cardiac Electrophysiology from Cell to Bedside, third edition. Philadelphia: WB Saunders Company, 1999:8–21.

9. Snyders DJ. Structure and function of cardiac potassium channels. Cardiovasc Res 1999; 42: 377–90.

10. Calloe K, Cordeiro JM, Di Diego JM, et al. A transient outward potassium current activator recapitulates the electrocardiographic manifestations of Brugada Syndrome. Cardiovasc Res 2009; 81(4):686–94.

11. Zareba W, Cygankiewicz I. Long QT syndrome and short QT syndrome. Prog Cardiovasc Dis 2008; 51:264–78.

12. Fedida D, Eldstrom J, Hesketh JC, et al. Kv1.5 is an important component of repolarizing K+ current in canine atrial myocytes. Circ Res 2003; 93:744–51.

13. Tristani-Firouzi M, Chen J, Mitcheson JS, et al. Molecular biology of K(+) channels and their role in cardiac arrhythmias. Am J Med 2001; 110:50–9.

14. Taggart P, Lab M. Cardiac mechano-electric feedback and electrical restitution in humans. Prog Biophys Mol Biol 2008; 97:452–60.

15. Viswanathan PC, Rudy Y. Cellular arrhythmogenic effects of congenital and acquired long-QT syndrome in the heterogeneous myocardium. Circulation 2000; 101:1192–8.

16. Tomaselli GF, Marban E. Electrophysiological remodeling in hypertrophy and heart failure. Cardiovasc Res 1999; 42:270–83.

17. Näbauer M, Beuckelmann DJ, Erdmann E. Characteristics of transient outward current in human ventricular myocytes from patients with terminal heart failure. Circ Res 1993; 73: 386–94.

18. Dhein S. Cardiovascular Gap Junctions. Basel: Karger, 2006.

19. van Rijen HV, Eckardt D, Degen J, et al. Slow conduction and enhanced anisotropy increase the propensity for ventricular tachyarrhythmias in adult mice with induced deletion of connexin43. Circulation 2004; 109:1048–55.

20. Van Rijen HVM, van Veen AB, van Kempen MJA, et al. Impaired conduction in the bundle branches of mouse hearts lacking the gap junction protein connexin40. Circulation 2001; 103: 1591–8.

21. Kreuzberg MM, Schrickel JW, Ghanem A, et al. Connexin30.2 containing gap junction channels decelerate impulse propagation through the atrioventricular node. Proc Natl Acad Sci U S A 2006; 103:5959–64.

22. Shaw RM, Rudy Y. Ionic mechanisms of propagation in cardiac tissue. Roles of the sodium and L-type calcium currents during reduced excitability and decreased gap junction coupling. Circ Res 1997; 81:727–41.

23. Rohr S, Kucera JP, Fast VG, et al. Paradoxical improvement of impulse conduction in cardiac tissue by partial cellular uncoupling. Science 1997; 275:841–4.

24. Elenes S, Martinez AD, Delmar M, et al. Heterotypic docking of Cx43 and Cx45 connexons blocks fast voltage gating of Cx43. Biophys J 2001; 81:1406–18.

25. Beauchamp P, Yamada KA, Baertschi AJ, et al. Relative contributions of connexins 40 and 43 to atrial impulse propagation in synthetic strands of neonatal and fetal murine cardiomyocytes. Circ Res 2006; 99:1216–24.

26. Severs NJ, Coppen SR, Dupont E, et al. Gap junction alterations in human cardiac disease. Cardiovasc Res 2004; 62:368–77.

27. Poelzing S, Rosenbaum DS. Altered connexin43 expression produces arrhythmia substrate in heart failure. Am J Physiol Heart Circ Physiol 2004; 287:H1762–70.

Chapter 4
Anatomy and Physiology of the Cardiac Conduction System

Paul A. Iaizzo and Timothy G. Laske

Abstract The intrinsic conduction system of the heart is comprised of several specialized subpopulations of cells that either spontaneously generate electrical activity (pacemaker cells) or preferentially conduct this excitation throughout the four chambers of the heart in a coordinated fashion. This chapter will discuss some of the details of this anatomy as well as physiological properties of the system. The cardiac action potential underlies signaling within the heart, and various myocyte populations elicit signature waveforms. The recording or active sensing of these action potentials is important in both research and clinical arenas. This chapter aims to provide a basic understanding of the cardiac conduction system, so the reader has a foundation for future research and reading on this topic. The information in this chapter is not comprehensive and should not be used to make decisions related to patient care.

4.1 Introduction

All myocytes within the heart have the capacity to conduct the cardiac impulse. A population of myocytes is specialized to generate the cardiac impulse and then to conduct it from the atrial to the ventricular chambers. This population has become known as the conduction system.[1] Orderly contractions of the atria and ventricles are regulated by the transmission of electrical impulses that pass through an intricate network of these modified cardiac muscle cells, and they are interposed within the contractile myocardium. This intrinsic conduction system is comprised of several specialized subpopulations of cells that spontaneously generate electrical activity (pacemaker cells) and/or preferentially conduct this activity throughout the heart. Following an initiating activation (or depolarization) within the myocardium, this electrical excitation spreads throughout the heart in a rapid and highly coordinated fashion. This system of cells also functionally

P.A. Iaizzo (✉)
Department of Surgery, University of Minnesota, Minneapolis, MN, USA
e-mail: iaizz001@umn.edu

D.C. Sigg et al. (eds.), *Cardiac Electrophysiology Methods and Models*,
DOI 10.1007/978-1-4419-6658-2_4, © Springer Science+Business Media, LLC 2010

controls the timing of the transfer of activity between the atrial and ventricular chambers, allowing for optimized hemodynamic performance. Interestingly, a common global architecture is present in mammals, but significant interspecies differences exist at the histological level.[2,3]

Discoveries related to the intrinsic conduction system within the heart are relatively recent and based on the overall knowledge of cardiac function and anatomy. For example, in 1845 Johannes E. von Purkinje first described the ventricular conduction system, and in 1882 Gaskell, an electrophysiologist, coined the phrase *heart block*. In addition, Gaskell also related the presence of a slow ventricular activation rate to disassociation with that of the atria.[4] A description of the mammalian sinoatrial node was reported by Sir Arthur Keith and Martin Flack in 1907 in the *Journal of Anatomy and Physiology*. Nevertheless, novel findings about the functionality of this node are still being discovered today.[1,5]

The elucidation of the connection from the atrioventricular node through the cardiac skeleton to the conduction system within the ventricles, known as the *bundle of His*, is attributed to Wilhelm His Jr.[6] Importantly, Tawara later verified the existence of the bundle of His in 1906.[7] Due to difficulty in distinguishing the atrioventricular nodal tissue from the surrounding tissue, he defined the beginning of the bundle of His as the point at which these specialized atrioventricular nodal cells enter the central fibrous body (which delineates the atria from the ventricles). Tawara is also credited with being the first person to clearly identify the specialized conduction tissues (modified myocytes) that span from the atrial septum to the ventricular apex, including the right and left bundle branches and Purkinje fibers.

Walter Karl Koch (1880–1962) was a distinguished German surgeon who discovered a triangular-shaped area in the right atrium of the heart that marks the atrioventricular node (known today as *Koch's triangle*). Among Koch's notable research accomplishments, based on detailed anatomical and histological studies of the hearts of animals and stillborn human fetuses, was the finding that the last part of the heart to lose activity when the whole organ dies is the pacemaker region (*ultimum moriens*). He postulated that the cardiac region near the opening of the wall of the coronary sinus was the true pacemaker of the heart[8,9]; note that the atrioventricular node will elicit an escape rhythm when the sinoatrial node in the right atrium fails (see below).

Early discoveries by distinguished researchers such as Koch, Tawara, and Aschoff have been immortalized in medical terminology (Koch's triangle, Tawara's node, and Aschoff's nodule).

4.2 Overview of Cardiac Conduction

The *sinoatrial node* is located in the upper part of the right atrium in the healthy heart, and serves as the natural pacemaker (Fig. 4.1). These nodal cells manifest spontaneous depolarizations and are thus responsible for generating the normal cardiac rhythm; such a heart rate can also be described as intrinsic or automatic.

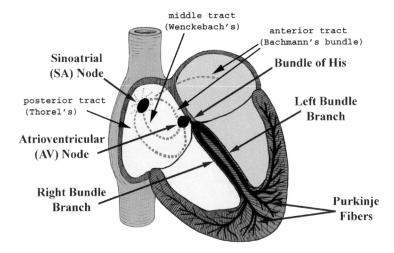

Fig. 4.1 The conduction system of the heart. Normal excitation originates in the sinoatrial (SA) node and then propagates through both atria (internodal tracts shown as *dashed lines*). The atrial depolarization spreads to the atrioventricular (AV) node, passes through the bundle of His, and then to the Purkinje fibers that make up the left and right bundle branches; subsequently, all ventricular muscle becomes activated

Importantly, the frequency of this earliest cardiac depolarization is well modulated by both sympathetic and parasympathetic efferent innervation. In addition, the nodal rate can also be modulated by local changes within perfusion and/or the chemical environment (i.e., neurohormonal, nutritional, oxygenation, etc.). Although the atrial rhythms normally emanate from the sinoatrial node, variations in the initiation site of atrial depolarization have been documented outside of the histological nodal tissues, particularly when high atrial rates are elicited, and may include paranodal tissue.[10–14]

One of the most conspicuous features of sinoatrial nodal cells is that they possess poorly developed contractile apparati (a common feature to all myocytes specialized for conduction), comprising only about 50% of the intracellular volume.[1,10,15] In general, although it typically cannot be seen grossly, the location of the sinoatrial node is on the *roof* of the right atrium at the approximate junction of the superior vena cava, the right atrial appendage, and the sulcus terminalis. In the adult human, the node is approximately 1 mm below the epicardium, 10–20 mm long, and up to 5-mm thick.[1,16]

After initial sinoatrial nodal excitation, depolarization spreads throughout the atria. The exact mechanisms involved in the spread of impulses (excitation) from the sinoatrial node across the atria are somewhat controversial.[1,17] However, it is generally accepted that (1) the spread of depolarizations from nodal cells can go directly to adjacent myocardial cells; and (2) preferentially ordered myofibril pathways allow this excitation to rapidly transverse the right atrium to both the left atrium and the atrioventricular node (Fig. 4.1). It is believed by some people that there are three preferential anatomic conduction pathways from the sinoatrial node to the atrioventricular node.[1,18] In general, these can be considered as the shortest electrical routes between the nodes. Nevertheless, there are microscopically identifiable structures, appearing to be preferentially oriented fibers that provide a direct node-to-node pathway. In some hearts, pale staining Purkinje-like fibers have also been reported in these regions. More specifically, the anterior tract is described as extending from the anterior part of the sinoatrial node, bifurcating into the so-called Bachmann's bundle (delivering impulses to the left atrium), with a second tract that descends along the interatrial septum that connects to the anterior part of the atrioventricular node. The middle (or Wenckebach's) pathway extends from the superior part of the sinoatrial node, runs posteriorly to the superior vena cava, then descends within the atrial septum, and may join the anterior bundle as it enters the atrioventricular node. The third pathway is described as being posterior (Thorel's) which, in general, is considered to extend from the inferior part of the sinoatrial node, passing through the crista terminalis and the Eustachian valve past the coronary sinus to enter the posterior portion of the atrioventricular node. In addition to excitation along these preferential conduction pathways, general excitation spreads from cell to cell throughout the entire atrial myocardium via the specialized connections between cells, the *gap junctions*, that exist between all myocardial cell types (see below).

It then follows that towards the end of atrial depolarization, the excitation reaches the atrioventricular node via the aforementioned atrial routes, with the final excitation of the atrioventricular node. These routes are known as the slow or fast pathways that are considered to be functionally and anatomically distinct. The *slow pathway* typically crosses the isthmus between the coronary sinus and the tricuspid annulus; it has a longer conduction time, but a shorter effective refractory period. The *fast pathway* is commonly a superior route, emanating from the interatrial septum, and has a faster conduction rate but, in turn, a longer effective refractory period. Normal conduction during sinus rhythm occurs along the fast pathway, but higher heart rates and/or premature beats are often conducted through the slow pathway, because the fast pathway may be refractory at these rates.

Though the primary function of the atrioventricular node may seem simple, that is to relay conduction between the atria and ventricles, its structure is very complex.[1] As a means to describe these complexities, mathematical arrays and finite element analysis models have been constructed to elucidate the underlying structure–function relationship of the node.[19]

In general, the atrioventricular node is located in the so-called *floor* of the right atrium, over the muscular part of the interventricular septum, inferior to the membranous septum, and within the triangle of Koch, which is bordered by the coronary sinus, the tricuspid valve annulus along the septal leaflet, and the tendon of Todaro (Fig. 4.2). Following atrioventricular nodal excitation, the slow pathway conducts impulses to the His bundle, indicated by a longer interval between atrial and His activation. Currently, there is interest in the ability to place pacing leads to preferentially activate the bundle of His; in such approaches, various modalities are used to map the characteristic electrical His potentials to position the pacing leads.[20]

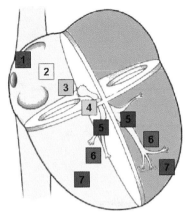

Normal Activation Sequence	Structure	Conduction velocity (m/sec)	Pacemaker rate (beats/min)
1	SA node	< 0.01	60 – 100
2	Atrial myocardium	1.0 – 1.2	None
3	AV node	0.02 – 0.05	40 – 55
4	Bundle of His	1.2 – 2.0	25 – 40
5	Bundle branches	2.0 – 4.0	25 – 40
6	Purkinje network	2.0 – 4.0	25 – 40
7	Ventricular myocardium	0.3 – 1.0	None

Fig. 4.2 The conduction system of the heart. *Left*: Normal excitation originates in the SA node and then propagates through both atria. The atrial depolarization spreads to the AV node, and passes through the bundle of His to the bundle branches/Purkinje fibers. *Right*: The table shows conduction velocities and intrinsic pacemaker rates of various structures within the cardiac conduction pathway. The structures are listed in the order of activation during a normal cardiac contraction, beginning with the SA node. Note that the intrinsic pacemaker rate is slower in structures further along the activation pathway. For example, the AV nodal rate is slower than the SA nodal rate. This prevents the AV node from generating a spontaneous rhythm under normal conditions, since it remains refractory at rates <55 bpm. If the SA node becomes inactive, the AV nodal rate will then determine the ventricular rate. Tabulation adapted from Katz AM. *Physiology of the Heart*, third edition. Philadelphia: Lippincott, Williams, and Wilkins, 2001

After leaving the bundle of His, the normal wave of cardiac depolarization spreads to both the left and right bundle branches; these pathways rapidly carry depolarization to the apical regions of the left and right ventricles, respectively (Fig. 4.1). Finally, the signal broadly travels through the remainder of the Purkinje fibers and ventricular myocardial depolarization spreads.

In certain pathological conditions, direct accessory connections from the atrioventricular node and the penetrating portion of the bundle of His to the ventricular myocardium have been described.[21] Yet, the function and prevalence of these connections, termed *Mahaim fibers*, is poorly understood. A rare *bundle of Kent*, an additional aberrant pathway when present, exists between the atria and ventricles and is associated with the clinical manifestation of ventricular tachycardias (also known as *Wolff–Parkinson–White syndrome*). Therapeutically, this accessory pathway is electrically identified and then commonly ablated as a curative procedure.

The left bundle branch splits into fascicles as it travels down the left side of the ventricular septum just below the endocardium. Its fascicles extend for a distance of 5–15 mm, fanning out over the left ventricle. Importantly, typically about midway to the apex of the left ventricle, the left bundle separates into two major divisions, the anterior and posterior branches (or fascicles). These divisions extend to the base of the two papillary muscles and the adjacent myocardium. In contrast, the right bundle branch continues inferiorly, as if it were a continuation of the bundle of His, traveling along the right side of the muscular interventricular septum. This bundle branch runs proximally just deep to the endocardium, and its course runs slightly inferior to the septal papillary muscle of the tricuspid valve before dividing into fibers that spread throughout the right ventricle. The complex network of conducting fibers that extends from either the right or left bundle branches is composed of the rapid conduction cells known as *Purkinje fibers*. Purkinje fibers in both the right and left ventricles act as preferential conduction pathways to provide rapid activation and coordinate the excitation pattern within the various regions of the ventricular myocardium. Most of these fibers travel within the trabeculations of the right and left ventricles, as well as within the myocardium. Due to tremendous variability in the degree and morphology of the trabeculations existing both within and between species, it is likely that variations in the left ventricular conduction patterns also exist. It should be noted that one of the most common and easily recognized conduction pathways found in mammalian hearts is the moderator band, which contains Purkinje fibers from the right bundle branch. Furthermore, in many human hearts, within both the right and left ventricles, one can identify conduction bands that are white in appearance (see *Atlas of Human Cardiac Anatomy*, www. vhlab.umn.edu/atlas).

In 1910, Aschoff and Monckeberg provided three criteria for considering a myocardial cell as a specialized conduction cell, including (1) the ability to histologically identify discrete features; (2) the ability to track cells from section to section; and (3) insulation of the cell by fibrous sheaths from the nonspecialized contractile myocardium.[22,23] It is noteworthy that only the cells within the bundle of His, left and right bundle branches, and Purkinje fibers satisfy all three criteria. No structure within the atria meets all three criteria, including the Bachmann's bundle, sinoatrial node, and atrioventricular node (which are all uninsulated tissues). Yet, with major advances in histomolecular techniques, it is likely that new criterion will follow that better define the uniqueness of specialized conduction structures.

4.3 Cardiac Rate Control

Under normal physiologic conditions, the dominant pacemaker cells of the heart lie within the sinoatrial node; in adults, these pacemaker cells fire at rates between 60 and 100 beats/minute (bpm) (i.e., faster than cells in any other cardiac region, Fig 4.3). Even at rest, modulation by the autonomic nervous system dominates, with the primary drive from the parasympathetics; at rest or during sleep, the sinoatrial nodal rate decreases to about 75 bpm or even slower.

In addition to pacemaker cells of the sinoatrial node, other cells within the conduction system are capable of developing autorhythmicity, specifically those within the atrioventricular node (junction region) and His–Purkinje system. Yet, rhythms generated within these cells are in a much lower range (25–55 bpm), hence not altering the intrinsic atrial rates (Fig. 4.2). These lower rate rhythms are commonly

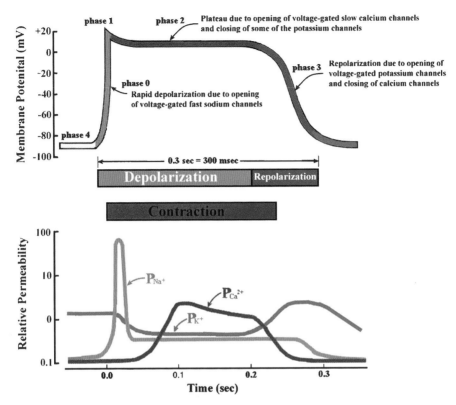

Fig. 4.3 A typical action potential of a ventricular myocyte and the underlying ion currents. The resting membrane potential is approximately −90 mV (phase 4). The rapid depolarization is primarily due to the voltage-gated Na⁺ current (phase 0), which results in a relatively sharp peak (phase 1) and transitions into the plateau (phase 2) until repolarization (phase 3). Also indicated are the refractory period and timing of the ventricular contraction. Modified from Tortora GJ, Grabowski SR. *Principles of Anatomy and Physiology*, ninth edition. New York: Wiley, 2000

referred to as *ventricular escape rhythms* and are important for patient survival, because they maintain some degree of cardiac output in situations when the sinoa-trial and/or atrioventricular nodes are functioning inappropriately (e.g., in a patient with atrial fibrillation). Note that the various populations of pacemaker myocytes (i.e., in the sinoatrial and atrioventricular nodes) elicit so-called slow type action potentials (slow response action potential, see below).

In addition to the normal sources of cardiac rhythms, myocardial tissue can also exhibit abnormal self-excitability; such a site is also called an *ectopic pacemaker* or *ectopic focus*. This pacemaker may operate only occasionally, producing extra beats, or it may induce a new cardiac rhythm for some period of time. Potentiators of ectopic activity include caffeine, nicotine, electrolyte imbalances, hypoxia, and/or toxic reactions to drugs such as digitalis. It should also be noted that any cell(s) in the heart can take over pacemaker function if driven to do so, such as in electrical pacing via an implanted electrode/lead.

4.4   Cardiac Action Potentials

Although cardiac myocytes branch and interconnect with each other (mechanically via the intercalated disc and electrically via the gap junctions, see below), under normal conditions the heart should be considered to form two separate functional networks of myocytes: the atria and the ventricles. This is due to the separation of atrial and ventricular tissues by the fibrous skeleton of the heart (the central fibrous body). This skeleton is comprised of dense connective tissue rings that surround the valves of the heart, fuse with one another, and also merge with the interventricular septum. More specifically, this fibrous structure can be thought to (1) form the foundation to which valves attach; (2) prevent overstretching of the valves; (3) serve as a point of insertion for cardiac muscle bundles; and (4) act as an electrical insulator that prevents the direct spread of action potential from the atria to the ventricles (normal spread is through the bundle of His).

A healthy myocardial cell has a resting membrane potential of approximately –90 mV (Fig. 4.3). This resting potential can be described by the Goldman–Hodgkin–Katz equation, which takes into account the permeability (P) as well as the intracellular and extracellular concentration of ions [X], where X is the ion.

$$V_m = (2.3R * T / F) * \log_{10} \frac{P_K [K]_o \pm P_{Na} [Na]_o \pm P_{Cl} [Cl]_i \pm P_{Ca} [Ca]_o + \dots}{P_K [K]_i + P_{Na} [Na]_i + P_{Cl} [Cl]_o + P_{Ca} [Ca]_i + \dots}$$

In the cardiac myocyte, the membrane potential is dominated by the K^+ equilibrium potential. An action potential is initiated when this resting potential becomes shifted towards a more positive value of approximately –60 to –70 mV (Fig. 4.3). At this threshold potential, the cell's voltage-gated Na^+ channels open and begin a cascade of events involving other ion channels. In artificial electrical stimulation, this shift of the resting potential and subsequent depolarization is produced by the excitation delivered through the pacing system. The typical ion concentrations for a mammalian cardiac myocyte are summarized in Table 4.1 and graphically depicted in Fig. 4.3.

When a potential of the myocyte is brought to the threshold, normally via transmitted activation from a neighboring cell, voltage-gated fast Na^+ channels actively open (activation gates), and the permeability of the sarcolemma (plasma membrane) to sodium ions (P_{Na}^+) dramatically increases. Because the cytosol is

Table 4.1 Ion concentrations for mammalian myocytes

Ion	Intracellular concentration (mM)	Extracellular concentration (mM)
Sodium (Na)	5–34	140
Potassium (K)	104–180	5.4
Chloride (Cl)	4.2	117
Calcium (Ca)		3

Adapted from Katz AM. *Physiology of the Heart*, third edition. Philadelphia: Lippincott, Williams, and Wilkins, 2001

electrically more negative than extracellular fluid and the Na^+ concentration is higher in the extracellular fluid, Na^+ rapidly crosses the cell membrane. Importantly, within a few milliseconds, these fast Na^+ channels automatically inactivate (via inactivation gates) and P_{Na}^+ decreases.

The membrane depolarization due to the activation of Na^+ induces the opening of the voltage-gated slow Ca^{2+} channels located within both the sarcolemma and sarcoplasmic reticulum (internal storage site for Ca^{2+}). Thus, there is an increase in the permeability of Ca^{2+} (P_{ca}^{2+}), which allows the concentration to dramatically increase intracellularly (Fig. 4.3). At the same time, the membrane permeability to K^+ ions decreases due to closing of K^+ channels. For approximately 200–250 ms, the membrane potential stays close to 0 mV (i.e., depolarized relative to at rest), as a small outflow of K^+ just balances the inflow of Ca^{2+}. After this fairly long delay, voltage-gated K^+ channels open and active repolarization is initiated. The opening of these K^+ channels (increased membrane permeability) allows for K^+ to diffuse out of the cell due to its concentration gradient. At this same time, Ca^{2+} channels begin to close and net charge movement is dominated by the outward flux of the positively charged K^+, restoring the negative resting membrane potential to approximately –90 mV (Fig. 4.3).

As mentioned above, not all action potentials that are elicited in the cardiac myocardium have the same time courses. More specifically, *slow* and *fast* response cells have different shaped action potentials with different electrical properties in each phase. Recall that the pacemaker cells (slow response type) have the ability to spontaneously depolarize (unstable resting potential) until they reach threshold and then elicit action potentials. Action potentials from such cells are also characterized by a slower initial depolarization phase, a lower amplitude overshoot, a shorter and less stable plateau phase, and repolarization to an unstable, slowly depolarizing resting potential (Fig. 4.4). In the pacemaker cells, at least three mechanisms are thought to underlie the slow depolarization that occurs during phase 4 (diastolic interval): (1) a progressive decrease in P_K^+; (2) a slight increase in P_{Na}^+; and (3) an increase in P_{Ca}^{2+}.

4.5   Gap Junctions (Cell-to-Cell Conduction)

In the heart, cardiac muscle cells (myocytes) are connected end to end by structures known as *intercalated disks*. These are irregular transverse thickenings of the sarcolemma, within which there are *desmosomes* that hold the cells together and to which the myofibrils are attached. Adjacent to the intercalated discs are the gap junctions that allow action potentials to directly spread from one myocyte to the next. More specifically, the disks join the cells together by both mechanical attachment and protein channels. The firm mechanical connections are created between the adjacent cell membranes by proteins. The electrical connections (low resistance pathways, gap junctions) between the myocytes are via the channels formed by the protein connexin. These channels allow ion movements between cells (Fig. 4.5). There are several different isoforms of connexins that can be identified within the various populations of myocytes (see below).

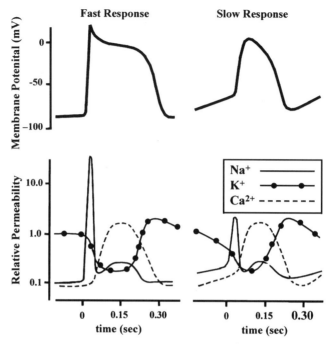

Fig. 4.4 The comparative time courses of membrane potentials and ion permeabilities that would typically occur in a fast response (*left*, e.g., ventricular myocyte) and a slow response cell (*right*, e.g., nodal myocyte). Modified from Mohrman DE, Heller LJ. *Cardiovascular Physiology*, fifth edition. New York: Langer Medical Books/McGraw-Hill, 2003

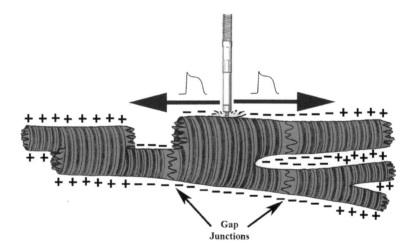

Fig. 4.5 Shown are several cardiac myocytes in different states of excitation. The initial depolarization that occurred within the centrally located cell was induced via a pacemaker lead (fixated into the cell). This then resulted in the spread of depolarization of adjacent cells, in both directions, through cell-to-cell conduction via the gap junctions (nexus). Eventually all adjoining cells will depolarize. In other words, action potentials initiated in any of these cells will be conducted from cell to cell in either direction

As noted above, not all cells elicit the same types of action potentials, even though excitation is propagated from cell to cell via their interconnections (gap junctions). Nevertheless, via gap junctions the slow response action potentials elicited in the sinoatrial nodal cells will trigger fast response action potentials in adjacent myocytes and then those within the remainder of the atria (Fig. 4.6).

In a healthy heart, it takes approximately 30 ms for excitation to spread between the sinoatrial and atrioventricular nodes, and the widespread atrial activation occurs over a period of approximately 70–90 ms (Figs. 4.2 and 4.3). The speed at which an action potential propagates through a given region of cardiac tissue can be described as the relative *conduction velocity* (Fig. 4.2). The propogation velocity varies considerably within regions of the heart and is directly dependent on the relative diameter of given myocyte populations. For example, action potential conduction is greatly slowed as it passes through the atrioventricular node, but is rapid in the bundle branches connected via the His bundle. This nodal slowing is

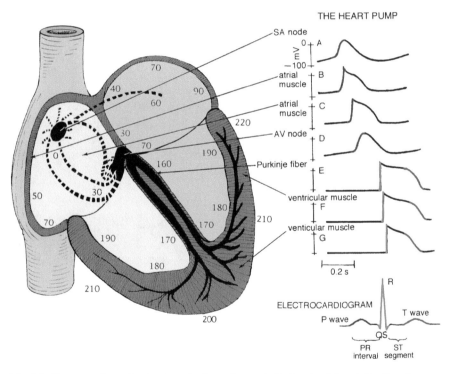

Fig. 4.6 Shown are the predominant conduction pathways in the heart and the relative time, in msec, that cells in these various regions become activated following an initial depolarization within the sinoatrial (SA) node. *To the right* are typical action potential waveforms that would be recorded from myocytes in these specific locations. The SA and atrioventricular (AV) nodal cells have similar shaped actions potentials. The nonpacemaker atrial cells elicit action potentials that have shapes somewhat between the slow response (nodal) and fast response cells (e.g., ventricular myocytes). The ventricular cells elicit fast response type action potentials; however, their durations vary in length. Due to the rapid excitation within the Purkinje fiber system, the initiation of depolarization of the ventricular myocytes occurs within 30–40 ms, and is recorded as the QRS complex in the electrocardiogram

due to the (1) small diameter of these cells; (2) tortuosity of the cellular pathway[3]; and (3) slower rates of rise of elicited action potentials. Nevertheless, this delay is essential to allow adequate time for ventricular filling.

Action potentials in the Purkinje fibers are of the fast response type (Fig. 4.4), i.e., rapid depolarization rates that, in part, are due to their large diameters. This feature allows the Purkinje system to transfer depolarization to the majority of cells in the ventricular myocardium nearly in unison. It is important to note that the ventricular cells that are last to depolarize (those near the base of the heart) have shorter duration action potentials (shorter Ca^{2+} current), and thus are typically the ones to repolarize first. The ventricular myocardium repolarizes within the time period represented by the T-wave in the electrocardiogram, thus a change in the duration of this wave indicates a change in the duration of functional repolarization of the ventricular cells.

4.6 The Atrioventricular Node and Bundle of His: Specific Features

The atrioventricular node and bundle of His play critical roles in the maintenance and control of ventricular rhythms. As mentioned above, the atrioventricular node is composed of heterogeneous gap junctions with electrical communication via the protein connexin. More specifically, within the human myocardium there are four connexin proteins identified to date: Cx43, Cx40, Cx45, and Cx30.2/31.9. Importantly, Cx43 and Cx40 are primarily associated with the fast conduction pathways, whereas Cx45 and Cx30.2/31.9 are generally expressed in the slow conduction pathways.[24] It should be noted that one study by Davis et al. reported that Cx43, Cx40, and Cx45 are expressed in the human atrioventricular junction.[25]

Additionally, during clinical cardiac catheterization procedures, frequent attempts are made to electrically identify both the atrioventricular node and the bundle of His in order to (1) provide anatomic landmarks; (2) gain insights on atrial–ventricular conduction behaviors; and/or (3) determine locations to ablate these structures or the surrounding tissues. Such ablations are commonly performed to terminate aberrant behaviors (e.g., reentrant tachycardias) or to prevent atrioventricular conduction in patients with chronic atrial fibrillation. There remains strong interest by medical device designers to understand details of the structural and functional properties of the atrioventricular node and the bundle of His in order to develop new therapies and/or avoid inducing complications. For example, in a recent study in our laboratory, we attempted to provide direct correlations between means to record and activate the bundle of His in an in vitro swine heart study.[26] In addition, several recent studies have explored 3D reconstruction of the human atrioventricular node,[27] but much more work on this topic needs to be performed.[1]

In general, the His bundle is located adjacent to the annulus of the tricuspid valve, distal to the atrioventricular node, and slightly proximal to the right bundle branch and left bundle branch. The functional origin may be ill defined, but as described above, it is typically considered to anatomically begin at the point where the atrioventricular nodal tissue enters the central fibrous body. The bundle of His is described as having three regions – the penetrating bundle, nonbranching bundle, and branching bundle. The penetrating bundle is the region that enters the central fibrous body. At this point, the His fascicles are insulated but are surrounded by atrial tissue (superiorly and anteriorly), the ventricular septum (inferiorly), and the central fibrous body (posteriorly). Thus, the exact point where the atrioventricular nodal tissues end and the bundle begins is difficult to define, because it occurs over a transitional region. The nonbranching bundle passes through the central fibrous body and is surrounded on all sides by the central fibrous body. In this cardiac region, the His bundle still has atrial tissue superior and anterior to it, the ventricular septum inferior to it, and now the aortic and mitral valves posterior to it. It should be noted that His myocytes are innervated, but to a lesser extent than those in the atrioventricular node. Unlike the sinoatrial and atrioventricular nodes, the His bundle has no large blood vessels that supply it specifically.

The common branching bundle is described to begin as the His exits the central fibrous body. At this point, it is inferior to the membranous septum and superior to the ventricular septum. After leaving the central fibrous body, it then bifurcates into the right and left bundle branches. The right bundle branch passes within the myocardium of the interventricular septum and the left bundle branch primarily travels subendocardially along the septum in the left ventricle (as noted above).

4.7 Recording the Spread of Excitation Through the Heart

Action potential waveforms can be actively monitored from the epicardial, endocardial, or transmural surfaces of the heart. Several methods exist for the acquisition of such signals such as (1) glass micropipette electrodes; (2) metal electrodes of various designs; (3) multielectrode arrays; (4) optical mapping; and (5) contact or noncontact endocardial mapping. Contact or noncontact endocardial mapping technologies measure the intracardiac endocardial electrograms rather than those from the epicardial surface, or globally from the whole myocardium as in a standard 12-lead ECG.

Typically today, glass micropipettes are produced from small diameter capillary tubing employing a commercially available micropipette puller, which reproducibly creates electrodes with tips of about 0.1 μm with resistances of 10–40 mΩ. The pipette is then filled with an electrolyte such as 3 M KCl and a silver, platinum, or stainless steel wire is then positioned inside the pipette until it is in contact with the electrolytic solution.[28] The ultimate goal of this recording approach is to impale the microelectrode through the cell membrane, so that the tip is into the myoplasm of a single cell while not inducing major damage to the cell; the membrane seals around the tip and the cell does not become depolarized.

On a more macro scale, there are various designs for metal recording electrodes which can be employed to monitor action potential waveforms extracellularly; such systems typically record focal potential changes from a small population of myocytes.

These electrode designs can be either bipolar (i.e., typically with a relatively small spacing between the active and reference conductors) or monopolar (i.e., the needle is a single shaft and the reference is taken from the subject ground).[29] Each of these designs can have needle tip diameters as small as 0.30 mm. Note that the morphology of a recorded signal will typically depend on (1) the configuration of the electrode employed (monopolar or bipolar); (2) the relative surface area that the electrode will monitor; (3) the anatomical placement (atrium or ventricle); and/or (4) the site specific myocardial wall recording location (endocardial, epicardial, or transmural).

Modern pacemaker leads, which can be positioned to touch the endocardial surface or actively fixed within it, can also be used to sense focal myocyte depolarization and repolarization; such leads have typical diameters ranging from 4 to 10 French (Fr; 1 Fr = one-third millimeter). These active or passive pacing leads can be used to detect action potential waveforms in either unipolar or bipolar configurations (i.e., with leads that have both a distal tip electrode and a distal ring electrode). Note that the leads' relative dimensions will ultimately dictate the size of the field from which they are sensing electrical potentials. As with any active fixation lead or metal electrode that is engaged into the myocardium, an initial injury potential can be associated with its placement.[30] It should also be noted that the current trend in the pacing lead industry is to continually decrease the diameter of both the body and tip dimensions (i.e., 2 Fr leads are currently in development and in clinical trials).

If one would like to record potential changes of excitation from a broader area of the heart, a multielectrode array would typically be employed. Such systems consist of an array of equally spaced electrodes supported by a base, and conducting wires are attached to the electrodes on the array. Depending on the design, one or more of the electrodes on the array can serve as the reference electrode, while the others become active electrodes. These arrays allow for the mapping of electrical potentials within a given region of the heart.[31] For example, electrophysiological studies of the bundle of His have most often been performed using catheters with polished electrodes and short interelectrode spacing (i.e., those with diameters of 2 mm). Due to the small amplitude of the His potential, special high-pass filtering must be used (>30 Hz) in order to separate the His signal from the low frequency shift in the isopotential line between the atrial depolarization and the atrial repolarization/ventricular depolarization. His potentials can commonly be mapped by deploying an electrode in one of three ways: (1) endocardially in the right atrium at a point on the tricuspid annulus near the membranous septum; (2) epicardially at the base of the aorta near the right atrial appendage; or (3) radially within the noncoronary cusp of the aortic valve.[32–36]

Today, His potentials are commonly mapped to provide a landmark for ablation of the atrioventricular node as well as to assess A-to-V conduction timing. In addition to direct electrical mapping, much can be learned about the general anatomical and functional properties of the cell lying within the bundle via attempts to directly stimulate it. For example, direct stimulation of the His produces normal ventricular activation due to the initiation of depolarization into the intrinsic conduction pathway.[32,33,37] Thus, if one frequently experiences failed attempts to selectively stimulate the His bundle, s/he may assume pathological changes.[35]

Beyond these positioned catheters, numerous other sophisticated mapping systems have been developed and are described in other chapters within this book.

4.8   Future Research on the Heart's Conduction System

Although much is already known, a great deal of supposition and controversy remains related to our understanding of the cardiac conduction system. More specifically, characterization of the anatomy and electrophysiology of the atrioventricular nodal region and the bundle of His continues to be an area of great scientific interest and debate.[38-40] For example, current clinical interest in the atrioventricular node and His bundle has focused research on their potential stimulation to ultimately improve hemodynamics in patients requiring pacing[32-35,37,41] and their use in treating atrioventricular nodal reentrant tachycardias.[2,3,31,42] In addition to these applied research investigations, there is a need for additional basic scientific investigation to improve our understanding of the fundamental anatomical and physiological features of the heart's conduction system and how they are modified by disease processes; such findings will provide a better foundation for future therapies.

4.9   Summary

This chapter reviewed the basic architecture and function of the cardiac conduction system in order to provide the reader with a working knowledge and pertinent vocabulary associated with this topic. While a great deal of literature exists regarding the cardiac conduction system, numerous questions remain related to the detailed histological anatomy and cellular physiology of these specialized conduction tissues and how they become modified in disease states. Future findings associated with the function and anatomy of the cardiac conduction system will likely lead to improvements in therapeutic approaches and medical devices.

Acknowledgements   We would like to thank Monica Mahre for her assistance with preparing this chapter and Gary Williams for his help with the figures.

References

1. Anderson RH, Yanni J, Boyett MR, et al. The anatomy of the cardiac conduction system. Clin Anat 2009; 22:99–113.
2. Ho SY, Kilpatrick L, Kanai T, et al. The architecture of the atrioventricular conduction axis in dog compared to man – its significance to ablation of the atrioventricular nodal approaches. J Cardiovasc Electrophysiol 1995; 6:26–39.
3. Racker DK, Kadish AH. Proximal atrioventricular bundle, atrioventricular node, and distal atrioventricular bundle are distinct anatomic structures with unique histological characteristics and innervation. Circulation 2000; 101:1049–59.
4. Furman S. A brief history of cardiac stimulation and electrophysiology – the past fifty years and the next century. NASPE Keynote Address, 1995.
5. Boyett D, Dobrzynski H. The sinoatrial node is still setting the pace 100 years after its discovery. Circ Res 2007; 100:1543–5.
6. His Jr W. Die Tatigkeit des embryonalen herzens und deren bedcutung fur die lehre von der herzbewegung beim erwachsenen. Artbeiten aus der Medizinischen Klinik zu Leipzig 1893; 1:14–49.

7. Tawara S. Das Reizleitungssystem des Saugetierherzens: Eine anatomisch-histologische Studie uber das Atrioventrikularbundel und die Purkinjeschen Faden. Jena, Germany: Gustav Fischer 1906; 9–70:114–56.
8. Conti AA, Giaccardi M, Yen Ho S, et al. Koch and the "ultimum moriens" theory – the last part to die of the heart. J Interv Card Electrophysiol 2006; 15:69–70.
9. Koch WK. Der funktionelle bau des menschlichen herzen. Berlin and Vienna: Urban und Schwarzenberg, 1922.
10. Yamamoto M, Dobrzynski H, Tellez J, et al. Extended atrial conduction system characterised by the expression of the HCN4 channel and connexin45. Cardiovasc Res 2006; 72:271–81
11. Betts TR, Roberts PR, Ho SY, et al. High density mapping of shifts in the site of earliest depolarization during sinus rhythm and sinus tachycardia. PACE 2003; 26:874–82.
12. Boineau JB, Schuessler RB, Hackel DB, et al. Widespread distribution and rate differentiation of the atrial pacemaker complex. Am J Physiol 1980; 239:H406–15.
13. Boineau JB, Schuessler RB, Mooney CR. Multicentric origin of the atrial depolarization wave: the pacemaker complex. Relation to the dynamics of atrial conduction, P-wave changes and heart rate control. Circulation 1978; 58:1036–48.
14. Lee RJ, Kalman JM, Fitzpatrick AP, et al. Radiofrequency catheter modification of the sinus node for 'inappropriate' sinus tachycardia. Circulation 1995; 92:2919–28.
15. Tranum-Jensen J. The fine structure of the atrial and atrio-ventricular (AV) junctional specialized tissues of the rabbit heart. In: Wellens HJJ, Lie KI, Janse MJ, editors. The conduction system of the heart: structure, function, and clinical implications. Philadelphia, PA: Lea & Febiger, 1976:55–81.
16. Waller BF, Gering LE, Branyas NA, et al. Anatomy, histology, and pathology of the cardiac conduction system: Part I. Clinical cardiology 1993; 16:249–52.
17. Boyett MR, Honjo H, Kodama I, et al. The sinoatrial node: cell size does matter. Circ Res 2007; 101:e81–2.
18. Garson AJ, Bricker JT, Fisher DJ, Neish SR, editors. The science and practice of pediatric cardiology. Volume I. Baltimore, MD: Williams & Williams, 1998:141–3.
19. Li JL, Greener ID, Inada S, et al. Computer three-dimensional reconstruction of the atrioventricular node. Circ Res 2008; 102:975–85.
20. Yin L, Laske TG, Rakow N, et al. Intracardiac echocardiography-guided his bundle pacing and atrioventricular nodal ablation. Pacing Clin Electrophysiol 2008; 31:536–42.
21. Becker AE, Anderson RH. The morphology of the human atrioventricular junctional area. In: Wellens HJJ, Lie KI, Janse MJ, editors. The conduction system of the heart: structure, function, and clinical implications. Philadelphia, PA: Lea & Febiger, 1976:263–86.
22. Aschoff L. Referat uber die herzstorungen in ihren bezeihungen zu den spezifischen muskelsystem des herzens. Verh Dtsch Ges Pathol 1910; 14:3–35.
23. Monckeberg JG. Beitrage zur normalen und pathologischen anatomie des herzens. Verh Dtsch Ges Pathol 1910; 14:64–71.
24. Hucker WJ, McCain ML, Laughner JI, et al. Connexin 43 expression delineates two discrete pathways in the human atrioventricular junction. Anat Rec 2008; 291:204–15.
25. Davis LM, Rodefeld ME, Green K, et al. Gap junction protein phenotypes of the human heart and conduction system. J Cardiovasc Electrophysiol 1995; 6:813–22.
26. Laske TG, Skadsberg ND, Hill AJet al., Excitation of the intrinsic conduction system through His and intraventricular septal pacing. Pacing Clin Electrophysiol 2006; 29:397–405.
27. Hucker WJ, Fedorov VV, Foyil KV, et al. Optical mapping of the human atrioventricular junction. Circulation 2008; 117:1474–7.
28. Webster JG. Bioinstrumentation. Hoboken, NJ: Wiley, 2004: xiv, p. 383.
29. Shrivastav M. Methods of ambulatory detection and treatment of cardiac arrhythmias using implantable cardioverter-defibrillators. Biomed Instrum Technol 1999; 33:505–21.
30. Webster JG. Design of Cardiac Pacemakers. IEEE Press, 1995.
31. Sahakian AV, Peterson MS, Shkurovich S, et al. A simultaneous multichannel monophasic action potential electrode array for in vivo epicardial repolarization mapping. IEEE Trans Biomed Eng 2001; 48:345–53.

32. Deshmukh P, Casavant DA, Romanyshyn M, et al. Permanent direct His-bundle pacing: a novel approach to cardiac pacing in patients with normal His-Purkinje activation. Circulation 2000; 101:869–77.
33. Karpawich P, Gates J, Stokes K. Septal His-Purkinje ventricular pacing in canines: a new endocardial electrode approach. Pacing Clin Electrophysiol 1992; 15:2011–5.
34. Karpawich PP, Gillette PC, Lewis RM, et al. Chronic epicardial His bundle recordings in awake nonsedated dogs: a new method. Am Heart J 1983; 105:16–21.
35. Williams DO, Sherlag BJ, Hope RR, et al. Selective versus non-selective His bundle pacing. Cardiovasc Res 1976; 10:91–100.
36. Zhang Y, Bharati S, Mowrey KA, et al. His Electrogram alternans reveal dual-wavefront inputs into and longitudinal dissociation within the bundle of His. Circulation 2001; 104:832–8.
37. Scheinman MM, Saxon LA. Long-term His-bundle pacing and cardiac function. Circulation 2000; 101:836–7.
38. Becker AE, Anderson RH. Proximal atrioventricular bundle, atrioventricular node, and distal atrioventricular bundle are distinct anatomic structures with unique histological characteristics and innervation – response. Circulation 2001; 103:e30–1.
39. Bharati S. Anatomy of the atrioventricular conduction system – response. Circulation 2001; 103:e63–4.
40. Magalev TN, Ho SY, Anderson RH. Special report: anatomic-electrophysiological correlations concerning the pathways for atrioventricular conduction. Circulation 2001; 103:2660–7.
41. Karpawich PP, Rabah R, Haas JE. Altered cardiac histology following apical right ventricular pacing in patients with congenital atrioventricular block. Pacing Clin Electrophysiol 1999; 22:1372–7.
42. Kucera JP, Rudy Y. Mechanistic insights into very slow conduction in branching cardiac tissue – a model study. Circulation Res 2001; 89:799–806.

Additional References

Mohrman DE, Heller LJ. Cardiovascular Physiology, fifth edition. New York: Langer Medical Books/McGraw-Hill, 2003.
Wellens HJJ, Lie KI, Janse MJ. The Conduction System of the Heart: Structure, Function, and Clinical Implications. Philadelphia: Lea & Febiger, 1976.
Alexander RW, Schlant RC, Fuster V. Hurst's: The Heart: Arteries and Veins, ninth edition. New York: McGraw-Hill, 1998.
Katz AM. Physiology of the Heart, third edition. Philadelphia: Lippincott, Williams, and Wilkins, 2001.
Tortora GJ, Grabowski SR. Principles of Anatomy and Physiology, ninth edition. New York: Wiley, 2000.

Chapter 5
The Electrocardiogram and Clinical Cardiac Electrophysiology

John T. Nguyen, Xiaohuan Li, and Fei Lü

Abstract Normal pacemaker cell and conduction system function is fundamentally important in maintaining cardiac mechanical performance. Cardiac arrhythmias consist of a group of electrical disturbances in the heart, including pacemaker cell firing and/or conduction abnormalities. The resultant fast, slow, or irregular heart rhythm can cause significant hemodynamic compromise and discomforts, and/or death. Importantly, a thorough understanding of cardiac electrophysiology is essential for management of any cardiac patient. The electrocardiogram, as recorded from electrodes placed on the surface of the chest and extremities, is a simple, yet important diagnostic technique for identification of cardiac arrhythmias. Nevertheless, it can also be useful in diagnoses of electrolyte abnormalities, medication toxicity, ischemic heart disease, and/or enlargement of cardiac chambers.

List of Abbreviations

AF	atrial fibrillation
APC	atrial premature complex
AV	atrioventricular
AVNRT	atrioventricular nodal reentry tachycardia
ECG	electrocardiogram
ICD	implantable cardioverter defibrillator
IHR	intrinsic heart rate
PSVT	paroxysmal supraventricular tachycardia
SA	sinoatrial
SVT	supraventricular tachycardia
TdP	Torsades de Pointes
VPC	ventricular premature complex
VT	ventricular tachycardia

F. Lü (✉)
Department of Medicine, Cardiovascular Division, University of Minnesota,
Minneapolis, MN, USA
e-mail: luxxx074@umn.edu

D.C. Sigg et al. (eds.), *Cardiac Electrophysiology Methods and Models*,
DOI 10.1007/978-1-4419-6658-2_5, © Springer Science+Business Media, LLC 2010

5.1 Introduction

Despite the invaluable usefulness of the surface electrocardiogram (ECG), it remains, in a broad sense, a tool only to describe electrical depolarization and repolarization of the atrial and ventricular tissue over time. Conclusions pertaining to the precise origins of impulse formation as well as conduction pathways from the atria to the ventricles can be inferred based on the relationship of their respective deflections on the ECG. In other words, invasive electrophysiologic study must be implemented by direct measurement of the electrical signals using small flexible electrode catheters placed into the heart via a transvenous approach, to provide the ability to interrogate the complex electrical system of the heart in more detail. Yet, surface ECGs and electrophysiologic studies together provide the essential tools in cardiac electrophysiology, i.e., in the science of describing, diagnosing, and treating electrical abnormalities of the heart. This chapter will focus on the basics of electrocardiography and cardiac electrophysiology.

5.2 The Specialized Cardiac Conduction System

Normally, electrical activation of the heart is initiated by a group of specialized pacemaker cells, termed the sinoatrial (SA) node, located on the epicardial surface of the heart at the junction of the right atrium and the superior vena cava. The intrinsic firing rate (automaticity) of these cells determines the rate and regularity of SA node activity and can be modulated by extrinsic factors such as autonomic neural tone, electrolytes, and medications. The normal resting sinus rate is variable, but is usually between 50 and 90 beats/min. However, rates as low as 40 beats/min are not uncommon in well-conditioned (athletic) individuals. Once generated by the sinus node cells, the cardiac electrical impulse traverses the atria by means of preferential conduction routes (determined by intra-atrial muscle band geography) to the atrioventricular (AV) node, located in the low interatrial septum near the tricuspid valve. The AV node is often considered to represent the beginning of the true anatomic specialized conduction system of the heart. Normally, impulses transit through the AV node at relatively slower rates than the remaining conduction system. Importantly, this delay allows time for mechanical transfer of blood from the atria to the ventricles prior to initiation of ventricular activation. Similar to the SA node, conduction through the AV node is influenced by sympathetic and parasympathetic neural tone, medications, and electrolytes. Once through the AV node, however, the electrical impulses travel more rapidly through the infranodal specialized conducting system comprised of the bundle of His, left and right bundle branches, and penetrating Purkinje fiber network. This concert of electrical activity ultimately results in coordinated mechanical contractions of both atria followed by the ventricles. (For more details on the conduction system, see Chap. 4.).

5.3 Electrocardiogram

The ECG is one representation of the electrical events of the cardiac cycle. Each event has associated waveforms, and careful analyses of these wave morphologies and their relationships to one another can provide insights on the electrophysiologic state of the heart. An ECG machine records atrial and ventricular depolarization and repolarization by inscribing deflections on a grid consisting of 1 mm squares. The width of these squares corresponds to duration, with standard values equal to 40 ms; the height of the squares denotes voltage amplitude of the deflection, usually representing 1 mV each centimeter.

5.3.1 ECG Leads

The ECG itself is recorded via electrodes (leads) placed on the body surface to measure the difference in electrical potential during impulse propagation. In general, when an impulse travels in the same direction as a lead (toward the positive electrode), it will result in a positive deflection on the ECG; conversely, an electrical impulse traveling in the opposite direction of a lead (away from the positive electrode) will be inscribed as a negative deflection.

There are two types of lead configurations: (1) *bipolar leads* measure electrical potential difference between two points on the body; and (2) *unipolar leads* compare a point on the body with a virtual reference located in the center of the chest. In general, a series of body surface electrodes can be placed at specific points on the arms, legs, and chest wall in order to record the electrical activity of the heart. Typically, there are six limb lead configurations that are used to view the heart in the frontal plane, three of which are standard bipolar (lead I, II, and III), while the remaining three limb leads are *augmented unipolar leads* (aVR, aVL, and aVF). The limb leads are created in the following manner:

I: positive – left arm; negative – right arm
II: positive – left leg; negative – right arm
III: positive – left leg; negative – left arm
aVR: positive – right arm; negative – left arm and leg
aVL: positive – left arm; negative – right arm and left leg
aVF: positive – left leg; negative – right and left arms

Together, these form Einthoven's triangle to determine an electrical axis in the frontal plane (Fig. 5.1a, b).

The precordial chest leads are used in a unipolar configuration and examine the heart in the horizontal plane, including leads V1, V2, V3, V4, V5, and V6 (Fig. 5.1c, d). The location of these leads is as follows:

V1: fourth intercostal space, right border of the sternum
V2: fourth intercostal space, left border of the sternum

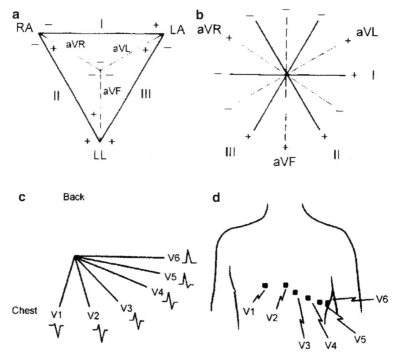

Fig. 5.1 Twelve ECG recording leads. The Einthoven's triangle (**a**) and the hexaxial reference system (**b**) depicting frontal plane ECG leads are shown at the *top*. Direction of chest lead axis (**c**) with corresponding recording sites on the chest (**d**) is shown at the *bottom* (*Source*: Dupre A, Vincent S, Iaizzo PA. Basic ECG theory, recordings, and interpretation. In: Iaizzo PA, editor. *Handbook of Cardiac Anatomy, Physiology, and Devices.* Totowa, NJ: Humana Press, 2005:191–201)

V3: right between leads V2 and V4
V4: fifth intercostal space in the midclavicular line
V5: lateral to V4 in the anterior axillary line
V6: lateral to V4 and V5 in the midaxillary line

5.3.2   Waves and Intervals

The basic ECG signal during a normal cardiac cycle consists of a *P-wave, QRS complex*, and *T-wave* (Fig. 5.2). Sometimes, the T-wave is followed by a small deflection called the *U-wave*, often associated with after-depolarizations in the ventricles. The baseline voltage of the ECG is referred to as the *isoelectric line*.

5.3.2.1   P-wave

The P-wave is the result of atrial depolarization. Normally, a sinus impulse initiates in the SA node (located in the high right atrium) and travels leftward and inferiorly,

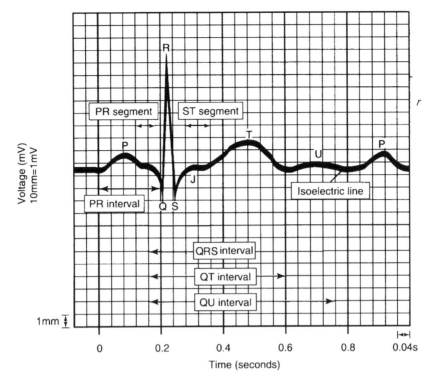

Fig. 5.2 ECG waves and intervals (modified from: Cecil RL, Goldman L, Bennett JC, editors. *Cecil Textbook of Medicine*, 21st edition. Philadelphia: W.B. Saunders, 2000)

thus the P-wave on the ECG during normal sinus rhythm is upright in II and aVF, and inverted in aVR. Normal P-wave duration is usually <100 ms with an amplitude between 2 and 3 mV.

5.3.2.2   PR Interval

The PR interval is the interval measured from the beginning of the P-wave to the beginning of the QRS complex. Normal PR intervals range between 120 and 200 ms. A prolonged PR interval suggests a "first-degree AV block," whereas a shorter PR interval is typically seen in ventricular pre-excitation such as Wolff–Parkinson–White syndrome.

5.3.2.3   QRS Complex

The deflection complex following the PR interval is the *QRS complex*, representing primarily ventricular depolarization. It is comprised of the Q (first downward deflection after the P-wave), R (the first positive deflection after the P-wave), and S waves (the first downward deflection after the R-wave). In the normal heart, its total duration is <110 ms. A prolonged QRS complex duration may suggest the presence of either left or right bundle branch block or some other pathology. Q-waves wider than 40 ms or deeper than 25% of the QRS complex will typically signify a prior myocardial infarction. Normally, the R-wave is small in lead V1, and gradually becomes larger across the precordial leads with maximum R-wave amplitude around lead V5. Poor R-wave progression often suggests a prior anterior myocardial infarction. Note that the R-wave height should normally not exceed 25 mm in leads V5 and V6, or 12 mm in lead aVL, otherwise disease such as left ventricular hypertrophy may be underlying.

5.3.2.4   ST Segment

This ST segment begins with the *J-point* (the point in which the ST segment takes off from the QRS) and terminates with initiation of the *T-wave*. This segment is usually isoelectric; a ST segment elevation may represent (1) myocardial injury if the pattern is consistent with a coronary distribution pattern; (2) pericarditis if the elevation is diffusely distributed among all the ECG leads; or (3) the presence of a ventricular aneurysm if persistent after an acute myocardial infarction.

5.3.2.5   T-wave

The T-wave is associated with ventricular repolarization. Atypically, it may be "peaked" with large pointed amplitude in the setting of hyperkalemia; a peaked T-wave can also be one of the earliest signs of an acute infarction.

5.3.2.6   QT Interval

QT interval is measured from the Q-wave to the end of the T-wave. It varies with gender and age, e.g., in adolescence, males and females have similar QT intervals, however, this value shortens in males as maturity is reached. It is important to note that the QT interval is heart rate dependent and is usually corrected by the square root of the preceding RR interval ($QTc = QT/\sqrt{RR}$). In adults, a corrected QT interval of >460 ms in females and >440 ms for males is considered prolonged. Additionally, common causes of prolonged QT durations include congenital channelopathies (long QT syndromes), medications, and electrolyte disturbances (such as hypokalemia and hypocalcemia).

5.4   Mechanisms of Arrhythmias

The term "arrhythmia" is mainly used to refer to disturbances of the normal heart rhythm, and is generally categorized as either bradycardia or tachycardia. *Bradycardia* is generally defined as a heart rate <60 beats/min, whereas *tachycardia*

Table 5.1 Mechanisms of tachycardias

- Abnormal impulse initiation
  - Automaticity
    - Enhanced normal automaticity: seen in inappropriate sinus tachycardia, some idiopathic ventricular tachycardias (VT)
    - Abnormal automaticity: presumed to be the case in ectopic atrial tachycardia, accelerated junctional rhythm, and possibly certain idiopathic VTs
  - Triggered activity
    - Early after-depolarization: presumed to be the case in torsades de pointes
    - Delayed after-depolarization: seen in digitalis-induced arrhythmias or presumed to occur in certain exercise-induced arrhythmias
- Abnormal impulse conduction
  - Ectopic escape after block: such as junctional escape
  - Unidirectional block and reentry
    - Orderly reentry: macro-reentry in atrial flutter and micro-reentry in atrial or VT
    - Random reentry: as seen in atrial fibrillation
- Other concepts (reflection, phase 2 reentry, and anisotropic reentry)

refers to heart rates >100 beats/min. Yet, bradycardia may be "physiologic" in some individuals, e.g., the endurance athlete. In an individual eliciting a disease state with an associated bradycardia, the typical cause is either in the SA node (sinus node dysfunction) or AV node (AV block). Most commonly, either of these conditions can be caused by intrinsic disease in the pacemaker cells or conduction system, or extrinsic factors such as medications or autonomic system disturbances.

The mechanisms underlying tachycardias are typically more numerous and complex than those causing bradycardias. Nevertheless, different tachycardias can generally be classified as being due to *abnormal impulse initiation, abnormal impulse conduction*, or a combination of both (Table 5.1). Importantly, intracardiac recordings can greatly facilitate interpretation of arrhythmias (Fig. 5.3).

5.5   Clinical Presentation and Diagnosis

Some arrhythmias can and often do occur in apparently healthy individuals with normal hearts, but they are more commonly associated with structural heart disease. Myocardial ischemia is the most important substrate for serious arrhythmias. However, other forms of cardiac dysfunction such as cardiomyopathies, valvular heart disease, and certain genetically determined disorders (e.g., long QT syndrome, Brugada syndrome) are also associated with arrhythmias in some patients.

In general, the clinical presentation of cardiac arrhythmias may range from completely asymptomatic or mild symptoms (palpitations and anxiety) to syncope (fainting) to even sudden cardiac death; the symptoms are largely dependent on the degree of arrhythmia-induced hemodynamic changes. The electrophysiologic and hemodynamic consequences of a particular arrhythmia are primarily determined by the rates, durations, and/or chambers of origin (atrial versus ventricular). Importantly,

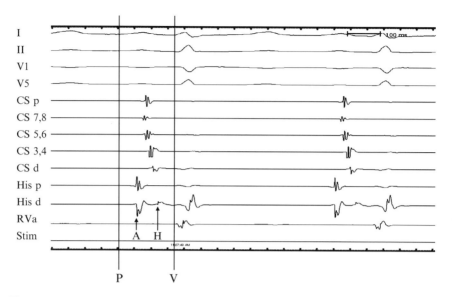

Fig. 5.3 Measurements in the His bundle electrogram. These measurements are important for evaluation of atrioventricular (AV) conduction. AH interval, measured from the earliest reproducible rapid deflection of the atrial electrogram in the His recording to the onset of the His deflection, represents conduction time from the low right atrium at the interatrial septum through the AV node to the His bundle (AV node function). The HV interval, measured from the beginning of the His deflection to the earliest onset of ventricular activation (surface leads or intracardiac recordings), represents conduction time from the proximal His bundle to the ventricular myocardium (infra-His conduction function). I = surface ECG lead I; II = surface ECG lead II; III = surface ECG lead III; V1 = surface ECG lead V1; V5 = surface ECG lead V5; CS d = distal coronary sinus; CS p = proximal coronary sinus; His d = distal His bundle; His p = proximal His bundle; RVa = right ventricular apex; Stim = stimulation; P = onset of P-wave; A = onset of atrial activation; H = onset of His activation; V = onset of ventricular activation

both underlying comorbidities and the patients' relative cardiovascular status also play large roles in clinical presentations.

A standard 12-lead ECG can be employed to readily diagnose some types of arrhythmias, however, it is limited by providing only a brief glance at rhythm abnormalities that are often short lived. Consequently, other techniques are frequently required in order to establish more accurate diagnoses: (1) prolonged ambulatory ECG monitoring (event monitor, Holter monitor, mobile outpatient cardiac telemetry from CardioNet®, Conshohocken, PA); (2) implantable loop recorders (Reveal®, Medtronic Inc., Minneapolis, MN; Confirm®, St Jude Medical Inc., St. Paul, MN; and Sleuth®, Transoma Medical Inc., St. Paul, MN); and/or (3) electrophysiologic testing. In selected cases, exercise stress testing or signal-averaged ECG recording may also be used for additional assessment regarding the precise nature of an arrhythmia or even the relative susceptibility of the patient to an arrhythmia. Other techniques such as analysis of heart rate variability, baroreflex sensitivity, assessment of QT dispersion, T-wave alternans, and body surface potential mapping have also been used to provide useful research information, but their value in daily practice remains to be fully defined at this time.

5.6 Treatment Considerations

The goals for treatment of arrhythmias are twofold: (1) to alleviate symptoms and improve quality of life; and (2) to prolong survival. Pharmacologic treatment has been the mainstay for management of most cardiac arrhythmias, although implantable devices and transcatheter ablation have become increasingly important in recent years. With regard to antiarrhythmic drugs, many clinicians find it convenient to group them according to the widely used *Vaughn–Williams classification.* This classification is simple and offers a means to keep the principal pharmacologic effects of drugs in mind (Table 5.2). A more comprehensive classification of antiarrhythmic drugs, termed the *Sicilian Gambit*, was introduced in 1991. Regardless, the selection of antiarrhythmic drugs for a given patient should be individualized based on the arrhythmia being treated, the nature and severity of any underlying heart disease, the proposed drug's antiarrhythmic and proarrhythmic actions, and/or its potential side effects.

In patients with tachycardias associated with ischemia or left ventricular dysfunction, class I antiarrhythmic agents should be avoided due to their potential

Table 5.2 Vaughn – Williams classification

- Class I: sodium channel blockers
    - Class Ia: drugs that reduce Vmax (phase 0 upstroke of action potential) and prolong action potential duration, such as quinidine, procainamide, and disopyramide
    - Class Ib: drugs that do not reduce V_{max} and shorten action potential duration, such as lidocaine, mexiletine, and phenytoin
    - Class Ic: drugs that predominantly slow conduction, moderately reduce V_{max}, and minimally prolong refractoriness, such as flecainide, propafenone, and moricizine

- Class II: β-adrenergic receptor blockers
    - β-blockers may be cardio- or $β_1$-selective (atenolol, esmolol, and metoprolol) or noncardioselective (carvedilol, pindolol, and propranolol)
    - Some exert intrinsic sympathomimetic activity (acebutolol, bucindolol, and pindolol)
    - Some have quinidine-like membrane stabilizing activity (acebutolol, carvedilol, and propranolol)
    - D-sotalol has a strong class III effect and has been regarded as a class III agent in many conditions

- Class III: potassium channel blockers that prolong refractoriness, such as amiodarone, bretylium, dofetilide, ibutilide, and sotalol; amiodarone has all the four class effects

- Class IV: calcium channel blockers
    - Dihydropyridine (amlodipine and nefedipine)
    - Nondihydropyridine drugs (diltiazem and verapamil)

As discussed in the text, the utility of this classification in terms of selection of therapy is limited, but the grouping permits important toxicity issues to be more readily kept in mind, an important factor in choosing drugs for individual patients

proarrhythmic risks and marked negative inotropic effects. Class III drugs, on the other hand (i.e., amiodarone, sotalol, dofetilide), appear to have neutral effects on survival in these patients and fewer negative inotropic concerns. β-blockers (Class II) have been proven to prolong survival in patients with structural heart disease, but in terms of use for suppression of symptomatic arrhythmias, they are mainly useful for the prevention of AV node-dependent reentrant supraventricular tachycardias (SVT) and/or catecholamine-sensitive arrhythmias. It is noteworthy that nonpharmacologic interventions, such as catheter ablation for SVTs and implantable cardioverter defibrillators (ICD) for primary and secondary prevention of sudden cardiac death, are currently considered as the treatments of choice in these clinical settings.

5.7   Bradyarrhythmias

As discussed earlier, *bradycardia* may result from either sinus node dysfunction or AV conduction block. Acute treatment options for symptomatic bradycardia include atropine, isoproterenol, and/or temporary pacing. When the underlying cause is reversible, such as in the case of drug toxicity (e.g., excess digitalis or β-blocker), temporary pacing and elimination of the offending agent is usually sufficient. However, if the cause is not reversible, a permanent electronic pacemaker is usually warranted.

5.7.1   Sinus Node Dysfunction

Sinus node dysfunction can be related to impaired impulse formation within the SA node (also often referred to as sick sinus syndrome), or due to impaired impulse conduction from the node into the atrium (termed SA block). The electrocardiographic manifestation may be excessive sinus bradycardia, or alternating periods of bradycardia and atrial tachycardia/fibrillation (*tachy-brady syndrome*). Patients with such symptoms often deteriorate further with age and/or age-related disease states. Additionally, the sinus node may simply become less responsive to physical exertion over time in terms of generating an appropriate heart rate (i.e., the patient will present with *chronotropic incompetence*).

In such patients, the typical resultant symptoms include fatigue, dizziness, confusion, exertional intolerance, diminished mental acuity, syncope, and/or congestive heart failure. Sinus node dysfunction may also present as various forms of SA exit block which may be classified into three general categories: (1) first-degree blocks; (2) second-degree type I and II blocks; and (3) third-degree blocks. Only the second-degree SA blocks can be recognized on the surface ECG.

Since sinus rate can be slowed by increased vagal tone, the *intrinsic heart rate* (IHR) after complete autonomic blockage is often used to assess integrity of sinus node function. Complete autonomic blockade can be achieved after the intravenous administration of propranolol (0.2 mg/kg) and atropine (0.04 mg/kg). Normal IHR is equal to 118.1 - (0.57 × age); an IHR < 80 beats/min in the elderly is usually suggestive of sinus node dysfunction. More specifically, sinus node recovery times (normal value <1,500 ms), corrected sinus node recovery times (normal value <550 ms), and less frequently, SA conduction times (normal value <125 ms) can be assessed within the electrophysiology laboratory to more precisely evaluate SA node function, i.e., when clinical diagnosis is uncertain.

5.7.2 AV Block

The term *first-degree AV block* is used to characterize a PR interval >0.20 s without loss of a QRS complex following each P-wave (Fig. 5.4a). *Second-degree AV block* is defined as when some atrial impulses fail to conduct to the ventricles. *Mobitz type I* second-degree AV block (Fig. 5.4b) is characterized by progressive PR interval prolongation until an atrial impulse is blocked (*Wenckebach phenomenon*). After an incomplete compensatory pause, the Wenckebach cycle starts again with a shorter PR interval compared with the last PR interval prior to block. Mobitz type I block is almost always located within the AV node and, importantly, the risk of developing complete AV block is low. In contrast, in *Mobitz type II* second-degree AV block (Fig. 5.4c), AV conduction fails suddenly without a change in the

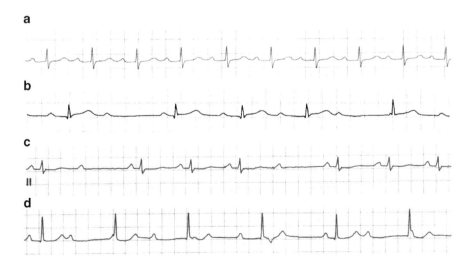

Fig. 5.4 AV block. The figures show (**a**) first-degree, (**b**) Mobitz type I second-degree, (**c**) Mobitz type II second-degree, and (**d**) third-degree AV block. See text for discussion

preceding PR interval. This type of block is usually due to His-Purkinje disease and is associated with a higher risk of progressing to complete AV block, with a slow and unreliable escape rhythm. When two or more consecutive atrial impulses fail to conduct, *high-degree AV block* is present and pacemaker implantation is often necessary. *Third-degree AV block* (complete AV block; Fig. 5.4d) occurs when no atrial impulses can conduct to the ventricles, resulting in no relationship between P-waves and QRS complexes on ECG.

The clinical significance of AV block depends on the (1) site of block; (2) risk of progression to complete block; and (3) subsidiary escape rate. When complete AV block occurs above the His bundle, the ventricular escape rhythm is believed to originate from the His bundle (40–60 beats/min); this is usually termed as a *junctional escape rhythm* and results in a narrow QRS complex. When AV block occurs below the His bundle, the escape is generated in the distal His-Purkinje fibers and the escape rhythm is much slower and less reliable (25–45 beats/min); this is referred to as a *ventricular escape rhythm* with a wide QRS complex. A permanent pacemaker is usually required in the third-degree AV block. In this regard, dual-chamber pacing (i.e., pacing both the atrium and ventricle) has become widely accepted as the approach of choice.

5.8 Tachyarrhythmias

5.8.1 Premature Complexes

Ectopic premature beats may originate from the atria, the AV junction, or the ventricles. Treatment of premature complexes is usually not necessary, however, if symptomatic, precipitating factors (such as alcohol, tobacco, and caffeine) should be identified and eliminated. Although anxiolytic agents and β-blockers may be tried therapeutically, they often produce more adverse side-effects than clinical benefits. Antiarrhythmic drugs may be used depending on the severity of symptoms and underlying cardiac disease. Further, catheter ablation may sometimes be used to eliminate symptomatic premature complexes.

5.8.1.1 Atrial Premature Complexes

Atrial premature complexes (APC) can typically be recognized on the ECG as early P-waves with a different morphology from that of sinus origin (Fig. 5.5a). The APCs may conduct to the ventricles with (1) a normal PR interval if they occur during the period when the AV junction is not refractory; (2) prolonged PR interval when they fall within the *relative refractory period*; or (3) they may be blocked entirely when the AV junction is in its *effective refractory period*. The appearance of bundle branch aberrancy may become evident if APCs occur when either bundle branch is refractory. APCs almost always enter the sinus node and reset the sinus cycle length,

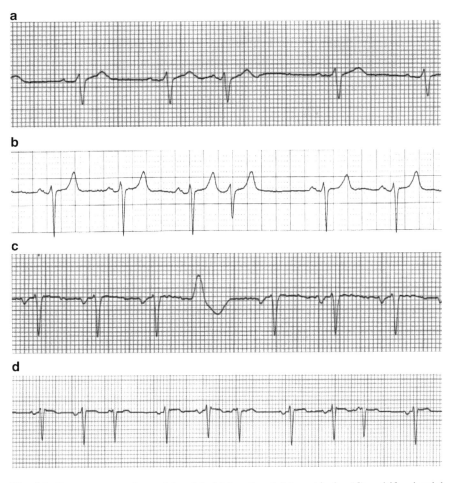

Fig. 5.5 Premature complexes. (**a**) atrial, (**b**) junctional, (**c**) ventricular, (**d**) multifocal atrial tachycardia

resulting in an *incomplete compensatory pause* (i.e., the sum of pre- and post-APC intervals is less than that of two normal sinus PP intervals).

5.8.1.2   Multifocal Atrial Tachycardia

Multifocal atrial tachycardia is a relatively uncommon arrhythmia characterized by atrial rates between 100 and 130 beats/min, with marked variations in P-wave morphology (arbitrarily defined as at least three different P-wave contours). In such patients, multifocal atrial tachycardia often manifests as a short burst of tachycardia (Fig. 5.5d), and typically occurs in older individuals with moderate to severe cardiopulmonary disease (especially during an exacerbation).

5.8.1.3 AV Junctional Premature Complexes

These complexes are recognized on the ECG as normal QRS complexes without a preceding P-wave (Fig. 5.5b); *retrograde P-waves* (inverted in II, III, and aVF) may be seen after the QRS complexes, further supporting the diagnosis. Atrioventricular junctional complexes are less common than APCs and are often associated with drug intoxication and cardiac diseases. Most junctional beats have an incomplete compensatory sinus pause (like an APC) because the atrium is activated retrogradely, i.e., resetting the sinus node in the process. On rare occasions, a junctional premature beat may fail to conduct to either the atria or ventricles (*concealed junctional beat*), but results in refractoriness in the AV junction and blocks subsequent supraventricular beats.

5.8.1.4 Ventricular Premature Complexes

Ventricular premature complexes (VPCs) are recognized as wide bizarre QRS complexes not preceded by P-waves (Fig. 5.5c). They often fail to conduct retrograde to the atria and thus do not typically reset the sinus node; this results in a *full compensatory pause* (the sum of pre- and post-APC intervals equals that of two normal sinus PP intervals). *An interpolated VPC* does not influence the following sinus beats (i.e., its occurrence is timed so as not to impair the next sinus beat from traversing the AV node and reaching the ventricles at the expected moment). The VPCs may occur as a single event, but may also occur in patterns of *bigeminy* (repeating pattern of sinus beat followed by a VPC) and *trigeminy* (two sinus beats coupled with a VPC). *Couplets* or *pairs* (two consecutive VPCs) and *nonsustained ventricular tachycardia* (VT, arbitrarily defined as three or more consecutive VPCs at a rate of >100 beats/min) are also relatively common observations during monitoring of patients with heart disease. The morphology may be *monomorphic* (uniform) or *polymorphic* (multiform).

The VPCs often bear a fixed *coupling interval*, i.e., a given period between the onset of VPC and the onset of its preceding sinus QRS complex. When there is a protected ventricular ectopic focus, the focus is constantly firing without being reset by sinus beats; this is clinically referred to as *ventricular parasystole* and is characterized by varying coupling intervals with relatively fixed inter-VPC intervals (i.e., variation <120 ms). Currently, pharmacologic treatment of VPCs is aimed at alleviating symptoms rather than prolongation of survival.

5.8.2 Sinus Tachycardias

5.8.2.1 Physiological Sinus Tachycardia

Physiologic sinus tachycardia represents a normal response to a variety of physiologic (anxiety and exercise) and/or pathologic stresses (fever, hypotension, thyrotoxicosis, hypoxemia, and congestive heart failure). Sinus tachycardia rarely exceeds 200 beats/min and, by itself, should not be the target of treatment; in other words, therapy should be directed towards the underlying etiology if warranted (e.g., fever, anemia, hyperthyroidism, sepsis).

5.8.2.2 Inappropriate Sinus Tachycardia

Inappropriate sinus tachycardia is characterized by an increased resting heart rate (often >100 beats/min) and an exaggerated heart rate response to minimal stress. The ECG for this arrhythmia is indistinguishable from physiologic sinus tachycardia, presenting with normal P-wave morphology. β-blockers and calcium channel blockers can be used for symptomatic treatment, although with imperfect results. Subsequently, radiofrequency therapeutic modifications of the sinus node can be considered if drug therapy fails, as is often the case.

5.8.3 Paroxysmal Supraventricular Tachycardias

Paroxysmal supraventricular tachycardias (PSVTs) are a group of SVTs with sudden onset and termination. They are usually recurrent and often occur in otherwise seemingly healthy individuals.

5.8.3.1 Sinus Node Reentry Tachycardia

Sinus node reentry tachycardias are relatively rare, accounting for approximately 3% of all PSVTs. The average heart rate ranges between 130 and 140 beats/min, yet it can be quite labile, suggesting autonomic influences may be at play. Sinus node reentry tachycardias should be suspected in "anxiety-related sinus tachycardia." β-blockers and/or calcium channel blockers (e.g., verapamil, dilti-azem) as well as ablation are common treatment options.

5.8.3.2 Atrial Tachycardias

Atrial tachycardias refer to those tachyarrhythmias that arise in atrial tissues due to abnormal automaticities or reentries. Typical atrial tachycardias have atrial rates between 150 and 200 beats/min, with P-wave morphologies that are usually different from those of P-waves with sinus node origins. Atrial tachycardias account for 5–10% of all PSVTs. Since atrial tachycardias arise within and are sustained by atrial tissues alone, AV block may develop without interrupting the tachycardia. The atrial rates often gradually accelerate after initiation until stabilizing between

100 and 175 beats/min, an observation termed *warm-up phenomenon*. Ablation is often the treatment of choice when feasible in such patients.

5.8.3.3 AV Nodal Reentry Tachycardia

AV nodal reentry tachycardias (AVNRTs) are the most common PSVTs (50–65%) and usually present with narrow QRS complexes with regular heart rates between 130 and 250 beats/min. A schematic of a typical AV nodal reentry circuit is shown in Fig. 5.6. In such patients, retrograde P-waves may not be apparent in many instances, due to being buried within the QRS complexes. P-waves may also appear as subtle distortions at the terminal portion of the QRS complexes. During electrophysiologic testing, the onset of an AVNRT is almost always associated with a prolonged AH interval, which produces sufficient conduction delay in the so-called slow pathway to ensure recovery of the fast pathway. This delay permits the fast pathway to conduct retrograde toward the atrium, thereby completing the reentry circuit. Importantly, a critical balance between conduction delay and recovery of refractoriness in the two pathways is required to sustain the tachycardia.

Acute treatments to terminate AVNRT include (1) vagal maneuvers (e.g., carotid sinus massage or Valsalva maneuver); (2) adenosine injection; (3) administration of verapamil, diltiazem, or β-blockers; and/or (4) electrical (direct current) cardioversion. The majority of these interventions are designed to interrupt AV nodal conductions transiently, thereby "breaking" the fragile reentry circuits. Drugs used for long-term prevention of AVNRT recurrences include digitalis (not currently recommended due to low efficacy), β-blockers, calcium channel blockers, and/or class Ia and Ic antiarrhythmic drugs. Nevertheless, the most important advance in the treatment of AVNRT is transcatheter ablation, principally of the "slow" pathway region. In experienced hands, catheter ablation of AVNRT is a safe and highly effective curative treatment (i.e., with nearly 100% success rates).

5.8.3.4 AV Reciprocating Tachycardia Using Concealed Accessory Pathway

AV reciprocating tachycardia is another common form of PSVT. In such patients, accessory conduction tissue remaining from embryonic development of the heart can create the substrate for reentry PSVT. The most common type of accessory pathway is the AV bypass tract connecting the atria to the ventricles. In many cases, accessory connections only conduct in the retrograde direction (termed "concealed" accessory connections). In these individuals, there are no apparent ECG footprints since ventricular pre-excitations do not occur. It is noteworthy that

Fig. 5.6 (continued) Since the atria and ventricles are activated near simultaneously by a circuit within the AV node, the time difference between ventricular and atrial activation is relatively short. The retrograde P-wave is often buried in QRS complex (RP interval is 0 ms), as shown in this case. Recording channels are the same as in Fig. 5.3

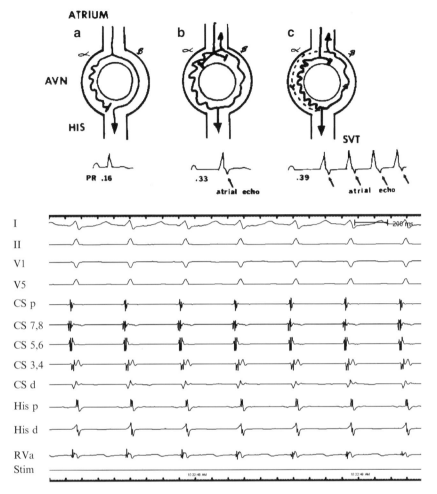

Fig. 5.6 (*Top*) Schematic of the typical AV nodal reentry tachycardia (AVNRT). The AV node has a slow pathway with short refractoriness and a fast pathway with long refractoriness. (**a**) During sinus rhythm, the impulse conducts the ventricles through the fast pathway, yielding a normal PR interval. The impulse simultaneously goes down the slow pathway, but cannot conduct to the His bundle antegradely or retrogradely to the fast pathway since they are rendered refractory by the prior beat. (**b**) An atrial premature complex (APC) reaches the effective refractory period of the fast pathway and is blocked in the fast pathway. This APC is able to conduct slowly down to the slow pathway, yielding a prolonged PR interval. The delay in conduction over the slow pathway provides enough time for the fast pathway to recover and allow the impulse conducted from the slow pathway to continue over the fast pathway retrogradely to the atria, producing an atrial echo beat. At same time, the returned impulse tries to conduct down over the slow pathway and fails due to unrecovered refractoriness of the slow pathway. (**c**) A sufficient early APC occurs, producing a similar echo beat as in **b**. However, the returned impulse is able to conduct down the slow pathway, repeatedly producing another ventricular beat and atrial echo, i.e., supraventricular tachycardia or SVT (*Source*: Josephson ME. *Clinical Cardiac Electrophysiology. Techniques and Interpretation*, third edition. Philadelphia, PA: Lippincott Williams & Wilkins, 2002). (*Bottom*) Intracardiac recordings of typical AVNRT.

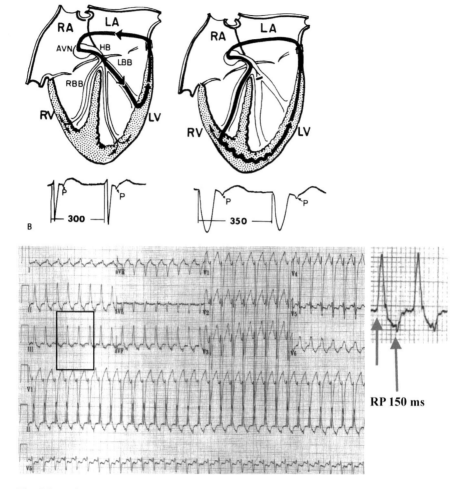

Fig. 5.7 Typical AV reentry tachycardia. (*Top*) Illustration of AV reciprocating tachycardia using a left-sided concealed accessory pathway. Left bundle branch block prolongs the tachycardia cycle length by 50 ms due to the conduction delay of the tachycardia circuit in the left ventricle. (*Bottom*) 12-lead ECG recording of AV reentry tachycardia. Note that the retrograde P-wave is 150 ms after the onset of QRS complex (RP interval is 150 ms). AVN = atrioventricular node; HB = His bundle; LA = left atrium; LBB = left bundle branch; LV = left ventricle; RA = right atrium; RBB = right bundle branch; RV = right ventricle

this form of accessory pathway accounts for approximately 30% of all PSVTs. The electrical impulses for this type of PSVT circulate antegrade through the AV nodes and retrograde through the concealed accessory pathways (Fig. 5.7); both the atria and ventricles are necessary components of the reentry circuit in this type of arrhythmia, distinguishing it from AVNRT.

Medical treatment of AV reciprocating tachycardia is similar to that of AVNRT. Nevertheless, catheter ablation is highly effective for eliminating accessory AV connections and is often the preferred approach, especially in younger individuals.

5.9 Wolff–Parkinson–White Syndrome

When there are one or more accessory AV pathways or connections that conduct in the antegrade direction, the ventricles may become overtly pre-excited to a varying degree. This condition is referred to as *Wolff–Parkinson–White syndrome*, i.e., when palpitations/tachyarrhythmias occur in the setting of pre-excitation. The ECG features of a typical AV connection in Wolff–Parkinson–White syndrome are (1) shortened PR interval <120 ms during sinus rhythm; (2) widened QRS duration; and (3) the presence of a delta wave (a slurred, slowly rising onset of the QRS) (Fig. 5.8). The terminal QRS portions are usually normal, and sometimes they are associated with secondary ST-T changes.

In addition to typical AV accessory pathways, other variants may exist in such patients, such as atriohisian, atriofascicular, nodofascicular, and nodoventricular fibers. More specifically, the *Lown–Ganong–Levine syndrome* is defined in patients with recurrent paroxysmal tachycardias or atrial fibrillation (AF) associated with short PR intervals and normal QRS complexes. Further, when present, the majority of *Mahaim fibers* are long right-sided atriofascicular or AV pathways between the lateral tricuspid and distal right bundle branches in the right ventricular free walls. These fibers almost represent a duplication of the AV node and are capable of only antegrade conduction with decremental conduction properties.

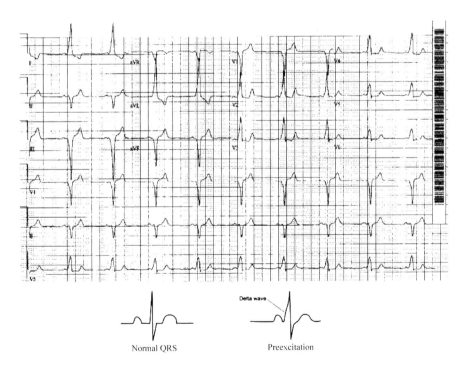

Fig. 5.8 ECG recording and delta wave of Wolff–Parkinson–White Syndrome. The vector of the delta waves suggests a right posterior septal accessory pathway. See text for discussion

5.10   Nonparoxysmal Junctional Tachycardia

Nonparoxysmal junctional tachycardia, also called *accelerated junctional rhythm*, is readily recognized by a narrow QRS complex without a consistent P-wave preceding each QRS complex, at heart rates between 70 and 130 beats/min; it is usually associated with a warm-up period at the onset. Nonparoxysmal junctional tachycardia frequently results from conditions that produce enhanced automaticity or triggered activities in the AV junction, such as those associated with inferior acute myocardial infarctions, digitalis intoxications, or postvalvular surgery. Typically, treatments in such cases should be directed toward the underlying diseases.

5.11   Atrial Flutter and Fibrillation

5.11.1   Atrial Flutter

Atrial flutter is characterized by atrial rates between 250 and 350 beats/min, usually accompanied with 2:1 AV conductions and resulting in ventricular rates of approximately 150 beats/min. Classical flutter waves (*F-waves*) are regular saw-tooth patterns on the ECG, most prominently detected in the inferior leads and sometimes V1 (Fig. 5.9). Although antiarrhythmic drugs may be useful to prevent recurrences of atrial flutter, they are less effective for the conversion to

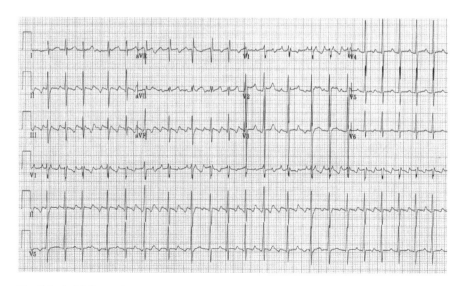

Fig. 5.9 Atrial flutter. See text for discussion

sinus rhythm. In such patients, cardioversion (50–100 J) is oftentimes the most effective method for termination of atrial flutter. Although systemic embolization is less common in atrial flutter than in AF (discussed later), such patients should be prescribed chronic anticoagulation for stroke prophylaxes according to standardized AF guidelines.

5.11.2   *Atrial Fibrillation*

Atrial fibrillation (AF) is an uncoordinated atrial tachyarrhythmia characterized on ECG by (1) the absence of distinct P-waves before each QRS complex; (2) the presence of rapid atrial oscillations (*F-waves*); and (3) irregular RR intervals (Fig. 5.10). The AF is considered *recurrent* when two or more episodes have occurred. Recurrent AF is designated *paroxysmal* if there is spontaneous termination of the arrhythmia. The term *persistent* is used when AF is present longer than seven days. If several attempts at cardioversion fail or are not indicated in long-standing cases (>1 year), AF is regarded as *permanent*. When no history is available, the term *recent or new onset* is often used.

The incidence of AF is highly age-dependent; other common cardiac precursors include a history of congestive heart failure, valvular heart disease, hypertension, and/or coronary artery disease. *Lone AF* is said to be present when this tachyarrhythmia occurs in the absence of underlying structural heart disease or transient precipitating factors.

The mechanisms underlying AF may include multiple wavelet reentry and focal enhanced automaticity. The atrial "rates" during AF can range from 350 to 600 beats/min.

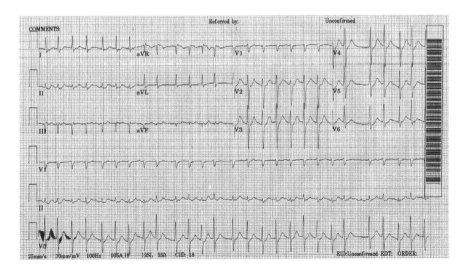

Fig. 5.10 Atrial fibrillation. See text for discussion

Due to *concealed AV nodal penetrations* and subsequent variable degrees of AV block, the characteristic *irregularly irregular* ventricular rates are usually between 100 and 160 beats/min in untreated patients with normal AV conduction properties.

The major adverse clinical consequences of AF include palpitations, impaired cardiac function, and/or thromboembolism. Typical physical findings in such patients include irregularly irregular ventricular rhythms, variations in the intensity of the first heart sounds, and/or the absence of "*a*" waves in jugular venous pulses. If the ventricular responses are too rapid, a peripheral *pulse deficit* (peripheral pulse rate less than heart rate) can result from insufficient diastolic filling time. Patients with chronic rapid ventricular rates are also at risk for developing *tachycardia-induced cardiomyopathies*. In addition to rheumatic mitral valve disease and prosthetic valves (mechanical or tissue), major risk factors for embolization in *nonvalvular AF* are often assessed using a $CHADS_2$ scheme (Cardiac Failure, Hypertension, Age, Diabetes, Stroke [Doubled]).

The goals of therapies for AF are improvement of symptoms, reduction of AF-associated morbidities, and improvement in prognoses. The three basic tenets of therapy for AF are (1) restoration and maintenance of sinus rhythm; (2) control of ventricular rate responses; and (3) prevention of thromboembolism.

5.12 Ventricular Tachyarrhythmias

5.12.1 Ventricular Tachycardias

Although VTs can occur in clinically normal hearts, they generally accompany some form of structural heart disease, particularly in patients with prior myocardial infarctions. A fixed substrate, such as an old infarct scar, is typically responsible for most episodes of recurrent monomorphic VT. Yet, acute ischemia may also play a more important role in the pathogenesis of polymorphic VT or ventricular fibrillation.

The VTs are characterized on ECG by a wide QRS complex and tachycardia at rates of >100 beats/min (Fig. 5.11). Like VPCs, VTs can be monomorphic (Fig. 5.11a) or polymorphic. A *sustained VT* is defined as a VT persisting >30 s or requiring termination due to hemodynamic compromise. A *nonsustained VT* is defined as lasting >3 consecutive beats but less than 30 s. *Bidirectional VT* refers to VT that shows an alternation in QRS amplitudes and axes. The key marker of VT on ECG is ventriculo-atrial dissociation; capture or fusion beats also strongly support the diagnosis of VT. Sustained VT is almost always symptomatic and the presentation, prognosis, and management of VT largely depend on the patient's underlying cardiovascular state.

Procainamide and amiodarone are commonly used medications for the pharmacological treatment of acute termination of VT. Yet, in patients with heart disease, sotalol, dofetilide, and amiodarone are the recommended drugs for chronic

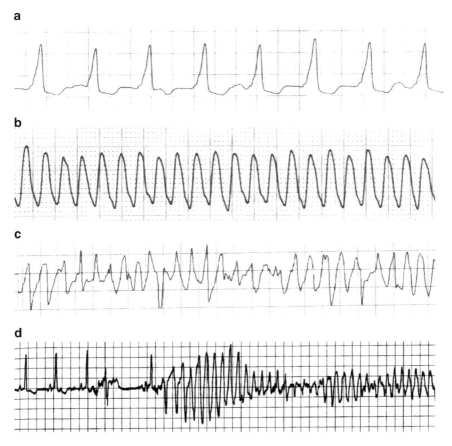

Fig. 5.11 Ventricular tachyarrhythmias. (**a**) ventricular tachycardia, (**b**) ventricular flutter, (**c**) ventricular fibrillation, and (**d**) torsades de pointes (TdP)

suppression. An ICD, with or without supplemental dosing with amiodarone, is the most established long-term therapy for VT. Nevertheless, catheter ablation may provide cures for some forms including (1) VT in those with structurally normal hearts (idiopathic VT); (2) those with bundle-branch reentry VT; and/or (3) selected cases of scar-related VT. However, in patients with diminished left ventricular function, it may be prudent to place an ICD even after an apparently successful ablation. A complete guideline for management of ventricular arrhythmias was published in 2006.

5.12.2   Ventricular Flutter and Ventricular Fibrillation

Electrocardiographically, *ventricular flutters* (Fig. 5.11b) usually appear as "sine waves" with a rate between 150 and 300 beats/min; it is essentially impossible to assign a specific morphology of these oscillations. *Ventricular fibrillation* (Fig. 5.11c) is recognized by grossly irregular undulations of varying amplitudes, contours, and rates, and is often preceded by a rapid repetitive sequence of VT. Spontaneous conversions of ventricular fibrillation to sinus rhythm are rare, and prompt electrical defibrillation is essential. Long-term prevention of sudden cardiac death in these patients predominately relies on ICDs.

5.12.3 Accelerated Idioventricular Rhythm

Accelerated idioventricular rhythm can be regarded as a type of slow VT with heart rates between 60 and 110 beats/min. These rhythms usually occur in settings such as acute myocardial infarction, particularly during reperfusion. Since these rhythms are usually transient without significant hemodynamic compromise, treatments are rarely required.

5.12.4 Torsades de Pointes

When polymorphic VT occurs in the presence of prolonged QT intervals (congenital or acquired), it is termed *Torsades de Pointes* (TdP). This arrhythmia is often preceded by VPCs with a *long-short sequence* (Fig. 5.11d). Oftentimes, TdP presents with multiple nonsustained episodes causing recurrent syncope, but also has a predilection to degenerate into ventricular fibrillation. Identification of TdP has important therapeutic implications because treatments are completely different from that of non-TdP polymorphic VT. Magnesium, pacing, and/or isoproterenolol can be used to treat TdP if required. It should be noted that a left cervicothoracic sympathectomy, involving resection of the lower half of the left stellate ganglion and portions of the thoracic sympathetic ganglia, has also been proposed as a form of therapy for TdP in patients with congenital long QT syndrome.

5.13 Summary

Cardiac arrhythmias encompass a wide spectrum of abnormalities in both electrical generation and conduction at all levels within the heart. These defects can manifest as either bradycardia or tachycardia. Clinical and basic laboratory research gained important insights into the mechanisms underlying these various arrhythmias (e.g., increased automaticity, triggered activity, micro- and/or macro-reentry), and has provided valuable tools for their treatment (medications, pacemakers, defibrillators, and catheter-based ablations). The clinical significance of these cardiac arrhythmias is predominantly related to hemodynamic outcomes and the risk of life-threatening consequences (e.g., ventricular fibrillation), in addition to associated symptoms.

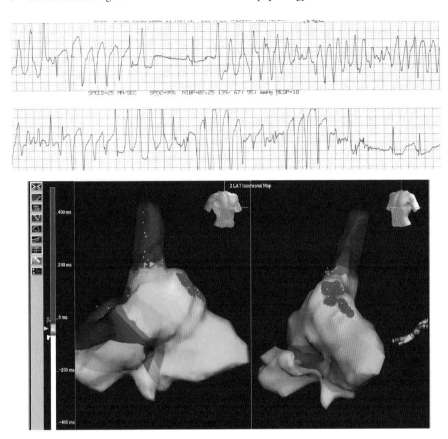

Fig. 5.12 TdP. Successful catheter ablation of premature ventricular ectopics in the anteroseptal wall of the right ventricular outflow tract eliminates frequent episodes of TdP (as shown on the *top*) that are refractory to medical management. The *bottom* shows an activation map using the Ensite NavX system. The *red areas* indicate the ablation lesions

Careful inspection of a patient's ECG recordings often makes it possible to correctly diagnose many rhythm disturbances and guide clinical management. It is important to note that recent technical advancements have enabled more complex arrhythmias to be ablated, thus providing a curative treatment (Fig. 5.12).

Further Readings

Benditt DG, Lü F. Atriofascicular pathways: fuzzy nomenclature or merely wishful thinking? J Cardiovasc Electrophysiol 2006; 17:261–5.

Blomström-Lundqvist C, Scheinman MM, Aliot EM, et al. ACC/AHA/ESC guidelines for the management of patients with supraventricular arrhythmias. J Am Coll Cardiol 2003; 42:1493–531.

Camm AJ, Lü F. Risk stratification after myocardial infarction. Pacing Clin Electrophysiol 1994; 17:401–16.

Camm AJ, Lü F. Chronotropic incompetence. Part I. Normal modulation of the heart rate. Clin Cardiol 1996; 19:424–8.

Camm AJ, Lü F. Chronotropic incompetence. Part II. Clinical significance. Clin Cardiol 1996; 19:424–8.

Epstein AE, DiMarco JP, Ellenbogen KA, et al. ACC/AHA/HRS 2008 guidelines for device-based therapy of cardiac rhythm abnormalities. J Am Coll Cardiol 2008; 51:1–62.

Lü F, Statters DJ, Hnatkova K, et al. Change of the autonomic influence on the heart immediately before the onset of spontaneous idiopathic ventricular tachycardia. J Am Coll Cardiol 1994; 24:1515–22.

Fuster V, Rydén LE, Cannom DS, et al. ACC/AHA/ESC 2006 guidelines for the management of patients with atrial fibrillation. J Am Coll Cardiol 2006; 48:854–906.

Hancock EW, Deal BJ, Mirvis DM, et al. AHA/ACCF/HRS recommendations for the standardization and interpretation of the electrocardiogram: Part V: electrocardiogram changes associated with cardiac chamber hypertrophy. J Am Coll Cardiol 2009; 53:992–1002.

Hjalmarson A, Goldstein S, Fagerberg B, et al. Effects of controlled-release metoprolol on total mortality, hospitalizations, and well-being in patients with heart failure: The metoprolol CR/XL randomized intervention trial in congestive heart failure (MERIT-HF). MERIT-HF study group. JAMA 2000; 283:1295–302.

Packer M, Bristow MR, Cohn JN, et al. The effect of carvedilol on morbidity and mortality in patients with chronic heart failure. U.S. Carvedilol Heart Failure Study Group. N Engl J Med 1996; 334:1349–55.

Preliminary report: Effect of encainide and flecainide on mortality in a randomized trial of arrhythmia suppression after myocardial infarction. The Cardiac Arrhythmia Suppression Trial (CAST) investigators. N Engl J Med 1989; 321:406–12.

Rautaharju PM, Surawicz B, Gettes LS, et al. AHA/ACCF/HRS recommendations for the standardization and interpretation of the electrocardiogram: Part IV: the ST segment, T and U waves, and the QT interval. J Am Coll Cardiol 2009; 53:982–91.

Surawicz B, Childers R, Deal BJ, et al. AHA/ACCF/HRS recommendations for the standardization and interpretation of the electrocardiogram: Part III: intraventricular conduction disturbances J Am Coll Cardiol 2009; 53:976–81.

Wagner GS, Macfarlane P, Wellens H, et al. AHA/ACCF/HRS recommendations for the standardization and interpretation of the electrocardiogram: Part VI: acute ischemia/infarction. J Am Coll Cardiol 2009; 53:1003–11.

Zipes DP, Camm AJ, Borggrefe M, et al. ACC/AHA/ESC 2006 guidelines for management of patients with ventricular arrhythmias and the prevention of sudden cardiac death. J Am Coll Cardiol 2006; 48:1064–108.

Part II
Methods and Models

Chapter 6
Principles of Electrophysiological In Vitro Measurements

Frank Lehmann-Horn, Michael Fauler, Boris Holzherr, and Karin Jurkat-Rott

Abstract A variety of in vitro electrophysiological techniques have been developed and enhanced over the last half century to study the membrane properties of excitable tissues such as skeletal or cardiac muscle. Each technique has its specific advantages and methodological requirements, and the proper use of these techniques is important to obtain accurate data. This chapter describes the origins and methodologies of the voltage clamp technique, which has revolutionized the field of cellular electrophysiology, and the patch clamp technique, which is the principal tool for studying ion channels. In addition, we provide an overview on the usage of voltage-sensitive fluorescence probes and ion-sensitive microelectrodes.

6.1 Introduction

Considerable progress in understanding the molecular basis of cardiac excitability and conduction has been made through a combined approach of genetics, molecular biology, and cellular electrophysiology. Over time, several specific electrophysiologic techniques have been developed and refined to study the properties of excitable tissues such as skeletal or cardiac muscle. More specifically, these techniques allow researchers to investigate action potentials in tissues and cells or ion channel currents even on the single channel level (Fig.6.1). Since an extracellularly recorded electrocardiogram (ECG) is only the second derivative over time of the action potential, an intracellularly measured potential provides more precise information relative to the electrical events, e.g., the resting membrane potential and/or the absolute voltage changes associated with an action potential. For example, the resting membrane potential of a ventricular cell can be permanently depolarized due to a reduced inwardly rectifying K^+ channel conductance, as in the Andersen syndrome. This alteration will not be visible in the ECG, and thus the resulting alteration in membrane excitability may or may not be reflected by changes in the extracellularly

F. Lehmann-Horn (✉)
Institute of Applied Physiology, Ulm University, Ulm, Germany
e-mail: frank.lehmann-horn@uni-ulm.de

D.C. Sigg et al. (eds.), *Cardiac Electrophysiology Methods and Models*,
DOI 10.1007/978-1-4419-6658-2_6, © Springer Science+Business Media, LLC 2010

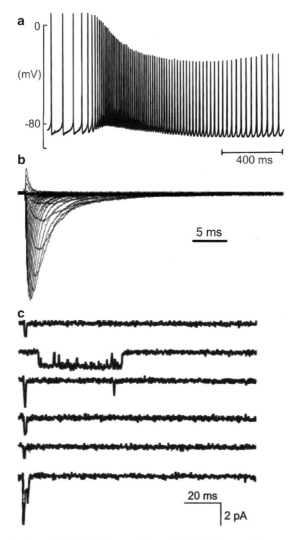

Fig. 6.1 Typical electrophysiological recordings obtained from various preparations using different recording techniques. (**a**) Action potentials recorded under current clamp. (**b**) Skeletal muscle sodium channel current recorded with the whole-cell patch clamp technique in HEK-293 cells. (**c**) Single channel recordings of sodium channels in cell-attached mode

recorded potentials. Similarly, in cardiac pacemaker cells, intracellular recordings will best define the relative prepotentials and thus infer the relationship between ion channel activities and ultimate rhythmicity.

While resting and action potentials can be simply recorded using a single intracellular microelectrode and a voltage amplifier, more efforts are needed to investigate the properties of specific ion channels. In general, it is considered that this research field was initiated by the pioneering work of Hodgkin and Huxley,[1] who originally utilized the voltage clamp technique by using two intracellular micro-electrodes and a feedback amplifier. Importantly, they provided the first detailed description of the *ionic basis* of the *action potential* in nerve axons. Their work and, in particular, their mathematical descriptions of the action potential provided novel insights into some of the functional properties of both *voltage-gated sodium* and potassium membrane *particles*; this is how ion conductances were described prior to knowledge of the existence of channel proteins. For the next 50 years, voltage clamp methodologies became the principal tool for the study of ion channels. More recently, the patch clamp technique has revolutionized the field of cellular electrophysiology. This experimental method was developed by Neher and colleagues[2] and can be considered as a specific application of voltage clamping, i.e., developed to record the currents through a membrane patch conducted by one or more channel molecules.

The magnitudes and selectivities of currents measured using patch clamp are dependent on the ionic gradients across the cell membrane. Therefore, a complete characterization of the channels cannot be performed without additional determination of the extracellular and intracellular ion activities as performed with ion-selective microelectrodes. Additionally, recent progress in fluorescence imaging techniques allows membrane potential measurements by using voltage-sensitive dyes. Yet, all methodologies have their shortcomings, as described in detail in this chapter.

In principle, there are two tasks that typically need to be performed by an electrophysiologist's equipment on cardiac tissues or cells under study: (1) the measurement of bio-potentials; and/or (2) the injection of current. Both tasks need special consideration relative to electrode properties and performance and the electronics used.

6.2 Electrodes

The basis for any methodology that measures electric potentials from (or that injects current into) a biological material is to make electrical contact between the tissue or cells and the electronic recording device. This is done by the electrode and an electrochemical half-cell which consists of a solid (metallic) conductor and an electrolyte. Typically there are two basic configurations of electrodes used in most electrophysiological practices: (1) a solid electrode which builds the electrochemical half-cell with the tissue as the electrolyte; and (2) a fluid-filled electrode that separates the electrochemical cell from the tissue. Note that solid electrodes are typically used for extracellular recordings and/or stimulation, while fluid-filled electrodes, especially glass microelectrodes, are used for intracellular applications.

There are important properties of electrochemical cells that must be considered for the correct usage of such electrodes. For example, there can be undesirable consequences by the electrochemical reaction occurring at the metal–electrolyte interface and/or capacitance changes that might occur at the junction; this is especially a concern for glass microelectrodes which alter tip potentials.

6.2.1 The Metal–Electrolyte Interface

The properties of the metal–electrolyte interface are most important for the stability of the electrode potential as well as when currents are passed through the electrode. To increase the stability of electrode potentials, the participants of the redox reactions in the half-cell must be saturated. This is easily achieved in Ag/AgCl-electrodes in which a silver (Ag) wire is coated with slightly soluble silver chloride (AgCl), providing the following redox reaction:

$$Ag(solid) + Cl^- \leftrightarrow AgCl(solid) + e^-.$$

It is important to note that AgCl will become diminished over time, drastically reducing electrode performance and the stability of the electrode potential. Therefore, it is necessary to routinely check such electrodes and regularly recoat them. Additionally, one should consider that silver is a biologic toxin. If altered cellular viabilities are observed, it is possible to separate the Ag/AgCl-electrode from the tissue or cells under investigation by the use of a bridge (e.g., agar bridge, typically glass capillaries filled with electrolyte in 2–3% agar). For other (metal) electrodes, especially when used for stimulation, dissolution of the electrode might occur:

$$M \rightarrow M^{n+} + n \cdot e^-.$$

It should also be noted that electrolysis of water can lead to serious problems due to gas formation and generation of free radicals, causing associated damage to tissues and cells:

$$2H_2O + 2e^- \rightarrow 2H_2 - +2OH^-.$$

Since the metal–electrolyte interface commonly induces a capacitance, it is possible to avoid such detrimental effects by employing appropriate electrode designs that increase this capacitance. In other words, if the stimulating current is kept small enough to avoid overcharging of the capacitance, electrolysis can be prevented.

6.2.2 Junction Potentials

Liquid junction potentials are due to different mobilities of ions at interfaces between different solutions. The result from a charge imbalance at the interface between two solutions is caused by a differing extent of diffusion among the various ions. Liquid junction potentials are usually in the range of several mV and can be approximated by the generalized Henderson Liquid Junction Potential Equation[3]:

$$E^{\mathrm{B}} - E^{\mathrm{P}} = \frac{RT}{F} \cdot S \cdot \ln \left(\frac{\displaystyle\sum_{i=1}^{N} z_i^2 u_i a_i^{\mathrm{P}}}{\displaystyle\sum_{i=1}^{N} z_i^2 u_i a_i^{\mathrm{B}}} \right)$$

$$S = \frac{\displaystyle\sum_{i=1}^{N} \left[(z_i u_i)(a_i^{\mathrm{B}} - a_i^{\mathrm{P}}) \right]}{\displaystyle\sum_{i=1}^{N} \left[(z_i^2 u_i)(a_i^{\mathrm{B}} - a_i^{\mathrm{P}}) \right]},$$

where $E^{\mathrm{B}} - E^{\mathrm{P}}$ represents the potential of the bath solution B relative to the pipette P. The variables u, a, and z represent the mobility, activity, and valence of the ionic species i. The constants R, T, and F represent the gas constant, absolute temperature, and the Faraday constant.

For intracellular recordings, high concentrations of KCl are commonly used because K and Cl have the same relative mobilities, and thus the resulting junction potentials will be very low.

6.2.3   Tip Potential

The so-called electrode *tip potential* is a distinct and practically unique feature of glass microelectrodes commonly used for intracellular measurements. It is elicited by the negatively charged glass surface which reduces anionic mobilities, thus altering the junction potentials. In other words, this change of junction potential induced by properties of the microelectrode tip influences the tip potential. It is typically negative and this can profoundly affect the accurate measurement of resting membrane potentials. The main problem arises from the fact that the size of the tip potential depends on the electrolyte composition in which the electrode is immersed. It is more negative in an extracellular solution (dominated by NaCl) compared to an intracellular solution (dominated by K salts). Nevertheless, the overall change of tip potential depends on many factors and is practically unpredictable. Note that an electrode with a tip potential of −5 mV in an extracellular solution typically reduces its tip potential to −3 mV when measured in a comparable intracellular solution; thus, this would introduce an error of 2 mV to the measurement of the resting membrane potential. The change of the tip potential depends on the size of the tip potential itself. Therefore, electrodes with larger tip potentials introduce larger inaccuracies to the measurements. To avoid significant changes of the tip potential under different conditions, only electrodes with tip potentials less than −5 mV should be used. It is recommended that only freshly made electrodes are used, since tip potentials get more negative with storage time. Note that acidification of the filling solution with HCl will reduce the tip potential.

6.2.4 Glass Microelectrodes

Besides employing low noise amplifiers and micromanipulators, the proper fabrication of microelectrodes plays a primary role in the success of such electrophysiologic methodologies. Depending on their application (e.g., intracellular recording, patch clamping, etc.), the shape of the employed microelectrodes differs accordingly. Figure 6.2 summarizes typical electrode shapes used in electrophysiology. As these microelectrodes are fabricated from glass, the melting temperature of the glass is an important property to obtain the desired electrode shape. The electrical properties of the glass are important for low noise recordings. The loss factor, a parameter used by manufacturers to describe the dielectric properties of glass, gives an estimate of the pipette suitability for microelectrodes.

It is important to note that the physical basis of gigaohm seals of patch clamp microelectrodes, at the interface of the glass and the cell membrane, is still not fully understood; several studies have shown that essentially any glass is capable of forming a seal with cell membranes. There is no solid evidence that one glass seals better than another. Yet, as a rough guide, thicker glass walls and a low loss factor are typically better, and additional coating with hydrophobic substances like Dow Corning Sylgard (R) 184 further improves the electrical properties.

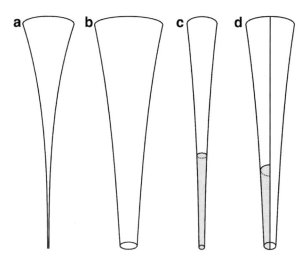

Fig. 6.2 Glass microelectrodes used for electrophysiological recordings: (**a**) sharp microelectrode for intracellular recordings; (**b**) patch clamp electrode used for whole-cell recordings; (**c**) ion-sensitive microelectrode filled with a liquid ion-sensitive membrane (*yellow*); (**d**) double-barreled ion-sensitive microelectrode; one barrel is filled with a liquid ion-sensitive membrane (*yellow*)

6.3 Measurement of Membrane Potentials

6.3.1 Electrophysiological Measurement of Membrane Potentials

Membrane potentials are commonly measured by connecting an intracellularly placed glass microelectrode (Fig. 6.2a) and an extracellular reference electrode to a voltmeter. Such a voltmeter must have a high input resistance to avoid current flow through the electrode. This is accomplished by using a so-called voltage-follower which connects the amplifier to an independent current source that drives the measurement circuit or by using a current clamp amplifier, which uses a feedback circuit which, in turn, reduces the current flowing through the electrode to virtually zero.

The glass microelectrodes used in these cases need to have small diameters (<1 μm) which will reduce damage to the given cell during the impalement process. Further, such electrodes are filled with 3 M KCl, which provides a small resistance and junction potential.[4] If such electrodes have resistances larger than 5–8 MΩ, disturbing effects by tip potentials must be considered.

Typically, to impale a living cell, the microelectrode is first lowered until it touches the cell surface, which is readily visible as a small artifact on a real-time monitor (e.g., oscilloscopes or computers with an A/D converter). Next, the electrode is advanced (forced) into the cell by either simply tapping on the microscope stage or quickly advancing the micromanipulator in the linear direction of the electrode. It is advisable to use a four-axis manipulator for such experiments, with the fourth axis oriented in the linear direction of the microelectrode.

A good cellular impalement is characterized by a rapid and continuous change of the measured potential to a stable value; if not stable, it is likely that the cell membrane was disrupted by the microelectrode tip and that sodium leaked into (and potassium out of) the cell, causing progressive depolarization.

The resting membrane potential is defined as the potential difference between intracellular and extracellular voltage, which is best estimated after the microelectrode has been withdrawn from the cell, to redetermine the baseline potential.

When fast changes of the membrane potential need to be captured (e.g., action potentials), it is important that the recording system has a high response time to follow the signal (i.e., minimal or adjustable high-pass filtering). Typically, one of the main problems arises from different sources of capacitances within a given experimental recording setup; these are primarily electrode and stray capacitances. The electrode capacitance is best reduced by keeping the level of the bath solution low. Stray capacitances can often be reduced by using amplifiers with a driven shield. If necessary, it is possible to compensate remaining capacitances by adjusting a so-called *negative capacitance*, which is an integral component of most commercial amplifiers. Yet, it must be noted that this will increase the noise and might produce oscillations that may cause damage to the cell being investigated. Note that if a second electrode is to be used to stimulate the cells of study, this electrode must be shielded from the recording electrode in order to avoid capacitive artifacts in the recorded potentials.

6.3.2   Fluorescence Techniques for Membrane Potential Measurement

To provide simple high-throughput examinations and/or visualizations of spatial dynamics of membrane potential changes within a single cell or a population of adjacent cells in tissue-like growth cultures, it can be very useful to employ voltage-sensitive fluorescent dyes. Many of these dyes produce either: (1) an electrochromic effect, i.e., the dye spectra are directly altered by voltage; or (2) an electrophoretic effect, i.e., the dye distribution is altered by voltage.[5,6] The relative voltage sensitivities of these dyes range from about 10–43% per 100 mV,[5] the latter for second harmonic generation signals. Using such methodologies, membrane potential changes are usually reported as relative fluorescence changes over a basal value. From these measurements, absolute membrane potentials can be estimated based on reported dye sensitivities and control curves. Recently, it has been shown that imaging using fluorescence resonance energy transfer (FRET) between a mobile voltage-sensing dye and a membrane-bound fluorophore can improve voltage sensitivity and reduce experimental error.[7]

Even though fluorescence techniques are less sensitive for the measurement of membrane potentials, they eliminate the membrane potential disturbances by impaling electrodes and the alteration potentially caused by unphysiological internal solutions. Additionally, using the dye approaches, small cells or cell protrusions (such as neuronal dendrites) can be studied that are especially difficult to patch with electrodes. Yet, one major disadvantage of optical methods that needs special consideration is the calibration of the dyes; this remains challenging and thus leads to difficulties in obtaining absolute values for membrane potentials.

6.4   Membrane Current Measurements

The voltage clamp technique, as developed by Cole and Marmont,[8,9] enables investigators to record currents through ion channels as well as additional electrical properties of excitable cells.

6.4.1   Classical Two-Electrode Voltage Clamp for the Measurement of Macroscopic Currents

In general, voltage clamp methodologies (Fig. 6.3a) allow for measurement of the ion flow across a cell membrane, while the membrane potential can be controlled at any potential by a feedback amplifier. It is of interest to note that Hodgkin and Huxley used this method to develop their ionic theory of membrane excitation,[1] for which they subsequently won the Nobel Prize in Physiology or Medicine in 1963 (along with Sir John Eccles).

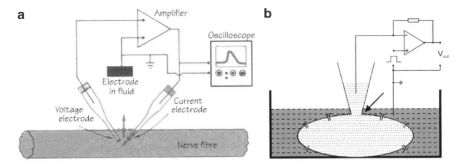

Fig. 6.3 (**a**) Classical two-electrode voltage clamp setup. (**b**) Patch clamp setup for whole-cell recordings

Briefly, the classical two-electrode voltage clamp is performed employing two intracellular "sharp" microelectrodes (Fig. 6.2a). One electrode, the so-called *voltage electrode*, records the voltage (see above), and the other electrode, the *current electrode*, allows one to inject current to adjust the membrane potential. The membrane potentials recorded by the voltage electrode are fed into a feedback amplifier. In other words, this amplifier compares the actual voltages (V_m) with the desired voltages (V_c), e.g., from a signal generator, and injects the appropriate amounts of current through the current electrode to remove the difference between V_m and V_c. The injected current corresponds to the current flowing across the cell membrane. It is important to note that, besides the currents through the membrane, there are currents resulting from capacitive charging, which can be compensated for by proper electronic circuits. Because of its simplicity, this technique is still commonly used, particularly for investigations of oocytes.

It should be noted that in classical voltage clamp experiments, incomplete space clamp distorts the recorded currents, rendering accurate analyses impossible. In general, space clamp is described as one's ability to control the voltage of every area of the cell properly. Insufficient space clamp is difficult to quantify, but there are several known factors that facilitate or impair space clamp. Specifically, the sizes and shapes of the given cells, and especially the relative resistances of the surrounding membranes, are the main determinants for sufficient space clamp.

The fact that the impalement of two electrodes is necessary to perform the above-mentioned recordings limits its application to certain types of preparations, e.g., those which have a minimum spatial extent like oocytes and muscle fibers. It is therefore extremely difficult or impossible to get recordings from small cells.

6.4.2 The Patch Clamp Technique

Several steps of development and improvements of the voltage clamp technique led to the patch clamp technique[10,11] for which Neher and Sakmann won the Nobel

Prize in Physiology or Medicine in 1991. Briefly, the patch clamp technique (Fig. 6.3b) can be considered as a further development of the classical two-electrode voltage clamp. Its main advantage relies on the use of a single electrode instead of two. Both voltage recording and current injection are done by a single glass electrode, yet when doing so there are some important factors that need to be kept in mind. At the same time, such electrodes need to have low resistances and the internal potentials need to be well isolated from bath potentials. Microelectrodes used for patch clamp are pulled from glass with openings considerably larger than the conventional intracellular microelectrodes (0.5–1 μm)(Fig. 6.2b). The formed tips of the pipettes are subsequently fire polished to ensure a smooth glass surface. The pipettes are then filled, in contrast to internal microelectrodes, with physiological saline instead of 3 M KCl. Next, the pipette tip is brought in contact with the cell membrane, then slight suction is applied to the pipette.[2,11] Thereby, a small patch of the cell membrane is sucked into the pipette interior, forming an omega-shaped semi-vesicle. The electrical resistance across the seal is then in the range of 10–100 GΩ, and ideally the membrane is firmly attached to the pipette walls.

The so-called *gigaseal* is the starting point for several variants of the patch clamp technique which will be discussed in more detail elsewhere in this book (see Chapter 16: Electrophysiology of Single Cardiomyocytes: Patch Clamp and Other Recording Methods). As several electrical aspects are important for qualitative patch clamping, Fig. 6.4 represents a scheme of the whole-cell configuration, as this is the most used configuration.[12,13] In the whole-cell configuration, the membrane patch under the pipette is ruptured by the application of slight suction or a voltage pulse, and this then leads to a direct contact between the pipette solution and the cell interior. This electric circuit includes all important electrical components that, in turn, have an impact on the quality of the recordings.

The electrical cell properties can be summarized as a membrane capacitance and resistance that consists of the passive membrane resistance and the conductivity of the incorporated channels. Technical limits allow for only the injection of small currents compared to classical two-electrode voltage clamp methods and, therefore, recordings are considered limited to small cells and/or small currents. The ultimate quality of the recordings is highly dependent on the quality of the formed seal; thus the leak resistance must be as large as possible. In whole cell recordings, the leak current is usually larger compared to the others, as the passive conductivity of the membrane needs to be considered. In this setting, to obtain good voltage clamp, the conductivity between pipette electrode and cell interior must be as high as possible. This conductivity is determined by the series resistance of the pipette and the access resistance of the opening; as the pipette resistance and access resistance are in series to the membrane, if not optimized, then voltage errors will occur. Yet, such voltage errors are often proportional to the current and the resistance, and thus can be compensated by special electrical circuits.

In conclusion, the whole-cell patch clamp mode measures the current through the total cell membrane superimposed with noise. This *macroscopic* current corresponds to the average of many simultaneously conducting channels. Because of the more simple and subsequent fast analyses, it is the configuration that is most frequently used. Also note that primary cultured cells or cell lines are usually preferred, as they

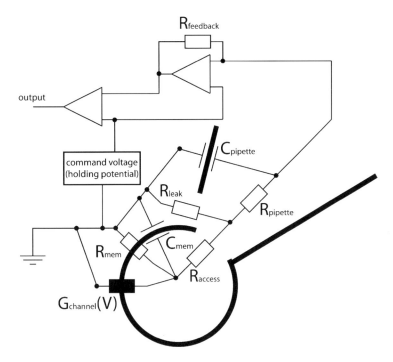

Fig. 6.4 The electric circuit representing the whole-cell patch clamp configuration consists of a set of resistors and capacitors describing the electrical properties of the cells. R_{mem}, the membrane resistance, is determined by nonselective conductances of the cell membrane (e.g., TRP channels); C_{mem}, the capacity of the cell membrane, reflects the size of the cell; $G_{channel}$ represents the voltage dependent conductances of the membrane (e.g., channels); $C_{pipette}$ is the capacity of the patch pipette; $R_{pipette}$ reflects the patch pipette resistance, mainly determined by the opening of the pipette and the containing solution, which describes the properties of the patch pipette; R_{access} is the access resistance that is determined by the size of the patch and the opening of the patch; R_{leak} reflects the quality of the gigaohm seal and the quality of the patch configuration

reveal a relatively clean surface membrane[14] and require no enzymatic treatment that may damage the plasma membranes. Importantly, the patch clamp technique is now the "gold standard" measurement for characterizing and studying ion channels and one of the most important methods applied to in vitro electrophysiology.

6.4.3 High-Throughput Screening for the Pharmaceutical Industry

Although very powerful, the patch clamp technique is generally considered extremely labor intensive and thereby typically limited to a throughput of 10–20 individual cell measurements per day. In an effort to reduce time-consuming single cell measurements, microchip-based patch clamping has been developed more recently. These methodologies are based on positioning a cell on a small hole separated by

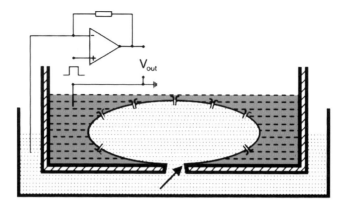

Fig. 6.5 Patch clamp chip and circuit. High-throughput setups consist of multiple units that allow automated parallel recordings. In addition, the arrangement allows scientists to install a second technique, e.g., fluorescence or force microscopy, from the upside of the setup

two isolated fluid chambers, in a manner that requires no manual intervention or micromanipulation (Fig. 6.5). Achieving this experimental goal requires more than just the automation of existing patch clamp techniques; rather, it requires the development of an entirely new paradigm for making electrophysiological measurements. For example, several chip-based devices use a planar patch clamp approach, where microchips are fabricated with apertures that serve as inverted patch electrode tips, allowing parallel processing of many cell recordings simultaneously.[13,15]

In order to perform whole-cell electrophysiological measurements within such a geometry, two criteria must be met: (1) a high-resistance seal must form between the cell membrane and peripheral region of the substrate pore (as in the case of patch clamp electrophysiology, this insures that the current measured between the two electrodes passes through the cell membrane); and (2) in order to be able to control the cell's membrane potential, a low-resistance electrical pathway must form through the cell wall that covers the pore. This latter requirement, in effect, places the associated electrode at the interior of the cell and allows one to clamp the membrane potential over the rest of the cell membrane. Once these criteria have been met, and assuming no manual intervention is required, it is then possible to conceive of a parallel format where many wells can be measured simultaneously. In contrast to standard patch clamp, large efforts need to be made to improve channel expression and to achieve homogeneity of the cell culture.[16]

6.5 Solution and Pharmacology

For electrophysiological measurements employing either patch clamp or other intracellular recording methodologies, Na^+ can be replaced by $NMGD^+$ or choline, K^+ by Cs^+, and Cl^- by aspartate, methanesulfonate or F^-. Yet it is important to note that the composition of the solution has a high impact on the junction potential

Table 6.1 Typical blockers used for specific ion channel block

Channel	Blocker
Voltage-gated K$^+$ channels	TEA$^+$, 4-aminopyridine (4-AP)
Inwardly rectifying K$^+$ channels	Ba^{2+} (at low concentrations)
Na$^+$ channels	Tetrodotoxin (TTX)
Ca^{2+} channels	Nifedipine
Cl$^-$ channels	9-anthracen carbonic acid (9-AC)

which has to be corrected properly (see Chap. 6). Besides very specific ion channel blockers, e.g., toxins from scorpions or spiders, several agents are deployed to block specific channels (Table 6.1).

6.6 Selective Measurements of Ion Activities

To allow for the direct characterization of the ion channels of interest, actual concentrations or activities of ions in the intracellular and extracellular space need to be well controlled. These ionic gradients across the membrane are important for two reasons: (1) the activity of primary and secondary active transporters and of many ion channels depends on the associated ion concentrations (e.g., Na/K-ATPase, Na/Ca-exchanger, inward-rectifying potassium channels); and (2) ionic homeostasis is a prerequisite for long-term cellular stability and function.[17] In such experiments, for example, important applications of ionic control include the monitoring of interstitial K$^+$ concentrations of the beating myocytes or the measurement of intracellular Na$^+$ concentrations, which secondarily affect Ca^{2+} dynamics and/or pH homeostasis.

For experimental approaches which aim to address physiological measurements in biological tissues, glass microelectrodes with liquid ion exchange membranes in their tips are used (Fig. 6.2c). More specifically, this membrane separates a reference electrolyte in the shank of the electrode from the test electrolyte (e.g., the cytoplasm); since the membrane is perm-selective, it only allows the selective ion species to equilibrate. The potential difference that is measured between test and reference solutions corresponds to the Nernst equilibrium potential of that ion.

It is most common that microelectrodes are pulled from borosilicate glass. They must be silanized to render the inner surface lipophilic, since the liquid ion exchange membrane is hydrophobic and must be sealed in the tip of the electrode. Typically, the liquid membrane is composed of an ion exchanger, a solvent, additives, and sometimes a matrix. Additionally, the ion exchanger can be a charged or neutral ion carrier; additives help to improve electrode performance and the matrix, e.g., PVC stabilizes the membrane. Liquid ion exchange membranes are available for most physiological relevant cations (Na$^+$, K$^+$, Mg^{2+}, Ca^{2+}) and some anions (Cl$^-$, HCO$_3^-$).[18] Microelectrodes are backfilled first with the liquid membrane and then with the reference electrolyte. Note that each electrode must be calibrated with solutions of an ionic strength similar to that of the test solution.

The resistances of such electrodes are very large, usually beyond 10^{11} Ω. Therefore, it is necessary to use amplifiers with a very high input resistance, which should be at least 100 times larger than the electrode resistance.[19] Microelectrodes for intracellular measurements have the smallest tip diameters (<1 μm) and the largest electrode resistances; these high resistances reduce ion selectivities.

It is important to note that ion-sensitive microelectrodes not only measure the equilibrium potentials of ions, but also measure the membrane potential. Therefore, it is necessary to correct the results for the actual membrane potential when intracellular ion activities are measured. This can be done by simultaneous impalement of the cell by a conventional microelectrode and the ion-sensitive electrode or by using a double-barreled ion-sensitive microelectrode. Double-barreled microelectrodes (Fig. 6.2d) are most often made from theta-style glass tubing in which a septum separates the tubing in two canals. After pulling such a microelectrode, only one of the canals is to be silanized and used as the ion-sensitive electrode, while the other is filled with an electrolyte and is used to measure the membrane potential.

6.7 Troubleshooting

6.7.1 Low Series Resistances

It is important to note that a patch clamp amplifier is a very sensitive current-to-voltage converter, converting small pipette currents (picoampere to nanoampere) into voltage signals that can be observed with an oscilloscope and/or recorded via a computer. The feedback amplifier compares the pipette voltage with the command voltage and injects current to equilibrate both. The injected current is proportional to the current measured through the pipette and therefore proportional to the current through the channels. Only cells with certain current amplitudes can be used for recordings, because small currents could be influenced by endogenous cell currents and extremely large currents cannot be clamped satisfactorily. Usually, the recordings are performed at a sampling rate of 100 kHz and filtered at 10 kHz using a low-pass Bessel filter.

Figure 6.4 shows a common scheme of the feedback circuit. Note that only recordings with a voltage error less than 2.5 or 5 mV should be considered appropriate for evaluation. In general, commercial patch clamp amplifiers are equipped with additional circuits for capacitive transient cancellation and series resistance compensation.

6.7.2 Avoidance of Ground Loops

For measurements of these low level voltage and current signals, the electrical ground system should have appropriate current-carrying capabilities in order to serve as an adequate zero-voltage level. In electronic circuit theory, a "ground" is usually idealized as an infinite source or sink for charge, i.e., it can absorb an unlimited amount of current without changing its potential. In the case where a ground connection has a significant resistance, the approximation of zero potential is no longer valid, a situation which can create noise in signals. In voltage clamp setups, a special signal ground known as a *technical ground* (or *technical earth*) is often installed to prevent ground loops. This is basically the same thing as an AC power ground, but no appliance ground wires are allowed any connection to it, as they may carry electrical interference. In such recording setups, the experimental cage, the rack, and all equipments should be directly connected to the technical ground with copper cables. Great care should also be taken that no AC-grounded appliances are placed on the racks, as a single AC ground connection to the technical ground will destroy its effectiveness. For particularly demanding applications, the main technical ground may consist of a heavy copper pipe, if necessary fitted by drilling through several concrete floors (an *earth ground*), such that all technical grounds may be connected by the shortest possible path to a grounding rod in the basement. All metal parts near the head-stage must be grounded according to the star grounding method, using the virtual ground input of the amplifier.

6.7.3   Stable Salt Bridges

For such in vitro electrophysiological measurements, a stable reference potential is also essential. Conventional electrodes are made of chlorinated silver wires. Yet, when the bath solution contains a low Cl^- concentration or even no Cl^- at all, the interface becomes non-reversible (polarized), and the electrode potential will drift with time. In order to overcome this problem, efforts have been made to build salt bridges that provide high concentrations of Cl^- interfacing the Ag/AgCl wire and are independent of the Cl^- concentrations in the bath solution. In addition to salt bridges for bath electrodes, efforts are made to build micro salt bridges for pipette electrodes.[20]

6.7.4   Summary

A variety of in vitro electrophysiological techniques have been developed and refined over the last half century to study the membrane properties of excitable cells. Each technique has its specific advantages and methodological requirements, and the proper use of these techniques is important to obtain accurate data. This chapter described some of the features of these methods and their relative applications relative to the study of cardiac myocytes.

References

1. Hodgkin AL, Huxley AF. A quantitative description of membrane current and its application to conduction and excitation in nerve. J Physiol 1952;117:500.
2. Hamill OP, Marty A, Neher E, et al. Improved patch-clamp techniques for high-resolution current recording from cells and cell-free membrane patches. Pflügers Arch 1981;391:85–100.
3. Perram JW, Stiles PJ. On the nature of liquid junction and membrane potentials. Phys Chem Chem Phys 2006;8:4200–13.
4. Ling G, Gerard RW. The normal membrane potential of frog sartorius fibers. J Cell Comp Physiol 1949;34:383–96.
5. Millard AC, Jin L, Wei MD, et al. Sensitivity of second harmonic generation from styryl Dyes to transmembrane potential. Biophys J 2004;86:1169–76.
6. Plasek J, Sigler K. Slow fluorescent indicators of membrane potential: a survey of different approaches to probe response analysis. J Photochem Photobiol B 1996;33:101–24.
7. Gonzalez JE, Tsien RY. Improved indicators of cell membrane potential that use fluorescence resonance energy transfer. Chem Biol 1997;4:269–77.
8. Cole KS. Some physical aspects of bioelectric phenomena. Proc Natl Acad Sci USA 1949; 35:558–66.
9. Marmont G. Studies on the axon membrane; a new method. J Cell Physiol 1949;34:351–82.
10. Neher E, Sakmann B. Single-channel currents recorded from membrane of denervated frog muscle fibres. Nature 1976;260:799–802.
11. Sigworth FJ, Neher E. Single Na^+ channel currents observed in cultured rat muscle cells. Nature 1980;287:447–9.
12. Jurkat-Rott K, Lehmann-Horn F. The patch clamp technique in ion channel research. Curr Pharm Biotechnol 2004;5:387–95.
13. Lehmann-Horn F, Jurkat-Rott K. Nanotechnology for neuronal ion channels. J Neurol Neurosurg Psychiatry 2003;74:1466–75.
14. Le Grimellec C, Lesniewska E, Giocondi MC, et al. Imaging of the surface of living cells by low-force contact-mode atomic force microscopy. Biophys J 1998;75:695–703.
15. Brüggemann A, Stoelzle S, George M, et al. Microchip technology for automated and parallel patch-clamp recording. Small 2006;2:840–6.
16. Milligan CJ, Li J, Sukumar P, et al. Robotic multiwell planar patch-clamp for native and primary mammalian cells. Nat Protoc 2009;4:244–55.
17. Hilgemann DW, Yaradanakul A, Wang Y, et al. Molecular sodium homeostasis in health and disease. J Cardiovasc Electrophysiol 2006;17 Suppl 1:S47–S56.
18. Carlini WG, Bruce RR. Fabrication and implementation of ion-selective microelectrodes. In: Boulton AA, Baker GB, Vanderwolf CH, editors. Neurophysiological Techniques: Basic Methods and Concepts. Clifton, NJ: The Humana Press Inc; 1990.
19. Voipio J, Pasternack M, Macleod K. Ion-sensitive microelectrodes. In: Odgen DC, editor. Microelectrode techniques—The Plymouth Workshop Handbook. 2nd ed. Cambridge: Company of Biologists Limited; 1994.
20. Shao XM, Feldman JL. Micro-agar salt bridge in patch-clamp electrode holder stabilizes electrode potentials. J Neuroscience Methods 2007;159:108–15.

Chapter 7
Cardiac Cellular Electrophysiological Modeling

David P. Nickerson and Peter J. Hunter

Abstract Mathematical models of cardiac cellular electrophysiology have evolved significantly over the last 50 years. Beginning with the initial four ODE models from Noble in 1962, models are now being developed with many tens of differential equations requiring hundreds of parameters and integrating multiple aspects of cellular physiology. Such increases in complexity inevitably result in significant barriers to the use of the models by independent scientists or even application of existing models in novel scenarios. Technologies are being developed which negate these barriers to some extent and provide tools to aid model developers and users in the reuse of previous models. In this chapter, we review some of the common cardiac cellular electrophysiology models and place them in the context of current model description technologies in order to illustrate the current state of the field.

7.1   Modeling Cardiac Cellular Electrophysiology

Detailed reviews of specific cardiac cellular electrophysiology models can be found elsewhere[1-4]; here, we provide a general outline of the field touching on some of the more common models. Integration of these models into tissue and organ cardiac models is discussed in Chap.11: Isolated Tissue Models and Chap.12: Isolated Heart Models. Figure 7.1 provides a summary of the development of modern cardiac cellular electrophysiological models illustrating the common ancestors of the models.

The Hodgkin and Huxley (1952) model is the ancestor model of all modern cardiac electrophysiology models.[5] As experimental techniques develop to provide higher resolution quantification of cellular physiology, modern models are more and more reflecting this basic model with complicated multi-state models of individual protein functions. It is still rare, however, to find a cellular model devoid of any "Hodgkin–Huxley" voltage-dependent gating kinetics.

D.P. Nickerson (✉)
Auckland Bioengineering Institute, The University of Auckland, New Zealand
e-mail: nickerson@auckland.ac.nz

D.C. Sigg et al. (eds.), *Cardiac Electrophysiology Methods and Models*,
DOI 10.1007/978-1-4419-6658-2_7, © Springer Science+Business Media, LLC 2010

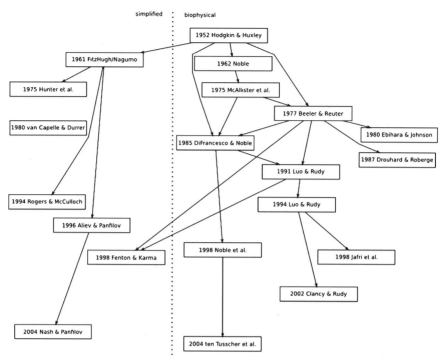

Fig. 7.1 Illustration of the development of cardiac electrophysiological models. While not a cardiac model, Hodgkin and Huxley[5] is included as the common ancestor for the vast majority of models

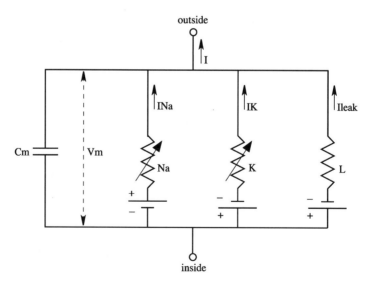

Fig. 7.2 The Hodgkin and Huxley equivalent electrical circuit representing the membrane of an electrically excitable cell with three distinct membrane transport mechanisms

Over the period from 1935 to 1952, Hodgkin and Huxley performed a series of experiments related to the flow of electric current through the surface membrane of a squid giant nerve fiber. These experiments led to the publication of the first biophysically based model of the electrophysiology of a single cell in 1952.[5] This model laid the foundation for much of the electrical modeling of cardiac cells.

In their model, Hodgkin and Huxley presented the idea that the electrical behavior of the axon membrane may be represented by the equivalent electrical circuit shown in Fig. 7.2. This analogy shows that current can be carried through the membrane by charging the membrane capacity or by the movement of ions through resistances in parallel to the capacity.

Hodgkin and Huxley break the membrane current into three components: sodium, potassium, and a leak current (made up of chloride and other ions). Each component current is determined by a driving force conveniently measured as an electrical potential difference and a permeability coefficient which has the dimensions of conductance. Their experiments suggested that the conductance for the sodium and potassium currents was a function of time and membrane potential, while that of the leakage current was constant, as were the equilibrium potentials for all three components of the membrane current. They also observed that changes in membrane permeability were dependent on membrane potential, not membrane current.

Possibly, the most significant contribution of their work was the suggestion that changes in ionic permeability depend on the movement of some component of the membrane which behaved as though it had a large charge or dipole moment. With this suggestion, they also stated that, for such components to exist, it would be necessary to suppose that their density was relatively low and that a number of ions cross the membrane at a single (selective) active patch, i.e., a selective transmembrane ion channel. In their model, Hodgkin and Huxley describe two such components – one sodium sensitive with both activation and inactivation molecules and one potassium sensitive with slower kinetics and no blocking or inactivation molecules.

This model and all the following electrophysiology models make extensive use of an ion's equilibrium, or Nernst, potential. An ion's equilibrium potential is calculated using the Nernst equation, which describes the relationship between the ratio of concentrations of an ion across a membrane and the electrical potential difference across the membrane when the ion is distributed in equilibrium. The Nernst potential for ion X is given by the equation:

$$E_X = \frac{RT}{z_X F} \ln\left(\frac{[X]_o}{[X]_i}\right)$$

where R is the natural gas constant, T is the absolute temperature, z_X is the ion's valence, $[X]_o$ denotes extracellular concentration of the ion, and $[X]_i$ is the intracellular concentration.

Cardiac specific models of cellular electrophysiology are usually divided into two main classifications. The first category is termed *simplified models* as they attempt to replicate certain key features of the electrophysiology without the inclusion of biophysical mechanisms. Key features typically replicated by such models are restitution behavior, propagation, and activation properties. The second category of models includes *biophysically based models*. These models are derived from extensive experimental observations and are designed to model the underlying physiological mechanisms (especially gated ion channels) rather than just reproduce features. Due to inclusion of the physiological detail, these models tend to have much greater predictive power than the simplified models, but that same detail leads to very large (and typically stiff) systems of ordinary differential equations, which is still a limiting factor in the use of this class of model in large-scale models.

7.1.1 Simplified Models of Cardiac Cellular Electrophysiology

FitzHugh[6] and Nagumo et al.[7] independently published a generalization of van der Pol's equation for a relaxation oscillator to provide a simplified unifying concept for the theoretical study of axon physiology. This model has become known as the FitzHugh–Nagumo (FHN) model of nerve membrane. By considering the Hodgkin and Huxley model[5] as one member of a large class of nonlinear systems showing excitable and oscillatory behavior and through the application of phase space methods, FitzHugh reduced the four-state variable Hodgkin and Huxley model to a two-state variable model. This model can be taken as representative of a wide class of nonlinear excitable–oscillatory systems which show threshold and refractory properties as well as oscillations or infinite trains of responses.

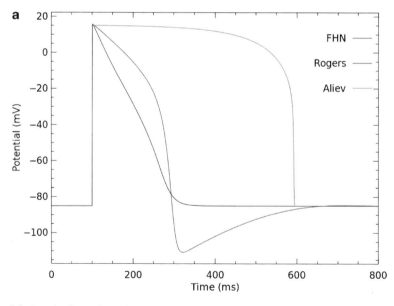

Fig. 7.3 Results from simplified models of cardiac cellular electrophysiology. (**a**) Simulated action potentials from the Rogers and McCulloch[8] and Aliev and Panfilov[9] modified FHN

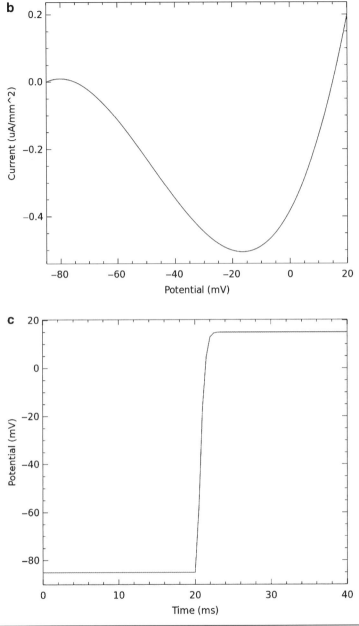

Fig. 7.3 (continued)   models plotted with that from the original FHN model.[6,7] For all models, a stimulus of 400 μA mm⁻³ is applied at 100 ms for 0.5 ms. (**b** and **c**) Results from the simulation of the Hunter et al. cubic polynomial model of activation.[10] The activation is initiated with an applied 1 ms duration stimulus of 100 μA mm⁻³. Complete descriptions of these simulation experiments are available at: http://models.cellml.org/workspace/a1

In 1994, Rogers and McCulloch published a modification of the FHN model designed to make the model more characteristic of cardiac electrical behavior.[8] As shown in Fig. 7.3a, the Rogers and McCulloch modified model removes the hyperpolarization from the refractory part of the action potential.

Aliev and Panfilov proposed another modification of the FHN model which simulates the restitution property of cardiac tissue, adequately represents the shape of the action potential, and can be used efficiently in computer simulations, particularly in whole heart modeling.[9] A simulated action potential is presented in Fig. 7.3a.

Hunter et al.[10] investigated the mathematics of electrical impulse propagation in excitable cells, namely conduction in fibers of uniform geometry. One motivation for this work was to establish a quantitative technique for calculation of conduction velocities in nerve fibers. The model developed by Hunter et al. built on earlier work which assumed that, at a given threshold potential, an instantaneous change in membrane electromotive force occurs, an assumption which is incorrect, as the ionic current was known to be a smooth (even if sometimes steep) function of potential. Thus, Hunter et al. proposed various continuous polynomial functions for the ionic current.[10] Polynomial functions were used as they could be chosen to give very good fits to current–voltage relations found in excitable cells without having to include more than a few powers in the polynomial equation.

Like the earlier discontinuous models, however, the polynomial models still model the ionic current as purely voltage-dependent, whereas in real cells the ionic current is also an independent function of time. Hunter et al. mentioned some contemporary models which include time dependence through the addition of a recovery variable.[10] However, for the purposes of reproducing the conduction process, Hunter et al. stated that this is an unnecessary modification since, at normal temperatures, it is the activation properties that limit conduction. Their third-order polynomial model has become known as the *cubic model of electrical activation* and is used in various studies of electrical propagation in continuum tissue models. Plotting the current–voltage relationship for this model illustrates the cubic nature of this model, as shown in Fig. 7.3b, and the continuous activation of the membrane potential is shown in Fig. 7.3c.

In a study of the role of spatial interaction among excitable elements in the mechanisms underlying cardiac arrhythmia, van Capelle and Durrer developed a simplified membrane electrical activation model.[11] Like the FHN type models, their model consisted of two variables of state – the transmembrane potential (V_m) and a generalized excitability variable (Y). Y can have any value between 0 (maximal excitability) and 1 (complete in-excitability). The state of a "cell" in this model is then completely determined at any time by V_m and Y. In this way, Y is essentially playing the role of the m, h, and n gating variables in the Hodgkin and Huxley kinetics.

While investigating reentry phenomenon in cardiac tissue, Fenton and Karma[12] developed an ionic activation model that retains the minimal ionic complexity necessary to reproduce quantitatively the restitution curves that describe how the pulse duration and its propagation velocity depend on the time interval after repolarization during which the membrane recovers its resting properties. They concentrate on the action potential duration and conduction velocity restitution curves because these dictate the dynamics of the depolarization wavefront and repolarization wave back, as well as the interaction between these two fronts – most important for modeling reentry. When modeling wave dynamics, these two properties are more fundamental quantities than the shape of the action potential.

The model consists of three "ionic" currents: (1) a fast inward current that is responsible for depolarization of the membrane and only depends on one inactivation–reactivation gate; (2) a slow, time-independent, outward current that is responsible for repolarization of the membrane; and (3) a slow inward current activated during the plateau phase of the action potential and only dependent on one inactivation–reactivation gate.

Fenton and Karma[12] chose their model parameters to fit the restitution curves from four sources. Three of the sources were previously published biophysical ventricular cell models: the Beeler and Reuter (BR) model,[13] and modified versions of the Beeler and Reuter (MBR) and Luo and Rudy (MLR-I)[14] models. The modification made to the models was to speed up the calcium dynamics by a factor of 2. The fourth source involved some experimental steady-state curves from optical recordings of membrane potentials on the epicardial surface of the left ventricle of a guinea pig during plane wave pacing at fixed cycle lengths (GP). The results of the model for each version are presented in Fig. 7.4. In Fig. 7.5,the action potential for the BR version of the Fenton and Karma (FK) model is plotted with that from the full Beeler and Reuter ventricular myocyte model.

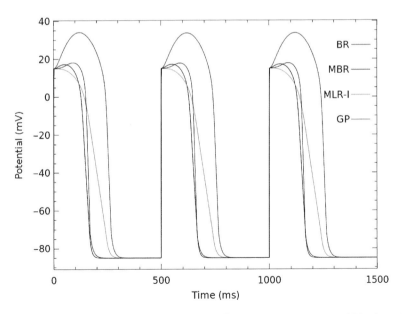

Fig. 7.4 Results from the Fenton and Karma model,[12] for an applied stimulus of 80 µA mm^{-3} at a frequency of 2 Hz with a duration of 1.0 ms. This shows the action potential for each of the four versions of the model – Beeler and Reuter (BR/MBR),[13] Luo and Rudy (MLR-I),[14] and the experimentally derived version (GP). A complete description of these simulation experiments can be found at: http://models.cellml.org/workspace/a1

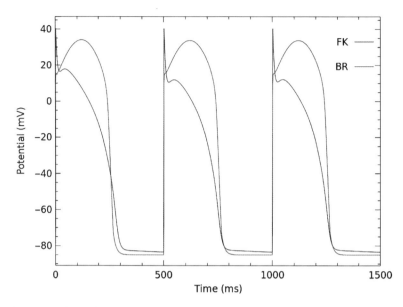

Fig. 7.5 Comparison of the action potentials calculated from the Beeler and Reuter (BR) version of the Fenton and Karma (FK) model and those from the original Beeler and Reuter model,[13] for an applied periodic stimulus current. The results show the ability of the FK model to reproduce the action potential duration of the BR model. A complete description of these simulation experiments can be found at: http://models.cellml.org/workspace/a1

7.1.2 Biophysically Based Models of Cardiac Cellular Electrophysiology

As mentioned previously, these models were largely based on the model of the squid axon by Hodgkin and Huxley.[5] But with ever improving experimental techniques, the models are gradually leaning more and more toward stochastic modeling of populations of individual channels governed by more biochemically oriented models. Differential equations can then be formulated from these stochastic channel population models to give approximations for inclusion into whole cell models.

Following the discovery that there were at least two K^+ conductances in the heart, I_{K1} and I_K (initially known as I_{K2}), Noble developed a model to test whether this combination of K^+ currents plus a Hodgkin and Huxley type Na^+ channel could be used to describe the long-lasting action and pacemaker potentials of the Purkinje fibers of the heart.[15] The sodium current equations in this model are very similar to the Hodgkin and Huxley description,[5] with the curves now fitted to voltage clamp data from Purkinje fiber experiments. The I_{K1} current is assumed to be an instantaneous function of the membrane potential and falls when the membrane is depolarized (a time-independent rectification current). The I_{K2} current slowly rises when the membrane is depolarized, described using Hodgkin and Huxley's potassium current equations,[5] with two main modifications: (1) the maximum value was made

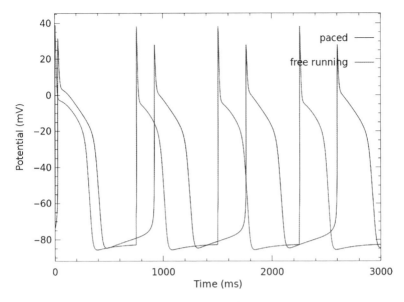

Fig. 7.6 Results from simulating the Noble model.[15] The two traces show the free running pacemaker variant of the model compared with the quiescent variant with an applied periodic stimulus current (paced). A complete description of these simulation experiments can be found at: http://models.cellml.org/workspace/a1

much smaller than in nerve; and (2) the rate constants were divided by 100 in order to take account of the much slower onset of this effect in Purkinje fibers. Results from simulating the model are presented in Fig. 7.6.

With the development of better and more extensive experiments on cardiac membranes, McAllister et al. found that previous cardiac models based on modifications to the Hodgkin and Huxley nerve model were inadequate in important ways.[16] Using the wealth of data then available, McAllister et al. developed a new model of cardiac Purkinje fibers containing many significant advances from the Noble model.[15] The model contains two time-dependent inward currents – a fast sodium current (I_{Na}, similar to that of Hodgkin and Huxley[5]) and a secondary inward current (I_{si}) with slower kinetics that was identified and is partly carried by calcium ions. There is a transient outward chloride current (I_{qr}) activated during strong depolarizations. Finally, instead of the single K+ current of Hodgkin and Huxley[5] and Noble[15] models, McAllister et al. found three distinguishable time-dependent potassium currents (I_{K2}, Ix_1, and Ix_2).[16] None of these potassium currents quantitatively resembled the squid potassium current.

In addition to these currents, McAllister et al. expanded the time-independent leakage current from the Hodgkin and Huxley nerve model into three distinct components, based on the possible ionic composition of the currents.[16] The outward background current is carried mainly by K+ (I_{K1}) and corresponds to the outward membrane current that may be recorded below the I_{x1} and I_{x2} threshold in Na+-free solutions. They also defined an inward background current carried by Na+ which gives the measured resting potential deviation from that of the potassium equilibrium potential (the primary cause of the resting potential value). The third component came from experimental evidence that Cl⁻ contributes to the current flow during the pacemaker and plateau phases of the action potential. While McAllister et al. formulated the three background time-independent currents in terms of specific ions, they noted that there was, at that time, no reliable means to experimentally dissect the total background current[16]; thus their formulation was rather tentative and does not imply that there necessarily exists such distinct membrane channels. Figure 7.7 presents the pacemaker action potentials of the McAllister model.[16]

In 1977, Beeler and Reuter published the first mathematical model of the cardiac ventricular action potential. This model formulated the cardiac ventricular action potential from transmembrane ionic currents using Hodgkin and Huxley type equations,[5] in a similar manner to the model by McAllister et al.[16] for the cardiac Purkinje fiber. The Beeler and Reuter model[13] became the framework for development of later more comprehensive models of cardiac ventricular action potentials and has been used extensively in simulations of action potential propagation in multicellular models of cardiac tissue such as Noble and Rudy.[1]

The model includes four individual components of ionic current. The two inward voltage- and time-dependent currents are the excitatory sodium current (I_{Na}) and a secondary or slow current primarily carried by calcium ions (I_s). For outward currents, there is a time-independent potassium current (I_{K1}) which exhibits inward-going rectification and a voltage- and time-dependent current primarily carried by potassium ions (I_{x1}). Both I_{K1} and I_{x1} were adopted from the McAllister[16] model, while the pacemaker current (I_{K2}) and I_{x2} were dropped as there was no convincing experimental evidence for the presence of these currents in ventricular myocardium.

The fast sodium current (I_{Na}) was adapted from Hodgkin and Huxley[5] with the addition of a slow inactivation gating variable (j) based on experimental evidence that reactivation of I_{Na} was much slower than inactivation. The secondary inward current (I_s) was the main focus of the Beeler and Reuter model[13] and included an initial model of intracellular calcium handling (Fig. 7.8). Results from simulation with this model are presented in Figs. 7.5 and 7.7.

In 1980, Ebihara and Johnson (with corrections later published in Spach and Heidlage[17]) published possibly the first mathematical model focused on a single cardiac transmembrane ionic current – the fast sodium channel (I_{Na}).[18] While previous models had been developed for this current, the lack of experimental data for the kinetics of the channel under physiological conditions led to ad hoc assumptions in such models. The aim of the Ebihara and Johnson model was to provide a quantitative description of the kinetics of the fast sodium channel using voltage clamp data obtained from small spherical clusters of tissue-cultured heart cells.[18] The kinetic data were fit to the Hodgkin and Huxley model[5] to facilitate comparison of the kinetics to those of other studies.

While the model given by Ebihara and Johnson[18] was only for the I_{Na} current, this model can be treated as a direct replacement for I_{Na} in the Beeler and Reuter ventricular myocyte model.[13] Figure 7.7 shows a comparison of the Ebihara and Johnson modified model with the original Beeler and Reuter model.

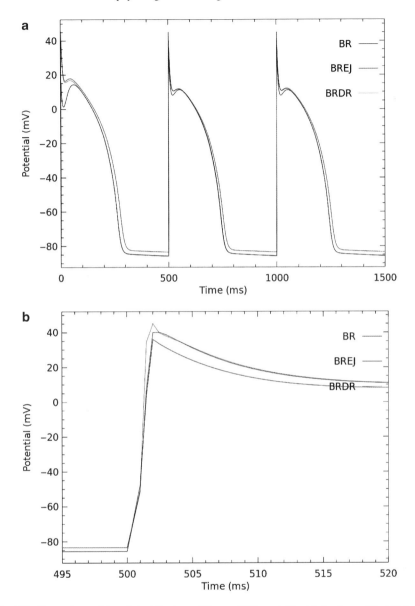

Fig. 7.7 Comparison of the original Beeler and Reuter (BR) model[13] with the I_{Na} modified Ebihara and Johnson (BREJ)[18] and Drouhard and Roberge (BRDR)[19] versions (cf. Fig. 6 of Drouhard and Roberge[19]). The stimuli used follow that specified by Drouhard and Roberge[19] (Table 2) – BR 64.8 μA mm⁻³, BREJ 80 μA mm⁻³, and BRDR 72 μA mm⁻³, all with a 2 ms duration. A complete description of these simulation experiments can be found at: http://models.cellml.org/workspace/a1

Using more recent and extensive voltage clamp data, Drouhard and Roberge[19] further revised the Hodgkin–Huxley formulation of the I_{Na} current for ventricular myocardial cells. They developed the kinetics of the fast sodium channel to represent

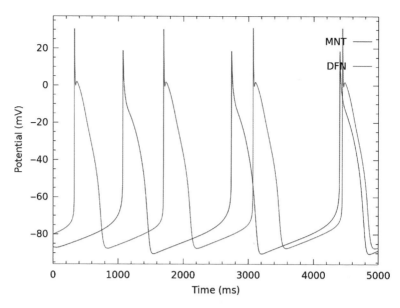

Fig. 7.8 Pacemaker action potentials from the McAllister et al. (MNT)[16] and DiFrancesco and Noble (DFN)[24] models. A complete description of these simulation experiments can be found at: http://models.cellml.org/workspace/a1

a good compromise between available experimental data and to lead to a reasonable average representation of the cardiac Na^+ current.

As with the Ebihara and Johnson model,[18] that of Drouhard and Roberge can be used as a replacement for the fast sodium channel in the original Beeler and Reuter ventricular myocyte model. Figure 7.7 compares this version of the Beeler and Reuter model with the previous Ebihara and Johnson version, as well as the original Beeler and Reuter model.[13] The Drouhard and Roberge modified Beeler and Reuter model[19] was further modified by Skouibine et al.[20] to handle potentials outside the normal physiological range, allowing the model to be used in defibrillation studies.

Making use of the extensive developments in experimental work since the development of the McAllister cardiac Purkinje model[16] (e.g., Fabiato and Fabiato,[21] Colatsky,[22] Gadsby[23]), DiFrancesco and Noble published a new model of cardiac Purkinje fiber electrophysiology[24] – a model which remains the most comprehensive of all Purkinje fiber ionic current models. Some results from model simulations are shown in Fig. 7.8.

This model provided the first description of ion exchangers in a cellular model – the sodium pump (Na^+–K^+ exchange), Na^+–$Ca2^+$ exchanger, and the sarcoplasmic reticulum (SR) calcium pump. The development of this model involved a modeling avalanche (i.e., Noble and Rudy[1]), in which the addition of Na^+–K^+ exchange to match experimental data for K^+ concentrations in the extracellular spaces led to the inclusion of other mechanisms to maintain the intracellular cation balances (Na⁺ and Ca²⁺), since they are all linked via the sodium pump and Na⁺–Ca²⁺ exchanger. In another first, the model also included intracellular events through the incorporation of a model of calcium release from the SR.

In a good example of the model's predictive power, the DiFrancesco and Noble model[24] showed that, in order to maintain a resting intracellular Ca²⁺ concentration below 1 μM, the Na⁺–Ca²⁺ exchanger must operate with a 3:1 (Na⁺:Ca²⁺) stoichiometry rather than the widely accepted (at that time) 2:1. This stoichiometry predicts that there must be a current carried by the Na⁺–Ca²⁺ exchanger and that, if dependent on intracellular calcium, it must be strongly time-dependent. Shortly after the publication of this model, experimental data showing the validity of these predictions was published (Kimura et al.[25]).

However, while the model keeps the resting calcium concentration within physiologically acceptable limits, the peak value reached (~7 μM) is outside those limits. This inaccuracy in the model was corrected in the development of the Hilgemann and Noble atrial cell model[26] and later versions of the Noble model (i.e., Noble et al.[27]) through the inclusion of intracellular calcium buffers.

In 1991, Luo and Rudy reformulated the Beeler and Reuter ventricular myocyte model[13] using new experimental data provided by single cell and single channel recordings. The model included formulations of the fast sodium current (I_{Na}), delayed rectifier potassium current (I_K), and the inward rectifier current (I_{K1}). The plateau potassium

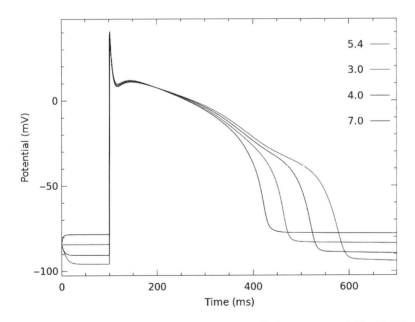

Fig. 7.9 Results from simulations of the Luo and Rudy ventricular myocyte model[14] with different values for extracellular potassium concentration ($[K^+]_o$) – cf. Luo and Rudy[14] (Fig. 4). The legend gives the $[K^+]_o$ values, in mM, used for the simulations. In all the simulations, a stimulus current of 100 μA mm⁻³ is applied with a duration of 1 ms. A complete description of these simulation experiments can be found at: http://models.cellml.org/workspace/a1

current (I_{Kp}) from Yue and Marban[28] was also included in the model. A summary of the results of simulating the Luo and Rudy model[14] is presented in Fig. 7.9.

Following the formulation of Beeler and Reuter, the Luo and Rudy model[14] also takes into account the changes in intracellular calcium concentration ($[Ca^{2+}]i$). The Luo and Rudy model, however, also incorporates the possibility of changing extracellular potassium concentration ($[K^+]_o$), an important factor in ischemic tissue. The action potential simulations of this model duplicate the experimentally observed effects of changes in $[K^+]_o$ on action potential duration and resting potential (Fig. 7.9).

Continuing the development of the Luo and Rudy cardiac ventricular action potential model,[14] Luo and Rudy introduced processes that control the dynamically changing concentrations of intracellular ions (Ca^{2+}, Na^+, and K^+) and their effects on transmembrane currents.[29] The model also included cell compartmentalization (myoplasm and junctional and network SR) and models the Ca^{2+} concentration in each of the three compartments with an initial model of calcium-induced calcium release from the junctional SR. Buffering of Ca^{2+} in the myoplasm (by calmodulin and troponin) and in the junctional SR (by calsequestrin) was also incorporated into the model. Some summary results from this model are presented in Fig. 7.10.

Due to the extent to which the membrane current formulations and model predictions have been validated against experimental data, the Luo and Rudy model[29] has become the most widely used model of cardiac ventricular myocyte

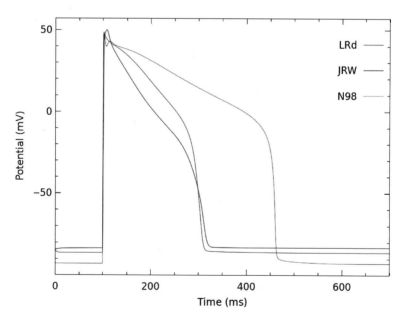

Fig. 7.10 Results from simulations with the Luo and Rudy (LRd),[29] Jafri et al. (JRW),[34] and Nobel et al. (N98)[27] ventricular myocyte models. A stimulus current of 250 μA mm⁻³ is applied with a duration of 1 ms for the Jafri et al.[34] and Noble et al.[27] models, and 100 μA mm⁻³ for the Luo and Rudy[29] model. A complete description of these simulation experiments can be found at: http://models.cellml.org/workspace/a1

electrophysiology.[30] While the model was originally formulated from guinea pig data, it has since been fitted to several species. Due to its prolific use, the base Luo and Rudy action potential model[29] has been, and continues to be, developed to remain consistent with accepted experimental data as it becomes available. Some of the advances in the model by Rudy and colleagues are described below.

Zeng et al.[31] split the delayed rectifier current (I_K) into two components – I_{Kr} (rapid) and I_{Ks} (slow), and added the T-type calcium channel $(I_{Ca(T)})$. I_{Kr} incorporated a $[K^+]_o$-dependent conductance, and the I_{Ks} conductance was $[Ca^{2+}]_i$-dependent. Viswanathan et al.[32] refined I_{Ks} with the addition of a second gating variable and reformulated the channel conductance and its $[Ca^{2+}]_i$ dependence. This version of the model also included a reformulation of the calcium-induced calcium release process to provide a graded response for even a small entry of Ca^{2+} into the cell. The Viswanathan et al. model[32] provided formulations for three different cell types (epi-, mid-, and endocardial cells) by scaling the I_{Ks} current to represent the differing density of these channels through the ventricular wall.

Faber and Rudy[33] studied the effect on the action potential and contraction with changes caused by intracellular sodium overload. This required several modifications to the previous version of the Luo and Rudy model. Calcium-induced calcium release was once again reformulated to give graded release without threshold, and calcium uptake into the network SR was increased. The $Na^+–K^+$ exchanger current (I_{NaK}) was increased and I_{NaCa} was also reformulated. For the case when the cell was experiencing sodium overload, a Na^+-activated K^+ channel was introduced.

The continual reformulation of the calcium-induced calcium release process used in the various Luo and Rudy models is related to the focus of these models being on whole cell electrophysiology rather than on biophysical details of the mechanisms involved in calcium handling. This allows for the best use of computational and numerical resources in modeling the electrophysiology at the cost of excluding possible effects of detailed calcium models.

The Jafri, Rice, and Winslow model[34] addresses this through the addition of a biophysically detailed calcium subsystem to the Luo and Rudy model.[29] In the Jafri et al. model, several modifications and additions are made:

- the L-type Ca^{2+} current is replaced with a new formulation based on the mode-switching Markov-state model of Imredy and Yue[35];
- the SR calcium release mechanism is replaced with the Markov-state model of ryanodine receptor Ca^{2+} release channels in the junctional SR membrane[36];
- ryanodine receptors and L-type Ca^{2+} channels are assumed to be empty in a restricted subspace located between the junctional SR and T-tubules;
- both high- and low-affinity Ca^{2+} binding sites for troponin are included; and
- the magnitudes of the I_{Kp}, I_{Na}, I_{NaCa}, $I_{ns(Ca)}$, and $I_{Ca,b}$ currents are scaled to preserve myoplasmic ionic concentrations and action potential shape.

Figure 7.10 provides a comparison of the action potentials between the original Luo and Rudy model[29] and the Jafri et al. model.[34]

When investigating excitation–contraction coupling, many of the phenomena of interest depend on the interval between stimuli and, hence, evolve over the time course of multiple action potentials. These phenomena are known as interval–force relations. Due to force generation in a myocyte being roughly proportional to intracellular Ca^{2+} concentration and the inclusion of a detailed calcium subsystem in their model, Jafri et al.[34] were able to investigate the effects of pacing rate on force generation. One of the simulations Jafri et al. presented examined the transition period between increasing and decreasing pacing frequency of the model. This simulation illustrated the extended range of applicability of the Jafri model over the Luo and Rudy model[29] by producing results comparable to those seen experimentally. The model also allowed a prediction to be made as to the mechanisms involved in producing the experimentally observed phenomena.

The Noble et al. guinea pig ventricular cell electrophysiology model[27] is an extension and update of the earlier Noble, Noble, Bett, Earm, Ho and So ventricular model[37] built from the initial Purkinje fiber (e.g., Noble,[15] McAllister et al.,[16] DiFrancesco and Noble[24]) and atrial (e.g., Hilgemann and Noble[26] and Earm and Noble[38]) cellular models.

This version of the Nobel model includes a dyadic space between the sarcolemma and junctional SR, equivalent to the restricted subspace of the Jafri et al. model.[34] In the Noble et al. model,[27] the L-type Ca^{2+} channels (or at least a large fraction of them) in the dyadic space are empty and the concentration of Ca^{2+} in the diadic space is used both to initiate calcium-induced calcium release from the SR and to terminate the L-type Ca^{2+} current ($I_{Ca(L)}$). Unlike the Jafri et al. model,[34] however, the Noble et al. model[27] assumes that activation of SR calcium release sites by the diadic space Ca^{2+} triggers the release into the bulk myoplasm.

In addition to the diadic space, the Noble et al. model[27] splits the delayed potassium current (I_K) into a rapidly activating component (I_{Kr}) and a slowly activating component (I_{Ks}). The rapidly activating component is divided into two further components: I_{Kr1} for the fast deactivation component and I_{Kr2} for the slow component. The slow component of the deactivation, I_{Kr2}, is slower than the deactivation rate of I_{Ks}.

The Noble et al. model[27] also includes mechanisms for cellular contraction and tension generation, stretch- and tension-dependent processes, and drug–receptor interactions. For the case of normal healthy myocytes, these processes have little or no effect on the bulk cellular electrophysiology. Some simulation results from this model are given in Fig. 7.10 for comparison with the Jafri et al.[34] and Luo and Rudy[29] models.

With the exception of the Jafri et al. model[34], the above biophysical models were formulated using the traditional Hodgkin and Huxley scheme,[5] i.e., the whole cell action potential is simulated from macroscopic descriptions of transmembrane currents generated by a large ensemble of ion channels. More recently, a large body of knowledge has been accumulated on the relationships between ion channel structure and function, on the kinetic properties of single ion channels, and on the modification of ion channel structure and function by genetic defects. Most of these data were obtained in expression systems (e.g., Xenopus oocyte), away from the actual physiological environment where the channel interacts with other types of channels and the dynamically changing ionic composition of its environment. Thus, a major challenge is the integration of this single channel information into the functioning cardiac cell in an effort to mechanistically relate molecular level findings to whole cell function (Noble and Rudy[1]).

Jafri et al.[34] used such information in the formulation of their calcium subsystem model for normal guinea pig ventricular myocytes. Clancy and Rudy[39] presented the first application of such molecular level data to the formulation of a state-specific Markov model of the cardiac sodium channel (I_{Na}). They formulated models for wild-type sodium channels and ΔKPQ mutant channels, a three amino-acid deletion that affects the channel inactivation and is associated with a congenital form of the long-QT syndrome, LQT3. The Clancy and Rudy study[39] showed how a genetic defect in a single type of ion channel could be incorporated into a whole cell model of electrophysiology.

The model of Clancy and Rudy[39] was then extended to include models of wild-type and mutant I_{Kr} channels, again using a Markovian state-based model (Clancy and Rudy[40]). This model was used to investigate the effect of HERG (the major subunit of the rapidly activating component of the cardiac delayed rectifier, I_{Kr}) mutations on the action potential and to provide insight into the mechanism by which each defect results in a net loss of repolarizing current and prolongation of the action potential duration.

In an excellent example of the usefulness of computational approaches in establishing a mechanistic link between genetic defects and functional abnormalities, Clancy and Rudy[41] performed simulations showing that a single sodium channel mutation can cause both LQT and Brugada syndromes. Coexistence of these two syndromes seems paradoxical, with LQT associated with enhanced sodium channel function, while Brugada is associated with reduced function. Clancy and Rudy[41] demonstrated in their study that the 1795insD mutation (1795insD results from the insertion of aspartic acid in the C terminus of SCN5A, the cardiac sodium channel gene) of the sodium channel can cause both LQT and Brugada syndromes through interaction with the heterogeneous myocardium in a rate-dependent manner. This result highlights the complexity and multiplicity of genotype–phenotype relationships.

Clancy and Rudy[41] conducted simulations of isolated epicardial, endocardial, and midmyocardial (M) cells using a model based on the Clancy and Rudy[40] modified version of the Luo and Rudy[29] ventricular cell model. The three cell types are defined by varying the maximum conductance of the slowly activating delayed rectifier current, I_{Ks}, as described by Viswanathan et al.[32] A transient outward current (I_{to}) was also added to the model with varying maximal conductances in the three cell types. The previous Markov formulation of I_{Na} from Clancy and Rudy[39] was extended to incorporate new experimental observations and to better represent various states in both the wild-type and mutant models (see Clancy and Rudy for the full models[41]).

In an attempt to move to a more clinically applicable cellular model, ten Tusscher et al. presented a modification of the Noble et al. model[27] suitable for use in simulations of electrical activation and propagation in human tissue.[42] Being designed for tissue and organ simulations requires that the model is computationally efficient while still being able to represent the underlying electrophysiology.

Most of the major ionic currents in the model (fast Na^+, L-type Ca^{2+}, transient outward, rapid delayed rectifier, slow delayed rectifier, and inward rectifier) are based on recent experimental data. The model includes a simple representation of intracellular Ca^{2+} dynamics with the removal of a separate diadic subspace and using a simplified buffering approximation in the cytosol and SR. This added a low computational cost to the model while allowing the realistic modeling of key experimental observations.

In their study, ten Tusscher et al.[42] compared their model to those of Priebe and Beuckelmann[43] and Courtemanche et al.[44] The Priebe and Beuckelmann model[43] was the only existing human ventricular model at that time and consists of a modified Luo and Rudy model[29] based partly on human data, and the Courtemanche et al. model[44] is an atrial model. Through the inclusion of much more recent and detailed experimental data from human studies, ten Tusscher et al. demonstrated the enhanced applicability of their model.[42]

The ten Tusscher et al. model[42] provides slight parameter and equation variations to model differences in epicardial, endocardial, and M cell types. Figure 7.11 presents results obtained from the model highlighting the differences between the three cell types described in the model.

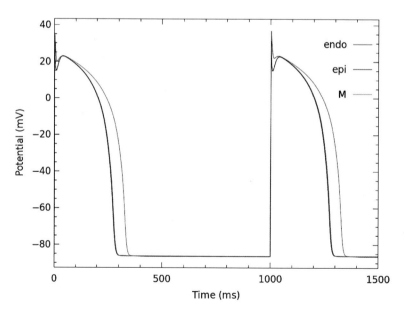

Fig. 7.11 Transmembrane action potentials for the three cell type variants of the ten Tusscher et al. human ventricular model.[42] A complete description of these simulation experiments can be found at: http://models.cellml.org/workspace/a1

7.2 Model Description

All of the models described in Sect. 7.1 were primarily made available to the scientific community as textural descriptions appearing in scientific journals, i.e., journal articles. These original articles may include: a listing of mathematical equations of which the model consists; various parameter sets and boundary conditions which reproduce the various simulation experiments presented in the article; plots illustrating certain outcomes from the simulation experiments; descriptions of the various numerical methods and algorithms used; descriptions of model changes required for specific outcomes, etc. In order to perform simulation experiments with, or based on, these original models, modelers must first translate the textural description into a computable format. This is traditionally a time-consuming and error-prone process. CellML is a model encoding format developed to alleviate this process and to address issues of model reuse and exchange.[45]

For example, each of the plots presented in Sect. 7.1 was generated directly from comprehensive descriptions of the various simulation experiments based on CellML. The original textural descriptions of each model have been encoded into CellML models.[46,47] These CellML-encoded models provide a machine readable and unambiguous description of the underlying mathematical models. The mathematical models were then annotated with comprehensive descriptions of each of the simulation experiments presented in Sect. 7.1.[48-50] Each result in Sect. 7.1 provides a link to the corresponding comprehensive description.

The integration of these comprehensive descriptions with the CellML model repository[51] provides an extremely powerful dissemination and reuse technology. Modelers wishing to make use of any of the models presented in Sect. 7.1 can directly access and reuse the models in the repository. As these model descriptions are further validated, tested, and curated, models developed from this collection will benefit from any corrections and improvements.

As mentioned above, each of the result figures in Sect. 7.1 specifies a link to an online and web browsable description. This comprehensive description defines the specific simulation experiment presented in the figure, including references to the underlying mathematical model(s). By providing such a comprehensive description of both the mathematical models and their application to specific simulations, modelers are provided with a large pool of information on which to base their decisions to reuse, modify, or replace any part of the models. As model annotation becomes more detailed[52] and tools which utilize this information are developed,[53] intelligent reasoning methods will be used to provide a high level interface by which modelers can interact with model collections such as the one accompanying this chapter.

7.2.1 Worked Examples

Nickerson and Buist provide a comprehensive example of the application of CellML-based methods and technology to a detailed model of a human ventricular myocyte model.[46] In that work, the ten Tusscher et al. human ventricular myocyte model[42] is extended through the addition of various mechanisms or the alteration of the kinetics of existing mechanisms in the model. Wimalaratne et al.[47] and Cooling et al.[54] provide further examples of the description of assembling models from modular building blocks. As all of these examples demonstrate, the form of the mathematical model description influences its ability to be reused. The following examples, taken from Sect. 7.1 above, illustrate this point as well as demonstrate the advantages of the model description approach described above.

7.2.1.1 One Model, Multiple Parameter Sets

The most applicable level of abstraction when describing a mathematical model of cellular electrophysiology is the separation of the mathematical model from any specific parameter set. Such separation allows the reuse of the mathematical model with many different parameter sets without needing to alter the mathematical model description itself. In this situation, the mathematical model is encapsulated behind an interface (Fig. 7.12a). The interface defines all the required parameters and boundary conditions and may also provide access to variables computed within the model (the current from a membrane transporter, for example). The model interface can be annotated in order to completely define the requirements of the required parameterization and provided outputs.

Most of the models described in Sect. 7.1 utilize this approach in order to separate the application of an electrical stimulus protocol from the model formulation. This allows for the rapid application of different protocols to the same model. Standard protocols can then be defined once and applied to a range of models (see http://models.cellml.org/workspace/a1 for example).

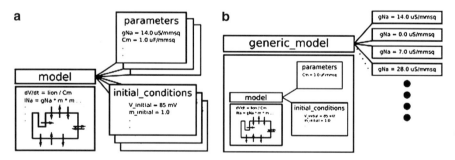

Fig. 7.12 (a) Illustration of the encapsulation of a mathematical model beneath an interface which defines the model's parameterization. The complexity of the model is "hidden" beneath the model interface and all external information must refer only to the model interface. (b) Specialization of the concept for the case when a limited subset of parameters are varying (the *gNa* parameter in this example). The generic model defines all required parameters and initial conditions except the *gNa* parameter which is defined externally for a range of values. See Nickerson and Buist for complete details[46]

This approach can be further refined in some circumstances whereby a subset of the complete parameter set is known a priori to vary. The Fenton and Karma model presented in Fig. 7.4 is such an example.[12] In this approach, the model is encapsulated as described above and then utilized in the definition of a generic simulation experiment. The generic experiment defines the stimulation protocol and the bulk of the model's parameterization. Then the generic experiment is reused in each of the Fenton and Karma variants which simply define the parameters specific to that variant (Fig. 7.12b).[12]

7.2.1.2   Model Evolution

As described in Sect. 7.1.2, the models of Ebihara and Johnson[18] and Drouhard and Roberge[19] describe refinements of the fast sodium current as defined in the Beeler and Reuter cellular model.[13] Using the model description framework described above, it is a straight forward process to substitute the Beeler and Reuter[13] sodium channel with either of the improved versions of the current. Figure 7.7 provides the observed outcome when this is done.

An extension to this example is the addition of new mechanisms to an existing model, which is described in detail in Nickerson and Buist.[46] While that article describes only the addition of electrophysiological mechanisms, the approach extends to other types of mechanisms, for example, the coupling of a cellular mechanics model to a detailed calcium dynamics model or the addition of mitochondrial dynamics to a cellular electrophysiological model.[55]

7.3   Conclusions

We have surveyed the development of cardiac cellular electrophysiology models originating with the Hodgkin and Huxley model[5] and evolving through the early Noble Purkinje fiber remodels and more recent Noble and Rudy ventricular myocyte models. Due to the increasing complexity of the models, we discussed the use of CellML to alleviate some common problems that arise in their implementation and application. The advantages for model robustness and reuse provided by the CellML model repository were also discussed.

As the amount of biophysical detail represented in these cellular models continues to increase, the technical overhead required to support and develop these models similarly rises. Tracking the provenance of model parameters, for example, is particularly problematic.[56] Adoption of the model description framework discussed in Sect. 7.2 provides the technology to unambiguously define and track all aspects of model provenance. Justification of model parameter choices, for example, can be linked directly to experimental data or extracted from a validated and curated parameter database.

The focus of this chapter is modeling of cardiac cellular electrophysiology. However, it is well known that the electrophysiology is just one of many constituent functional components in a living cell. In reflection of this, models integrating several of these functional components are being developed. Such integrated models can be used in studies investigating, for example, the effects of beta-adrenergic signaling[57,58] or the regulation of mitochondrial energetics[59] on cardiomyocyte function. The process of integrating these various functional units into a single model is significantly improved when utilizing the model description framework presented above. In particular, the modular nature of CellML lends itself to this type of model development.[46,47]

References

1. Noble D, Rudy Y. Models of cardiac ventricular action potentials: iterative interaction between experiment and simulation. Phil Trans R Soc Lond A 2001;359:1127–42.
2. Nickerson DP, Hunter PJ. The Noble cardiac ventricular electrophysiology models in CellML. Prog Biophys Mol Biol 2006;90:346–59. URL: http://dx.doi.org/10.1016/j.pbiomolbio. 2005.05.007.
3. Rudy Y, Silva JR. Computational biology in the study of cardiac ion channels and cell electrophysiology. Q Rev Biophys 2006;39:57–116. URL: http://dx.doi.org/10.1017/S0033583506004227.
4. ten Tusscher KHWJ, Bernus O, Hren R, et al. Comparison of electrophysiological models for human ventricular cells and tissues. Prog Biophys Mol Biol 2006;90:326–45. URL: http:// dx.doi.org/10.1016/j.pbiomolbio.2005.05.015.
5. Hodgkin AL, Huxley AF. A quantitative description of membrane current and its application to conductance and excitation in nerve. J Physiol 1952;117:500–44.
6. FitzHugh R. Impulses and physiological states in theoretical models of nerve membrane. Biophys J 1961;1:445–66.
7. Nagumo J, Animoto S, Yoshizawa S. An active pulse transmission line simulating nerve axon. Proc Inst Radio Engineers 1962;50:2061–70.
8. Rogers JM, McCulloch A. A collocation-Galerkin finite element model of cardiac action potential propagation. IEEE Trans Biomed Eng 1994;41:743–57.
9. Aliev RR, Panfilov AV. A simple two-variable model of cardiac excitation, Chaos Solitons Fractals 1996;7:293–301.
10. Hunter PJ, McNaughton PA, Noble D. Analytical models of propagation in excitable cells. Prog Biophys Molec Biol 1975;30:99–144.
11. van Capelle FJL, Durrer D. Computer simulation of arrhythmias in a network of coupled excitable elements. Circ Res 1980;47:454–66.
12. Fenton F, Karma A. Vortex dynamics in three-dimensional continuous myocardium with fiber rotation: filament instability and fibrillation. Chaos 1998;8:20–47.
13. Beeler GW, Reuter H. Reconstruction of the action potential of ventricular myocardial fibres. J Physiol 1977;268:177–210.
14. Luo CH, Rudy Y. A model of the ventricular cardiac action potential. Depolarisation, repolarisation, and their interaction. Circ Res 1991;68:1501–26.
15. Noble D. A modification of the Hodgkin-Huxley equation applicable to Purkinje fibre action and pacemaker potentials. J Physiol 1962;160:317–52.
16. McAllister RE, Noble D, Tsien RW. Reconstruction of the electrical activity of cardiac Purkinje fibres. J Physiol 1975;251:1–59.
17. Spach MS, Heidlage JF. A multidimensional model of cellular effects on the spread of electronic currents and on propagating action potentials. In: Pilkington TC, Loftis B, Thompson JF, Woo SLY, Palmer TC, Budinger TF, editors. High-performance computing in biomedical research. Boca Raton, FL: CRC Press Inc., 1993; p. 289–317.

18. Ebihara L, Johnson EA. Fast sodium current in cardiac muscle. A quantitative description. Biophys J 1980;32:779–90.
19. Drouhard JP, Roberge FA. Revised formulation of the Hodgkin-Huxley representation of the sodium current in cardiac cells. Comput Biomed Res 1987;20:333–50.
20. Skouibine KB, Trayanova NA, Moore PK. A numerically efficient model for simulation of defibrillation in an active bidomain sheet of myocardium. Math Biosci 2000;166:85–100.
21. Fabiato A, Fabiato F. Contractions induced by a calcium-triggered release of calcium from the sarcoplasmic reticulum of single skinned cardiac cells. J Physiol Lond 1975;249:469–95.
22. Colatsky TJ. Voltage clamp measurement of sodium channel properties in rabbit cardiac Purkinje fibre. J Physiol Lond 1980;305:215–34.
23. Gadsby DC. Activation of electrogenic Na+/K+ exchange by extracellular K+ in canine cardiac Purkinje fibers. Proc Natl Acad Sci USA 1980;77:4035–9.
24. DiFrancesco D. Noble D. A model of cardiac electrical activity incorporating ionic pumps and concentration changes. Phil Trans R Soc Lond B 1985;307:353–98.
25. Kimura J, Noma A, Irisawa H. Na–Ca exchange current in mammalian heart cells. Nature 1986;319:596–7.
26. Hilgemann DW, Noble D. Excitation-contraction coupling and extracellular calcium transients in rabbit atrium: reconstruction of basic cellular mechanisms. Proc R Soc Lond B 1987;230:163–205.
27. Noble D, Varghese A, Kohl P, et al. Improved guinea-pig ventricular cell model incorporating a diadic space, i_{Kr} and i_{Ks}, length- and tension-dependent processes. Can J Cardiol 1998; 14:123–34.
28. Yue DT, Marban E. A novel cardiac potassium channel that is active and conductive at depolarized potentials. Pflueg Arch 1988;413:127–33.
29. Luo CH, Rudy Y. A dynamic model of the cardiac ventricular action potential. I. Simulations of ionic currents and concentration changes. Circ Res 1994;74:1071–96.
30. Winslow RL, Scollan DF, Holmes A, et al. Electrophysiological modeling of cardiac ventricular function: from cell to organ. Annu Rev Biomed Eng 2000;2:119–55.
31. Zeng J, Laurita KR, Rosenbaum DS, et al. Two components of the delayed rectifier k+ current in ventricular myocytes of the guinea pig type: theoretical formulation and their role in repolarization. Circ Res 1995;77:140–52.
32. Viswanathan PC, Shaw RM, Rudy Y. Effects of i_{Kr} and i_{Ks} heterogeneity on action potential duration and its rate dependence. Circulation 1999;99:2466–74.
33. Faber GM, Rudy Y. Action potential and contractility changes in $[Na^+]_i$ overloaded cardiac myocytes: a simulation study. Biophys J 2000;78:2392–404.
34. Jafri MS, Rice JJ, Winslow RL. Cardiac Ca^{2+} dynamics: the role of ryanodine receptor adaptation and sarcoplasmic reticulum load. Biophys J 1998;74:1149–68.
35. Imredy JP, Yue DT. Mechanism of Ca^{2+}-sensitive inactivation of L-type Ca^{2+} channels. Neuron 1994;12:1301–18.
36. Keizer J, Levine L. Ryanodine receptor adaptation and Ca^{2+}-induced Ca^{2+} release-dependent Ca^{2+} oscillations. Biophys J 1996;71:3477–87.
37. Noble D, Noble SJ, Bett GCL, et al. The role of sodium–calcium exchange during the cardiac action potential. Ann NY Acad Sci 1991;639:334–53.
38. Earm YE, Noble D. A model of the single atrial cell: relation between calcium current and calcium release. Proc R Soc Lond B 1990;240:83–96.
39. Clancy CE, Rudy Y. Linking a genetic defect to its cellular phenotype in a cardiac arrhythmia. Nature 1999;400:566–9.
40. Clancy CE, Rudy Y. Cellular consequences of HERG mutations in the long QT syndrome: precursors to sudden cardiac death. Cardiovasc Res 2001;50:301–13.
41. Clancy CE, Rudy Y. Na+ channel mutation that causes both Brugada and long-QT syndrome phenotypes: a simulation study of mechanism, Circulation 2002;105:1208–13.
42. ten Tusscher KHWJ, Noble D, Noble PJ, et al. A model for human ventricular tissue. Am J Physiol Heart Circ Physiol 2004;286:H1573–89. URL: http://dx.doi.org/10.1152/ajpheart.00794.2003.
43. Priebe L, Beuckelmann DJ. Simulation study of cellular electric properties in heart failure. Circ Res 1998;82:1206–23.

44. Courtemanche M, Ramirez RJ, Nattel S. Ionic mechanisms underlying human atrial action potential properties: insights from a mathematical model. Am J Physiol Heart Circ Physiol 1998;275:H301–21.

45. Cuellar AA, Lloyd CM, Nielsen PF, et al. An overview of CellML 1.1, a biological model description language. Simulation 2003;79:740–7.

46. Nickerson D, Buist M. Practical application of CellML 1.1: the integration of new mechanisms into a human ventricular myocyte model. Prog Biophys Mol Biol 2008;98:38–51. URL: http://dx.doi.org/10.1016/j.pbiomolbio.2008.05.006.

47. Wimalaratne SM, Halstead MDB, Lloyd CM, et al. Facilitating modularity and reuse: guidelines for structuring cellml 1.1 models by isolating common biophysical concepts. Exp Physiol 2009;94:472–85. URL: http://dx.doi.org/10.1113/expphysiol.2008.045161.

48. Nickerson DP, Corrias A, Buist ML. Reference descriptions of cellular electrophysiology models. Bioinformatics 2008;24:1112–4. URL: http://dx.doi.org/10.1093/bioinformatics/btn080.

49. Nickerson D, Buist M. Interactive reference descriptions of cellular electrophysiology models. Conf Proc IEEE Eng Med Biol Soc 2008;2008:2427–30. URL: http://dx.doi.org/10.1109/IEMBS.2008.4649689.

50. Nickerson DP, Buist ML. A physiome standards-based model publication paradigm. Philos Transact A Math Phys Eng Sci 2009;367:1823–44. URL: http://dx.doi.org/10.1098/rsta.2008.0296.

51. Lloyd CM, Lawson JR, Hunter PJ, et al. The cellml model repository. Bioinformatics 2008;24:2122–3. URL: http://dx.doi.org/10.1093/bioinformatics/btn390.

52. Beard DA, Britten R, Cooling MT, et al. Cellml metadata standards, associated tools and repositories. Philos Transact A Math Phys Eng Sci 2009;67:1845–67. URL: http://dx.doi.org/10.1098/rsta.2008.0310.

53. Garny A, Nickerson DP, Cooper J, et al. Cellml and associated tools and techniques. Philos Transact A Math Phys Eng Sci 2008;366:3017–43. URL: http://dx.doi.org/10.1098/rsta.2008.0094.

54. Cooling MT, Hunter P, Crampin EJ. Modelling biological modularity with cellml. IET Syst Biol 2008;2:73–9. URL: http://dx.doi.org/10.1049/iet-syb:20070020.

55. Terkildsen JR, Niederer S, Crampin EJ, et al. Using physiome standards to couple cellular functions for rat cardiac excitation–contraction. Exp Physiol 2008;93:919–29. URL: http://dx.doi.org/10.1113/expphysiol.2007.041871.

56. Niederer SA, Fink M, Noble, D, et al. A meta-analysis of cardiac electrophysiology computational models. Exp Physiol 2009;94:486–95. URL: http://dx.doi.org/10.1113/expphysiol.2008.044610.

57. Saucerman JJ, Brunton LL, Michailova AP, et al. Modeling beta-adrenergic control of cardiac myocyte contractility in silico. J Biol Chem 2003;278:47997–8003. URL: http://dx.doi.org/10.1074/jbc.M308362200.

58. Saucerman JJ, McCulloch AD. Cardiac beta-adrenergic signaling: from subcellular microdomains to heart failure. Ann NY Acad Sci 2006;1080:348–61. URL: http://dx.doi.org/10.1196/annals.1380.026.

59. Cortassa S, O'Rourke B, Winslow RL, Aon MA. Control and regulation of mitochondrial energetics in an integrated model of cardiomyocyte function. Biophys J 2009;96:2466–78. URL: http://dx.doi.org/10.1016/j.bpj.2008.12.3893.

Chapter 8
Computer Modeling of Electrical Activation: From Cellular Dynamics to the Whole Heart

Bruce H. Smaill and Peter J. Hunter

Abstract This chapter is intended to: (1) serve as an overview of the current state of computer modeling of cardiac electrical activation at the tissue and whole organ levels; (2) indicate some of the issues that will need to be addressed over the next 5–10 years; and (3) provide a reference list that will guide the reader toward more thorough reading in this field. Limitations on space mean that it cannot be a comprehensive review, and we apologize for omissions or apparent bias that may have occurred as a result. However, we hope to persuade you that computer modeling, which has contributed so much already to our knowledge of the electrical function of the heart, will be a critical tool for enhancing scientific understanding of the field and facilitating clinical utilization of that understanding in the future.

8.1 Introduction

Computer modeling has made a key contribution to the development of our understanding of the electrical behavior of cardiac cells over the past 40 years. Experimental studies have provided detailed information about the time-varying function of a bewildering array of transmembrane ion channels, pumps, transporters, and intracellular processes that govern ionic homeostasis, and these have been incorporated into biophysically based models of increasing sophistication. The capacity of these models to replicate electrical behavior at the whole-cell level provides a quantitative basis for assessing the role of these sub-cellular components in cardiac electrophysiology. That is, biophysically based computer modeling provides the logical framework for integrating and understanding the results of detailed experimental study of cardiac cellular electrophysiology.

The motivation for translating this approach to specific myocardial tissues or to the whole heart is very similar. Electrical function at this level is not simply a function of cellular electrophysiology, but it also depends on anatomy – the organization

B.H. Smaill (✉)
Auckland Bioengineering Institute and Department of Physiology, University of Auckland, Auckland, New Zealand
e-mail: b.smaill@auckland.ac.nz

D.C. Sigg et al. (eds.), *Cardiac Electrophysiology Methods and Models*, DOI 10.1007/978-1-4419-6658-2_8, © Springer Science+Business Media, LLC 2010 of cells and resultant tissue conductivities. Within this context, modeling again provides a physical basis for understanding and interpreting observed electrical behaviors. However, modeling is also used to make inferences about phenomena that cannot readily be measured. Although electrical activity can be mapped with relatively high spatial resolution on the surfaces of the cardiac chambers, it is not possible to make comparable intramural measurements. Also, it is difficult to investigate structural mechanisms that underlie reentrant arrhythmias such as tachycardia and fibrillation reproducibly in animal preparations, because these rhythm disturbances progressively influence the substrate for reentry through their effects on metabolism. At the tissue level, therefore, computer modeling is used to provide information that cannot be acquired directly, and also plays a crucial role in the processes of hypothesis formation and testing.

Whole heart models also provide a means to aid interpretation of widely used clinical measures of cardiac electrical activity. These include the heart surface potentials that are reconstructed in intracardiac electrical mapping and body surface potentials, which are sampled during electrocardiographic (ECG) recording. The relationship between body surface potentials and cardiac electrical activity is covered in detail in other chapters.

In a general sense, the approaches that are used to model electrical activity at tissue and whole heart levels are straightforward. First, it is necessary to set up an appropriate continuum representation of cardiac anatomy, and the finite element method has been used almost exclusively for this purpose. The reaction-diffusion equations are then solved within this framework, with current sources associated with membrane ion channels and externally applied stimulation. This progression informs the order in which topics are dealt with here. We begin with a brief outline of the finite element method and then review models of cardiac anatomy that have been developed over the past 25 years. We then move on to the mathematical representation of cardiac electrophysiology in a 3D continuum and review techniques that have been used to address this problem. A survey of specific models of cardiac electrical behavior is the largest section of this chapter and emphasis is given to cases in which (in the authors' view) modeling has made, or is making, significant contributions to understanding in the field. Finally, we review some of the problems that are associated with this discipline and speculate on its future directions.

As stated at the outset, our treatment of this topic is necessarily brief and, as a result, cannot deal with it in the depth that is warranted. For a more detailed outline of the field, the reader is referred to the recently published monograph by Pullan et al.[1]

8.2   Finite Elements and Material Coordinate Systems

The finite element method seeks to describe complex structures by representing them as an assembly of elements that are defined by nodes. The shape of the ventricular walls of the heart can be efficiently modeled with a small number of elements using high order finite element interpolation functions. Figure 8.1a shows a 60-element model of the right and left ventricles (LV) using tricubic Hermite

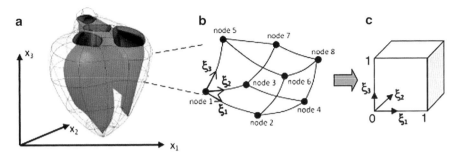

Fig. 8.1 Finite elements. A region of the myocardium (**a**) is defined by interpolation of nodal parameters (**b**) within an element using ξ_i -coordinates (**c**) that range from 0 to 1

elements. A system of rectangular Cartesian coordinates $\{x_1, x_2, x_3\}$ is used as a global reference coordinate system.

The myocardium is divided into subdomains or elements with corner nodes as shown in Fig. 8.1b. Any field within an element can be defined by interpolating field values defined at the element nodes using local coordinates $\{\xi_1, \xi_2, \xi_3\}$ that are defined to range from 0 to 1 along each element edge as shown in Fig. 8.1c. The geometry of the whole myocardium can therefore be defined by specifying the values of $\{x_1, x_2, x_3\}$ at each node and interpolating the eight element node values via *basis functions* (see below) defined in the element ξ_i- coordinates.

In fact, four nodes on an element face are shared by the two elements abutting that face. Therefore, if a mapping is defined which associates each vertex node of an element with its corresponding global node number, the geometric information at a node can be defined once and reused for multiple elements via the global node to element node mapping. We use the convention that element nodes are numbered 1–8 in the order of first increasing ξ_1, then ξ_2, and then ξ_3, as shown in Fig. 8.1b.

The 3D interpolating polynomial basis functions are generated as tensor products of 1D basis functions. For example, the 1D polynomials $1 - \xi$ and ξ can be used to generate the 3D trilinear basis functions $\psi_n(\xi_1, \xi_2, \xi_3)$ as follows:

$$\psi_1(\xi_1, \xi_2, \xi_3) = (1 - \xi_1)(1 - \xi_2)(1 - \xi_3)$$

$$\psi_2(\xi_1, \xi_2, \xi_3) = \xi_1(1 - \xi_2)(1 - \xi_3)$$

$$\psi_3(\xi_1, \xi_2, \xi_3) = (1 - \xi_1)\xi_2(1 - \xi_3)$$

$$\psi_4(\xi_1, \xi_2, \xi_3) = \xi_1\xi_2(1 - \xi_3).$$

$$\psi_5(\xi_1, \xi_2, \xi_3) = (1 - \xi_1)(1 - \xi_2)\xi_3$$

$$\psi_6(\xi_1, \xi_2, \xi_3) = \xi_1(1 - \xi_2)\xi_3$$

$$\psi_7(\xi_1, \xi_2, \xi_3) = (1 - \xi_1)\xi_2\xi_3$$

$$\psi_8(\xi_1,\xi_2,\xi_3) = \xi_1\xi_2\xi_3$$

Note that every basis function, when evaluated at an element node (where the ξ_i coordinates are 0 or 1), has the value 0 or 1 to ensure that the interpolated field value takes on the value of the nodal value. Any field variable can then be interpolated over $\{\xi_1, \xi_2, \xi_3\}$ – space using nodal parameters u_n for $n = 1$–8:

$$u(\xi_1,\xi_2,\xi_3) = \sum_{n=1,8} \psi_n(\xi_1,\xi_2,\xi_3) u_n \qquad (8.1)$$

One-dimensional cubic Hermite basis functions are illustrated in Fig. 8.2 and given by (8.2):

$$\psi_0^1(\xi) = 1 - 3\xi^2 + 2\xi^3$$
$$\psi_1^1(\xi) = \xi(\xi - 1)^2$$
$$\psi_2^0(\xi) = \xi^2(3 - 2\xi)$$
$$\psi_2^1(\xi) = \xi^2(\xi - 1) \qquad (8.2)$$

These are used to interpolate both nodal values of the dependent variable u_n and its first derivatives $(du / d\xi)_n$ as follows:

$$u = \psi_1^0(\xi)u_1 + \psi_1^1(\xi)\left(\frac{du}{d\xi}\right)_1 + \psi_2^1(\xi)u_2 + \psi_2^1(\xi)\left(\frac{du}{d\xi}\right)_2 \qquad (8.3)$$

Extending this to 3D using tensor products of the basis functions given in (8.2) gives the tricubic Hermite elements shown in Fig. 8.1a.

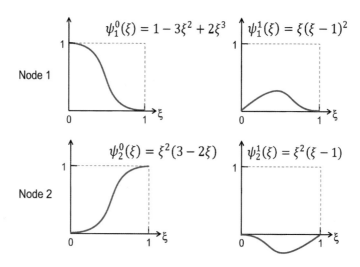

Fig. 8.2 The four cubic Hermite interpolating polynomials

8.3 Models of Cardiac Anatomy

Early models of cardiac anatomy focused on the LV and sought to capture its most fundamental architectural features. Thus the LV was commonly represented as a thick-walled ellipsoid of resolution, and the transmural rotation of myofiber orientation was represented by relatively simple functions.[2]

The first model based directly on the geometry and muscular architecture of an actual heart was reported by Hunter and Smaill,[3] and is outlined more fully in an article by Nielsen et al.[4] This has become known as the Auckland heart model – a misnomer because it represents the canine right and left ventricles only. Ventricular epi- and endo-cardial surfaces were mapped in fixed dog hearts and myofiber orientations were painstakingly measured throughout the ventricular walls with a purpose-built measurement rig. Prolate spheroidal coordinates were used to define ventricular geometry. This coordinate system has the advantage that relatively few elements are needed to represent the complex 3D geometry of the ventricles, and it is necessary to fit only one geometric coordinate (the radial coordinate) to match surface geometry. The initial Auckland heart model was an assembly of 24 3D elements with 96 degrees of freedom employing a mix of cubic Hermite and linear Lagrange basis functions. Epicardial geometry was faithfully reproduced with an RMS error of 0.9 mm. Fitted cavity geometry accurately represented papillary muscles, but could not resolve endocardial trabeculations (RMS errors typically on the order of 1.8–2.7 mm). Myofiber orientations measured throughout the walls of both ventricles were incorporated into the model.

A similar approach was also used to develop a representative anatomic model of the rabbit ventricles,[5] also known as the San Diego rabbit heart model. It should be noted that a prolate spheroid coordinate system limits the accuracy with which the geometry of the atrioventricular ring and left ventricular apex can be modeled. A rectangular Cartesian coordinate system with full cubic Hermite polynomial interpolation provides a more flexible, though less compact, description of ventricular geometry and was used more recently to model the ventricular anatomy of the pig heart.[6]

The standard view of ventricular cellular architecture has been that myocytes have a well-defined orientation at all points within the myocardium, but are uniformly coupled transverse to this axis. This notion lends itself to the representation of ventricular myocardium as a continuum that is inherently axially anisotropic. It is not consistent, however, with the laminar model of ventricular myocardium that has resulted from detailed morphometric investigations of 3D cardiac tissue architecture.[7] Ventricular myocardium is described as having a laminar organization in which myocytes are arranged in layers (myolaminae) with four to six cells' thickness. Adjacent layers branch and interconnect, but are separated by cleavage planes across which there can be little direct cell-to-cell coupling. The laminar model of myocardial architecture is supported by analyses of cardiac mechanical function.[8–10] Therefore, at any point within the ventricular wall, it is possible to define three distinct structural axes (fiber orientation, myolaminar orientation, and laminar-normal). On this basis, it has been argued that the electrical properties of ventricular myocardium would be expected to be fully orthotropic rather than axially anisotropic, and the Auckland heart model has been extended to accommodate this.[11] Recently microscopy techniques have also been developed that enable relatively large specimens of ventricular myocardium to be reconstructed in 3D at high spatial resolution.[12,13] Image-based finite element models that explicitly incorporate the discontinuities introduced by interlaminar clefts have been set up, and the effects of this microstructure on electrical behavior have been investigated.[14]

The orientation of fibers and layers is illustrated in Fig. 8.3a. The muscle fibers lie substantially parallel to the wall tangent plane at any point between the inner (endocardial) and outer (epicardial) surfaces. A material axis aligned with the fiber direction at any point is given a coordinate η_1. Myolaminae can be defined by another material axis with coordinate η_2 that is orthogonal to the fiber axis in the unloaded reference state of the tissue. A third material axis, orthogonal to the fiber-sheet plane, is defined with coordinate η_3. On the epicardial surface of the ventricle, the fiber-layer plane is tangent to this surface so that η_3 points out from the wall as shown in Fig. 8.3b.

The angle that the fiber axis makes with the circumferential direction of the ventricle is called the *fiber angle* and this varies from about −60° on the epicardial surface to +80° on the endocardial surface. Note that the fiber angle is shown as zero in Fig. 8.2. The sheet axis rotates through the wall from being tangential to the wall at the epicardium, to approximately transmural in the center of the wall, to again tangential to the wall at the endocardium. The spatial variation in fiber and sheet angles throughout the myocardium can be defined by finite element fields.

Accurate 3D representations of the specialized conduction system are necessary to model reentrant arrhythmia and ventricular fibrillation in the intact heart. Berenfeld and Jalife[15] added a representation of the Purkinje network to the Auckland heart model for this purpose (Sect. 8.4) while Vigmond and Clements[16] recently developed an anatomically based Purkinje system for the San Diego rabbit heart model. For a more comprehensive review of this topic, the reader is referred

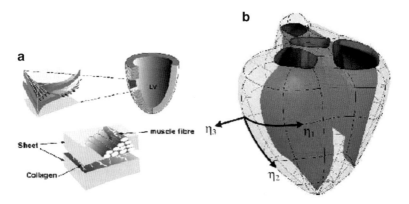

Fig. 8.3 The muscular architecture of the ventricular myocardium. (**a**) Schematic of the organization of fibers and layers. (**b**) Illustration of the fiber-layer material axes defined by the coordinates (h_1, h_2, h_3) in relation to the heart model (see text)

to ten Tusscher and Panfilov.[17] Realistic models of human heart anatomy are also essential for studies of electrical reentry, and one of the most recent such models is reported in ten Tusscher and Panfilov.[18] Here generalized information on the distribution of myofiber orientation derived from diffusion tensor MR imaging (DT-MRI)[19] and other modalities was incorporated into a detailed 3D reconstruction of the structurally normal human ventricles.[20] A 3D representation of the Purkinje system was subsequently added to this model.[21]

Over the past three years, new tissue-specific approaches that have the capacity to provide much more detailed models of ventricular anatomy have been developed; for an up-to-date account, see Plank.[22] Cardiac geometry is characterized using MRI, and ventricular surfaces have been fitted using spatially adaptive, unstructured mesh generation techniques that preserve mesh conformity, while minimizing degrees of freedom. Myofiber orientation throughout the heart walls is characterized using DT-MRI. The first eigenvector of the diffusion tensor is aligned with myofiber direction, and it is argued (but has not yet been directly confirmed histologically) that the second eigenvector can be used to characterize laminar orientation.[19,23] Finally, high-resolution 3D histologic data are being merged with corresponding MR image volumes to develop models that contain precise information on the distribution of the specialized tissue structures.[22]

In comparison to the work described above, the development of anatomically detailed atrial models has been much slower, possibly reflecting the inherent complexity of atrial structure. In one of the earliest computer models of cardiac electrical activity, Moe and co-workers[24] represented atrial tissue as a sheet of interconnected cells. Subsequently, membrane models that incorporate important features of 3D atrial structure have been used with some success to simulate atrial electrical activity.[25–28] One problem with this approach is that the fast conducting pathways which determine the spread of atrial activation – crista terminalis, pectinate muscles, and Bachmann's bundle – are not represented. Harrild and Henriquez[29] presented the first real 3D model of atrial structure. It provides a realistic description of the epicardial geometry of the human atria. While endocardial geometry is less accurately described, the model incorporates stylized representations of the principal conduction pathways. More recently, Seemann and colleagues[30] presented a more detailed model of atrial anatomy based on the Visible Female dataset.[31] With a resolution of 330 μm, this model provides the most detailed representation of atrial surface geometry and cellular architecture available to date.

The detailed 3D reconstructions of the sinoatrial node (SAN) and atrioventricular node (AVN) developed by Boyett and his research group[32,33] provide an objective lesson of what can be achieved with tissue-level anatomic models. For example, to construct a model of the AVN, serial sections were cut throughout a rabbit AVN and alternately stained for histology or immunolabeled to identify nodal cells and gap junction proteins. Different structures associated with the AVN – nodal tissue, transitional tissue, His bundle, atrial and ventricular myocardium, etc. – were identified. On this basis, the cellular architecture of the AVN was reconstructed in 3D and incorporated into an anatomic model consisting of 13 million elements on which electrical activation could be simulated.

8.4   Tissue Electrodynamics

Cellular-level models can be incorporated into larger-scale models either as a discrete set of cells or tissue bundles or as a continuum. The latter approach treats the tissue as a syncytium and assumes that, at any given point, there exists both intra- and extracellular space. A fundamental assumption here is that the length scales of the physically observable phenomena (e.g., the spatial gradients of voltage and transmembrane current) are sufficiently large in comparison with the underlying discrete structures for the myocardium to be considered as a continuum.

Fundamental electrical relationships for a 3D continuum are:

$$\mathbf{E} = -\nabla\Phi \tag{8.4}$$

and

$$\mathbf{J} = \sigma\mathbf{E} \tag{8.5}$$

where $\mathbf{E}$ is the electric field, the scalar Φ is potential, $\mathbf{J}$ is current density, and σ is the conductivity of the medium through which current is flowing (in general, an orthogonal tensor).

Where a current source of density I_v is present,

$$\nabla \cdot \mathbf{J} = I_v \tag{8.6}$$

Poisson's equation

$$\nabla^2\Phi = -\frac{I_v}{\sigma} \tag{8.7}$$

can be obtained (for spatially constant s) by combining (8.4)–(8.6) above.

Laplace's equation

$$\nabla^2\Phi = 0 \tag{8.8}$$

relates to the particular case in which the conducting region is free of sources.

8.4.1   The Bidomain Equations

The *bidomain* formulation recognizes that cardiac tissue is electrically anisotropic and that, during activation, current flows in both extracellular and intracellular domains. Bidomain models are necessary to simulate defibrillation and pacing where current is injected into the heart via the extracellular domain, and have the further advantage that the most commonly measured cardiac electrical signals, extracellular potential, and transmembrane potential are direct model outputs. The bidomain equations were formulated mathematically by Tung[34] and are extensively reviewed by Pullan et al.[1] A very brief outline of the derivation of these equations is given below.

We define macroscopic potentials Φ_i and Φ_e in intra- and extracellular spaces, respectively. Thus the transmembrane potential V_m is given by:

$$V_m = \Phi_i - \Phi_e \tag{8.9}$$

The basis of the bidomain equations is the assumption that net current flux between intra- and extracellular domains is zero everywhere, that is,

$$-\nabla \bullet \mathbf{J}_i = \nabla \bullet \mathbf{J}_e \tag{8.10}$$

The first of the bidomain equations can be derived from (8.4), (8.5), (8.9), and (8.10).

$$\nabla \bullet (\sigma_i \nabla V_m) = -\nabla \bullet ((\sigma_i + \sigma_e)\nabla \Phi_e) \tag{8.11}$$

In addition,

$$-\nabla \bullet \mathbf{J}_i = A_m I_m - I_s \tag{8.12}$$

where A_m is the surface-to-volume ratio of the cell membrane, I_m the transmembrane current density per unit area, and I_s an externally imposed source current density. From this expression, it can be shown that:

$$\nabla \bullet (\sigma_i \nabla V_m) + \nabla \bullet (\sigma_i \nabla \Phi_e) = A_m I_m - I_s \tag{8.13}$$

$$I_m = C_m \frac{\partial V_m}{\partial t} + I_{ion} \tag{8.14}$$

where I_{ion} is the net current carried by transmembrane ion channels.

Combining (8.13) and (8.14), we obtain the second bidomain equation

$$\nabla \bullet (\sigma_i \nabla V_m) + \nabla \bullet (\sigma_i \nabla \Phi_e) = A_m \left(C_m \frac{\partial V_m}{\partial t} + I_{ion} \right) - I_s \tag{8.15}$$

The boundary condition generally used to solve the bidomain equations in cardiac tissue is that there is no current flow out of the intracellular domain at the surface of the heart. That is,

$$(\sigma_i \nabla \Phi_i) \bullet \mathbf{n} = 0 \tag{8.16}$$

where $\mathbf{n}$ is a unit vector outwardly normal to the myocardial surface.

This can be rewritten in terms of Φ_e and V_m so that it matches the formulation of the bidomain (8.11) and (8.15):

$$(\sigma_i \nabla V_m) \bullet \mathbf{n} = -(\sigma_i \nabla \Phi_e) \bullet \mathbf{n} \tag{8.17}$$

8.4.2   The Monodomain Equations

The monodomain equation,

$$\nabla \bullet (\sigma_i \nabla V_m) = A_m \left(C_m \frac{\partial V_m}{\partial t} + I_{ion} \right) \tag{8.18}$$

is a simplification of the bidomain equations in which it is assumed that the extracellular field is infinitely conducting (or the two domains are equally anisotropic). While the monodomain equation is often used in large-scale simulations, it does not yield direct estimates of extracellular potential, and it cannot be used to model the response to stimuli such as defibrillation shocks that are delivered extracellularly.

The monodomain equation above has been used to analyze factors that influence the propagation of electrical activation in the heart. Consider the 1D case in which electrical activation propagates along a cylindrical fiber of radius a. V_m is a function of the z coordinate (along the axis of propagation) alone and A_m the surface volume ratio per unit length is $2/a$. Therefore, (8.18) reduces to:

$$\frac{a}{2R_i} \frac{\partial^2 V_m}{\partial z^2} = C_m \frac{\partial V_m}{\partial t} + I_{ion} \tag{8.19}$$

This 1D reaction-diffusion equation provides some insight into the mechanisms that sustain and influence the spread of excitation in excitable tissues.

As a wavefront of depolarization propagates, potential-sensitive membrane cation channels reach threshold and open transiently (in the heart, inward current is carried by fast sodium channels, but also by L-type Ca^{2+} channels). Sodium (and calcium) ions not only cross the cell membrane at the wavefront and behind it, but also diffuse forward bringing the cell membrane ahead of the activation wavefront toward threshold. The magnitude of the transmembrane ion flux triggered by activation affects the time taken for tissue ahead of the wavefront to reach threshold and therefore determines the rate of propagation.

For uniform propagation, V_m must satisfy the wave equation

$$V_m(z,t) = V_m(z - \theta t) \tag{8.20}$$

where θ is the axial propagation velocity. Application of the chain rule gives:

$$\frac{a}{2R_i \theta^2} \frac{d^2 V_m}{dt^2} = C_m \frac{dV_m}{dt} + I_{ion} \tag{8.21}$$

Any solution of (8.21) will be a solution everywhere, provided:

$$\frac{a}{2R_i\theta^2} = \text{constant} \tag{8.22}$$

For this to hold, q must be proportional to both $\sqrt{a}$ and to $\sqrt{1/R_i}$.

This analysis indicates that the velocity at which electrical activation spreads in heart tissue is influenced by: (1) cell dimension; (2) intracellular resistance, which is affected by gap junction density; and (3) the extent and rate of net inward current flow across the cell membrane during depolarization.

The final point also provides a qualitative explanation of how and why the curvature of activation wavefront affects the spread of electrical activation in 2D and 3D tissue domains. The rate of propagation increases when the activation wavefront is concave because the area or volume of active tissue behind the wavefront is greater than that in front. That is, the supply of transmembrane ion current is greater than the current load. As a result, net inward ion flux is increased and propagation is more rapid. The opposite applies when the activation wavefront is convex. The area or volume of active tissue behind the wavefront is less than that in front and propagation reduces. For a more complete analysis of these issues see Kleber and Rudy.[35]

8.5   Models of Cardiac Electrical Activation

8.5.1   Computational Issues

For the computer modeling of a discontinuous myocardial structure with no-flux boundaries, methods based on the weak or integral forms of the bidomain or monodomain equations are desirable. Finite difference, finite element, collocation, and finite volume methods have been used for this purpose (for a more detailed account of this topic, see Pullan et al.[1]). Each of these approaches has advantages and disadvantages. Finite difference techniques are numerically straightforward, but require a uniformly spaced solution grid. This does not lend itself to the investigation of problems in which the deformation of the heart during the activation cycle must be taken into account. With the finite element method, solution variables are interpolated across each element using basis functions such as those introduced in Sect. 8.2. This procedure readily accommodates material deformation, but is computationally expensive, particularly for structurally complex problems. The collocation method is a hybrid approach which seeks to exploit the strengths of both of its components; a finite element mesh is used to describe the geometry and material deformation of the heart and a finite difference grid is then defined with respect to this.[36] With the finite volume method,[37,38] the solution divided into an array of volume elements and solutions is obtained by calculating the current flow across the six faces of each of the individual volumes. This approach is efficient and well suited to image-based modeling. However, it should be noted that the use of structured meshes in finite difference, finite element, and finite volume methods introduces specific problems. The use of "jagged" edges to represent complex boundaries or discontinuities may lead to errors in the estimation of current flow due to misalignment of conductivity tensors that should be parallel to anatomic surfaces.[1,22]

An alternative large-scale modeling approach is to assume that the upstroke of the action potential is sufficiently rapid, both temporally and spatially, that it can be modeled as a step jump. This is known as the *eikonal method* and details can be found in Colli Franzone et al.[39] However, such models cannot capture fully the factors that influence transmembrane current flux during activation and are not appropriate for modeling repolarization or reentrant phenomena.

8.5.2 2D Tissue Models

One- and two-dimensional computer models have been used widely to investigate the effects of specific structural features on electrical activity in the heart and have provided considerable insight into the ways in which discontinuities at cell and tissue levels influence propagation. Structurally simple models that incorporate realistic cellular kinetics have been used to analyze: (1) the effects of gap junction uncoupling on propagation and action potential characteristics[40]; (2) the role of gap junction distribution and cardiomyocyte boundary topology on the spread of activation within and between cells[41]; and (3) propagation and propagation safety at the boundaries between different tissue domains[42] among many other applications. A strength of computer modeling at this level is that predictions can be compared with closely related experimental studies carried out using patterned cell culture.[43]

A similar application of 2D computer modeling has been to investigate the effects of nonconducting discontinuities (for instance, representing interstitial fibrosis) on the stability of electrical propagation. These studies suggest that the risk of wavebreak is exacerbated by structural discontinuities that spread across a range of spatial scales[44] and that interstitial fibrosis is more likely to give rise to reentry and fibrillation if it is patchy and nonuniformly distributed.[18,45,46] Two-dimensional computer models have also indicated that both structural discontinuities[47] and heterogeneous electrophysiological properties[48] can give rise to alternans rhythm (beat-to-beat instability in action potential duration) which is widely viewed as a precursor to reentrant activation and wavebreak.[49]

Computer modeling has also made an invaluable contribution to the general understanding of the heart's response to externally applied electric fields. The current flows set up by external point or field stimulation generate complex potential distributions in myocardial tissue with adjacent regions of depolarization and hyperpolarization (virtual electrodes). This cannot be explained by simple 1D cable models or by 2D monodomain formulations. Wikswo et al.[50] showed that a bidomain tissue model with unequal intra- and extracellular anisotropy predicted virtual electrodes adjacent to a point stimulus that explained observed responses to anodal and cathodal unipolar stimulation, and matched potential distributions recorded experimentally using optical mapping. The generation of complex virtual electrodes by external fields also offered possible explanations for an apparent conundrum associated with cardiac defibrillation. First, it is evident that defibrillation-strength shocks reverse ventricular fibrillation by "resetting" myocardial tissue across the ventricular wall, and this occurs despite the fact that measured electrical space constants for cardiac tissue[51] are consistent with rapid decay of induced potentials intramurally. Second, during normal rhythm, external shocks of sufficient strength to induce cardioversion can give rise to reentrant electrical activity. It was initially suggested[52] that application of external field stimulation generates a "saw tooth" distribution of polarization across the ventricle as a result of the resistance to current flow between cardiac cells at gap junctions. However, this was not demonstrated experimentally.[53] Computer modeling has been used to show that a wide range of factors could be responsible for diffuse virtual electrode formation.[54] These include tissue heterogeneity, myofiber curvature,[55] and myocardial disconti-nuities.[14,56] Induction of reentrant activation by virtual electrodes adjacent to stimulus electrodes has also been predicted with computer models and confirmed experimentally.[57,58]

8.5.3 3D Tissue Models

Three-dimensional tissue models that incorporate detailed structural information can also provide information about local electrical behavior that would not otherwise be available. The model of the AVN already described[33] provides an excellent example. The spread of electrical activation in the AVN has been simulated in this anatomic model employing a monodomain formulation and using specialized, biophysically based activation models for atrial and ventricular myocardium as well as N, transitional, and NH nodal cells. The results shown in Fig. 8.4 predict the existence of slow and fast pathways in the AVN, and these were demonstrated experimentally using optical mapping techniques. Activation was also modeled during S1 S2 stimulation – stimulus pairs with a relatively short coupling interval between them. Atrial and ventricular cells, as well as the three classes of nodal cells listed above, were represented as cellular automata, and initiation of electrical reentry within the AVN was demonstrated.

A detailed microstructure-based tissue model has been used to address three specific hypotheses relating to the electrical properties of ventricular myocardium.[14] These are that: (1) early propagation from a focal activation can be accurately described only by a discontinuous model of myocardium; (2) the laminar organiza-tion of myocytes determines unique propagation velocities in three microstructurally defined directions at any point in the myocardium; and (3) interlaminar clefts, or cleavage planes, provide a means by which an externally applied shock can influ-ence a sufficient volume of heart tissue to terminate cardiac fibrillation. The studies

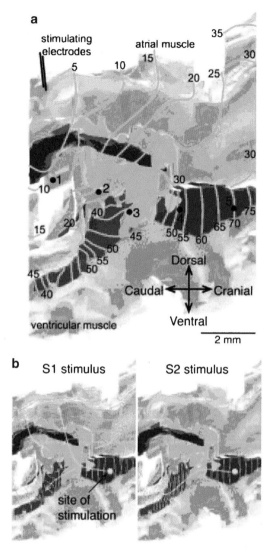

Fig. 8.4 Structure–function relationships of the atrioventricular node. (**a**) Anterograde conduction as calculated using a monodomain model. The preparation was stimulated at the crista terminalis. The activation sequence is shown as isochrones at 5 ms intervals. *Arrows* highlight conduction pathway. (**b**) Fast–slow reentry as calculated using the cellular automaton model. Preparation was stimulated at the His bundle (*yellow spot*) using an S1–S2 protocol (S1–S2 interval, 96 ms). The activation sequence (isochrones at 5 ms intervals) in response to S1 and S2 stimuli is shown. *Arrows* highlight the conduction pathway. Reproduced with permission from Li et al.[33]

were carried out using an extended volume image acquired from a transmural segment of rat LV free wall ($0.8 \times 0.8 \times 3.7$ mm) and consisted of 6.07×10^8 cubic voxels at 1.56 μm resolution[13] (Fig. 8.5). The spatial arrangement of muscle layers

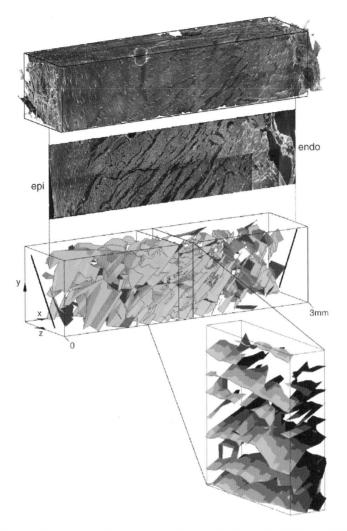

Fig. 8.5 (*Top panel*) Reconstructed volume of rat left ventricular free-wall. (*Middle panel*) Transmural slice from the reconstructed volume showing a complex network of cleavage planes which course between myocyte laminae. (*Bottom panel*) Bilinear finite element description of cleavage planes through the entire tissue block and a smaller midwall subsection. Myofiber orientation is shown on the epi- and endocardial surfaces. Reproduced with permission from Hooks et al.[14]

was quantified as follows: cleavage planes were manually segmented and represented as bilinear finite element surface patches, while the transmural variation of myocyte orientation was characterized throughout the volume and represented as a linear function. A bidomain formulation was used to model the spread of electrical activation in this tissue volume. Ventricular myocytes and extracellular space were represented as overlapping domains, while cleavage planes were modeled as boundaries to current flow in the intracellular domain.

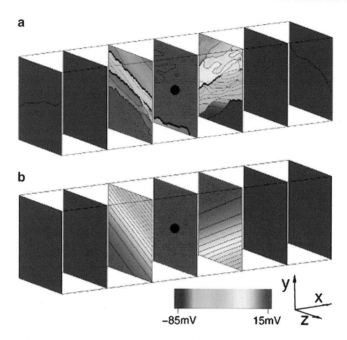

Fig. 8.6 Ectopic activation of (**a**) discontinuous model and (**b**) continuous model. Transmembrane potentials are mapped on seven equi-spaced surfaces through the reconstructed tissue volume, at 8 ms following midwall stimulation. Isopotential lines at 5-mV intervals are shown in *black*. Site of stimulation is shown with *black dot* at center of volume. The cleavage plane obstacles in (**a**) lead to a highly discontinuous form of propagation which is, however, well approximated by the continuous model. Reproduced with permission from Smaill et al.[86]

The isopotential regions in Fig. 8.6 indicate the spread of electrical activation from a point stimulus at the center of the tissue segment. Activation was simulated using a simple cubic ionic current model.[59] Two cases were considered. In Fig. 8.6a, we present the results for the spread of activation where the discontinuities due to cleavage planes were explicitly represented. It was assumed that electrical conductivity in intra- and extracellular domains is transversely isotropic with respect to local myocyte orientation. Comparable data, presented in Fig. 8.6b, were obtained using a continuous model in which it was assumed that conductivity is orthotropic with respect to three microstructurally defined material axes. These three conductivity parameters were adjusted to best fit the propagation patterns predicted by the discontinuous model. This analysis suggests that the spread of electrical activation from an intramural point stimulus in the LV is highly anisotropic due to discontinuities associated with cleavage planes between muscle layers. Propagation is most rapid along the myocyte axis, somewhat slower transverse to the cell axis in muscle layers, but much slower again in the direction perpendicular to the muscle layers.

Despite this global correspondence between the discontinuous and continuous orthotropic model, the latter cannot reproduce the complex local patterns of activation that occur along the activation wavefront. Nearly all signals from the discontinuous model show some degree of fractionation, which is greatest in extent adjacent to the stimulus site. Moreover, the downstroke duration of signals recorded close to the stimulus site was considerably longer in the discontinuous model than in the continuous model. The model predictions that the laminar architecture of ventricular myocardium will give rise to orthotropic electric properties have been tested by two recent studies,[60,61] in which a combination of high-resolution intramural mapping detailed structural measurement and structure-based modeling was employed in pig hearts. Hooks and coworkers[61] analyzed the passive response to current injection and showed that bulk conductivity transverse to the fiber axis divided in a ratio of approximately 2:1, with maximum bulk conductivity in the direction of myolaminae and minimum conductivity perpendicular to this. Caldwell et al.[60] demonstrated that maximum and minimum velocities transverse to the fiber direction separate in a similar ratio. Maximum velocity aligned with myolaminae with minimum velocity perpendicular to it. These results are not consistent with the widely held view that the electric properties of ventricular myocardium are isotropic transverse to the fiber axis.

The effects of applying defibrillation-strength shocks on the discontinuous tissue model have also been investigated.[14,56] This produced a series of sharp intra-mural voltage steps centered on the cleavage planes that separate muscle layers. These local potential gradients were generated by current in the extracellular space adjacent to cleavage planes and acted as secondary sources to "seed" near-synchronous activation. Transmural activation of the ventricular wall was most rapid for shock strengths in the range of 5–10 V/cm, with an absence of secondary source forma-tion for shocks <5 V/cm. Shock strengths >10 V/cm induced virtual anodes that persisted for the duration of the shock, suppressing virtual electrode propagation and delaying activation. These results were consistent with the findings of experi-mental studies in which optical techniques were used to map membrane potential across the surface of a perfused, transmural segment removed from the LV free wall of the pig heart.[62,63]

8.5.4   3D Ventricular Models

Colli Franzone et al.[64] have used modeling to investigate the development of intra-mural potentials in the LV during activation and to analyze the extent to which extracellular electrograms measured on the epicardial surface of the LV reflect intramural electrical activity. They employed the eikonal method to solve the bidomain equations for models that represent the LV: (1) as a slab[64]; and (2) as a truncated, thick-walled ellipsoid of revolution.[39] In both cases, it was assumed that conductivities were axially anisotropic and the models incorporated realistic transmural myofiber rotation. Activation was simulated by injecting current at a series of different intramural sites, and extracellular potential fields were constructed throughout these tissue volumes at various intervals after stimulation. Closed regions of positive potential were observed ahead of the wavefront of depolarization which propagated preferentially in the myofiber direction. The line intersecting the two regions of positive potential on the epicardial surface initially coincided with fiber orientation at the site of stimulation, but rotated clockwise as activation developed and spread toward the epicardial surface. In a closely related study, Muzikant and coworkers[65] mapped the time course of activation on the LV epicardial surface of dog hearts due to point stimulation at different intramural depths. Myofiber orientation was measured in each of these hearts using DT-MRI, and these data were incorporated into a bidomain model in which the LV wall was represented as a $3 \times 3 \times 0.75$ cm slab and axially anisotropic electrical properties were assumed. Extracellular potentials were simulated using a simple FitzHugh-Nagumo ionic current model, and the results were compared directly with corresponding experimental data. The predicted epicardial potentials matched those reported previously,[64] and were qualitatively similar to experimental findings. However, there were significant quantitative differences between predicted and observed results. In particular, the predicted downstroke of epicardial electrograms during activation was substantially more rapid than observed experimentally and the effects of myofiber rotation were less pronounced. Subsequently, the effects of axial anisotropy and full orthotropy were compared by Colli Franzone and colleagues for the ellipsoid model.[66] They found that the effects of intramural fiber rotation masked the orthotropic nature of the medium, particularly for epicardial activation maps, and stated that, from a qualitative point of view, both axially anisotropic and orthotropic models are compatible with the experimental findings "… and only a quantitative comparison with the experimental data could provide a means for validating one of the two assumptions."

The Auckland heart model has been used by a number of research groups to study mechanisms of electrical reentry, wavebreak, and fibrillation. Berenfeld and Jalife[15] added a representation of the Purkinje network to this 3D anatomic model to demonstrate that the Purkinje system may play a role in initiating focal subendocardial activation and also subsequently in the establishment of intramyocardial reentry. Panfilov and colleagues also used the Auckland heart model to investigate mechanisms associated with the progression from spiral wave formation, through wavebreak to the "turbulent" electrical rhythm that characterizes ventricular fibrillation (Fig. 8.7).[67–69] More recently, this group has extended its focus to the human heart. It has used a description of 3D human ventricular anatomy (Sect. 8.3) and an ionic current model developed for human ventricular myocytes[70] to investigate the organization of human ventricular fibrillation. The characteristics of their simulated ventricular fibrillation were similar to clinical studies,[71] but they demonstrated that human ventricular fibrillation exhibits greater spatial organization than animal hearts of equivalent dimension. For further detail on this work, the readers are referred to the following sources: Clayton and Panfilov,[72] Keldermann and colleagues,[73] and ten Tusscher et al.[21]

It is clear from our discussion earlier on the formation of virtual electrodes in cardiac tissue that there is a close link between defibrillation and cardiac vulnerability to electric shocks. Strong external shocks are effective in defibrillating

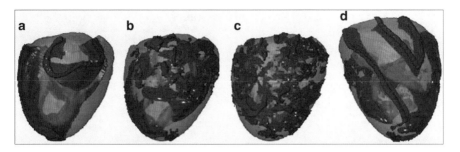

Fig. 8.7 Spiral breakup in the Auckland heart model. Posterior views of 3D excitation (**a**) 500 ms, (**b**) 1,000 ms, and (**c**) 2,500 ms after initiation of spiral wave. Anterior view in (**d**) 1,000 ms after spiral wave initiation. Reproduced with permission from Panfilov and Pertsov[69]

the heart because they generate virtual electrodes through the ventricular wall, but virtual electrodes may also induce reentrant activation and, therefore, give rise to fibrillation. In fact, the upper limit of vulnerability (the maximum shock strength at which sustained reentrant activity may occur) is very close to the defibrillation threshold, and understanding of the processes involved is of considerable importance in programming implantable cardioverter/defibrillators. An elegant combination of 3D modeling and experimentation has been undertaken by Trayanova and colleagues to address this issue.[74] This work was carried out using the San Diego model of rabbit ventricular anatomy with ionic current models modified to produce realistic results in the presence of defibrillation-strength fields. The bidomain formulation was solved using finite element methods.[74]

Figure 8.8 demonstrates the effects of anatomy on the response to external shocks. Excitation occurs within the thick LV wall in both cases – in the interventricular septum for a LV shock and in the LV free wall for a right ventricular (RV) shock. This results in different patterns of reentry that qualitatively match the experimental results obtained using optical mapping.[75] There is reasonable correspondence also between predicted and observed conditions (shock strength and coupling interval) for which sustained tachyarrhythmia could be induced.[76] A closely related study confirmed that the vulnerable window shifts to lower coupling intervals with global ischemia[76]; for a recent review of this research, see Trayanova's work.[74]

8.5.5   3D Atrial Models

Anatomically based computer models offer a quantitative framework for understanding the mechanisms that give rise to atrial tachycardia and atrial fibrillation. They also provide a means of exploring the likely success of different ablation strategies, in a systematic fashion. The many variables that determine ablation outcome can be more readily controlled in such a model "test-bed," compared with animal or clinical studies. A recent model-based study by Dang et al.[77] revealed that a three-line connection

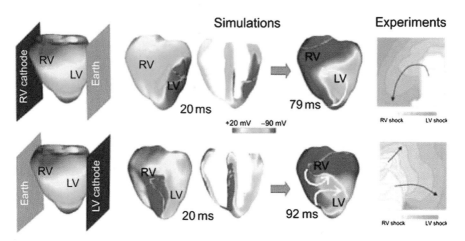

Fig. 8.8 Evolution of post-shock activity for right ventricular or RV (*top panel*) and left ventricular or LV (*bottom panel*) shocks. Anterior epicardial and some transmural views of transmembrane potential distribution are shown. *White arrows* represent direction of propagation; see color scale as indicated. The experiments show optical maps of electrical activation on the anterior surface of a rabbit heart for RV and LV shocks within the vulnerable area. *Black arrows* indicate direction of propagation. In both simulations and experiments, RV shocks result in a single spiral wave, while LV shocks generate figure-of-eight reentry on the anterior epicardium. This is based on figures from Rodriguez et al.[76] Reproduced with permission from Trayanova[74]

of the pulmonary veins in conjunction with a superior-to-inferior vena cava ablation line was the most simple configuration that terminated established atrial fibrillation in 100% of cases. However, the model simplified atrial geometry to a sheet. The thoracic veins, which are thought to play a major role in the initiation of atrial fibrillation, were included as no more than holes in the mesh. Moreover, specialized conduction tracts, such as the crista terminalis, Bachmann's bundle, and the pectinate muscles, were not explicitly included in the model. A more complete study of ablation strategies awaits inclusion of appropriate microstructural complexity, particularly at the junction of the pulmonary valve and the left atrium, where atrial fibrillation may be triggered.

Atrial activation in the human atria has been simulated by Harrild and Henriquez[29] using the more realistic finite-element model outlined in Sect. 8.3. This was solved as a monodomain problem using the Nuygen human atrial cell activation model[78] and the results demonstrate that it is necessary to include key atrial conduction bundles to reproduce normal patterns of activation. More recently, Fenton and coworkers[79] used this anatomic model to investigate the role of focal pulmonary vein activity in generating atrial fibrillation. In this case, a bidomain formulation was employed and the Fenton-Karma activation model[80] was adapted to best match the different electrophysiologic properties of atria and pulmonary veins. In Fig. 8.9, we represent one instant during the development of reentrant activation in this model; this simulation was carried out in our laboratory. We also solved the bidomain equations and used a Fenton-Karma activation model.

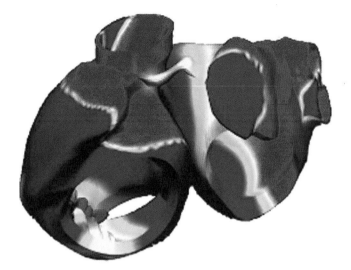

Fig. 8.9 Development of reentrant activation in a 3D model of the human atria (Harrild and Henriquez[29]). A bidomain formulation was used with a Fenton-Karma activation model. Reentrant activation was generated by applying an ectopic stimulus with a short coupling interval to the Bachmann's bundle. Image courtesy of Dr. Gregory Sands, University of Auckland

Reentrant activation was generated by applying an ectopic stimulus with a short coupling interval to the Bachmann's bundle.

8.6 Problems and Future Directions

Current state-of-the-art 3D myocardial activation models are now extremely complex. Highly detailed ion channel cell models (see Chap. 5: The Electrocardiogram and Clinical Cardiac Electrophysiology) are being coupled with finely resolved cardiac architecture and anisotropic tissue conductivity. The problem with these models is that a resolution of 0.1 mm is needed to obtain spatially converged solutions of the reaction-diffusion bidomain equations, and the meshes required for a normal human heart are of the order of 100 million nodes. Moreover, time steps of 0.01 ms are required to achieve temporal convergence because the upstroke of the cardiac action potential is very rapid. A more detailed analysis of these issues is given by Plank and colleagues[22] who report that simulation of 1 ms activity for their bidomain formulation took 70.6 s using 64 processors. They noted that this exercise should therefore be viewed as a proof of concept. It is certainly not feasible at this stage to use such complex models to study rhythm disturbances in which it is necessary to simulate multiple cycles of activation.

The good news is that computational power is continuing to increase, and the super computer of today will be on our desktops within five years. In the meantime, we need to develop new approaches. It seems fair comment that the methods currently used to solve complex whole heart models are inefficient. The solutions exhibit smooth activation wavefronts that, under normal physiological circumstances, occupy less than 1% of the volume of the myocardium. One approach is to use adaptive meshing, where the mesh is kept at a coarse level of spatial resolution except in the active region, where a finely resolved mesh is used. Adaptive meshing is expensive, however, and it may be that there are much better approaches involving wavefront algorithms that are closer in spirit to the eikonal equation approach discussed earlier. An alternative approach is to use reduced models that capture key features of the problem addressed. Recent work from Zhao and colleagues[81] provides a successful example of this. Electrical activation was modeled in a detailed 3D reconstruction of the pig right atrial appendage acquired using high-resolution serial imaging. Activation was simulated using a bidomain formulation, and it was assumed that the ratio of axial to transverse conductivity for crista terminalis and large pectinate muscles was 10:1, while small pectinate muscles and the thin atrial wall were assumed to be isotropic. A Courtemanche cell model[82] was used for the crista terminalis, while a modified Luo Rudy model[83] was used for pectinate muscles and other atrial cells. Despite the structural complexity of the 3D model, activation was quite uniform at normal rates of stimulation (Fig. 8.10). Moreover, these results were reproduced with surprising accuracy using a 2D model that captured the organization of the crista terminalis and pectinate muscles. It took many hours to model a single cycle of activation for the 3D model using a high performance computer, but solutions with the 2D model were around 30 times faster. Using the 2D model, it was possible to investigate mechanisms of reentry in the right atrial appendage using stimulus trains in which the cycle length was progressively reduced (Fig. 8.10). With stimulation from the crista terminalis at its junction with a large pectinate muscle, conduction block was observed within the crista terminalis due to a reduced safety factor, as well as unidirectional block and reentry due to its high anisotropy. These results are consistent with previous experimental studies of reentry in the right atrial appendage.[84,85]

In addition to the need for better numerical algorithms or realistic reduced-order models, there are other major challenges for future cardiac electrical modeling that must be addressed, and some of these are introduced very briefly below. One of the problems of whole heart modeling is how to represent structures that are inherently discontinuous within a continuum framework. This issue is particularly important in studies of structural heart disease, where interstitial fibrosis and/or tortuous conduction pathways in the border zone surrounding a myocardial infarct provide a substrate for electrical instability. Other structural factors that are thought to play an important role in cardiac rhythm disturbance are: (1) the Purkinje fiber network and, in particular, the junctions of Purkinje cells with ventricular myocardium; (2) the distribution of autonomic nerve terminals in the heart, which appears to become more heterogeneous in heart failure; and (3) the architecture and intrinsic electrophysiology of tissue at the junction of the left atrium and the pulmonary veins. There is an evident need for improved structural and functional models in each of these areas. Finally, none of the models discussed above accounts for the

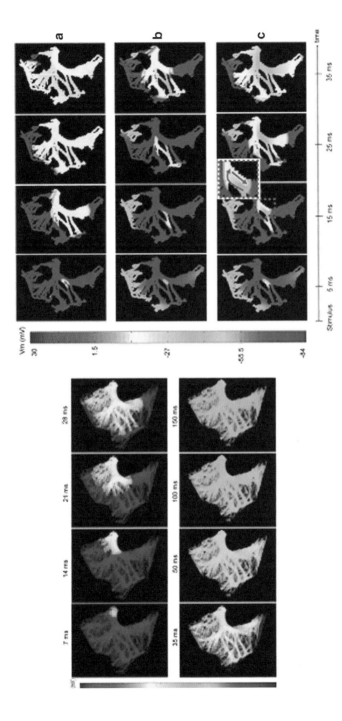

Fig. 8.10 (*Left panel*) Spread of electrical activation in 3D right atrial appendage model. Membrane potentials are rendered on a semi-transparent representation of the 3D structure. (*Right panel*) Conduction block and reentry with repeated cycles of activation at reducing cycle length. (**a**) Normal spread of activation cycle length 600 ms, (**b**) Conduction block in the crista terminalis (CT) (cycle length 70 ms, 38th cycle), (**c**) Unidirectional block and reentry within the CT (cycle length of 70 ms, 38th cycle, increased stimulus strength). Reproduced with permission from Zhao et al.[81]

fact that the heart deforms substantially through the normal cycle of electrical activity (from activation to repolarization). Electromechanical interactions certainly play an important role in the maintenance of many arrhythmias and this also needs to be a focus in the future development of this field.

References

1. Pullan AJ, Cheng LK, Buist ML. Mathematically Modeling the Electrical Activity of the Heart: FromCell to Body Surface and Back Again. Hackensack NJ: World Scientific Publishing Co. Pvt. Ltd., 2005.
2. Streeter DDJ. Gross morphology and fiber geometry of the heart. In: Berne RM, Sperilakis N, Geigert SR, editors. Handbook of Physiology. Baltimore: Williams Wilkins, 1979: 61–112.
3. Hunter PJ, Smaill BH. The analysis of cardiac function: a continuum approach. Prog Biophys Mol Biol 1989; 52:101–64.
4. Nielsen PM, Le Grice IJ, Smaill BH, et al. Mathematical model of geometry and fibrous structure of the heart. Am J Physiol Heart Circ Physiol 1991; 260:H1365–78.
5. Vetter FJ, McCulloch AD. Three dimensional analysis of regional cardiac function: a model of rabbit ventricular anatomy. Prog Biophys Mol Biol 1998; 69:157–83.
6. Stevens C, Hunter PJ. Sarcomere length changes in a 3D mathematical model of the pig ventricles. Prog Biophys Mol Biol 2003; 82:229–41.
7. LeGrice I, Smaill B, Chai L, et al. Laminar structure of the heart: ventricular myocyte arrangment and connective tissue architecture in the dog. Am J Physiol Heart Circ Physiol 1995; 269:H571–82.
8. Arts T, Costa K, Covell J, et al. Relating myocardial laminar architecture to shear strain and muscle fiber orientation. Am J Physiol Heart Circ Physiol 2001; 280:H2222–9.
9. Costa K, May-Newman K, Farr D, et al. Three-dimensional residual strain in midanterior canine left ventricle. Am J Physiol Heart Circ Physiol 1997; 42:H1968–76.
10. LeGrice I, Takayama, Y, Covell, JW. Transverse shear along myocardial cleavage planes provides a mechanism for normal systolic wall thickening. Circ Res 1995; 77:182–93.
11. LeGrice I, Hunter P, Smaill B. Laminar structure of the heart: a mathematical model. Am J Physiol Heart Circ Physiol 1997; 272:H2466–76.
12. Sands G, Gerneke D, Hooks D, et al. Automated imaging of extended tissue volumes using confocal microscopy. Microsc Res Tech 2005; 67:227–39.
13. Young A, LeGrice I, Young M, et al. Extended confocal microscopy of myocardial laminae and collagen network. J Microsc 1998; 192:139–50.
14. Hooks DA, Tomlinson KA, Marsden SG, et al. Cardiac microstructure: implications for electrical propagation and defibrillation in the heart. Circ Res 2002; 91:331–8.
15. Berenfeld O, Jalife J. Purkinje-muscle reentry as a mechanism of poly-morphic ventricular arrhythmias in a 3-dimensional model of the ventricles. Circ Res 1998; 82:1063–77.
16. Vigmond EJ, Clements CJ. Construction of a computer model to investigate sawtooth effects in the Purkinje system. IEEE Trans Biomed Eng 2007; 54:389–99.
17. ten Tusscher KHWJ, Panfilov AV. Modelling of the ventricular conduction system. Prog Biophys Mol Biol 2008; 96:152–70.
18. ten Tusscher K, Panfilov A. Reentry in heterogeneous cardiac tissue described by the Luo-Rudy ventricular action potential model. Am J Physiol Heart Circ Physiol 2003; 284:H542–48.
19. Helm P, Tseng HJ, Younes L, et al. Ex vivo 3D diffusion tensor imaging and quantification of cardiac laminar structure. Magn Reson Med 2005; 54:850–9.
20. Hren RA. Realistic model of the human ventricular myocardium: application to the study of ectopic activation (PhD Thesis). Halifax, Nova Scotia: Dalhousie University, 1996.
21. ten Tusscher KHWJ, Mourad A, Nash MP, et al. Organization of ventricular fibrillation in the human heart: experiments and models. Exp Physiol 2009; 94:553–62.

22. Plank G, Burton RAB, Hales P, et al. Generation of histo-anatomically representative models of the individual heart: tools and application. Philos Trans R Soc Lond A 2009; 367: 2257–92.
23. Chen J, Liu W, Zhang H, et al. Regional ventricular wall thickening reflects changes in cardiac fiber and sheet structure during contraction: quantification with diffusion tensor MRI. Am J Physiol Heart Circ Physiol 2005; 289:H1898–907.
24. Moe GK, Rheinboldt WC, Abildskov JA. A computer model of atrial fibrillation. Am Heart J 1964; 67:200–20.
25. Blanc O, Virag N, Vesin J-M, et al. A computer model of human atria with reasonable computation load and realistic anatomical properties. IEEE Trans Biomed Eng 2001; 48:1229–37.
26. Jacquemet V, Virag N, Ihara Z, et al. Study of unipolar electrogram morphology in a computer model of atrial fibrillation. J Cardiovasc Electrophysiol 2003; 14:S172–9.
27. Vigmond EJ, Ruckdeschel R, Trayanova NA. Reentry in a morphologically realistic atrial model. J Cardiovasc Electrophysiol 2001; 12:1046–54.
28. Virag N, Jacquemet V, Henriquez CS, et al. Study of atrial arrhythmias in a computer model based on magnetic resonance images of human atria. Chaos 2002; 12:754–63.
29. Harrild DM, Henriquez CS. A computer model of normal conduction in the human atria. Circ Res 2000; 87:E25–36.
30. Seemann G, Hoper C, Sache FB, et al. Heterogeneous three-dimensional anatomical and electrophysiological model of human atria. Philos Trans R Soc London A 2006; 364:1465–81.
31. Sachse FB, Werner CD, Stenroos MH, et al. Modeling the anatomy of the human heart using the cryosection images of the Visible Female dataset. In: Patrias K, editor. Visible Human Project: January 1987 Through August 2000. Bethesda, MD: U.S. Dept of Health and Human Services, Public Health Service, NIH.
32. Dobrzynski H, Li J, Tellez J, Greener ID, Nikolski VP, Wright SE, Parson SH, Jones SA, Lancaster MK, Yamamoto M, Honjo H, Takagishi Y, Kodama I, Efimov IR, Billeter R, and Boyett MR. Computer Three-Dimensional Reconstruction of the Sinoatrial Node. Circulation 111: 846–854, 2005.
33. Li J, Greener ID, Inada S, Nikolski VP, Yamamoto M, Hancox JC, Zhang H, Billeter R, Efimov IR, Dobrzynski H, and Boyett MR. Computer Three-Dimensional Reconstruction of the Atrioventricular Node. Circulation Research 102: 975–985, 2008.
34. Tung L. A biodomain model for describing ischemic myocardial DC potentials (PhD Thesis). MIT, 1978.
35. Kleber AG, Rudy Y. Basic mechanisms of cardiac impulse propagation and associated arrhythmias. Physiol Rev 2004; 84:431–88.
36. Buist ML, Sands GB, Hunter PJ, et al. A deformable finite element derived finite difference method for cardiac activation problems. Ann Biomed Eng 2003; 31:577–88.
37. Harrild DM, Henriquez CS. A finite volume model of cardiac propagation. Ann Biomed Eng 1997; 25:315–34.
38. Trew M, LeGrice I, Smaill B, et al. A finite volume method for modeling discontinuous electrical activation in cardiac tissue. Ann Biomed Eng 2005; 33:590–602.
39. Colli Franzone P, Guerri L, Pennacchio M, et al. Spread of excitation in 3D models of anisotropic cardiac tissue. II. Effects of fiber fiber architecture and ventricular geometry. Math Biosci 1998; 147:131–71.
40. Shaw R, Rudy Y. Ionic mechanisms of propagation in cardiac tissue. Roles of the sodium and L-type calcium currents during reduced excitability and decreased gap junction coupling. Circ Res 1997; 81:727–41.
41. Spach MS, Heidlage JF. The stochastic nature of cardiac propagation at a microscopic level: electrical description of myocardial architecture and its application to conduction. Circ Res 1995; 76:366–80.
42. Kucera JP, Rudy Y. Mechanistic insights into very slow conduction in branching cardiac tissue: a model study. Circ Res 2001; 89:799–806.
43. Rohr S, Schölly D, Kléber A. Patterned growth of neonatal rat heart cells in culture: morphological and electrophysiological characterization. Circ Res 1991; 68:114–30.

44. Pertsov AM. Scale of geometric structures responsible for discontinuous propagation in myocardial tissue. In: Spooner P, Joyner R, Jalife J, editors. Discontinuous conduction in the heart. Armonk, NY: Futura Publishing Company, 1997.

45. Tanaka K, Zlochiver S, Vikstrom KL, et al. Spatial distribution of fibrosis governs fibrillation wave dynamics in the posterior left atrium during heart failure. Circ Res 2007; 101:839–47.

46. ten Tusscher KH, Hren R, Panifilov AV. Organization of ventricular fibrillation in the human heart. Circ Res 2007; 100:e87–101.

47. Krogh-Madsen T, Christini DJ. Action potential duration dispersion and alternans in simulated heterogeneous cardiac tissue with a structural barrier. Biophys J 2007; 92:1138–49.

48. Clayton R, Taggart P. Regional differences in APD restitution can initiate wavebreak and re-entry in cardiac tissue: a computational study. Biomed Eng 2005; 4:54.

49. Weiss J, Karma A, Shiferaw Y, et al. From pulsus to pulseless: the saga of cardiac alternans. Circ Res 2006; 98:1244–53.

50. Wikswo JP, Lin, SF, Abbas, RA. Virtual electrodes in cardiac tissue: a common mechanism for anodal and cathodal stimulation. Biophys J 1995; 69:2195–210.

51. Weidmann S. Electrical constants of trabecular muscle for mammalian heart. J Physiol 1970; 210:1041–54.

52. Plonsey R, Barr R. Effect of microscopic and macroscopic discontinuities on the response of cardiac tissue to defibrillating (stimulating) currents. Med Biol Eng Comput 1986; 24:130–6.

53. Zhou X, Knisley S, Smith W, et al. Spatial changes in the transmembrane potential during extracellular electric stimulation. Circ Res 1998; 83:1003–14.

54. Sobie EA, Susil RC, Tung L. A generalized activating function for predicting virtual electrodes in cardiac tissue. Biophys J 1997; 73:1410–23.

55. Trayanova N, Skouibine K. Modeling defibrillation: effects of fiber curvature. J Electrocardiol 1998; 31(Suppl):23–9.

56. Hooks D, Trew M, LeGrice I, et al. Evidence that intramural virtual electrodes facilitate successful fibrillation: do transmural boundaries obscure the view? J Cardiovasc Electrophysiol 2006; 17:305–11.

57. Efimov I, Gray R, Roth B. Virtual electrodes and deexcitation: new insights into fibrillation induction and defibrillation. J Cardiovasc Electrophysiol 2000; 11:339–53.

58. Lin S, Roth B, Wikswo J. Quatrefoil reentry in myocardium: an optical imaging study of the induction mechanism. J Cardiovasc Electrophysiol 1999; 10:574–86.

59. Hunter PJ, McNaughton PA, Noble D. Analytical models of propagation in excitable cells. Prog Biophys Mol Biol 1975; 30:99–144.

60. Caldwell BJ, Trew ML, Sands GB, et al. Three distinct directions of intramural activation reveal nonuniform side-to-side electrical coupling of ventricular myocytes. Circ Arrhythm Electrophysiol 2009; 2:433–40.

61. Hooks DA, Trew ML, Caldwell BJ, et al. Laminar arrangement of ventricular myocytes influences electrical behavior of the heart. Circ Res 2007; 107:e103–12.

62. Sharifov O, Fast V. Intramural virtual electrodes in ventricular wall: effects on epicardial polarizations. Circulation 2004; 109:2349–56.

63. Sharifov O, Ideker R, Fast V. High-resolution optical mapping of intramural virtual electrodes in porcine left ventricular wall. Cardiovasc Res 2004; 64:448–56.

64. Colli Franzone P, Guerri L, Taccardi B. Potential distributions generated by point stimulation in a myocardial volume: simulation studies in a model of anisotropic ventricular muscle. J Cardiovasc Electrophysiol 1993; 4:438–58.

65. Muzikant AL, Hsu EW, Wolf PD, et al. Region specific modeling of cardiac muscle: comparison of simulated and experimental potentials. Ann Biomed Eng 2002; 30:867–83.

66. Colli Franzone P, Guerri L, Taccardi B. Modeling ventricular activation: axial and orthotropic anisotropy effects on wavefronts and potentials. Math Biosci 2004; 188:191–205.

67. Panfilov A. Modeling of re-entrant patterns in an anatomical model of the heart. In: Panfilov A, Holden A, editors. Computational Biology of the Heart. Chichester, UK: Wiley, 1997:259–76.

68. Panfilov AV. Three-dimensional organization of electrical turbulence in the heart. Phys Rev E 1999; 59:R6251–4.

69. Panfilov AV, Pertsov AM. Ventricular fibrillation: evolution of the multiple wavelet hypothesis. Philos Trans R Soc London A 2001; 359:1315–25.
70. ten Tusscher K, Noble D, Noble P, et al. A model for human ventricular tissue. Am J Physiol Heart Circ Physiol 2004; 286:H1573–89.
71. Nash MP, Bradley CP, Sutton PM, et al. Whole heart action potential duration restitution properties in cardiac patients: a combined clinical and modelling study. Exp Physiol 2006; 9:339–54.
72. Clayton RH, Panfilov AV. A guide to modelling cardiac electrical activity in anatomically detailed ventricles. Prog Biophys Mol Biol 2008; 96:19–43.
73. Keldermann RH, Ten Tusscher KHWJ, Nash MP, et al. A computational study of mother rotor VF in the human ventricles. Am J Physiol Heart Circ Physiol 2009; 296:H370–9.
74. Trayanova N. Defibrillation of the heart: insights into mechanisms from modelling studies. Exp Physiol 2006; 91:323–37.
75. Eason J, Malkin RA. A simulation study evaluating the performance of high-density electrode arrays on myocardial tissue. IEEE Trans Biomed Eng 2000; 47:893–901.
76. Rodríguez B, Li L, Eason JC, et al. Differences between left and right ventricular chamber geometry affect cardiac vulnerability to electric shocks. Circ Res 2005; 97:168–75.
77. Dang L, Virag N, Ihara Z, et al. Evaluation of ablation patterns using a biophysical model of atrial fibrillation. Ann Biomed Eng 2005; 33:465–74.
78. Nygren A, Fiset C, Firek L, et al. Mathematical model of an adult human atrial cell: the role of K^+ currents in repolarization. Circ Res 1998; 82:63–81.
79. Fenton FH, Cherry EM, Ehrlich JR, et al. A simulation study of atrial fibrillation initiation: differences in resting membrane potential can produce spontaneous activation at the pulmonary vein-left atrial junction. Heart Rhythm 2004; 1:S187–88.
80. Fenton FH, Karma A. Vortex dynamics in three-dimensional continuous myocardium with fiber rotation: filament instability and fibrillation. Chaos 1998; 8:20–47.
81. Zhao J, Trew M, LeGrice I, et al. A tissue specific model of reentry in the right atrial appendage. J Cardiovasc Electrophysiol 2009; 20:675–84.
82. Courtemanche M, Ramirez RJ, Nattel S. Ionic mechanisms underlying human atrial action potential properties: insights from a mathematical model. Am J Physiol Heart Circ Physiol 1998; 275:H301–21.
83. Luo CH, Rudy Y. A model of the ventricular cardiac action potential. Depolarization, repolarization, and their interaction. Circ Res 1991; 68:1501–26.
84. Becker R, Bauer A, Metz S, et al. Intercaval block in normal canine hearts: role of the terminal crest. Circ Res 2001; 103:2521–6.
85. Cosío F. The right atrium as an anatomic set-up for re-entry: electrophysiology goes back to anatomy. Heart 2002; 88:325–7.
86. Smaill B, LeGrice I, Hooks D, et al. Cardiac structure and electrical activation: models and measurement. Clin Exp Pharmacol Physiol 2004; 31:913–9.

Chapter 9
Detection and Measurement
of Cardiac Ion Channels

**Gwilym M. Morris, Mark R. Boyett, Joseph Yanni, Rudolf Billeter,
and Halina Dobrzynski**

Abstract Since the 1950s, technological advances have forged molecular biology
into one of the most powerful fields of science. The primary molecular specializations of the cardiac conduction system are a lower expression of the fast Na^+
channel ($Na_v1.5$), the background K^+ channel ($K_{ir}2.1$), and the high conductance
connexin (Cx43), but with a higher expression of the pacemaker channel (HCN4)
and the alternative L-type Ca^{2+} channel ($Ca_v1.3$). Therefore, it is possible to investigate gene transcription and protein expression for these channels. This chapter
describes the use of *in situ* hybridization, qPCR, and immunohistochemistry to
study cardiac ion channel expression.

Abbreviations

BCIP	5-bromo-4-chloro-3-indolyl phosphate
BSA	bovine serum albumin
$Ca_v1.3$	L-type Ca^{2+} channel in the heart, mainly found in the cardiac conduction system
cDNA	complementary DNA
CT	critical threshold
Cx43	main gap junction channel in the heart
DAPI	4′,6-diamidino-2-phenylindole
DNA	deoxyribonucleic acid
DNAse	deoxyribonuclease
EDTA	ethylenediaminetetraacetic acid
FITC	fluorescein isothiocyanate
HCN4	main ion channel responsible for the pacemaker current in the heart, I_f
IgG	immunoglobulin G
IgM	immunoglobulin M

H. Dobrzynski (✉)
Cardiovascular Medicine, School of Medicine, University of Manchester, Manchester, UK
e-mail: halina.dobrzynski@manchester.ac.uk

D.C. Sigg et al. (eds.), *Cardiac Electrophysiology Methods and Models*,
DOI 10.1007/978-1-4419-6658-2_9, © Springer Science+Business Media, LLC 2010

$K_{ir}2.1$	inward rectifier K^+ channel, responsible for the resting potential in the heart
mRNA	messenger RNA
$Na_v1.5$	cardiac Na^+ channel
N-BT	nitro blue tetrazolium
OCT	optimal cutting temperature compound
PBS	phosphate-buffered saline
PFA	paraformaldehyde
PVA	polyvinylalcohol
qPCR	quantitative polymerase chain reaction
RNA	ribonucleic acid
RNAse	ribonuclease
rRNA	ribosomal RNA
RyR2	sarcoplasmic reticulum Ca^{2+} release channel in heart
SSC	sodium chloride and sodium citrate solution
T_m	melting temperature
UTP	uridine-5′-triphosphate

9.1 Introduction

William Astbury first coined the term "molecular biology" in 1950 and, in the intervening six decades, advances in technology have forged molecular biology into one of the most powerful fields of science.[1] We have applied molecular biology techniques (namely *in situ* hybridization and quantitative polymerase chain reaction or qPCR) along with immunohistochemistry to elucidate: (1) the molecular details of the cardiac conduction system and its surrounding working myocardium; (2) how a unique pattern of expression of ion channels, connexins, and Ca^{2+}-handling proteins imparts the specialized functions of these tissues; and (3) how this expression pattern may change in response to cardiac diseases and cause cardiac arrhythmias.[2-7] The primary molecular specializations of the cardiac conduction system are a lower expression of the fast Na^+ channel ($Na_v1.5$), the background K^+ channel ($K_{ir}2.1$), and the high conductance connexin (Cx43), but with a higher expression of the pacemaker channel (HCN4) and the alternative L-type Ca^{2+} channel ($Ca_v1.3$). It is possible to investigate gene transcription and protein expression for these channels. The presence of messenger ribonucleic acid (mRNA) indicates gene transcription; mRNA can be detected using *in situ* hybridization and qPCR. It must be remembered that post-transcriptional regulation may prevent the translation of the mRNA and, therefore, it is necessary to test for the presence of the protein; this can be achieved, for example, by immunohistochemistry. This chapter describes the use of *in situ* hybridization, qPCR, and immunohistochemistry to study cardiac ion channel expression.

9.2   Apparatus

There is a plethora of commercially available equipment, kits, and reagents for the techniques described in this chapter. The ones described here have proved effective for our purpose; however, others may be equivalent. For qPCR, we use the ABI 7900 HT system (Applied Biosystems, Foster City, CA, USA). For visualization of the immunohistochemistry results, a confocal laser scanning microscope is optimal such as the LSM5 PASCAL (Carl Zeiss, Inc., Thornwood, NY, USA). Where we use specific kits or reagents, this is mentioned in the text.

9.3   Methodology and Pitfalls

9.3.1   In Situ Hybridization with Digoxigenin-Labelled RNA Probes

This method is used to show the distribution of mRNAs (e.g., for ion channels) in tissue sections; it localizes an mRNA by the use of complementary probes carrying a label that permits their detection. The focus of this chapter is a method using digoxigenin-labelled RNA probes, which we have found is the most successful method for localizing ion channel mRNAs in cardiac tissue. This method is semi-quantitative, but is remarkably sensitive. There are a number of excellent review articles detailing alternative methods,[8] as well as methods allowing quantitative analysis.[9] Additionally, there are a number of companies that sell kits for some steps of this method (e.g., Ambion, Applied Biosystems). The method using digoxigenin-labelled RNA probes is shown schematically in Fig. 9.1, and it involves four major steps:

1. *Hybridization.* Pretreated tissue is incubated with excess digoxigenin-labelled RNA probe in conditions that drive specific hybrid formation. The probe consists of a stretch (or stretches) of RNA that are complementary to the target RNA to be localized. It is labelled with digoxigenin attached to deoxyuridines in the probe RNA (Fig. 9.1a).
2. *Ribonuclease A (RNAse A) digestion (optional).* Non-hybridized probe (not bound to the target RNA) and single-stranded portions of other RNAs are digested by RNAse A. This enzyme cuts single-stranded RNA (i.e., excess digoxigenin-labelled probe) and leaves double-stranded RNA (i.e., probe/target hybrids) intact. This step reduces non-specific background (Fig. 9.1c).
3. *Incubation with labelled anti-digoxigenin antibody.* After washing away the remaining fragments of the excess probe with a specific wash and blocking of non-specific protein-binding sites, phosphatase-labelled anti-digoxigenin Fab is applied, which binds digoxigenin with high specificity and affinity (Fig. 9.1d).

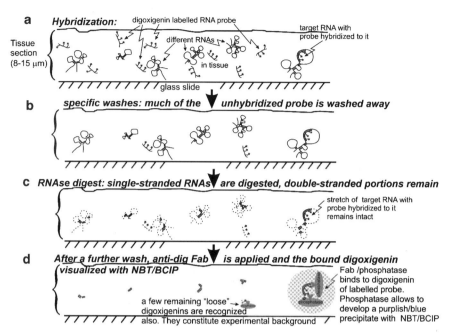

Fig. 9.1 Principle steps of *in situ* hybridization. See text for further details. *BCIP* 5-bromo-4-chloro-3-indolyl phosphate, *NBT* nitro blue tetrazolium

4. *Development of signal.* Phosphatase, bound to the double-stranded probe/target hybrids via the anti-digoxigenin Fab, generates a purple-blue precipitate from BCIP (5-bromo-4-chloro-3-indolyl phosphate; Roche, Basel, Switzerland) and N-BT (nitro blue tetrazolium, Roche). High concentrations of polyvinylalcohol (PVA) increase virtual concentrations of the precipitants and thus the signal.

9.3.1.1 Protocol Details

Our protocol for *in situ* hybridization[2] was adapted from Braissant and Wahli,[10] and the individual steps are as follows:

1. Cut 8–15 μm cryostat sections and apply them to Superfrost Plus slides.
2. Fix in 4% paraformaldehyde (PFA) in phosphate-buffered saline (PBS) for 10 min at room temperature.
3. Incubate twice in 0.25% acetic anhydride in 0.1-M triethanolamine (pH 8) for 10 min each time.
4. Incubate in 5× sodium chloride and sodium citrate solution (SSC; 20× SSC is 3-M NaCl and 0.3-M Na-citrate solution, pH 7) for 15 min.
5. Prehybridize for 2 h in 50% formamide, 5× SSC and 40 μg/ml sheared herring sperm DNA at 58°C in a sealed moist chamber.
6. Hybridize for 12–72 h in 50% formamide, 5× SSC, 40 μg/ml sheared herring sperm DNA and 0.3 ng/μl digoxigenin-labelled probe at 58°C in a sealed moist chamber.
7. Incubate in 2× SSC at room temperature for 30 min.

8. Incubate in 2× SSC at 65°C for 1 h.
9. Incubate in 0.1× SSC at 65°C for 1 h.
10. Digest with 0.5 µg/ml RNAse A (Sigma-Aldrich, St. Louis, MO, USA) in 2× SSC at 37°C for 30 min.
11. Incubate twice in 2× SSC for 5 min each time.
12. Incubate in 20% formamide and 0.5× SSC at 60°C for 10 min.
13. Incubate twice in 2× SSC for 5 min each time.
14. Incubate in dig buffer 1 (100-mM Tris, 150-mM NaCl, pH 7.5) for 5 min.
15. Block in dig buffer 1 with 1% blocking reagent (Roche) for 1 h.
16. Incubate in dig buffer 1, 1% blocking reagent and anti-dig Fab-phosphatase (1:5000) for 2 h.
17. Incubate twice in dig buffer 1 for 15 min each time.
18. Incubate in dig buffer 3 (100-mM Tris, 100-mM NaCl, 50-mM $MgCl_2$, pH 9.5) for 5 min.
19. Develop signal in dig buffer 3, 10% PVA (Sigma), 0.2-mM N-BT (Roche) and 0.2-mM BCIP (Roche) for between 10 min and 36 h at room temperature in darkness.
20. Stop color reaction by washing 3× in 0.1-M Tris and 1-mM ethylenediaminetetraacetic acid (EDTA; pH 8).
21. Embed in Kaiser's gelatin.

Crucial aspects of the individual steps are discussed below:

Pretreatment (Steps 1–4). For cardiac tissue, cryostat sections of 8–15 µm thickness have proven to be good for *in situ* hybridization. Immediate formaldehyde fixation gives the best results; however, the sections can be stored at −80°C. For such stored sections, we obtain improved signals if we take them through the equivalent of an antigen retrieval step by microwaving in diluted citrate buffer after the acetic anhydride (step 3). The reader should be aware that acetic anhydride is not stable in water and must be prepared fresh. In our hands, incubation in acetic anhydride instead of diethyl pyrocarbonate, as in the original protocol from Braissant and Wahli,[10] produces the same results, but it is easier to make up and less toxic.

Prehybridization and hybridization (steps 5 and 6). Hybridization (step 6) is carried out in 50% formamide and 5× SSC with DNA carrier (sheared herring sperm) for 12–72 h at 58°C (or at the melting temperature, T_m, minus 25°C, if this difference is lower than 58°C). We have not tested higher hybridization temperatures, but suggest that these might be problematic. Tissue sections (especially skeletal and cardiac muscle) can easily be detached. Fifty percent formamide and 5× SSC as the hybridization buffer yields better signal-to-noise ratios than hybridization buffers containing Denhardts, but it necessitates prehybridization with hybridization buffer-lacking probe, to reduce background (step 5). It is of paramount importance that the slides do not dry out during hybridization. Therefore, during hybridization, the sections are covered with a small piece of Parafilm and kept in a moist chamber containing tissue soaked in hybridization buffer (without probe) sealed with broad Tesa tape.

Washes and RNAse A digestion (steps 7–13). The most specific wash is in 0.1× SSC at 65°C (or T_m minus 15°C, if this difference results in a value lower than 60°C; step 9).

An RNAse A digestion step (step 10) distinctly reduces non-specific background. There is a danger of contaminating the laboratory with low level RNAse, therefore, we use a separate set of Coplin jars, beakers, and pipettes for the RNAse A step and the ensuing washes.

Visualization of bound digoxigenin-labelled probes (steps 14–21). The blocker sold by Roche (blocking reagent, 1096176) reduces background in comparison to serum, probably due to non-specific binding of the Fab by serum (step 15). Development of the N-BT precipitate in buffer containing 10% PVA (step 19) gives better results.[11] Polyvinylalcohol leads to an increased signal by several fold (up to 20×). Preparation of incubation buffer with 10% PVA is difficult and requires heating the buffer to boiling point in a microwave and adding small amounts of PVA under constant stirring. Re-heating is required to keep the solution close to boiling point, and water that evaporates during this process must be regularly replaced. Constant stirring must continue while the solution cools to room temperature, before the addition of N-BT (freshly dissolved in 70% dimethylformamide) and BCIP (freshly dissolved in 100% dimethylformamide). Development of signal (purple-blue) is performed for 10 min (strong signals, such as 28S rRNA) to 48 h (weak signals) at room temperature in darkness. For the majority of mRNAs, over-night incubation is sufficient. Development of the signal can be checked under a microscope and the reaction stopped when required. After incubation in stop buffer (step 20), we embed the sections in Kaiser's gelatin, and the signal is stable for many years. An example of an *in situ* hybridized section is shown in Fig. 9.2.

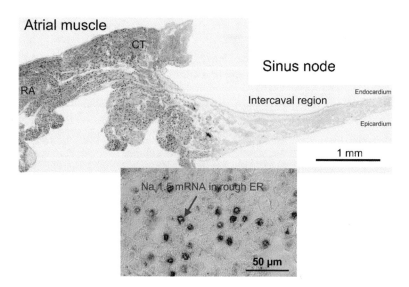

Fig. 9.2 *In situ* hybridization – mRNA for the Na[+] channel (Na$_v$1.5). This is the distribution of mRNA for the cardiac Na[+] channel (Na$_v$1.5) in a section through the rabbit sinus node and its surrounding atrial muscle as revealed by *in situ* hybridization. *Dark spots* indicate Na$_v$1.5 mRNA labelling in the rough endoplasmic reticulum (ER). There is abundant Na$_v$1.5 mRNA in the atrial muscle; in contrast, there is no Na$_v$1.5 mRNA in the sinus node. *CT* crista terminalis, *RA* right atrium. Modified from Tellez et al.[2]

9.3.1.2 Generation of Digoxigenin-Labelled RNA Probes

In situ hybridization requires probes (analogous to antibodies in immunohisto-chemistry). Compared to the other approaches discussed here, *in situ* hybridization is laborious, because each probe must be generated individually. This, together with a fair number of potential pitfalls, is the reason why *in situ* hybridization is not widely used. This section outlines the major steps in probe generation (outlined in Fig. 9.3).

9.3.1.3 Probe Design

Probe design is probably the most important step in *in situ* hybridization. A good probe must be complementary only to the target RNA. Genome sequences are available in public databases for a large number of species and, therefore, the specificities of probes can be assessed by BLAST searches (http://blast.ncbi.nlm.nih.gov/Blast.cgi). It is easier to BLAST against a complete set of mRNAs; BLASTs against whole genomes often reveal stretches of complementarities in non-coding regions, which should not interfere. However, genomic repeat sequences (e.g., alu-repeats) should be avoided. Furthermore, if the target sequence has closely related isoforms (e.g., α- or β-myosin heavy chains), the design of an isoform-specific probe can be difficult. In this situation,

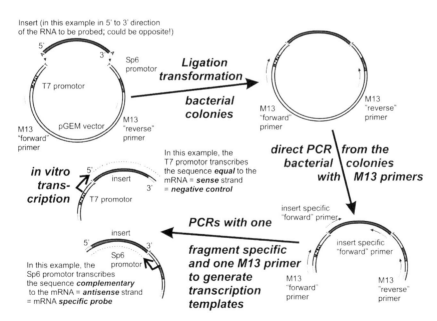

Fig. 9.3 Probe generation for *in situ* hybridization. PCR fragments are used to generate digoxigenin-labelled RNA probes. To generate complementary RNA, the fragments are subcloned in a vector between a T7 and a Sp6 promoter. From these subclones, specific fragments are isolated by PCR that contain either only the Sp6 promoter and the fragment in a given orientation or only the T7 promoter and the fragment. This allows *in vitro* transcription of the sequence complementary to the target RNA (antisense strand-specific probe) or equal to the target RNA (sense strand-negative control)

the probe should be long enough to allow hybridization to the target at 50°C while 25°C below the T_m (i.e., the probe T_m should be at least 75°C), but chosen such that the cross hybridization to the RNAs of the other isoforms is not above the hybridization temperature (i.e., ~50°C or below). The T_m can be estimated as:

$$T_m(\text{RNA/RNA}) = 78°C + 16.6 \times \log_{10}([\text{Na}^+]/(1.0 + 0.7[\text{Na}^+])) + 0.7 \times (\%\text{GC})$$
$$- 0.35 \times (\%\text{formamide}) - 500/(\text{duplex-length}) \qquad (9.1)$$

where $[\text{Na}^+]$ is the molar Na^+ concentration, %GC is the percentage of G and C in the sequence of the hybrid, and duplex-length is the length of the hybrid as a number of base pairs.

9.3.1.4   Probe Length

We have not observed reduced signals with probes of up to 500 bases long; however, probes with many strong secondary structures tend to give more background. A better signal-to-noise ratio is achieved when a greater sequence length of a RNA is covered; this can be achieved using several non-overlapping probes. Using this technique, we have obtained better signals when compared to using individual probes alone. Given that RNA in tissue is in a folded state and stabilized by RNA binding proteins, it is unlikely that the relationship between percentage "coverage" of a RNA by different probes and the signal obtained is linear. This adds an element of chance to probe design.

9.3.1.5   Generation of Probe

Digoxigenin-labelled RNA probes are generated by *in vitro* transcription using RNA polymerases (Sp6, T7, T3) and a given percentage of UTP carrying a digoxigenin label (usually 25%). Probe templates, therefore, contain an RNAse polymerase promoter (Sp6, T7, T3) linked to the probe sequence. One approach to template generation is subcloning the probe into a vector that carries RNA polymerase promotors at either side of the insert (for example, the Promega pGEM®-T kit, Madison, WI, USA; Fig. 9.3). This allows the generation of a labelled probe that is complementary to the RNA of choice to hybridize (antisense probe) and, from the opposite promoter, the generation of a probe that is identical to the RNA of choice as a negative control (sense probe). The antisense probe should produce labelling (if the target mRNA is present), whereas the sense probe should not.

9.3.1.6   Isolation of Insert (Probe) Sequences

The most convenient way of isolating the insert (probe) sequence for insertion into the vector is often by normal PCR. The easiest source of DNA is a plasmid containing the relevant complementary DNA (cDNA) as an insert. If that is not available, the fragment can be isolated from cDNA of a tissue in which the transcript is reasonably frequent, or from genomic DNA if the sequence is contained in a single exon. There are many programs (free or commercially available) for primer design; one of the most popular is "Primer 3" (http://frodo.wi.mit.edu/primer3/). The parameters are the same as used for the design of qPCR primers (see below), except that the probe length should be 100–500 bases. When using cDNA as the source, strong RNA secondary structures should be avoided.[12] These can inhibit reverse transcriptase and thus lead to under-representations of such fragments. To predict DNA and RNA folding (and thus the secondary structures), we use "Mfold" (http://www.bioinfo.rpi.edu/applications/mfold/).

9.3.1.7 Generation of Probe Template with RNA Polymerase Promoters

Direct PCR from the bacterial colonies with M13 primers allows the isolation of fragments containing the insert linked to RNA polymerase promoters on either side. The identity of the resulting fragment can be confirmed by sequencing, nested PCR, and/or restriction endonuclease digestion. Subfragments are isolated that contain only one of the RNA polymerase promoters (Sp6 or T7) by using one of the M13 and one of the specific insert primers. This prevents hybridization of complementary vector sequences by minimizing the proportion of vector sequences in the resulting probes. These subfragments are purified from primers and nucleotides (MinElute PCR Purification Kit, Qiagen, Valencia, CA, USA) and used as templates for probe synthesis by *in vitro* transcription (see below). The scheme of Fig. 9.3 was drawn for a hypothetical probe sequence that is inserted in the 5' to 3' direction into the vector. Most PCR fragments have an equal chance of being inserted in either direction. The direction of the insert is determined by sequencing, nested PCR, or restriction endonuclease digestion. The concentration of the transcription templates is determined by agarose gel electrophoresis in comparison to a DNA marker of known concentration. Ethidium bromide fluorescence can be assessed using "Image J" (http://rsbweb.nih.gov/ij/).

9.3.1.8 In Vitro Transcription

We use the Mega-Script or Maxi-Script systems from Ambion (Applied Biosystems) and digoxigenin-11-uridine-5'triphosphate (UTP; Roche) with a ratio of unlabelled UTP/digoxigenin-labelled UTP of 4:1. T7 transcriptions result in better yields than Sp6 transcriptions. The resulting RNA probes are purified from free nucleotides by RNA cleanup (e.g., Qiagen RNeasy Micro columns). Their integrity and concentration is determined by formaldehyde gel electrophoresis in comparison with a RNA marker of known concentration using "Image J."

9.3.2   Quantitative PCR (qPCR)

The advantage of qPCR is that the abundance of a large number of mRNAs can be determined quantitatively in tissue samples. Thus, qPCR has become a routine method, with most reagents available as commercial kits. Complementary DNA derived from RNA is exponentially amplified by PCR and the generated products monitored as fluorescence generated by a compound (SyBr Green or TaqMan) bound to it. This chapter presents a procedure that works well for cardiac tissue; there are equivalent alternatives for many of the steps and this is a steadily progressing field.

9.3.2.1   Protocol Details

The procedure involves the following steps: (1) total RNA isolation from the tissue of interest; (2) determination of the quantity and quality of the RNA isolated; (3) cDNA synthesis; (4) qPCR with primers specific for the target mRNA; and (5) calculation of the relative abundance of the target mRNA.

Total RNA isolation. First, a sample of the tissue of interest must be obtained; in the case of atrial or ventricular muscle, this is straightforward. The tissue can be cut in 10–20 μm sections on a cryostat as a form of "homogenization." We work on the cardiac conduction system and the tissues are small and scattered. In two studies, we successfully obtained samples of conducting tissue uncontaminated by working myocardium. In one study,[6] we lyophilized cryosections (up to 60 μm thickness) in order to inactivate RNAses in the tissue, whereas in the second study,[5] we did not lyophilize the cryosections (30–60 μm in thickness; collected on Superfrost slides). Sections stained with quick Haematoxylin and Eosin stain were used, and the specialized tissues were microdissected by hand using a fine surgical needle under a dissecting microscope. The microdissected tissues were directly homogenized in guanidine buffer (RLT; provided in the Qiagen RNeasy Mini or Micro system).

For cardiac tissue, we isolate total RNA with the Qiagen RNeasy Mini or Micro system (for fibrous tissues with minor modifications of the manufacturer's protocol). The RNA isolation method involves digestion of the cellular proteins with proteinase K after dilution of the RLT. Following proteinase K digestion, we add an extra volume of RLT buffer to the sample in order to increase its salt content towards the original RLT concentration. Note that the larger volume necessitates the addition of proportionally more alcohol. The higher salt leads to more consistent yields when the tissue input is small. Performing a deoxyribonuclease (DNAse) digestion on the column, following the manufacturers' guidelines, reduces the genomic DNA content to a level that is several hundred to several thousand times less than the cDNA content of an average ion channel generated by the reverse transcriptase. This is not the case for mitochondrial DNA, which can still interfere in some samples even after DNAse digestion. By using Micro columns, the sample can be eluted in a smaller volume (10 µl). This is advantageous when working with small amounts of input tissue.

Determination of RNA quantity and quality. The quantity and quality of the total RNA isolated must be determined. The RNA quality can be assessed by formaldehyde gel electrophoresis or capillary electrophoresis (e.g., nano- or pico-chips from Agilent Technologies, Inc., Santa Clara, CA, USA), from which concentrations can also be derived. RNA concentrations can also be determined with Quant-iT™ RiboGreen® (Molecular probes, Invitrogen Corp., Carlsbad, CA, USA), which is advantageous for samples with low concentrations due to low input tissue. The Nano-Drop system can also be used to determine the quantity of RNA.

cDNA synthesis. cDNA is generated from the RNA by reverse transcription. There are many different RT-PCR kits offered by a variety of manufacturers. We have used the Superscript reverse transcriptases (Superscript II or III) from Invitrogen with random hexamer priming. Using the same kit allows a rough comparison of the results from different experiments, when using the same amount of total RNA. More than 90% of total RNA is rRNA (ribosomal RNA) and, therefore, it is often assumed that the ribosomal content of different samples is the same. For this reason, rRNA is often used as a housekeeper (see below). However, the assumption may not always be true, which necessitates the use of several housekeepers.

Different reverse transcriptases and different priming procedures can yield very different quantities of cDNA for the sequence stretch quantitated with a given qPCR amplicon. Figure 9.4 shows an example of two aliquots of the same skeletal muscle

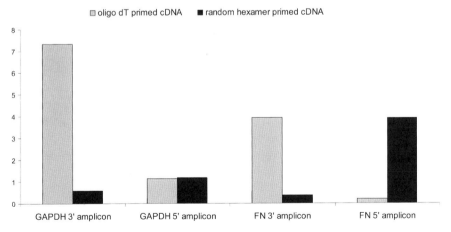

Fig. 9.4 Relative quantities of cDNA generated from aliquot of same total RNA (from rat gastrocnemius skeletal muscle). cDNA aliquots derived from equal amounts of input RNA were amplified with primer pairs specific for amplicons in the 3′ and 5′ region of GAPDH (glyceraldehyde phosphate dehydrogenase) and fibronectin (FN) on a Light Cycler (Roche) with SyBr Green detection. No primer dimers were detectable. Note the vastly different fragment proportions generated by the two different priming methods. *cDNA* complementary DNA

RNA that have been transcribed using either oligo dT priming or random hexamer priming. The relative content of cDNA fragments from the 3′ and the 5′ region of GAPDH (glyceraldehyde phosphate dehydrogenase) and fibronectin mRNA was determined by qPCR on a Light Cycler (Roche). Vastly different proportions between the fragments generated from the same mRNA were obtained; this is to be kept in mind when one tries to compare results from different studies. The increased proportion of 3′ end fragments after oligo dT priming is thought to be due to the reverse transcriptase not transcribing many RNA molecules fully. This may be due to: (1) strong RNA secondary structures[12]; (2) termination where RNA strands are cut ("nicked") by RNAse; and (3) detachment of the reverse transcriptase enzyme for other reasons.

Quantitative polymerase chain reaction. qPCR is an established technique for which many companies sell reliable equipment and reagents. However, compared to other areas of experimental biology, it is expensive. One source of expense is that many laboratories tend to carry out qPCR measurements in triplicate; we suggest that this is often not necessary. With a good pair of primers and accurate pipetting, the standard error of qPCR is between 3% and 10%. This is often smaller than the average standard error of cDNA synthesis (reverse transcription step), which is normally between 5% and 15%. Depending on the species from which the tissue yielding the RNA was derived (i.e., inbred rodent strains versus human), the inter-individual (biological) variability in the expression of a given RNA may be in or well above the range of the standard error of the reverse transcription step. Thus the additional cost of making triplicate measurements, instead of duplicate or single measurements, is often not justified. Instead, an increased number of tissue samples would enable improved detection of small differences. "Do more (samples) less well (less precisely measured)" is an old guideline from electron microscope stereology, which is also applicable to qPCR.

Calculation of the relative abundance of the target RNA – the ΔCT technique. During the qPCR, the target cDNA is amplified in an exponential fashion and, therefore, the measured fluorescence increases in an exponential fashion (Fig. 9.5a). To quantify the amount of target cDNA (and therefore the amount of target RNA) in the original sample, the critical threshold (CT) value is measured (Fig. 9.5a), i.e., the number of PCR cycles taken for the level of target cDNA and, therefore, fluorescence to reach a CT. The higher the amount of target cDNA (and therefore target RNA) in the original sample, the lower the CT value, i.e., the number of cycles to reach the CT. During each PCR cycle, the number of copies of the cDNA is ideally doubled, i.e., increased by a factor of 2; in practice the value (known as the efficiency) may be close to but less than 2 (see Fig. 9.5a for measurement of the efficiency). Note that the efficiency will vary for each target cDNA. At the CT, the amount of target cDNA is:

$$A_{t,s}E_t^{CT_t} \qquad (9.2)$$

where $A_{t,s}$ is the amount of the target cDNA in the original sample, E_t is the efficiency for the target cDNA, and CT_t is the CT value for the target cDNA.

In practice, the abundance of a target cDNA is expressed as a ratio to the abundance of a housekeeper cDNA. At the CT (same as for the target cDNA), the amount of housekeeper cDNA (h) will be:

$$A_{h,s} E_h^{CT_h} \tag{9.3}$$

At the CT, the amount of target and housekeeper cDNAs will be the same:

$$A_{t,s} E_t^{CT_t} = A_{h,s} E_h^{CT_h} \tag{9.4}$$

Rearranging (9.4) gives:

$$\frac{A_{t,s}}{A_{h,s}} = \frac{E_h^{CT_h}}{E_t^{CT_t}} \tag{9.5}$$

The abundance of the target cDNA relative to the housekeeper cDNA ($A_{t,s} / A_{h,s}$) can be calculated using (9.5).

If the abundance of a target mRNA in different samples is being compared, the amount of total RNA in the different samples reverse transcribed into cDNA should be the same; however, it is unlikely that it will be exactly the same. Calculation of the abundance of the target cDNA relative to the housekeeper cDNA has the advantage that variations in input RNA are corrected for. GAPDH, 18S and 28S rRNA, or β-actin are often used as housekeepers. A housekeeper should always be expressed at the same level. However, housekeepers are a contentious issue, because they are not always expressed at a constant level,[13] and thus this type of normalization (9.5) could introduce systematic errors. If a study involves the determination of several dozen mRNAs by qPCR, the approach described in Vandesompele et al.[14] can be used; they used an aggregate of different housekeepers. It is also our experience that an aggregate of three housekeepers leads to less variability in the calculated relative abundance of a target cDNA than a single or two housekeepers. It is, therefore, recommended to plan for three to five housekeepers when setting up a qPCR study. When performing the calculations using several housekeepers, the ratios to each of them are determined individually for each sample and then the average of these ratios is determined.

Equation (9.5) gives the relative abundance of a target cDNA. Does it give the relative abundance of the target mRNA? If the relative abundance of a single target is being compared in different samples, the answer is yes. It can be used to compare the relative abundance of *different* target mRNAs, but the results must be viewed with caution. This is because the efficiency of the reverse transcription varies for different mRNAs. Therefore, because there is a difference in the abundance of two target cDNAs does not necessarily mean that there is a difference in the abundance of the two target mRNAs. We assume that if the abundance of two target mRNAs apparently differs (in the same sample) by more than a factor of 10, then there is likely a real difference in the mRNA abundance.

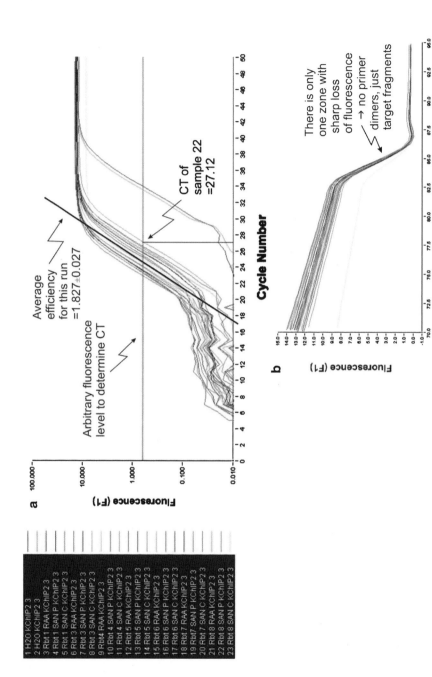

Fig. 9.5 Raw data from a qPCR run for cDNA for KChIP2 (an accessory K⁺ channel protein involved in the regulation of transient outward K⁺ channels) in 23 samples from the center (SAN C) and periphery (SAN P) of the sinus node and atrial muscle (RAA) from eight rabbits (Rbt 1-Rbt 8). (**a**) Amplification curves. During qPCR, the measured fluorescence increases as the cDNA of interest is amplified. Fluorescence is plotted on a log scale against the cycle number. Between cycles 20 and 28, the increase in fluorescence is linear on the log scale; this indicates an exponential amplification of the cDNA. The reaction runs exponentially from the beginning, but the machine can only detect the fluorescence above background beyond cycle 20. The slope of this "linear" phase is equivalent to the efficiency of this PCR. The average efficiency for all samples is shown. Critical threshold (CT) values are determined for each sample; this is the number of cycles taken for the fluorescence to reach an arbitrarily chosen fluorescence "critical threshold" in the linear zone. The CT value of sample 22 is shown. (**b**) Melting curves. To obtain a melting curve, the DNA generated during the 50 cycles of amplification is subjected to a linear rise in temperature. After a slow linear decline, there is one sudden sharp drop in fluorescence between 83 and 87°C. This indicates the separation (melting) of the two strands in the PCR amplicon, which leads to sharply diminished Sybr Green fluorescence. There is no evidence of primer dimers, which would manifest themselves in another zone of sharp fluorescence decline, generally at a lower (melting) temperature. A Light Cycler (Roche) was used

Calculation of the relative abundance of the target RNA – the ΔΔCT technique. The ΔCT technique involves a single normalization, and the ΔΔCT technique involves a double normalization. Some investigators run an identical "calibrator" sample in every run. The relative abundance of a target in a sample (calculated using (9.5)) is expressed as a ratio of its relative abundance in the calibrator (again calculated using (9.5)). The resulting ratio-of-ratios will be ~1. Because the same calibrator is used during every run, this technique allows for variations between runs. In practice, we have found that the ΔCT and ΔΔCT techniques produce similar data with similar standard errors.

Other investigators obtain "standard curves" using aliquots of the target cDNA at known concentrations. This has the advantage that the absolute abundance of a target can be determined. However, we do not obtain standard curves, because the precision of the aliquots (at very high dilutions at or below the range of most of our samples) is not sufficient.

If carefully controlled according to the above guidelines, qPCR can be remarkably precise and is able to demonstrate differences down to 10% or 20%. Figure 9.6 shows an example of qPCR data calculated using the ΔCT technique.

9.3.2.2   Primer Design

Primer design is the most important step in qPCR. One of the main problems in qPCR is primer dimer formation. Theoretically, the use of specific probes that hybridize to a given amplicon and yield a proportional fluorescent signal should ameliorate this problem. If there is much primer dimer formation, however, it can distinctly reduce the amount of fragment generated. There are many companies selling qPCR assays that should generate no dimers or few dimers for a number of species. For much of our work, we have designed the primer pairs ourselves. There are many companies selling software for primer design, but there are also publicly available programs. We use mostly "Primer 3" (http://frodo.wi.mit.edu/primer3/). When designing a primer, try to avoid:

- stretches that are homologous to other RNAs and thus could cross hybridize with a primer. These are found *in silico* by a BLAST search over the transcriptome (i.e., mRNA sequences) of the species in question.
- placing primers on either side of a stretch of a potentially strong RNA stem according to the criteria of Pallansch et al.[12] To predict RNA folding, we use "Mfold" (http://www.bioinfo.rpi.edu/applications/mfold/).
- placing a primer on an area that is potentially part of a DNA stem under the annealing conditions of the qPCR (i.e., 2 mM Mg^{2+}, 50 mM monovalent cations, 55–60°C).

In the "Primer 3" program, we do not use the default parameters; instead, we try to adhere as closely as possible to those defined by Beasley et al.[15] These are as follows:

1. amplicon size of ~ 100 base pairs;
2. ideal primer length of 23 bases;

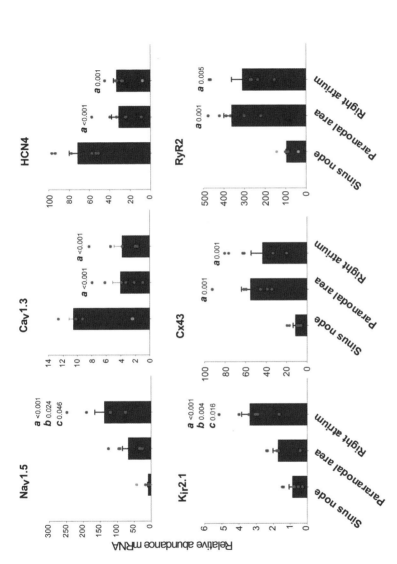

Fig. 9.6 Relative abundance of ion channel mRNAs as measured by qPCR (normalized to ribosomal 28S; ΔCT technique used) for $Na_v1.5$, $Ca_v1.3$, HCN4, $K_{ir}2.1$, Cx43, and RyR2 in human atrial muscle, paranodal area and sinus node. Mean + SEM ($n = 6$) shown. (**a**) and (**b**) Significantly different from sinus node (**a**) or paranodal area (**b**) (one-way ANOVA); (**c**) significantly different from paranodal area (paired t-test). Individual data for all six subjects are shown by the *red points* and the outliers are shown by the *grey points*. $Ca_v1.3$ = L-type Ca^{2+} channel; HCN4 = main ion channel responsible for I_f $K_{ir}2.1$ = inward rectifier K^+ channel; $Na_v1.5$ = cardiac Na^+ channel; Cx43 = main gap junction channel in the heart; RyR2 = sarcoplasmic reticulum Ca^{2+} release channel in the heart. Modified from Chandler et al.[5]

3. optimum T_m of 62°C (65°C for use in an ABI machine at a standard annealing temperature of 60°C, which is 5°C below the theoretical T_m);
4. ~50% G/C content;
5. no GC clamp; and
6. minimal 3′ self complementarity (if ever possible, choose 0).

This yields primer pairs that can be used reliably with SyBr Green detection. It is advisable, though, to use specific probes for rare transcripts or low input cDNA and for primer pairs that tend to infrequently yield primer dimers. We have seen distinct differences in primer dimer formation between different batches of same brand qPCR mixes.

9.3.3 Immunohistochemistry with Fluorescent Conjugated Secondary Antibodies

There are many excellent books, articles, and websites that explain the principle of this technique. In our laboratory, we use Smith and Burton[16] as an introduction. The principle of immunohistochemistry (shown in Fig. 9.7) is to use specific primary

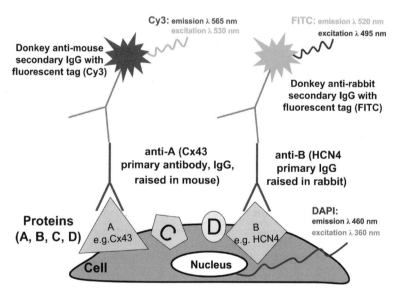

Fig. 9.7 Principle of immunofluorescence. Two primary antibodies are shown bound to their respective antigens on the surface of a cell. The anti-A primary antibody (assumed to be raised in mouse) binds to antigen A (e.g., Cx43), whereas the anti-B primary antibody (assumed to be raised in rabbit) binds to antigen B (e.g., HCN4). The primary antibody binds to the antigen with its Fab fragment. The secondary antibody normally binds to the Fc portion of the primary antibody molecule in a species-specific manner. The secondary antibody, therefore, binds to antibodies raised in a particular species (e.g., anti-mouse and anti-rabbit). The secondary antibodies contain fluorescent tags such as Cy3 and FITC (fluorescein isothiocyanate), which can be visualized using an epifluorescence or confocal laser scanning microscope

antibodies to determine the sub-cellular location of proteins of interest in tissue sections. To locate a protein of interest, the primary antibody binds specifically to the protein (the antigen) at the epitope (site on the protein at which the binding occurs). The primary antibody can then be detected by a selected secondary antibody conjugated, for example, to a fluorochrome (Fig. 9.7), which can be visualized by fluorescence microscopy. Poly- or monoclonal antibodies can be used. A polyclonal antibody is produced by injecting the protein of interest into a host laboratory animal (e.g., rabbit) and collecting serum samples. The collected serum contains antibodies to several regions of the molecule as well as other antibodies not specific to the protein. The serum is then purified to reduce non-specific binding. A monoclonal antibody is produced by hybridoma cells (a hybrid cell line that is created by fusing a mortal antibody-producing B-lymphocyte with an immortalized myeloma line; the hybridoma line is immortal and produces a continuous supply of a particular mono-clonal antibody). Hybridoma cells produce only one antibody to one region of the molecule, hence the term monoclonal. A polyclonal antibody can produce stronger labelling, because it contains multiple antibodies to several regions of the molecule. However, there is more risk of non-specific labelling with polyclonal antibodies (e.g., connective tissues seem to attract and hold antibodies non-specifically).

9.3.3.1 Protocol Details

There are seven major steps of the protocol:

1. *Preparation of tissue samples.* After dissection of a tissue sample of interest (e.g., the sinus node region of a rodent heart), the sample needs to be secured on a square of silicone rubber using insect pins or small gauge needles. The orientation of the sample is noted (e.g., by cutting a corner of the silicone) and the sample is covered in optimal cutting temperature compound (OCT) and frozen using isopentane cooled in liquid N_2 to $-152°C$. Isopentane is a cryo-protectant reagent and its use means that the tissue will only be cooled to $-152°C$ (lower temperatures will cause the tissue to crack). Please note that the tissue is not preserved in any common laboratory fixative at this stage. The sample is then stored at $-80°C$ until needed. The frozen tissue is cut using a cryostat and mounted onto microscope slides. In order to ascertain that there is good attachment of tissue sections to the microscope slides and, therefore, no loss of tissue sections during the rigorous steps of immunohistochemistry, which involves many washing steps, we use Superfrost Plus slides. For the best detection of ion channels, the sections should be 10–30 μm in thickness. The tissue sections are stored at $-80°C$ until needed.
2. *Preparation of tissue sections.* Tissue sections are taken from $-80°C$, and single, double, or triple labelling is performed. If different antibodies are to be applied to two tissue sections adjacent on a slide, the sections are separated by drawing a circle around each tissue section using a Pap Pen (water repellent), leaving a gap of ~5 mm at the edge of the tissue. This step must be performed quickly to ensure that tissue sections do not dry (a vital component of the whole protocol in order to avoid generation of unwanted background fluorescence).

3. *Fixation*. Tissue sections are fixed in 10% buffered formalin (equivalent to 4% paraformaldehyde, PFA) for 30 min and washed three times in 0.01 M phosphate-buffered saline (PBS) for 10–20 min each wash.

4. *Permeabilization and blocking of non-specific binding sites*. Tissue sections are permeabilized by treatment with 0.1% Triton X-100 for 30 min. This allows penetration of the antibodies to cytoplasmic epitopes. Following three PBS washes (10 min each time), the sections are treated with a universal blocker such as bovine serum albumin (1% BSA in 0.01 M PBS for 30 min) in order to block non-specific binding sites and reduce background fluorescence. If an antibody produces high background fluorescence, 10–20% normal serum can be added to the blocking solution. The selection of the normal serum is dictated by the host animal in which the secondary antibody was raised (e.g., if the anti-rabbit secondary antibody was raised in donkey, normal donkey serum is used).

5. *Application of primary antibodies*. Sufficient solution containing diluted primary antibody is added to cover each section within the Pap Pen ring so that a meniscus is formed. The slides are placed in a sealed humid chamber to prevent evaporation of the antibody mixture. Tissue sections are incubated with primary antibody either overnight at 4°C or at room temperature. For ion channels, tissue sections from species other than human are best incubated at 4°C overnight; for human tissue sections, we have obtained the best results with overnight incubation at room temperature.

(a) To allow exclusive binding of the secondary fluorescent conjugated antibody (see below) to the primary antibody only, the primary antibody should not have been raised in the same species as the tissue of interest. However, if no primary antibody raised in a different species is available, it is possible to use the primary antibody raised in the same species as the tissue of interest.[7] However, in this case, background fluorescence due to the secondary antibody is high and cannot be avoided. Provided that each primary antibody is raised in a different species (e.g., in our work, we may use Cx43 antibody raised in mouse, HCN4 antibody raised in goat, and $Na_v1.5$ antibody raised in rabbit) for double or triple labelling, the antibodies can be mixed and applied together in 1% BSA in 0.01 M PBS (with or without 0.1% Triton X-100). It is also possible to use primary antibodies raised in the same species in the same mixture if one is IgG (immunoglobulin G) and the other IgM (immunoglobulin M). Each antibody should be diluted to its individual optimal concentration in the final mixture; for ion channels 1 in 50 and connexins 1 in 1000 to 1 in 50, depending on the animal species used. It is important to empirically determine the optimal concentration of each primary antibody in order to obtain a good signal-to-background fluorescence ratio and to avoid non-specific staining. For example, in our hands all antibodies when used on human heart tissue are used at a dilution of 1 in 50. Figure 9.8 shows an experiment in which we applied Cx43 antibody to human right atrium at different dilutions and the strongest specific signal was obtained at a dilution of 1 in 50. Please note the diluted primary antibodies can be recycled several times. Before applying the secondary

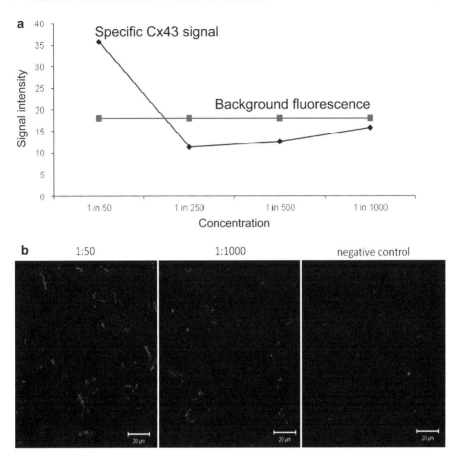

Fig. 9.8 Optimization of primary antibody concentration. (**a**) Intensity of specific Cx43 labelling (*diamonds*) and background fluorescence (*squares*) at different primary antibody dilutions. Signal intensity was measured using "Volocity" (Improvision) from images such as those in (**b**). It is concluded that a 1 in 50 dilution is the best; there is a strong specific signal related to Cx43. (**b**) Immunolabelling of Cx43 (*red signal*) in human right atrium with different primary antibody dilutions: 1 in 50 (*left*) and 1 in 1,000 (*middle*). In the "negative control" (*right*), the primary antibody was omitted. The Cx43 antibody (IgG) used was raised in rabbit and the anti-rabbit secondary antibody (IgG) used was raised in donkey and conjugated to Cy3. The images were captured using a confocal laser scanning microscope (Zeiss LSM5 PASCAL). From Ms. Mary-Anne Taube, medical student at the University of Manchester (unpublished data)

antibody solution the following day, the unbound primary antibodies should be thoroughly washed away with three to four washes in 1 × PBS for 10 min each.

(b) Over the years, we have successfully applied primary antibodies from the following companies to cardiac tissue: Alomone Labs, Sigma, Chemicon, Cambridge Bioscience, BD Biosciences, Invitrogen, Badrilla, Molecular Probes, Santa Cruz, Cell Signalling, Affinity BioReagents, Biogenesis, Progen and DSHB (Developmental Studies Hybridoma Bank).

Table 9.1 Excitation and emission spectra of commonly used fluorochromes

Fluorochrome	Absorption peak (nm)	Emission peak (nm)
Fluorescein, FITC	495	520
Indocarbocyanine, Cy3	530	565
Indodicarbocyanine, Cy5	650	670

FITC fluorescein isothiocyanate

6. *Application of secondary antibodies.* Sufficient solution containing diluted secondary antibody is added to cover each section within the Pap Pen ring. It might be necessary to reapply the Pap Pen following the washes. The tissue sections are incubated with the secondary antibody for 1–2 h. The secondary antibodies are reconstituted according to the manufacturer's instructions and then diluted in 1% BSA in 0.01 M PBS to their working concentration.

   (a) The secondary antibody binds to the primary antibody with specificity for species and immunoglobulin type, e.g., if the primary antibody is IgG raised in rabbit, the secondary antibody will be anti-rabbit IgG and if the primary antibody is IgM raised in mouse, the secondary antibody will be anti-mouse IgM. The secondary antibody is conjugated to a fluorochrome, which enables the visualization of the bound antibody using epifluorescence or confocal laser scanning microscopy (Table 9.1).

   (b) As previously stated, it is possible to label more than one protein in a tissue sample by using primary antibodies raised in different species or antibodies of different immunoglobulin types. Secondary antibodies can be selected to have differing excitation and emission spectra (Table 9.1). For example, a triple labelling experiment on a tissue section cut through the atrial muscle and sinus node of the human heart could involve labelling an ion channel (e.g., HCN4, labelled with anti-HCN4 IgG raised in rabbit), a connexin (e.g., Cx43, labelled with anti-Cx43 IgG raised in mouse), and a Ca^{2+}-handling protein (e.g., NCX1, the Na^+-Ca^{2+} exchanger, labelled with anti-NCX1 IgM raised in mouse). The secondary antibodies applied are then anti-rabbit IgG conjugated to fluorescein isothiocyanate (FITC), anti-mouse IgG conjugated to Cy3, and anti-mouse IgM conjugated to Cy5. Each can be viewed separately by confocal laser scanning microscopy using different excitation lasers and band pass filter sets (Table 9.1). There are many companies that specialize in secondary antibodies. In our laboratory, we routinely use affinity purified and absorbed secondary antibodies from Chemicon (Millipore, Billerica, MA, USA) and Molecular Probes (Invitrogen). Figures 9.9 and 9.10 show two examples of multiple labelling immunohistochemical experiments.

7. *Mounting and storage.* To avoid photo-bleaching during scanning, we recommend mounting the tissue sections in Vectashield mounting medium (seal the edges of the cover slips with nail varnish). Mounting medium is available without or with propidium iodide or 4′,6-diamidino-2-phenylindole (DAPI), if nuclear staining is

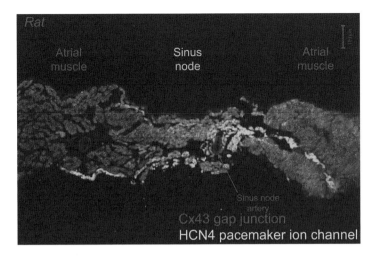

Fig. 9.9 The distribution of Cx43 (*red signal*) and HCN4 (*green signal*) in the rat sinus node as revealed by immunohistochemistry. The primary antibodies used were mouse anti-Cx43 IgG and rabbit anti-HCN4 IgG; the secondary antibodies were donkey anti-mouse IgG conjugated to Cy3 and donkey anti-rabbit IgG conjugated to FITC. The image was captured using a confocal laser scanning microscope (Zeiss LSM5 PASCAL). Cx43 (the major gap junction channel in the heart) is abundant in the atrial muscle; Cx43 is located at the intercalated disc. In the sinus node, Cx43 is absent, but HCN4 (the major ion channel responsible for the pacemaker current, I_f, in the sinus node) is abundant; HCN4 is located at the cell membrane. From Dr. J. Yanni (unpublished data)

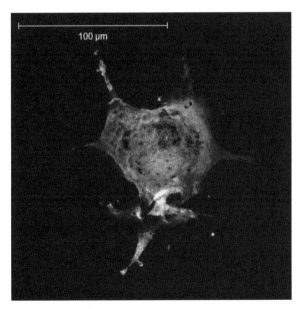

Fig. 9.10 Adenovirus mediated expression of HCN4 in a Cos7 cell. Cos7 cells were infected with a recombinant adenovirus (Ad5-GFP-HCN4) containing an internal ribosomal entry site allowing the expression of green fluorescent protein (GFP) and HCN4 under the control of the same CMV promoter. The cell was labelled with a primary antibody to HCN4 (mouse anti-HCN4 IgG) and a secondary antibody (donkey anti-mouse IgG conjugated to Cy3). HCN4 labelling is indicated by the *red signal*. The nucleus was stained using DAPI (*blue signal*); the GFP gives the *green signal*. The image was captured using a confocal laser scanning microscope (Zeiss LSM5 PASCAL)

required. Propidium iodide has a wide excitation range, peaking around 535 nm, and emits red fluorescence at 615 nm when bound to DNA, whereas peak excitation for DAPI is 360 nm with emission at 460 nm, producing a blue fluorescence when bound to DNA (e.g., Fig. 9.10). Due to the instability of fluorochromes, immuno-fluorescence signals should be captured as soon as the experiment is finished, but if this is not possible, the tissue sections should be stored in the dark at 4°C until use. The intensity of signals (above background fluorescence) can be measured using "Volocity" (Improvision, Waltham, MA, USA) or equivalent software.

9.4   New Emerging Techniques

9.4.1   Laser Capture Microdissection

The tissues making up the cardiac conduction system are small and scattered throughout the heart. Collection of the cardiac conduction system tissues for analysis is difficult; previously, we have microdissected the tissues by hand.[5] Laser capture microdissection allows the semi-automated collection of defined groups of cells or even individual cells.[17] Cryosections are applied onto special slides (e.g., from Leica, Germany) and stained, generally with histochemical stains such as Haematoxylin and Eosin; however, tissue sections can be immunolabelled under RNAse inhibiting conditions. The desired regions or cells are then cut out by a guided laser beam under a microscope, and total RNA can then be collected from the tissue. This procedure yields less RNA than the ones described above, but advances in the quality of cDNA synthesis kits combined with the extraordinary amplification power of PCR enable the quantitation of rare RNA species. For very small amounts of RNA isolated from individual single cells, cDNA amplification is normally used. The drawback with this procedure is that during the application of the section to the slide, the section thaws which, temporarily until inhibitors are applied, allows RNAse activity, as do staining steps in some of the protocols. This is difficult to control. Laser capture microdissection (plus qPCR) can complement *in situ* hybridization, because it is quantitative, whereas *in situ* hybridization is semi-quantitative at best.

9.4.2   qPCR Arrays

Modern experimental biology pays more and more homage to the complexities of cellular regulatory networks. The recognition that a measurable physiological change is accompanied by a myriad of changes in gene expression in the cells of the tissues affected has increased the demand for larger, more encompassing data sets to describe such changes. This is possible for the investigation of gene expression changes in the form of microarrays. Microarrays are sold by a number of companies, however, they are all noisy, i.e., the results have large standard errors, especially in the case of mRNAs expressed at a low level (which is true in the case of ion channels), and they require larger amounts of RNA or cDNA. qPCR arrays require much less input (i.e., cDNA generated from RNA) and are more precise. There are a number of companies that sell qPCR arrays with tried and tested qPCR reactions already in the wells. These come as 96 or 384 well plates (e.g., SABiosciences, Frederick, MD, USA) or microfluidics cards (TaqMan arrays, Applied Biosystems) with either a given set of qPCR reactions or a set of reactions chosen by the user from a large collection (in the case of Applied Biosystems, currently 47,000). These qPCR primers and probes are chosen such that they all work well under identical cycling conditions. There are also qPCR arrays for micro-RNAs. A big advantage of qPCR arrays is speed, as one can generate results several fold faster than with pipetting individual qPCR reactions. In the case of the microfluidics cards from Applied Biosystems, the diluted cDNA is simultaneously applied to many individual 1-μl wells. This eliminates the pipetting error generated when pipetting cDNA aliquots into individual qPCR reaction wells or capillaries. In the case of the custom-designed arrays, the challenge is to pick the right target mRNAs.

9.4.3 Protein Arrays

These are the analogues of DNA/RNA microarrays and are an emerging set of tools with large potential. The principle format is a capture array in which ligand-binding reagents (normally antibodies, but also alternative protein scaffolds, peptides, or nucleic acid aptamers) are used to detect target molecules in, for example, tissue extracts. The advantage is that they allow the quick acquisition of large amounts of protein data, which should give a better picture of the multitude of cellular changes upon, for example, a physiological stress. An example is the study by Murray et al.[18]

References

1. Astbury WT. Molecular biology or ultrastructural biology? Nature 1961; 190:1124.
2. Tellez JO, Dobrzynski H, Greener ID, et al. Differential expression of ion channel transcripts in atrial muscle and sinoatrial node in rabbit. Circ Res 2006; 319:105–114.
3. Dobrzynski H, Boyett MR, Anderson RH. New insights into pacemaker activity. Promoting understanding of sick sinus syndrome. Circulation 2007; 115:1921–1932.
4. Boyett MR, Tellez JO, Dobrzynski H. The sinoatrial node: its complex structure and unique ion channel gene program. Chapter 12: Cardiac Electrophysiology: From cell to bedside. 5th edition. Zipes DP, Jalife J, editors. Philadelphia: Saunders, Elsevier Science 2009; 127–138.
5. Chandler NJ, Greener ID, Tellez JO, et al. Molecular architecture of the human sinus node: insights into the function of the cardiac pacemaker. Circulation 2009; 119:1562–1575.
6. Greener ID, Tellez J, Dobrzynski H, et al. Ion channel transcript expression at the rabbit atrioventricular conduction axis. Circulation (Arrhythmia and Electrophysiology) 2009; 2:305–315.

7. Yanni J, Boyett MR, Anderson RH, et al. The extent of the specialized atrioventricular ring tissues. Heart Rhythm 2009; 6:672–680.

8. Mahmood R, Mason I. In-situ hybridization of radioactive riboprobes to RNA in tissue sections. Methods Mol Biol 2008; 461:675–686.

9. Küpper H, Seib LO, Sivaguru M, et al. A method for cellular localization of gene expression via quantitative in situ hybridization in plants. Plant J 2007; 50:159–175.

10. Braissant O, Wahli W. A simplified in situ hybridization protocol using non radioactively labelled probes to detect abundant and rare mRNAs on tissue sections. Biochemica 1998; 1:10–16.

11. De Block M, Debrouwer D. RNA-RNA in situ hybridization using digoxigenin-labelled probes: the use of high molecular weight polyvinyl alcohol in the alkaline phosphatise indoxyl-nitroblue tetrazolium reaction. Anal Biochem 1993; 215:86–89.

12. Pallansch L, Beswick H, Talian J, et al. Use of an RNA folding algorithm to choose regions for amplification by the polymerase chain reaction. Anal Biochem 1990; 185:57–62.

13. Brattelid T, Tvwit K, Birkeland JAK, et al. Expression of mRNA encoding G protein-coupled receptors involved in congestive heart failure. A quantitative RT-PCR study and the question of normalisation. Basic Res Cardiol 2007; 102:198–208.

14. Vandesompele J, De Preter K, Pattyn F, et al. Accurate normalization of real-time quantitative RT-PCR data by geometric averaging of multiple internal control genes. Genome Biol 2002; 3:1–12.

15. Beasley EM, Myers RM, Cox DR, et al. Statistical refinement of primer design parameters. In: Innis MA, Gelfand DH, Sninssky JJ, editors. PCR applications: protocols for functional genomics. London: Academic Press, 1999; 55–71.

16. Smith A, Burton JA Colour atlas of histological staining techniques. London: Wolfe Medical Publications Ltd., Sackville Press Billericay Ltd., 1977.

17. Kuhn DE, Roy S, Radtke J, et al. Laser microdissection and capture of pure cardiomyocytes and fibroblasts from infarcted heart regions: perceived hyperoxia induces p21 in peri-infarct myocytes. Am J Physiol 2007; 292:H1245–1253.

18. Murray J, Oquendo CE, Willis JH, et al. Monitoring oxidative and nitrative modification of cellular proteins; a paradigm for identifying key disease related markers of oxidative stress. Adv Drug Deliv Rev 2008; 60:1497–1503.

Chapter 10
Cell Culture Models and Methods

Alena Nikolskaya and Vinod Sharma

Abstract This chapter reviews methods to harvest and culture several different cell systems commonly employed in cardiac electrophysiology research. The cell systems covered fall into three main categories: (1) primary cell culture; (2) cell lines; and (3) stem cell-derived cardiomyocytes. Each cell system has its own set of advantages and disadvantages. Often the best choice depends on the question an investigator is attempting to answer and the specific experiments involved. The information provided in this chapter is intended to help investigators make such decisions.

10.1 Introduction

Model systems in all fields of science serve as powerful tools to investigate complex questions and gain mechanistic insights that would otherwise not be possible. In biological sciences, specifically cardiac electrophysiology as it pertains to the focus of this book, several cell culture systems are routinely employed by investigators as research tools. Several important questions would be much more difficult or impossible to answer if these model systems were unavailable and we were required to go directly to a more complex in vivo setting. Cell systems also are amenable to experimental measurements that may not be feasible in whole animals. For example, it is relatively easy to perform several sequential high-resolution spatiotemporal measurements in the cell culture system as opposed to an in vivo system. However, this advantage can also be viewed as a shortcoming since lack of recapitulating complex biology may mean that certain intersystem interactions that are important in whole animals (e.g., autonomic effects) may not be captured in cell systems. Nevertheless, the advantages far outweigh the disadvantages of using cell systems in terms of their simplicity, cost, and speed at which results can be produced.

V. Sharma (✉)
Cardiac Rhythm Disease Management, Medtronic Inc., Minneapolis, MN, USA
e-mail: vinod.sharma@medtronic.com

This chapter reviews methods to culture several cell systems commonly employed in cardiac electrophysiology research. The emphasis of our discussion is on methods involved in establishing and maintaining these culture systems. Although the applications of these cell culture systems are broad, we also provide a few examples of their usage wherever appropriate. The cell systems we cover broadly fall into three main categories: (1) *primary cell culture*, cells isolated from neonatal and adult hearts of various species; (2) *cell lines*, cells that proliferate and hence can be propagated in culture; and (3) *stem cell-derived cardiomyocytes*, cells derived from adult or embryonic stem cells (ESCs), or recently reported induced pluripotent cells. As will become apparent during the course of this chapter, each cell system has its own set of advantages and disadvantages. Often the best choice depends on the question an investigator is attempting to answer and the specific experiments involved. The information provided in this chapter is intended to help investigators make such decisions.

10.2 Primary Cardiac Cell Culture

10.2.1 Adult Cardiomyocytes

Isolated adult cardiac myocytes represent an exceptional model system for investigating cardiac electrophysiology on the cellular level.[1–3] Although the basic procedure for isolation of cardiac myocytes was established several decades ago, improvements and modifications to the procedure are constantly being made with advances in biological sciences.[4–8]

The methods for single cell isolation use enzymes to disrupt intercellular connections and release cells from the extracellular matrix.[9] The extracellular matrix of cardiac tissue is composed of a variety of proteins, glycoproteins, lipids, and glycolipids, which are species and age dependent. Generally used crude enzyme preparations contain several proteases, polysaccharidases, lipases, and nucleases.[9] A brief description of various enzymes and their action is provided in Table 10.1. Finally, the integrity of cell adhesion proteins (such as N-cadherin) requires calcium and can be broken down by calcium-free media.

Different enzymes dissociate tissue by different mechanisms, leading to the rationale of using enzymatic combinations rather than a single enzyme for cell isolation. But protease molecules, being proteins themselves, could be cleaved by other proteases, even of the same variety. This issue should be taken into account while considering the use of enzyme combinations. This effect can be mitigated by dissolving enzymes immediately before use, using multistep dissociation procedures, and starting digestion using one enzyme and subsequently replacing it with the others.

The most popular enzymatic combinations for cardiac tissue include trypsin and collagenase, sometimes with the addition of hyaluronidase and elastase.

Table 10.1 Enzymes

Enzyme	Description
Proteases	These are the enzymes that break down proteins by hydrolysis of the peptide bonds that link amino acids together in the polypeptide chain. Each protease has specificity for a particular peptide bond
Trypsin	This protease has specificity for peptide bonds involving the carboxyl group of the basic amino acids, arginine and lysine. Trypsin mainly disrupts an adhesive bonding protein responsible for the attachment of cells to their substratum
Collagenase	This protease is specific for the X–Gly bond in the Pro–X–Gly–Pro sequence, where X is usually some neutral amino acid. Such sequences are characteristic for collagen, but very rare in other proteins. The unique property of collagenase is the ability to degrade the triple-helical native collagen fibrils
Elastase	Elastase has specificity for peptide bonds adjacent to neutral amino acids. It has a unique ability to hydrolyze native elastin fibers that, together with collagen, determine the mechanical properties of the extracellular matrix
Hyaluronidase	It is a polysaccharidase with specificity for endo-N-acetylhexosamic bonds between 2-acetoamido-2-deoxy-beta-D-glucose and D-glucuronate. These bonds are common in hyaluronic acid, a major constituent of the interstitial barrier. The hyaluronidase catalyzes the hydrolysis of hyaluronic acid, thereby increasing tissue permeability

Isolation of viable adult cardiac cells is often challenging because of the strong connections with each other and attachments to the extracellular matrix. Cells can be dissociated from cardiac tissue quite effectively by perfusing enzyme containing solution through the arteries, which readily allows enzymes to access the interstitial space via the capillary bed. Perfusion can be performed either in a whole heart (retrograde aortic perfusion via Langendorff apparatus) or a piece of cardiac tissue (via a cannulated supply artery with tied off branch leaks).

Before administrating enzymatic solution, the heart should be first flushed with heparin (or citrate) to prevent formation of blood clots. The heart is then typically flushed with ice cold Ca^{2+}-free cardioplegic or Tyrode solution to disrupt intercellular connections and stop cell contractions. Working with ice cold solution allows the time spent between harvesting the heart and perfusion to be less stringent. It is also common to flush the heart with solution at room temperature, but then the transition to perfusion should happen rapidly (within a few minutes), otherwise the yield of myocyte isolation may drastically decrease. Typical composition of the Tyrode solution is as follows (all in mM): 135 NaCl, 5.4 KCl, 1 $MgCl_2$, 0.33 NaH_2PO_4, 5 Hepes, 5 glucose (adjusted to pH 7.4 with NaOH).[10] Note that other types of solutions (e.g., Krebs–Ringers, Krebs–Henseleit, and Hank's Buffered Salt Solution) can also be used during the isolation procedure. The enzymatic perfusion is usually performed at 37°C and lasts up to 25–30 min until tissue becomes well saturated with enzymes. Discoloration, softening, and slight enlargement of the heart are signs that enzymes are successfully degrading the extracellular matrix and loosening cardiac cells. The softened tissue could be abraded with a scalpel, minced, suspended in enzymatic perfusate, agitated and incubated at 37°C for several more minutes. Then myocytes are mechanically dispersed by triturating, or gently pumping the tissue pieces back and forward through a *wide-tip* pipette for better cell separation. The undigested masses are discarded after filtering through a sterile mesh or cell strainer. The enzymes can be deactivated by adding medium containing serum or special enzyme inhibitors to the cells. In a few laboratories, the cells are maintained in a high K^+ intracellular type solution initially and then slowly transitioned to an extracellular type solution with low K^+. Often Ca^{2+} is also lowered during this recovery period.[10] High K^+ depolarizes the membrane and therefore reduces metabolism of the cells. Along with low extracellular Ca^{2+}, it also helps prevent influx of Ca^{2+} into the cells, and thus improves cell viability. A yield of 90% and above is not uncommon. The next steps typically involve centrifugation and resuspension of cells in incubation or cultivation medium, depending on the future use of isolated cells.

While the above method describes a generic method to obtain viable cells, several modifications can be made to increase the cell yield. One key modification pertains to Ca^{2+} concentration during the course of the isolation procedure. Adult cardiomyocytes are very sensitive to changes in Ca^{2+} concentration. Perfusion with Ca^{2+}-free cardioplegic or Tyrode solution aids in breaking links between cells and the extracellular matrix. Thus, the cell yield can suffer if this step is not executed properly (e.g., solution contains trace amounts of Ca^{2+} and/or heart is not perfused for sufficient duration). Furthermore, the two most important enzymes used in isolation – trypsin and collagenase – work optimally under different Ca^{2+} conditions. While trypsin works best in the absence of Ca^{2+}, collagenase works best in the presence of Ca^{2+}. Although perfusion solution with varying amounts of Ca^{2+} with both trypsin and collagenase present simultaneously can be used, the best approach is to start with Ca^{2+}-free trypsin, and then gradually replace it with collagenase-containing solution supplemented with Ca^{2+} and trypsin inhibitor. Manipulations in Ca^{2+}, enzyme composition, and timing of perfusion can also be altered to obtain two or more coupled cells, which can serve as an elegant model system to investigate various questions (e.g., magnitude of intercellular coupling between cells, and its effect on modifying the electric field-induced response of the cardiac tissue).[11]

Although the arterial perfusion dissociation method described above is the most effective and commonly used method for obtaining single cells, sometimes it may not be feasible to use this approach. For example, if cells are to be isolated from human cardiac biopsy fragments obtained during a surgical procedure (e.g., valve repair and bypass surgery), access to a major artery via which enzymatic solution can be perfused may not be possible. In such a situation, an alternative method of *chunk* isolation can be used.[3] In this method, tissue pieces are collected in Ca^{2+}-free cardioplegia solution, washed with heparin-containing solution, minced or cut into 1–2 mm^3 pieces, washed, and enzymatically dissociated into single cell suspension via repeated digestions with gentle shaking or stirring. Unfortunately, the yield of viable myocytes after such a procedure is very low. Poor cell dissociation is attributed to the fact that enzymes are unable to penetrate and saturate the tissue fast enough, i.e., enzymes only act on the top layer of cells that leads to prolonged isolation time and unavoidable cell damage.

Human adult cardiomyocytes are the most suitable in vitro model to study normal and abnormal physiology of human myocardium, but have the obvious sourcing challenges. Since the human tissue is precious, often additional methodological adjustments are needed to maximize the cell yield. The fact the tissue often comes from elderly patients with significantly remodeled hearts (e.g., larger extent of fibrosis and less tolerant myocytes) is another contributing factor that necessitates adjustments in isolation procedure. These adjustments include enzyme concentration, duration of digestion, use of advanced cardioplegia solution, additional media supplements (e.g., vitamins, serum, antioxidants, and cardioprotective agents) during recovery, and further improvements in chunk isolation as described below.

In addition to the above described adjustments to the routine "chunk" isolation procedure, it is possible to employ a radically different and more extensive isolation procedure to obtain significantly higher cell yield. The method essentially leverages the fact that cardiac tissue can be preserved for at least 18 h in cold cardioplegia solution without the loss of cell viability. In this improved chunk isolation method, minced tissue is placed in cardioplegia solution, supplemented with dissociation enzymes, and incubated overnight at 4°C. In this overnight incubation step, enzymes are relatively inactive but they are able to gradually penetrate deep into the tissue. The next step is to bring the solution temperature to 37°C to start enzymatic activation, while stirring the solution for approximately 15 min. In this step, trypsin is able to act on the tissue as the solution is Ca^{2+} free. The solution is then gradually supplemented with Ca^{2+} and trypsin inhibitor to deactivate trypsin and is then finally replaced with collagenase-containing solution. The rest of the procedure is similar to what has been described above, i.e., stirring the solution at 37°C, triturating the tissue to isolate cells, filtering to remove undigested tissue, deactivating the enzymes by adding serum-containing medium, centrifugation, and resuspension of cells in fresh medium. Figure 10.1 provides a stepwise description of the chunk isolation procedure.

Adult cardiac myocytes are considered as terminally differentiated, postmitotic, nondividing cells. After isolation they have a distinct rod shape with rectangular ends, clear cross-striations, and many of them appear as bi-nuclear (Fig. 10.2). Multinucleation occurs because cardiac cells lose complete mitotic activity during development whereas DNA continues to replicate without accompanying cytokinesis. This process highly depends on age and species.[12, 13]

Electrophysiological experiments with acutely isolated adult cardiomyocytes include such techniques as microelectrode or patch-pipette voltage-clamp, field stimulation, measurements of changes in intracellular ion concentrations using fluorescent indicators, and membrane potentials using voltage-sensitive dyes (see Chaps. 11, 15, 16).

Primary isolated adult cardiac cells are the most valuable for comparative studies of the electrophysiological properties of cells from different areas of the heart (left, right atrial versus left, right ventricular) especially for acute and relatively short-term studies when there is no need to maintain cardiac cells in culture.

```
┌─────────────────────────────────────────────────────┐
│ Collect a small piece of cardiac tissue in the      │
│ appropriate buffer or balanced salt solution, wash  │
│ with heparin and place in ice cold cardioplegia.    │
│ Keep at 4°C before processing.                      │
└─────────────────────────────────────────────────────┘
```
⇩
```
┌─────────────────────────────────────────────────────┐
│ Cut the isolated piece of tissue into 1-2 mm³       │
│ pieces, wash 2-3 times, and add enzyme mixture      │
│ based on Ca²⁺-free ice cold cardioplegia.           │
└─────────────────────────────────────────────────────┘
```
⇩
```
┌─────────────────────────────────────────────────────┐
│ Incubate at 4°C overnight, mixing slowly, to        │
│ saturate the interstitial space with dissociation   │
│ enzymes.                                            │
└─────────────────────────────────────────────────────┘
```
⇩
```
┌─────────────────────────────────────────────────────┐
│ Gradually bring temperature to 37°C, incubate for   │
│ about 15 min with gentle agitation.                 │
└─────────────────────────────────────────────────────┘
```
⇩
```
┌─────────────────────────────────────────────────────┐
│ Gradually supplement enzymatic solution with        │
│ incremental addition of Ca²⁺ and trypsin inhibitor  │
│ to deactivate trypsin and activate collagenase.     │
│ Incubate for about 15 min with gentle agitation,    │
│ collect and discard first supernatant containing    │
│ mostly blood and damaged cells.                     │
└─────────────────────────────────────────────────────┘
```
⇩
```
┌─────────────────────────────────────────────────────┐
│ Add enzymatic solution containing collagenase to    │
│ the residual tissue, incubate for about 15 min,     │
│ with gentle agitation, disperse the cells by        │
│ triturating, and collect cell suspension in         │
│ supernatant. Repeat several times until viable      │
│ cells are being released from the tissue chunks.    │
└─────────────────────────────────────────────────────┘
```
⇩
```
┌─────────────────────────────────────────────────────┐
│ Filter the cell suspension through 100-200μm mesh;  │
│ deactivate the enzymes by adding medium containing  │
│ serum or enzyme inhibitors.                         │
└─────────────────────────────────────────────────────┘
```
⇩
```
┌─────────────────────────────────────────────────────┐
│ Allow the cells to settle by gentle centrifugation, │
│ aspirate the excess liquid containing enzymes, and  │
│ resuspend cells in appropriate medium or buffer.    │
└─────────────────────────────────────────────────────┘
```
⇩
```
┌─────────────────────────────────────────────────────┐
│ Estimate cell yield and viability, plate them or    │
│ use for acute experiments.                          │
└─────────────────────────────────────────────────────┘
```

Fig. 10.1 Stepwise description of chunk isolation procedure of primary atrial and ventricular cardiac myocytes

10.2.2 Cultured Neonatal Cardiomyocytes

Although isolated adult cardiac cells present an extremely valuable experimental model for a wide spectrum of cardiac electrophysiological studies, they do have

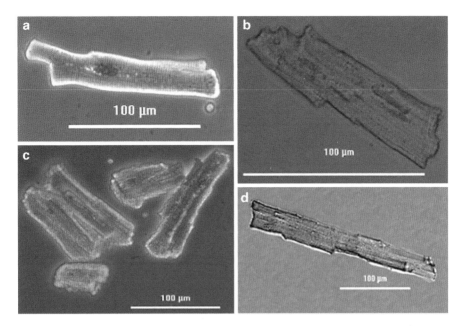

Fig. 10.2 Freshly isolated adult cardiomyocytes. (**a**) A ventricular myocyte derived from a human heart obtained from an elderly patient. A large fraction of myocytes from aged human hearts have one nucleus. (**b**) An adult canine cardiac myocyte. Note two nuclei, which is typical of the vast majority of cells. (**c**) A group of freshly isolated canine myocytes. Not all cells are healthy and one cell in the bottom portion of *panel c* is in the hypercontracted state. (**d**) A cell pair, with each cell in the pair having two nuclei. Often a small fraction of cells during single cell isolation can be coupled. The yield of coupled cells can be improved by modifying the cell isolation procedure (see text for details)

several limitations. One characteristic of isolated adult cardiomyocytes is that they tend not to easily attach to cell culture substrates. Isolated unattached adult cardiac cells stay viable for only a few hours after isolation after which they begin to degrade (Fig. 10.3). Attempts to culture adult cells have had limited success and, even though cells can stay viable in culture after elaborate procedures involving facilitated attachment and mechanical, electrical, or chemical stimulations, the cells tend to undergo substantial morphological and electrophysiological remodeling, thus raising questions about their utility. Specifically, attached adult cells tend to dedifferentiate and take on a neonatal-like phenotype when maintained in culture, while unattached cells suffer significant metabolic degradation (Fig. 10.3). In addition, isolated cells do not easily capture the syncytial nature of cardiac tissue, wherein all cells interconnect to form an electrical continuous structure. Thus, single cells are a bit removed from tissue-like structures. A better model that is more akin to tissue is two-dimensional or three-dimensional cultured cell systems that will be discussed below.

Although cells can be derived from several species (e.g., rat,[14–16] mouse,[17] rabbit,[18] guinea pig,[19] hamster,[20] chick,[21] canine,[13] feline,[22] and porcine[23]) to

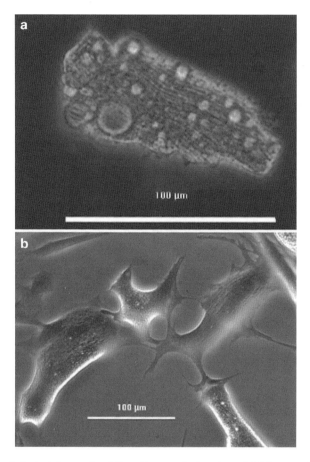

Fig. 10.3 Morphological changes in adult cardiomyocytes in culture. (**a**) A human adult ventricular cardiomyocyte maintained in culture for a week. The culture surface was not modified to have any cell attachment factors. The cell developed numerous small vesicles. (**b**) Morphological changes in human cardiomyocytes plated on the culture surface pretreated with attachment factors and maintained in culture. The cells started to send out pseudopodia-like projections toward neighboring cell. The cells appear to be "dedifferenting" and taking neonatal-like phenotype

create cardiac cell structures, the primary neonatal rat cardiomyocytes have become the most widely used experimental model.[16] More specifically, neonatal rat *ventricular* myocytes (NRVM) are routinely cultured by several laboratories worldwide because they are easy to isolate and cells can be obtained in abundance. In contrast, other neonatal cardiac cell types (e.g., atria cells) are significantly more difficult to isolate, purify, concentrate, and culture.

Cell isolation from neonatal rats is efficient and relatively inexpensive because pregnant rats with a specified gestation period are readily available commercially (e.g., Harlan, Indianapolis, IN, USA). A typical rat litter of 12–15 neonatal pups provides up to 70–80 million viable ventricular cardiomyocytes. Another advantage of rat neonatal cardiomyocytes is that they are relatively insensitive to changes in Ca^{2+} concentration, which makes the procedure for their isolation straightforward and less demanding. To maximize the success of isolation, the rat pups should ideally be 1–4 days old; the quality of cardiomyocyte preparations tends to decrease with the age of pups.[15]

Usually newborn rats are sacrificed by decapitation and their hearts are rapidly excised and washed in Ca^{2+}-free balanced salt solution. The ventricles are then minced into 1–2 mm^3 pieces and dissociated into single cell suspension by repeated digestion using proteolytic enzymes. Each digestion lasts 15–20 min and is typically enhanced with gentle shaking or stirring. This is followed by steps similar to those described above for adult cell isolation, including trituration and filtering through a cell strainer to remove undigested tissue. Usually, the first few digestion fractions are discarded because they mostly contain blood and endocardial/epicardial cells as well as cell debris. Collected cell suspension is mixed with serum for enzyme deactivation, centrifuged, and the cell pellet is resuspended in culturing media.

Careful examination of initial cell isolates would reveal that this cell population is not homogeneous. Instead, it contains a mixture of cardiomyocytes, fibroblasts, endothelial, smooth muscle, and other mesenchymal cells (Fig. 10.4). For some applications, such heterogeneous cell population containing a small yet measurable fraction of other cells may not be acceptable mainly because of their high proliferative potential. For such applications, cardiomyocytes can be significantly purified by the removal of nonmyocyte cells via selective preplating.[24] This method exploits a significantly faster rate of attachment of fibroblasts and mesenchymal cells to the plastic surface of cell-culture vehicles compared to cardiomyocytes. The majority of fibroblasts are attached within an hour, while cardiomyocytes remain floating in suspension for up to several hours. Repeated preplating steps can be used in succession to purify and concentrate cardiomyocytes. After preplating steps, cardiomyocyte-enriched suspension is collected. If necessary, the attached cells could be used to cultivate cardiac fibroblasts which, in contrast to cardiac myocytes, are highly proliferative in culture (Fig. 10.5). Purified cardiomyocytes are counted, diluted to desirable concentration, and plated into cell culture dishes generally pretreated with attachment factors such as collagen, laminin, and fibronectin.[15]

To maintain cell health, it is important that cells be periodically supplied with fresh media. The media should be changed a day after culture is started and then at least every second day thereafter. On the first 2–3 changes, media should be supplemented with cell proliferation inhibitors (such as 5-bromo-2′-deoxyuridine) to reduce the growth of residual fibroblasts. A β-adrenergic agonist such as norepinephrine, epinephrine, or isoproterenol should be added to the media to stimulate stable cell beating.[25]

Cultured NRVMs are nonproliferating, but they do grow in size. Thus, if plated at the correct cell density (at about 125,000 cardiomyocytes per cm^2 of culture vehicle), they grow within days to form a confluent monolayer in which all cells beat synchronously. Under appropriate conditions, the cell monolayer

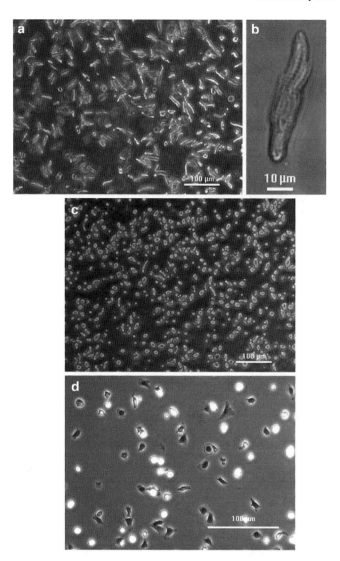

Fig. 10.4 Freshly isolated neonatal ventricular myocytes. (**a**) Initial isolated cell mixture of cardiac myocytes and nonmyocyte cells. Cardiomyocytes are mostly rod shaped. (**b**) A single isolated neonatal myocyte magnified. (**c**) Cells isolated during preplating step. Note that myocytes have become rounded. Nonmyocytes cells begin to attach first. (**d**) Nonmyocyte cells attached to culture surface during preplating step

can last for several months, allowing an investigator to perform long-lasting experiments such as long-term electrophysiological effects of drugs or exogenous gene expression.[26]

The morphology and physiology of cultured cardiomyocytes can be widely manipulated by controlling different factors, such as heterogeneity and density of cell plating,[27] concentration of companion cell (e.g., fibroblast),[24] attachment

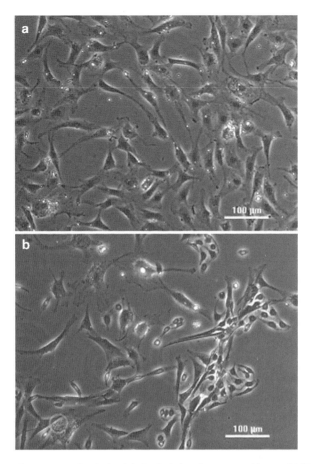

Fig. 10.5 Noncardiomyocyte cells obtained during isolation from neonatal hearts. (**a**) Noncardiac cells preplated during the process of isolating ventricular cells mostly take a fibroblast-like phenotype. (**b**) Noncardiac cells obtained during the atrial cardiomyocyte isolation are relatively less uniform, and exhibit fibroblast- and endothelial-like phenotype

substrates,[28–31] media composition,[32] external stimulation,[33] and timing of cells in culture.[34, 35] By appropriately controlling these factors, cultures can be controllably formed as homogeneous, well coupled, uniformly conducting monolyers (Fig. 10.6), as well as intentionally heterogeneous pro-arrhythmical structures, strands, or clusters (Fig. 10.7).[36]

It is also possible to grow monolayers of neonatal rat *atrial* myocyte, although the methodology to harvest cells, purify them, and accumulate them in large enough numbers is much more extensive compared to the ventricular cells.[33, 37] This is primarily because neonatal rat atria are quite small, and hence a much larger quantity of rat pups is needed to obtain a sufficient number of cells. Furthermore, it is much more difficult to separate nonmyocyte cells from atrial myocytes because the concentration of residual companion cells in atrial isolation even after careful preplating steps is significantly higher than that in ventricular isolation. Consequently,

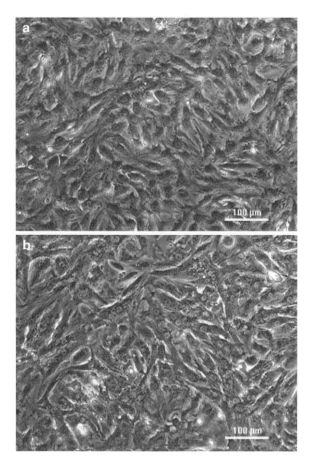

Fig. 10.6 Cultured neonatal rat ventricular myocytes (NRVMs). (**a**) A confluent NRVM monolayer after one week in culture. (**b**) A confluent NRVM monolayer after three weeks in culture

atrial cell monolyers are much more susceptible to reentrant arrhythmias because of unavoidable culture heterogeneity (Fig. 10.8). Overall, in our experience the atrial cell cultures are relatively less stable and controllable, and hence more challenging to initiate and maintain than their ventricular counterpart.

10.3 Cardiac Cell Lines

Cardiac cell lines provide investigators with a replenishable supply of cardiomyocytes, and are a convenient and reproducible cell system for a variety of electrophysiological experiments.[38]

The first successful cardiomyocyte cell line, HL-1, was developed in the laboratory of William Claycomb.[39] Later similar HL cell lines (e.g., HL-1P, HL-2, and HL-5)

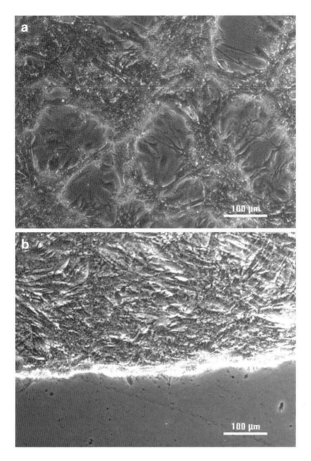

Fig. 10.7 Patterned NRVM culture system. (**a**) A cultured monolayer having a net-like structure. (**b**) A cell strand with defined boundary. Such patterned and well-defined systems, when combined with recording techniques such as multisite optical mapping, provide an ideal setting for understanding arrhythmia mechanisms

were derived. These cell lines were obtained from AT-1 mouse atrial cardiomyocyte tumor lineage developed in Loren J. Field's laboratory.[40] AT-1 cells are cultured atrial cardiomyocytes from transgenic mice in which expression of the Simian virus 40 (SV40) large T-antigen is controlled by atrial natriuretic factor (ANF) promoter. AT-1 cells in their native unmodified form do not proliferate and cannot be passaged. They keep cardiomyocyte phenotype in culture and contract spontaneously, but can be maintained only as a subcutaneous tumor lineage in transgenic mice; furthermore, they need to be freshly isolated from these tumors. The modified HL cells spontaneously contract under appropriate culture conditions but, unlike AT-1 cells, they proliferate and hence can be repeatedly passaged or frozen for later use (Fig. 10.9).

The HL cardiomyocytes have been carefully studied using electrophysiological, morphological, pharmacological, genetic, and immunohistochemical techniques.[41-43]

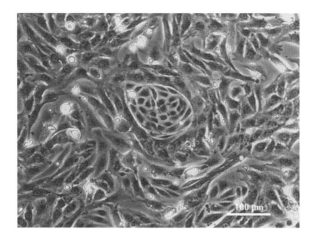

Fig. 10.8 Cultured neonatal rat atrial myocytes. *Panel* shows a confluent NRAM monolayer. The mono-layer contains a small region of proliferative nonmyocytes cells that can serve as pro-arrhythmical substrate

They express cardiac ion channels, gap junction proteins (e.g., connexin 43), α-MHC, α-cardiac actin, desmin, and other cardiomyocyte specific genes similar to that of adult atrial cardiomyocytes.[39] Moreover, they spontaneously depolarize and generate action potentials similar to the primary atrial cardiomyocytes, have organized sarcomeres essential for cell contraction, contain intracellular ANF granules distinctive for atrial myocytes, and respond appropriately to inotropic and chronotropic agonists, signifying the expression of signaling proteins and functional receptors.[42] Once plated on fibronectin–gelatin substrate and maintained in a specially formulated growth medium (e.g., Claycomb Medium, JRH Biosciences, Kansas, USA), HL cells can preserve a differentiated contractile cardiac phenotype through serial passaging in culture.

Despite its numerous advantages primarily related to ease of use, HL cells have some pitfalls. Some of the shortcomings especially relate to interpretation of results of electrophysiological studies performed on confluent monolyers of HL cells. As is the case for any tumor originated cell culture line, they continuously and rapidly proliferate in culture doubling approximately at every 48 h. Furthermore, their proliferation is not inhibited even after cells come in contact with one another. Thus, electrophysiological properties of cell monolayers strongly depend on initial plating density, plating homogeneity, and stage of the culture development.

It should be noted that in the early stage after the initial cell plating, the majority of HL cells do not beat spontaneously. After 1–2 days in culture, a few randomly scattered cells start to contract weakly at 60–180 beats/min. With time as the culture matures, the cell density increases, the culture reaches confluency, and the intercellular connectivity of cells results in synchronous and regular contraction of the entire monolayer. However, the three- or four-day-old monolayer becomes susceptible to high frequency reentries – self-rotating spiral waves, which might

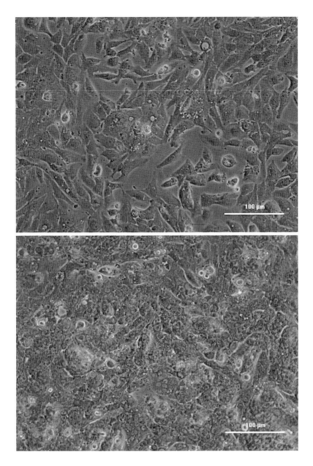

Fig. 10.9   HL cell monolayers. (*Top panel*) A subconfluent cell monolayer of HL cells. (*Bottom panel*) An overgrown monolayer. Compare the density of cells in the two monolayers

result in rapid degradation of the culture.[43, 44] It is possible that the reentrant activity at such high frequency can induce cellular remodeling similar to the situation of cells being subject to high frequency electrical field stimulations.[33] During the culture maturation, HL-cells go through the process of myolysis and membrane blebbing. The immunostaining shows a steady increase in the number of nuclei but a fast decline in the amount of motor proteins, cardiac myosin, possibly because myocytes become deficient in their motor system since they have been activated at very high frequency.

On one hand, susceptibility of HL cell cultures to long-lasting reentries makes them useful for studying wave dynamics of cardiac reentries, which could be helpful for modeling cardiac fibrillation.[44] However, on the other hand, susceptibility to reentrant activity can also be a confounding factor in electrophysiological experiments focusing on or involving automaticity. For example, HL cell cultures usually present a very regular fast spontaneous rhythm, which is in contrast to the intrinsic rhythm generated by pacemaker cells that is usually not as stable and has much lower frequency. Thus, it is unclear whether the spontaneous beating in HL is the result of well-documented funny current (I_f) found in HL cells[41] or self-sustaining micro-reentry. Finally, because of the tumorous origin of HL cell, they have major differences in energy metabolism as compared to native cardiomyocytes.[45]

Thus, HL cell cultures may be very useful models for electrophysiological studies, but investigators should be aware of all essential limitations associated with these cells. Only when plated at similar densities and producing cell monolayers with similar densities at the appropriate maturation stages can the HL cells provide relatively reproducible results.

10.4   Stem Cell-Derived Myocytes

10.4.1   Embryonic Stem Cell-Derived Cardiomyocytes

Embryonic stem cells were first derived from the mouse,[46, 47] and then years later human embryonic stem cells (hESC) were derived from unused human embryos.[48, 49] These pluripotent cells are capable of differentiating into cells of multiple lineages when appropriate conditions are provided. One method to derive cardiomyocytes is by generating embryoid bodies (Fig. 10.10). While straightforward to implement, this method is limited by the yield of cardiomyocytes; it also requires steps to purify cardiomyocytes from other cell types. Other methods employ a combination of growth factors and culture media to obtain higher yield and much purer populations of cardiomyocytes.

Irrespective of the methods used to coax the cells into cardiac differentiation, the source of ESCs is the same – the inner cell mass (ICM) in a developing embryo. To derive ESCs, the following steps are employed. The outer layer of a blastocyst is removed to isolate the ICM. The outer layer is referred to as trophectoderm and is destined to become the supporting tissue layer in the organism, while ICM mass cells give rise to the various tissue types in the developing organism. The inner mass cells are isolated and plated on a feeder layer of embryonic fibroblasts. The ESCs grown on the feeder cell layer can be propagated for multiple passages. Typical culture media consists of 80% knockout Dulbecco's modified Eagle's medium (KO-DMEM) (Invitrogen, Carlsbad, CA, USA) containing the following: 1 mM L-glutamine, 0.1 mM β-mercaptoethanol, 1% nonessential amino acids stock (Invitrogen), 20% Serum Replacement (Invitrogen), and 4 ng/ml hbFGF (Invitrogen). The ESCs can be dissociated from the feeder layer by incubating in enzyme solution containing 200 units/ml of collagenase IV for 5–10 min at 37°C. The dissociated cells can then be plated on Matrigel®-coated plates, maintained in media conditioned by embryonic fibroblasts, and used to generate cardiomycytes via embryoid bodies or direct differentiation approach.

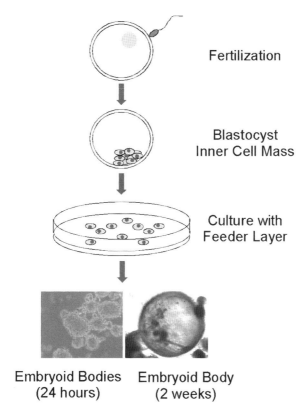

Fertilization

Blastocyst Inner Cell Mass

Culture with Feeder Layer

**Embryoid Bodies   Embryoid Body
(24 hours)   (2 weeks)**

Fig. 10.10 Differentiation of human embryonic stem cells into cardiomyocytes. The starting material for cardiomyocytes is the inner cell mass of a blastocyst. These are cultured to obtain embryoid bodies (see text). Some embryoid bodies have an outer bearing mass of cells containing a heterogeneous population of cardiac cells

To initiate differentiation of the ESCs into embryoid bodies, ESCs are removed from the feeder cell layer, which provides the cell signals necessary for self-renewal. Once removed, the cells are cultivated in suspension wherein they aggregate to form three-dimensional masses of cells referred to as embryoid bodies. For hESCs, the cell suspension cultivation needs to be maintained for a period of 7–10 days before cell aggregation can occur and result in embryoid bodies. Typically, 10% of embryoid bodies are spontaneously beating. The beating embryoid bodies consist of a heterogeneous cell mass and contain an outer beating layer from which various types of cardiac cells (e.g., nodal- and ventricular-like cardiomyocytes) can be isolated.[50] The cells isolated from the outer layer also express cardiac specific genes (e.g., myosin heavy chain) and cardiac transcription factors. In addition to the low and heterogeneous yield of cardiomyocytes, another disadvantage of this differentiation approach is that not all hESC lines are capable of generating embryoid bodies. A key challenge in ESC research is to generate high purity cardiomyocytes with well-defined molecular and electrophysiological composition using an animal free product.

A second approach to differentiate ESCs into cells of various lineages has borrowed lessons from developmental biology. Various muscular and vascular components of the heart are derived from the mesoderm of developing embryos, and it appears that several growth factors can enhance the formation of mesoderm and hence can lead to cardiomyogenesis in hESCs. One class of growth factors that seems to be common to several different species belongs to the class of TGF-β superfamily. BMP2, BMP4, TGFβ, and Activin are a few examples of the growth factors that belong to this pathway. We specifically elaborate on one method below for differentiating hESCs into cardiomyocytes, a method adapted from Laflamme and colleagues.[51] For a complete review of various growth factors affecting cardiac differentiation of hESCs, refer to Table 10.2.[52]

The human cell line used for cardiomyocyte generation in the following method was the female derived H7 human embryonic stem cell line. The following steps were employed:

1. Undifferentiated hESCs growing as a monolayer are detached using 10-min incubation with 0.5 mM EDTA or 200 U/ml collagenase IV and seed on matrigel coated plates. The density of cells is preferably maintained to ~100,000 cells/cm^2.
2. Cells are fed daily with special media conditioned with mouse embryonic fibroblast (MEF-CM). The same media is, in fact, used to maintain hESCs in their undifferentiated state. Media is enriched with 8 ng/ml basic fibroblast growth factor. The cells are fed with this media for six days.
3. To induce cardiac differentiation, MEF-CM media is removed and replaced with RPMI-B27 medium (Invitrogen) containing 100 ng/ml human recombinant activin A. The cells are maintained in activin A medium for two days.
4. Following this period, the activin A medium is removed and replaced with another fresh aliquot of RPMI-B27 medium containing 10 ng/ml of human recombinant BMP4. The cells are maintained in this medium for four days.
5. Following day 7, the BMP4 medium is removed and cells are fed with cytokine-free RPMI-B27 medium and cultured for several days.

With the above protocol, which is just one example of growth factor/cytokine utilization to induce cardiac differentiation, widespread beating cells can be observed typically by day 12. To improve the yield of cardiomyocytes, an additional step using Percoll gradient is employed. To achieve purification, cells are suspended in regular culture medium (supplementation with growth factors such as IGF1, ~100 ng/ml, is beneficial). Percoll (GE Healthcare, United Kingdom) is diluted in a buffer containing HEPES (20 mM) and NaCl (150 mM) to create discontinuous gradient: 40.5% Percoll over a layer of 58.5% Percoll. The cells are centrifuged for 30 min at $1,500 \times g$ to separate into distinct layers. The cells in different layers are collected, washed, and resuspended in the differentiation medium. Further analysis on these cells can be performed using immunostaining and RT-PCR techniques to confirm their cardiac phenotype.

Table 10.2 Advantages and disadvantages of using various cell systems

Cell type	Advantages	Disadvantages
Primary adult cardiomyocytes (e.g., ventricular cells or atrial cells derived from various species, including humans)	• Most relevant in vitro model of fully differentiated adult myocardium muscle cell • Suitable for single cell electrophysiological studies such as patch clamp, optical measurements of contractility, changes in intracellular ion concentrations with fluorescent indicators, and membrane potentials using voltage-sensitive dyes • Valuable for short-term comparative studies of the electrophysiological properties of cells from different areas of the heart (left, right atrial versus left, right ventricular) or cells from diseased myocardium	• Complicated isolation procedure • Cells stay viable for only a few hours after isolation • Slow recovery of cell membrane proteins, such as receptors and ion channels. • Cells may get damaged during isolation, which could compromise some electrophysiological studies • Not suitable for cell culturing because of poor attachment and lack of propensity to form synchronously beating monolayers • Fast morphological and electrophysiological remodeling under standard culture conditions
Primary neonatal cardiomyocytes (e.g., ventricular cells or atrial cells derived from various species)	• Routine, reliable, and well-established isolation procedure • Fast recovery and re-expression of damaged membrane proteins after isolation • Ability to form synchronous monolayers or cell structures directed by controlled culturing conditions • Endurance of cultured cell layers allowing long-lasting experiments	• Cells do not proliferate and cannot be passaged • Changes in expression of ion channels and contractile proteins during cell development under culture conditions do not completely correspond to in vivo differentiated myocardium • Special care is required to prevent overgrows by nonmyocytes • Cells do not replicate the adult myocardium morphologically (e.g., cell size) and electrophysiologically (e.g., ion channel expression)
Cardiac cell lines (e.g., HL-1, HL-5, AT-1)	• Can be passaged, frozen, and recovered from frozen stocks • Easily form synchronously beating monolayers • Maintain contractile activity over extensive passaging (> 240 times) • Retain majority of differentiated cardiac myocyte markers • Capitulate long-lasting reentries useful for modeling and studying wave dynamics of cardiac fibrillations	• Not suitable for long-lasting experiments; cell proliferation is not contact inhibited which leads to overgrowth and degradation of cell culture • Morphologically, electrophysiologically, and metabolically cell lines only partially resemble in vivo adult cardiomyocytes • Self-sustained reentries could mask the intrinsic rhythms in electrophysiological experiments

(continued)

Table 10.2 (continued)

Cell type	Advantages	Disadvantages
Stem cell-derived cardiomyocytes	• Stem cells provide a renewable source (does not require sacrificing animals) • Ability to create pure population if directed differentiation is used	• Efficient ways to induce cardiac progenitors from embryonic stem cells have not been well established • Cells may differ from adult cardiomyocytes both in morphology (e.g., size) and electrophysiology

10.4.2 Emerging Model: Induced-Pluripotent Stem Cells

Recently another source of cardiomyocytes has become available in the form of induced pluripotent stem (iPS) cells.[53, 54] iPS cells are obtained by introducing a few transcription factors in the somatic fibroblast cells. More specifically, three to four transcription factors have been introduced in the mouse and human skin fibroblasts to obtain pluripotent embryonic-like cells. The iPS cells can also be used to obtain cardiomyocytes in a manner similar to the derivation of cardiomyocytes from ESCs. However, since these are relatively new and their detailed molecular and electrophysiological characteristics are still being elucidated, we will not discuss the induction strategies in detail here. Nevertheless, it is important to be aware of this important cell source because iPS cells circumvent the ethical issues that surround conventional ESCs.

10.5 Conclusion

In this chapter, we reviewed various cardiac cell systems that are commonly used by investigators for research purposes. As is probably clear from the text above, none of the cell systems are perfect, and each has its own set of advantages and disadvantages. The best cell system is often chosen based on the specific application and other variables such as preference of the investigators and resource constraints. Often experimentation provides learning and a new set of questions that require the investigator to adjust course; hence, the best strategy often is not to be fixated on a given system and instead adapt the methodology to original and emerging questions.

References

1. Vahouny GV, Wei R, Starkweather R, et al. Preparation of beating heart cells from adult rats. Science 1970; 167:1616–8.
2. Welder AA, Grant R, Bradlaw J, et al. A primary culture system of adult rat heart cells for the study of toxicologic agents. In Vitro Cell Dev Biol 1991; 27A:921–6.

3. Peeters GA, Sanguinetti MC, Eki Y, et al. Method for isolation of human ventricular myocytes from single endocardial and epicardial biopsies. Am J Physiol 1995; 268:H1757–64.
4. Mitcheson JS, Hancox JC, Levi AJ. Cultured adult cardiac myocytes: future applications, culture methods, morphological and electrophysiological properties. Cardiovasc Res 1998; 39:280–300.
5. O'Connell TD, Rodrigo MC, Simpson PC. Isolation and culture of adult mouse cardiac myocytes. Methods Mol Biol 2007; 357:271–96.
6. Liao R, Jain M. Isolation, culture, and functional analysis of adult mouse cardiomyocytes. Methods Mol Med 2007; 139:251–62.
7. Bistola V, Nikolopoulou M, Derventzi A, et al. Long-term primary cultures of human adult atrial cardiac myocytes: cell viability, structural properties and BNP secretion in vitro. Int J Cardiol 2008; 131:113–22.
8. Viero C, Kraushaar U, Ruppenthal S, et al. A primary culture system for sustained expression of a calcium sensor in preserved adult rat ventricular myocytes. Cell Calcium 2008; 43:59–71.
9. Worthington Biochemical C. Tissue Dissociation Guide, Worthington Biochemical Corporation. 730 Vassar Ave., Lakewood, NJ 08701, http://www.tissuedissociation.com.
10. Sharma V, Tung L. Spatial heterogeneity of transmembrane potential responses of single guinea-pig cardiac cells during electric field stimulation. J Physiol 2002; 542:477–92.
11. Sharma V, Tung L. Theoretical and experimental study of sawtooth effect in isolated cardiac cell-pairs. J Cardiovasc Electrophysiol 2001; 12:1164–73.
12. Kajstura J, Pertoldi B, Leri A, et al. Telomere shortening is an in vivo marker of myocyte replication and aging. Am J Pathol 2000; 156:813–9.
13. Bishop SP, Hine P. Cardiac muscle cytoplasmic and nuclear development during canine neonatal growth. Recent Adv Stud Cardiac Struct Metab 1975; 8:77–98.
14. Harary I, Farley B. In vitro studies of single isolated beating heart cells. Science 1960; 131:1674–5.
15. Chlopčíková S, Psotová J, Miketová P. Neonatal rat cardiomyocytes—a model for the study of morphological, biochemical and electrophysiological characteristics of the heart. Biomed Pap Med Fac Univ Palacky Olomouc Czech Repub 2001; 145:49–55.
16. Maass AH, Buvoli M. Cardiomyocyte preparation, culture, and gene transfer. Methods Mol Biol 2007; 366:321–30.
17. Sreejit P, Kumar S, Verma RS. An improved protocol for primary culture of cardiomyocyte from neonatal mice. In Vitro Cell Dev Biol Anim 2008; 44:45–50.
18. Huang J, Hove-Madsen L, Tibbits GF. Na^+/Ca^{2+} exchange activity in neonatal rabbit ventricular myocytes. Am J Physiol Cell Physiol 2005; 288:C195–203.
19. Eigel BN, Gursahani H, Hadley RW. Na^+/Ca^{2+} exchanger plays a key role in inducing apoptosis after hypoxia in cultured guinea pig ventricular myocytes. Am J Physiol Heart Circ Physiol 2004; 287:H1466–75.
20. Zhang C, Osinska HE, Lemanski SL, et al. Changes in myofibrils and cytoskeleton of neonatal hamster myocardial cells in culture: an immunofluorescence study. Tissue Cell 2005; 37:435–45.
21. González H, Nagai Y, Bub G, et al. Reentrant waves in a ring of embryonic chick ventricular cells imaged with a Ca^{2+} sensitive dye. Biosystems 2003; 71:71–80.
22. Clark WA, Decker ML, Behnke-Barclay M, et al. Cell contact as an independent factor modulating cardiac myocyte hypertrophy and survival in long-term primary culture. J Mol Cell Cardiol 1998; 30:139–55.
23. Hohl CM, Livingston B, Hensley J, et al. Calcium handling by sarcoplasmic reticulum of neonatal swine cardiac myocytes. Am J Physiol 1997; 273:H192–9.
24. Simpson P, Savion S. Differentiation of rat myocytes in single cell cultures with and without proliferating nonmyocardial cells. Cross-striations, ultrastructure, and chronotropic response to isoproterenol. Circ Res 1982; 50:101–16.
25. Simpson P. Stimulation of hypertrophy of cultured neonatal rat heart cells through an alpha 1-adrenergic receptor and induction of beating through an alpha 1- and beta 1-adrenergic receptor interaction. Evidence for independent regulation of growth and beating. Circ Res 1985; 56:884–94.

26. Nikolskaya AV, Nikolski VP, Efimov IR. Gene printer: laser-scanning targeted transfection of cultured cardiac neonatal rat cells. Cell Commun Adhes 2006; 13:217–22.

27. Steinberg BE, Glass L, Shrier A, et al. The role of heterogeneities and intercellular coupling in wave propagation in cardiac tissue. Philos Transact A Math Phys Eng Sci 2006; 364:1299–311.

28. Davis RA, van Winkle WB, Buja LM, et al. Effect of a simple versus a complex matrix on the polarity of cardiomyocytes in culture. J Burns Wounds 2006; 5:e3.

29. Engler AJ, Carag-Krieger C, Johnson CP, et al. Embryonic cardiomyocytes beat best on a matrix with heart-like elasticity: scar-like rigidity inhibits beating. J Cell Sci 2008; 121:3794–802.

30. Shanker AJ, Yamada K, Green KG, et al. Matrix-protein-specific regulation of Cx43 expression in cardiac myocytes subjected to mechanical load. Circ Res 2005; 96:558–66.

31. Zajac AL, Discher DE. Cell differentiation through tissue elasticity-coupled, myosin-driven remodeling. Curr Opin Cell Biol 2008; 20:609–15.

32. Grynberg A, Athias P, Degois M. Effect of change in growth environment on cultured myocardial cells investigated in a standardized medium. In Vitro Cell Dev Biol 1986; 22:44–50.

33. Yang Z, Shen W, Rottman JN, et al. Rapid stimulation causes electrical remodeling in cultured atrial myocytes. J Mol Cell Cardiol 2005; 38:299–308.

34. Kamiya K, Guo W, Toyama J. Effects of chronic hypoxia on the developmental changes in action potential of cultured neonatal rat ventricular myocytes. Environ Med 1996; 40:163–6.

35. Meiry G, Reisner Y, Feld Y, et al. Evolution of action potential propagation and repolarization in cultured neonatal rat ventricular myocytes. J Cardiovasc Electrophysiol 2001; 12:1269–77.

36. Fast VG, Cheek ER. Optical mapping of arrhythmias induced by strong electrical shocks in myocyte cultures. Circ Res 2002; 90:664–70.

37. Suto F, Habuchi Y, Yamamoto T, et al. Increased sensitivity of neonate atrial myocytes to adenosine A1 receptor stimulation in regulation of the L-type Ca^{2+} current. Eur J Pharmacol 2000; 409:213–21.

38. Beuckelmann DJ, Näbauer M, Erdmann E. Characteristics of calcium-current in isolated human ventricular myocytes from patients with terminal heart failure. J Mol Cell Cardiol 1991; 23:929–37.

39. Claycomb WC, Lanson NA, Jr., Stallworth BS, et al. HL-1 cells: a cardiac muscle cell line that contracts and retains phenotypic characteristics of the adult cardiomyocyte. Proc Natl Acad Sci USA 1998; 95:2979–84.

40. Delcarpio JB, Lanson NA, Jr., Field LJ, et al. Morphological characterization of cardiomyocytes isolated from a transplantable cardiac tumor derived from transgenic mouse atria (AT-1 cells). Circ Res 1991; 69:1591–600.

41. Xiao Y-F, TenBroek EM, Wilhelm JJ, et al. Electrophysiological characterization of murine HL-5 atrial cardiomyocytes. Am J Physiol Cell Physiol 2006; 291:C407–16.

42. White SM, Constantin PE, Claycomb WC. Cardiac physiology at the cellular level: use of cultured HL-1 cardiomyocytes for studies of cardiac muscle cell structure and function. Am J Physiol Heart Circ Physiol 2004; 286:H823–9.

43. Umapathy K, Masse S, Kolodziejska K, et al. Electrogram fractionation in murine HL-1 atrial monolayer model. Heart Rhythm 2008; 5:1029–35.

44. Hong JH, Choi JH, Kim TY, et al. Spiral reentry waves in confluent layer of HL-1 cardiomyocyte cell lines. Biochem Biophys Res Commun 2008; 377:1269–73.

45. Eimre M, Paju K, Pelloux S, et al. Distinct organization of energy metabolism in HL-1 cardiac cell line and cardiomyocytes. Biochim Biophys Acta 2008; 1777:514–24.

46. Evans MJ, Kaufman MH. Establishment in culture of pluripotential cells from mouse embryos. Nature 1981; 292:154–6.

47. Martin GR. Isolation of a pluripotent cell line from early mouse embryos cultured in medium conditioned by teratocarcinoma stem cells. Proc Natl Acad Sci USA 1981; 78:7634–8.

48. Reubinoff BE, Pera MF, Fong CY, et al. Embryonic stem cell lines from human blastocysts: somatic differentiation in vitro. Nat Biotechnol 2000; 18:399–404.

49. Thomson JA, Itskovitz-Eldor J, Shapiro SS, et al. Embryonic stem cell lines derived from human blastocysts. Science 1998; 282:1145–7.
50. He JQ, Ma Y, Lee Y, et al. Human embryonic stem cells develop into multiple types of cardiac myocytes: action potential characterization. Circ Res 2003; 93:32–9.
51. Laflamme MA, Chen KY, Naumova AV, et al. Cardiomyocytes derived from human embryonic stem cells in pro-survival factors enhance function of infarcted rat hearts. Nat Biotechnol 2007; 25:1015–24.
52. Habib M, Caspi O, Gepstein L. Human embryonic stem cells for cardiomyogenesis. J Mol Cell Cardiol 2008; 45:462–74.
53. Takahashi K, Tanabe K, Ohnuki M, et al. Induction of pluripotent stem cells from adult human fibroblasts by defined factors. Cell 2007; 131:861–72.
54. Yu J, Vodyanik MA, Smuga-Otto K, et al. Induced pluripotent stem cell lines derived from human somatic cells. Science 2007; 318:1917–20.

Chapter 11
Isolated Tissue Models

Rodolphe P. Katra

Abstract This chapter covers large isolated cardiac tissue models and a partial listing of commonly used isolated cardiac tissue preparations. Perfusion and superperfusion techniques for delivering necessary nutrients to isolated tissue are described in detail, along with their advantages and disadvantages. Furthermore, various experimental implementations are discussed including isolated trabeculae and papillary muscle preparations, isolated ventricular preparations, isolated atrioventricular node preparations, and isolated atrial preparations.

11.1 Introduction

It is a long held belief in the scientific community that any experimental data are only as good and relevant as the animal model or preparation from which they were derived. To that end, investigators around the world have continually developed, modified, researched, and perfected large tissue preparations using a variety of animal species over a span of many decades. The result – major breakthroughs in the understanding of human basic electrophysiology and pathophysiology – has been possible only through some of these models. In this chapter, we will cover some commonly used isolated large cardiac tissue models, as well as some less commonly used ones.

11.2 Description of Models

Before discussing different animal models, a brief discussion on techniques of delivering necessary nutrients to isolated tissue is warranted. Large multicellular preparations are maintained viable after isolation throughout an experimental procedure by either perfusion techniques (through vasculature) or superfusion techniques

R.P. Katra (✉)
Department of Biomedical Engineering, College of Engineering, University of Alabama at Birmingham, Birmingham, AL, USA
e-mail: rkatra@uab.edu

(external bathing) with an iso-osmotic, electrolyte- and pH-balanced, buffered and oxygenated buffered solution. This solution is also known by many other names (e.g., Tyrode, Ringer, Locke, Krebs–Henseleit) with many electrolyte composition variations that are usually tailored to the experimental procedure and the animal species. As an alternative to these solutions, blood can be perfused or superfused through external mechanical pumps or through circulation mediated by another animal (an old technique known as cross-circulation that is nowadays less common for numerous experimental, ethical, and economic reasons) to ensure proper oxygenation, warming, and buffering. When external pumps are used instead of cross-circulation, blood or buffered solutions need to be artificially and continuously warmed and oxygenated throughout the experimental procedure. Compared to intravascular perfusion, superfusion is a relatively simple technique that can be used on small isolated preparations and relies on diffusion of electrolytes and nutrients along their concentration gradient (i.e., from the outside-in). On the other hand, perfusion techniques deliver the electrolytes and nutrients by utilizing vascular and capillary networks within the preparation (i.e., from the inside-out). The practical implementation and advantages/limitations of each technique will be discussed in a later section.

11.2.1   Isolated Trabeculae and Papillary Muscle Preparations

For over five decades, investigators have used and continually developed isolated trabeculae and papillary muscle preparations.[1-3] Trabeculae are irregular muscle structures with complex architecture that line the inner surface of the heart. They provide structural support and help in cardiac function. Papillary muscles are tubular or conical structures that anchor the heart valves to the ventricles, preventing backflow of blood to the atria. Trabeculae and papillary preparations can be isolated from a variety of animal species ranging from frogs to dogs. They can also be isolated from live human hearts through biopsy or from explanted hearts after transplant.

Anesthetized animals are usually anticoagulated to prevent blood clotting, and their hearts are subsequently excised. Harvested hearts are then bathed in a chilled buffer solution (about 5°C) to slow metabolic processes and reduce ischemic injury while the tissue is being processed. Small trabeculae muscle preparations from either the atria or ventricles can be isolated by sectioning the heart around the area of interest. Trabeculae structures are cut and the ends are ligated with fine surgical thread; they are then transferred to the experimental chamber or dish, and superfused with a buffer solution at a sufficient flow rate that prevents superfusate stagnation. The superfusate can be easily changed during the course of the experiment, allowing study of the effects of a variety of chemicals. Figure 11.1 shows an example of a superfused trabecular structure (*left*) mounted on a study chamber. Both edges of the preparation are fixed to allow for study of muscle mechanics. Figure 11.1 (*right*) shows a magnified view of a rat trabecula.

Larger preparations that are not amenable to superfusion are usually perfused; the surgical skills required to produce these models become a bit more

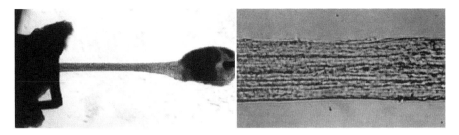

Fig. 11.1 Superfused trabecula preparation. *Left panel* shows trabecula mounted on a study chamber where it is continuously superfused with a buffered solution. Both edges of the preparation are fixed to create isometric tension of the muscle, one pinned and the other connected to a strain gauge. *Right panel* shows a magnified view of a rat trabecular preparation. Photographs courtesy of Professors Pieter DeTombe and John Solaro

involved. Since the heart is inherently heterogeneous anatomically and since the pathophysiology to be studied in an experiment can be part of either ventricle, isolating the left and/or right ventricle may be desired. To isolate large left ventricular trabeculae or papillary muscles for study, the right ventricular wall is surgically removed to expose the interventricular septum. The anterior septal artery is carefully isolated and instrumented with a cannula. All branches and collaterals, except for the arteries to the anterior papillary muscle, are ligated by suture. If using blood as the perfusate, a dye is mixed with the blood to demark the perfused areas and to localize the papillary muscle arteries; all unstained areas are surgically cut away from the papillary muscle. If using a clear buffer solution instead of blood, the perfused areas will be demarked by a blanching in color. Similar color changes will help identify the papillary muscle arteries. The preparation is then transferred to a special chamber or dish to start the experimental procedures. Isolating right ventricular trabeculae or papillary muscles is possible by reversing the procedure and surgically removing the left ventricular wall instead of the right ventricular wall. Usually, the distal end of the papillary muscle is loaded by attaching the tendinous part to a force transducer or weights. Depending on the goals of the study, a variety of compounds with small molecular structure and membrane permeable agents can be introduced to the preparation via the cannula. If performed properly, this preparation typically remains viable for many hours and retains local adrenergic and cholinergic activity through viable nerve fibers.[2] It can be electrically stimulated with external stimulators to mimic physiologic electrical function via fine, conductive electrodes placed on the muscle surface or plunged into the muscle. Figure 11.2 shows an experimental setup that uses cross-circulation to study papillary muscles.

11.2.2 Isolated Ventricular Preparation

Isolated ventricular preparations can be either superfused or perfused depending on preparation size, and can be prepared from a variety of animal species. Lamb and

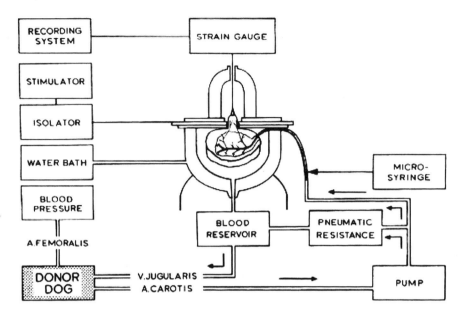

Fig. 11.2 Papillary muscle experimental setup. The papillary preparation is blood perfused through a cross-circulation approach using a donor dog. It is placed in a temperature-controlled reservoir that collects effluent blood for recirculation. The strain gauge is tethered to the tissue via fine suture, and the pacing electrodes are in contact with the tissue as the papillary muscle is passed through the hole in the reservoir cover. The microsyringe is used to introduce chemicals to the system quickly. Adapted from Endoh and Hashimoto[2]

McGuigan developed a half-ventricle superfused preparation from frog hearts[4]; the atria and aortas of excised hearts are removed surgically at the basal level of the ventricle. The resulting ventricle is then placed cut-side down and sectioned vertically to yield two semiconical ventricular structures. The sections are then bathed in a buffer solution to wash off residual blood. Each section can be studied independently by transferring it to the experimental chamber or dish, where it gets superfused with a buffer solution that can easily and quickly be changed. As with papillary muscle preparations, the half-ventricles can be loaded by a pressure transducer or weights. Figure 11.3 shows the experimental setup of the half-ventricle frog superfused preparation; this preparation can easily be adapted to other species (e.g., mice, rats) with relatively small hearts, or miniaturized by sectioning the hearts further to yield even smaller ventricular slices.

For larger ventricular preparations, intravascular perfusion is required. Yan and Antzelevitch developed a canine, arterially perfused ventricular wedge preparation that can be used to study transmembrane electrical function of cell types spanning the ventricle from epicardium to endocardium using microelectrodes.[5, 6] This model was later adapted for use with fluorescence-based optical mapping (refer to Chap. 15). The model preparation process is as follows. Hearts are harvested via a left thoracotomy from anesthetized and anticoagulated canines. Excised hearts are then placed in chilled cardioplegia (about 5°C) buffer solution to arrest the heart, slow the metabolic

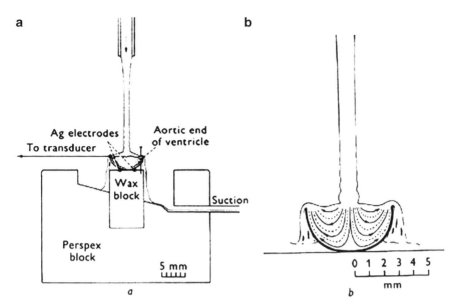

Fig. 11.3 Semiventricle experimental setup. (**a**) Preparation is pinned down to a wax block using a fine needle through the base, and the apex is connected to a transducer using fine thread. Effluent solution is suctioned out of the collection chamber. (**b**) Superfusate flow pattern through the semiventricle preparation is illustrated. Adapted from Lamb and McGuigan[4]

processes, and subsequently reduce ischemic injury while the tissue is being prepared. Transmural wedges of ventricular tissue around the left anterior descending artery, circumflex, or other major coronary arteries are isolated, cannulated, and perfused with buffer solution. The ventricular wedges blanch at areas of adequate perfusion; all nonperfused or poorly perfused areas are surgically cut with a sharp razor blade. Any major shunting of perfusate through the tissue or collaterals is reduced by ligation using fine suture. The cannulated wedge preparation is then transferred to an experimental chamber or dish where it is immersed in buffer solution to prevent surface desiccation. A variety of compounds or chemical agents can be introduced to the preparation through the perfusate. If properly prepared, the ventricular wedge preparation can remain viable for several hours. It can be electrically stimulated with fine electrodes placed on the surface or plunged into the preparation. Figure 11.4 illustrates the isolation of a ventricular wedge from a canine heart around arteries branching off the left anterior descending artery and a photograph of the cannulated wedge.

11.2.3   Isolated Atrioventricular Node Preparation

Investigating the function of the AV node requires unique and rather difficult large models. Needless to say, AV node large animal preparations are not amenable to

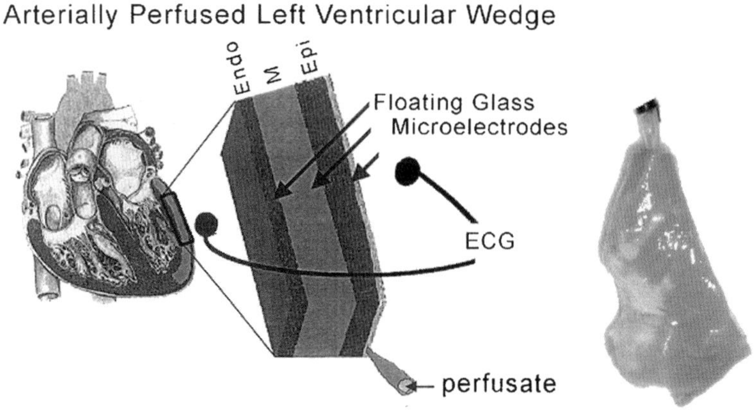

Arterially Perfused Left Ventricular Wedge

Fig. 11.4 Arterially perfused wedge preparation. (*Left*) Schematic describes the isolation of the wedge from the ventricular wall exposing the endocardial, epicardial, and transmural surfaces. Electrodes can be placed at different regions of the wedge to study different cell types and to produce a volume-conducted pseudo-ECG. Adapted from Yan et al.[6] (*Right*) Photograph of an arterially perfused wedge preparation with a subendocardial microinfarct

superfusion techniques, since the AV node is recessed within the muscle and spans the transition between the atrial and ventricular chambers. One elegant and surgically involved perfused AV node model was developed about four decades ago by skilled investigators using canine hearts.[7] In this model, hearts are harvested as described previously and arrested in chilled cardioplegia (about 5°C) buffer solution. Three cannulation sites are required to ensure proper perfusion of the AV node region and the encompassing muscle tissue:

1. The anterior septal artery supplying blood to the anterior ventricular septum is cannulated a few millimeters proximal to the branching of the septal artery from the anterior descending artery, close to the base of the ventricle. A few millimeters distal to the cannulation site, the anterior descending artery is ligated with fine suture.
2. The posterior descending artery, which branches from the left circumflex artery, and other branches feeding the left atrial and ventricular wall are ligated. The remaining posterior septal artery is cannulated.
3. The right coronary artery is dissected and cannulated, however, all the branches feeding the right ventricular wall are ligated. The left atrium, left ventricle, and right ventricle are then surgically dissected out. Next, the right atrium is incised to expose the endocardial surface of the right atrium and the interatrial wall (i.e., septum). The three cannulas feeding the anterior septal artery, the posterior septal artery, and the right coronary artery are then coupled to a single rubber tube or cannula to maintain uniform perfusion pressure across them. The AV node preparation is then supplied blood though cross-circulation or by using a buffer solution setup. Figure 11.5 shows an illustration of the AV node preparation.

A more recent AV node preparation was developed using rabbit hearts that were isolated and retrograde perfused with buffer solution.[8] After a stabilization period

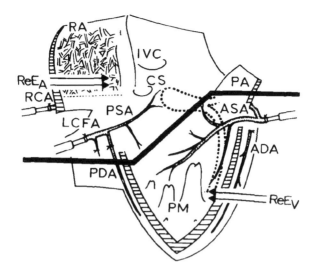

Fig. 11.5 Schematic representation of the isolated atrioventricular (AV) node model. *ADA* anterior descending artery; *ASA* anterior septal artery; *CS* coronary sinus; *IVC* inferior vena cava; *LCFA* left circumflex artery; *PA* pulmonary artery; *PDA* posterior descending artery; *PM* papillary muscle; *PSA* posterior septal artery; *RA* right atrium; *RCA* right coronary artery; *ReE*$_A$ arterial recording electrodes; *ReE*$_V$ ventricular recording electrodes. Adapted from Motomura et al.[7]

(about 30–60 min) in the study chamber, the isolated heart is transferred to a dissecting chamber filled with perfusate. The apex of the heart is surgically removed in a cross-sectional cut. A probe is introduced through the apical opening of the right ventricle, past the tricuspid valve, and to the superior vena cava. A longitudinal cut is then done with scissors using the probe as a guide, exposing the endocardial surface of the right atrium. Along the base of the heart, below the AV ring, all ventricular tissue is removed; the left atrium is also removed. The preparation that remains is comprised of ventricular septal tissue just below the His bundle, interatrial septum, right atrial tissue, right atrial appendage, septal leaflet of the tricuspid valve, and other attached tissue. The preparation is then returned to the study chamber.

11.2.4 Isolated Atrial Preparation

Small atrial sections can be studied by surgically isolating them from the intact atria and superfusing them with buffer solution. Sectioned atrial preparations lend themselves perfectly to superfusion techniques, because they have a limited thickness and generally are not as dense as ventricular tissue, thus permitting efficient nutrient and electrolyte diffusion. Studying large intact atrial preparations, however, requires a bit more surgical skill and more model preparation, because superfusion may not be adequate for nutrients and electrolyte delivery. Intact left atrial preparation, right

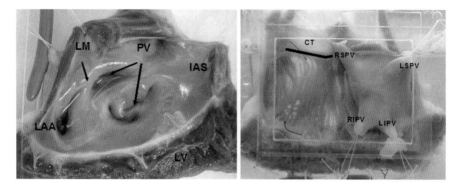

Fig. 11.6 Isolated atrial preparations. (*Left*) Photograph of the isolated, arterially perfused left atrial preparation. The orange tube is cannulated to the left coronary artery. (*Right*) Photograph of the isolated dual atrial preparation mounted on a custom frame. The orange tubes are cannulated to the left and right coronary arteries, respectively. Photographs courtesy of Dr. Masamichi Hirose. *CT* crista terminalis; *IAS* intraatrial septum; *LAA* left atrial appendage; *LIPV* left inferior pulmonary vein; *LM* ligament of Marshall; *LSPV* left superior pulmonary vein; *LV* left ventricle; *PV* pulmonary vein; *RIPV* right inferior pulmonary vein; *RSPV* right superior pulmonary vein

atrial preparation, or dual atrial preparation can be isolated from the excised heart at ventricular basal levels and perfused with buffer solution. The left and right atrial preparation are perfused via the left and right coronary arteries, respectively, while the dual atrial preparation requires cannulation of both coronary arteries. In all the three preparations, any leaking arteries need to be ligated with fine sutures. The preparations are then mounted on a special frame that stretches along the ventricular margin, crista terminalis, and borders of the atrial tissue, permitting electrophysiology studies. The preparation can be perfused with blood through a cross-circulation setup[9] or with buffer solution using external pumps.[10] The atrial preparations are then immersed in blood or perfusate depending on the experimental setup, and stimulated using fine electrodes applied to the tissue surface. Figure 11.6 shows photos of the left atrial preparation (*left*) and dual atrial preparation (*right*).

11.3   Advantages, Limitations, and Pitfalls

It is important to mention that no isolated tissue model truly replaces in vivo models, under all physiologic and pathophysiologic circumstances. Excised and isolated tissue loses the natural environment in which it operates. Cardiac hemodynamics, hydrostatic and ambient pressure gradients, physiologic homeostasis and chemical reactions, muscle tone and stretch properties, tissue–tissue interaction and system level dynamics, enervation pathways and reflex arcs, to name a few, are different, despite an investigator's attempt to replicate the native environment. However, because it is extremely difficult to control for all experimental parameters in vivo, isolated large tissue models are an acceptable surrogate and a powerful experimental

Table 11.1 Advantages and disadvantages of perfusion techniques

Perfusion technique	Advantages	Disadvantages
Superfusion	• Preparation is easy to isolate and prepare • Preparation can be isolated from any location in the heart • Ability to quickly switch experimental solution	• Preparation must be small to be adequately nourished via solution diffusion • Buffer solution cannot contain large or hydrophilic molecules • Preparation can develop a necrotic core
Vascular Perfusion	• Preparation can be large in size • Perfusion is more physiologic • Ability to study tissue with dense myocardial organization and matrix • Ability to study a preparation with different tissue types	• Preparation must be isolated from a region containing vasculature • Difficulty in perfusing the preparation adequately and homogenously • Solution cannot be too viscous or contain sediments/air bubbles • Perfusion is subject to vascular reactions like constriction or dilation • Difficulty in switching perfusion solution quickly • Requires greater surgical skills to prepare

tool to investigate physiological and mechanistic behavior. Conducting relevant mechanistic experiments and translating the physiology and pathophysiology to general scientific principles and applications requires the appropriate model studied in the appropriate way under the appropriate conditions. Table 11.1 summarizes major advantages and disadvantages for studying isolated tissue preparations using superfusion and perfusion techniques.

11.3.1 Advantages and Limitations of Superfused Tissue Models

Superfusion is a powerful method for nutrient and electrolyte delivery to small tissue preparations from the outside-in along the concentration gradient. The main advantage of this technique is the ability to study tissue isolated from practically any region of the heart without regard to availability of any vascular network. Another experimental advantage is the ability to quickly switch superfusion solutions containing different water-soluble chemical agents, electrolytes, or compounds, and to explore the preparation's response to different superfusates. This makes the technique ideal for studying mechanistic relationships in physiology and drug interactions with cardiac function.

The major drawback of this technique is that it relies on diffusion and, therefore, the size of the preparation must be small enough to allow for adequate and homogenous penetration of electrolytes and nutrients. In addition, the preparation cannot be very dense and should have a large surface area with small cross-section. This technique becomes less effective, as well, if the superfusate contains large or very hydrophilic molecules that need to be delivered. A major concern when using superfusion is preparation viability over time, which is usually plagued by a malnourished core. The superfusate, therefore, must have a high enough flow rate to ensure that the preparation is continually bathed with fresh, oxygenated, buffered, and warmed solution. Nonetheless, when used properly, superfusion is a powerful experimental technique that allows for the study of a variety of isolated tissue models.

11.3.2   Advantages and Limitations of Perfused Tissue Models

Perfusion is a powerful technique for delivery of nutrients and electrolytes in large isolated tissue preparations. Perfusion occurs from the inside-out along the concentration gradient, relying on the vascular and capillary networks of the preparation. The main advantage of the perfusion technique is the ability to use larger preparations than what is permissible with superfusion techniques, with little regard to the surface area to cross-section balance and diffusion concerns. Another advantage is the fact that perfusion is more physiologic since the nutrients, electrolytes, or drugs are delivered in a manner that is comparable to the native environment of the tissue in vivo (i.e., through the vascular network).

Despite these advantages, perfusion techniques have major limitations. The preparation must be isolated from an area that is nourished by vasculature; this limits the regions from which tissue can be isolated. Preparation stability and viability is also a concern when relying on vasculature, since actual delivery of perfusion solution depends on vascular resistance. The preparation may not be adequately and homogeneously perfused throughout an experiment, since the perfusate takes the path of least resistance, i.e., any un-ligated collaterals or lesions may shunt perfusate out of the preparation. In addition, if a perfusion solution includes large partially dissolved particles, develops sediment, contains air bubbles, or has compounds with vasoconstrictive properties, small vessels and capillaries may clog and result in poor and irregular tissue perfusion across the preparation. Therefore, a balance between constant perfusion flow and constant perfusion pressure needs to be maintained. Constant perfusion flow ensures the constant delivery of perfusate to a preparation at all times regardless of vasoconstriction, vascular occlusion, or rising in-line pressure. In extreme cases, this may rupture or damage delicate vascular networks by forcing perfusate through constricted vessels. On the other hand, constant perfusion pressure ensures that the pressure in the vascular network is maintained within a desired range throughout the course of the experiment, regardless of whether enough perfusate is being delivered to the preparation. In extreme cases and as a result of vasoconstriction or occlusion, the perfusate flow drops dramatically for a given pressure and certain regions of the preparation become ischemic due to low nutrient and electrolyte supply. Furthermore, the larger the tissue model, the more difficult it is to quickly switch between solutions and achieve uniform perfusion. This makes studies requiring complete solution washout more challenging. Lastly but equally important, perfusion models require far greater surgical skills than superfused models, making it difficult for relatively novice investigators to prepare reliable and viable perfused tissue models with a high level of reproducibility.

11.4 Conclusion

This chapter discussed large isolated tissue models and covered a partial listing of isolated cardiac tissue preparations that are commonly used. The models have been covered in context of the nutrient delivery methods that can be used to sustain their viability (i.e., superfusion or vascular perfusion). Experimental implementations, as well as advantages and limitations of isolated cardiac tissue models are also discussed to convey to the reader some practical subtleties of their utilization.

References

1. Chapman RA, Tunstall J. The relationship between the external calcium concentration and the contracture tension developed by auricular trabeculae isolated from the heart of the frog, *Rana pipiens*. J Physiol 1970; 210:147P–8P.
2. Endoh M, Hashimoto K. Pharmacological evidence of autonomic nerve activities in canine papillary muscle. Am J Physiol 1970; 218:1459–63.
3. Whalen WJ, Fishman N, Erickson R. Nature of the potentiating substance in cardiac muscle. Am J Physiol 1958; 194:573–80.
4. Lamb JF, McGuigan JA. Contractures in a superfused frog's ventricle. J Physiol 1966; 186:261–83.
5. Yan GX, Antzelevitch C. Cellular basis for the electrocardiographic J wave. Circulation 1996; 93:372–79.
6. Yan GX, Shimizu W, Antzelevitch C. Characteristics and distribution of M cells in arterially perfused canine left ventricular wedge preparations. Circulation 1998; 98:1921–27.
7. Motomura S, Iijima T, Taira N, et al. Effects of neurotransmitters injected into the posterior and the anterior septal artery on the automaticity of the atrioventricular junctional area of the dog heart. Circ Res 1975; 37:146–55.
8. Efimov IR, Fahy GJ, Cheng Y, et al. High-resolution fluorescent imaging does not reveal a distinct atrioventricular nodal anterior input channel (fast pathway) in the rabbit heart during sinus rhythm. J Cardiovasc Electrophysiol 1997; 8:295–306.
9. Chiba S, Kubota K, Hashimoto K. Double peaked positive chronotropic response of the isolated blood-perfused S-A node to caffeine. Tohoku J Exp Med 1972; 107:101–2.
10. Hirose M, Imamura H. Mechanisms of atrial tachyarrhythmia induction in a canine model of autonomic tone fluctuation. Basic Res Cardiol 2007; 102:52–62.

Chapter 12
Isolated Heart Models

Nicholas D. Skadsberg, Alexander J. Hill, and Paul A. Iaizzo

Abstract Cardiovascular research employs a milieu of experimental models to investigate various conditions of health and disease ranging from cellular and whole organ preparations to computer modeling simulations. Uniquely, the isolated perfused heart model allows for the separation of cardiac and systemic variables, yet one can still explore typical measures used in cardiac research including myocardial function, metabolism, and/or responses to pharmacological, mechanical, and electrical components. A survey of the literature reveals that such preparations can vary greatly in design including choice of animal model, perfusion modes, perfusate compositions, and/or procedural techniques. Further, the wide array of measurements are made in the denervated heart, allowing one to conduct research in the absence of the confounding effects of sympathetic and vagal stimulations. Recently, there have been several groups employing high-resolution imaging and monitoring technologies to gain further insight into the intracardiac environment and/or the impact of various surgical procedures and implant techniques on the device–tissue interface. This chapter summarizes the major methodologies used to support these models, provides examples of usage, and clarifies the advantages and disadvantages of isolated hearts in comparison with other types of cardiovascular research.

12.1 Introduction

There have been numerous isolated in vivo, in situ, in vitro, and postmortem heart studies conducted after Langendorff first described his work in 1895,[1] each based on various and different assumptions to better approximate normal physiological conditions and allow for eventual correlation to human function. Notably, the selection of an experimental model depends on many factors, including (1) costs; (2) ease of data collection; (3) relevance to the human condition; and/or (4) the experimental questions to be answered.[2] Yet, costs and ease of data collection have

N.D. Skadsberg (✉)
Medtronic, Inc., Mounds View, MN, USA
e-mail: nick.skadsberg@medtronic.com

D.C. Sigg et al. (eds.), *Cardiac Electrophysiology Methods and Models*,
DOI 10.1007/978-1-4419-6658-2_12, © Springer Science+Business Media, LLC 2010

been the primary reasons for the widespread use of small mammalian rather than large mammalian heart models. More specifically, small isolated animal heart models (i.e., rat, guinea pig, rabbit) have primarily found use in pharmacological, respiration, and crystalloid perfusate effects,[3–5] while larger animal heart models (i.e., pig, dog, calf) provide further benefit by better approximating human hemodynamic characteristics both within the heart and for modeling circulation characteristics.[6] Regarding large animal heart models, cardiac size, musculature, and geometry typically better approximate human function (cardiac output, coronary flow, etc.) compared to developed biventricular rat or guinea pig models.

In vitro models have specific advantages over in vivo models, specifically the separation of cardiac responses from systemic responses. This allows for characterization of pharmacological, electrical, and hemodynamic (blood flow and pressure) parameters specific to the heart. Additionally, characterizations of mechanical, electrical, and chemical variables are possible, with little compromise in contractility associated with denervation.[7] More recently, human hearts deemed not viable for transplantation have been successfully studied using these methodologies.[8–10] Utilizing human hearts would seem to be the ideal isolated heart model for the study of human physiology, however, the hearts available for such studies usually have severely compromised function and associated pathologies (fortunately, this means that all viable hearts are likely transplanted). Nevertheless, isolated human hearts are ideal for the study of anatomy, pathology, and device–tissue interactions. In fact, our laboratory recently reanimated a human heart on a portable apparatus, allowing for the study of function within a MRI unit (unpublished data).

12.2 Experimental Model and Methods

12.2.1 Species

In most laboratories, the model objectives are to develop the ability to represent in situ physiological cardiac function ex vivo. For example, our laboratory has primarily chosen to study swine hearts rather than smaller rat or guinea pig models, due to their notably similar anatomical and physiological similarities to humans. Nevertheless, canine and ovine hearts have also been studied using this preparation, as they are uniquely different from the swine heart and are therefore utilized in cardiovascular research for specific purposes. Canine hearts are considered the traditional pacing and defibrillation model and ovine hearts are the classic valve model. For example, our laboratory recently reported on the use of an isolated canine heart model in which chronically implanted pacing leads were evaluated employing various methodologies for lead extraction using direct visualization.[11] Nevertheless, if and when possible, the use of an isolated human heart is the ideal model to perform device placements. For example, Quill and coworkers described the deployment of a Melody™ valve (Medtronic, Inc., Minneapolis, MN) in the pulmonic position within a beating human heart,[8] and Laske et al. described the device–tissue interface during pacing lead fixation.[12]

12.2.2   Perfusion Method

Although many laboratories have described numerous methodologies to reanimate isolated hearts in vitro, in the following text we will focus on the methods that our lab has developed over the past 12 years. The original methods used to reanimate swine hearts in our laboratory were described in Chinchoy et al.[13] A subsequent publication detailed an updated methodology facilitating all large mammalian hearts, including human hearts.[14] Therefore, an overview of the methods, including updates since these publications, is provided in the following section.

Isolated swine, mini-pig, canine, ovine, and human hearts are studied within our laboratory, with heart weights ranging from several hundred grams to more than one thousand grams (i.e., severely diseased human hearts). Animal hearts are explanted using standard cardioplegia procedures and standardized or investigational buffers.[15,16] Human hearts are explanted using standard transplantation procedures, placed on ice, and then transported to our laboratory within 2–6 h of cross-clamp. Following explantation, the major vessels of all hearts are cannulated while hearts are maintained in a hypothermic state. In several hearts, an additional cannula is sewn into the right atrial appendage (RAA) to facilitate endoscopic imaging. Often, the major arteries arising off the arch of the aorta are cannulated to allow additional access for cameras or device delivery systems.

After cannulation, the hearts are placed on an in vitro apparatus capable of supporting Langendorff, right-side working, and four-chamber working modes.[13,14] We routinely employ a modified, clear, Krebs–Henseleit perfusate as a blood substitute throughout the in vitro portion of such experiments. The most common additives to this buffer used to maintain cardiac performance are: (1) ethylenedi-aminetetraacetic acid (0.32 mmol/L) to chelate calcium and toxic metal ions; (2) insulin (10.0 U/L) to aid in glucose utilization; (3) sodium pyruvate (2.27 mmol/L) as an additional energy substrate; and (4) mannitol (16.0 mmol/L) to increase perfusate osmolarity and ultimately reduce cardiac edema. It should also be noted that we have employed heparinated blood as a periodic perfusate.

To maintain proper perfusate and myocardial temperatures, water jackets surrounding the arterial compliance chambers and both preload chambers are employed and maintained at 38–39°C (Model 370 Bio-Cal, Medtronic, Inc.), resulting in measured myocardial temperatures of 37°C ± 0.5°C. It should be noted that swine core temperatures are typically around 38°C, whereas human core temperatures are commonly 37°C.

In the classic *Langendorff perfusion mode*, the perfusate is pumped via a left-side pump in a retrograde direction down the aortic cannula and through the coronary system, primarily emptying into the right atrium (RA) via the coronary sinus. *Right-side working mode* consists of physiologic flow (>3 L/min) through the right side of the heart, in concert with Langendorff perfusion of the coronaries. In *four-chamber working mode*, perfusate is circulated through the heart in a normal physiological manner, and two pumps provide input flows to the RA and left atrium (LA) simultaneously.

The relative heights of fluid columns in the preload chambers, above entry into the heart, determine the amount of preload placed on the heart and are kept at near physiological values. Similarly, afterloads are simulated by adjusting the heights of the tubing leading from the aortic and pulmonic cannulae to the appropriate reservoirs. Arterial compliance is simulated by employing an air-filled closed chamber in line between the aortic cannula and the reservoir. With this combination of preloads and afterloads, stroke work and oxygen consumption are relatively maintained, given the differences in ejecting versus isovolumetric and isobaric models.[17–19] It is important to note that several experimental systems have identified influences from various sources (e.g., a preserved pericardium in vitro), and thus improved upon the previous definition of *working* as sole left ventricular (LV) ejection affecting filling rates, given the interaction between both left and right sides.[20–22]

As needed, defibrillation and pacing support is provided by internal or external pacing/defibrillatory leads. Hemodynamic monitoring is typically accomplished via pressure-tip catheters inserted into the right ventricle (RV) and LV and/or ultrasonic flow probes placed in line with the aorta, pulmonary vein, and/or inferior vena cava. In addition, one can simply employ a bipolar configuration of surface electrodes to continuously record electrocardiograms.

12.2.3 Intracardiac Visualization

To obtain direct, real-time visualization of the intracardiac environment, we employ simultaneous endoscopic cameras (4 or 6 mm in diameter) and intracardiac echocardiography via access through the superior vena cava, RAA, aortic trunk arteries, pulmonary trunk, pulmonary veins, descending aorta, and/or the LV or RV apices (see www.vhlab.umn.edu/atlas). In addition, smaller diameter (1.5–2.5 mm) fiberscopes are used to image small areas of the hearts such as the lumens of coronary arteries. Simultaneously, we also employ fluoroscopy and/or external echocardiography (Figs. 12.1 and 12.2). Coupled with the use of a modified Krebs–Henseleit perfusate, this technique allows for visual depiction with variations of input to the heart (e.g., loading conditions) as well as investigation of device interactions.

Several investigators have recently employed isolated cardiac models for the observation of transient valve motion and resultant movement as a consequence of valvular interventions and/or surgeries.[8,23,24] Common to all studies was the use of a high-speed digital video camera to allow for careful observation of the motion of the valve leaflets and annulus prior to and after the intervention.

12.2.4 Electrophysiological Studies

For over a century, isolated heart models have provided insight into many important phenomena including the all-or-none law, the absolute refractory period, and the origin of cardiac automaticity.[25] More recently, isolated human and large mammalian heart models offer the potential for a wide variety of electrophysiological studies to

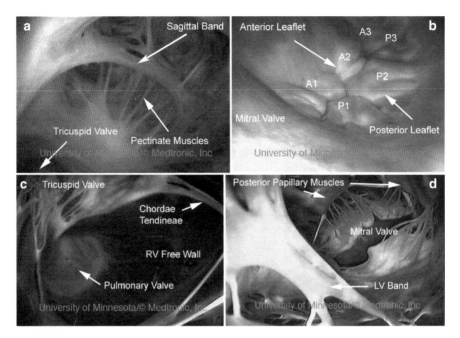

Fig. 12.1 Representative figure demonstrating direct visualization within the four chambers of a reanimated, isolated human heart. Shown in series are (**a**) right atrium, (**b**) left atrium, (**c**) right ventricle, and (**d**) left ventricle

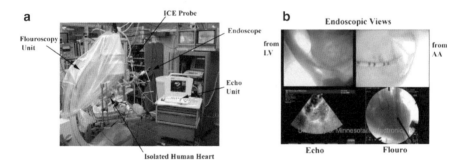

Fig. 12.2 Example of comparative imaging modalities employed in an isolated heart preparation. Shown are (**a**) laboratory with all imaging systems in place, (**b**) a quad-split view of simultaneous imaging: endoscopic views of the aortic valve (*upper images*), echo image (*lower left*) and a fluoroscopic view in anterior-to-posterior orientation. *AA* aortic arch; *ICE* intracardiac echocardiography; *LV* left ventricle

be performed. For example, Banville and colleagues studied restitution dynamics in isolated swine hearts in an effort to predict the development of alternans and reentrant arrhythmias during pacing.[26] Unfortunately, in the isolated swine heart, it was found that acute memory effects act to damp out proarrhythmic alternans in action potential durations that have been proposed to lead to wavebreak.

Using the previously reported methodology,[13] our group has reported on several studies investigating the electrophysiologic effects of various pacing strategies and anatomical locations. Such efforts stem from the increased interest in determining alternative pacing sites that minimize or eliminate the deleterious effects associated with RV apical pacing, including LV electrical and mechanical dyssynchrony, LV dysfunction (systolic and diastolic), and the possible promotion of ventricular arrhythmias.[27-31] Theoretically, pacing from the heart's intrinsic conduction system results in rapid, synchronous ventricular activation and performance. Employing high-resolution noncontact mapping, we evaluated pacing/sensing performance and endocardial activation sequences using custom designed plunge electrodes providing pacing at various depths relative to the His bundle.[32] It was demonstrated that LV activation patterns similar to sinus rhythm may be achieved without direct activation of the His bundle, while maintaining acceptable pacing and sensing performance. These data indicated that pacing systems designed to stimulate the tissues below the point at which the His bundle penetrates the central fibrous body may provide improved system efficiency and LV performance in comparison to both direct His bundle pacing and traditional pacing sites.

In acute animal studies, pacing from the RV outflow tract (RVOT) has demonstrated beneficial effects,[33] yet clinical experience has yielded inconsistent results.[34] Extensive hemodynamic measurements coupled with noncontact mapping have allowed for acute assessment of RVOT pacing in our lab, where we have demonstrated normal, physiological activation patterns and preserved systolic and diastolic performance when pacing from this anatomical site (Fig. 12.3).[35] The advantage of using an isolated heart model to perform such studies is that the precise pacing site can be visualized and subsequently studied using histological analyses.

12.2.5 Device–Tissue Interaction

Using a large mammalian isolated heart, the ability to obtain direct, intracardiac visualization provides the unique capability to investigate the interactions between medical device technology/therapies and the endocardial tissue. More specifically, employing a clear perfusate allows for recording images of internal cardiac structure, and also enables internal transient cardiac motion visualization during contraction and relaxation with varying cardiac inputs. Recently, we demonstrated that variations in measured impedances at the time of implant were associated with the nature of the fixation in both isolated swine and human hearts (Fig. 12.4).[10] Intracardiac visualization demonstrated that overtorquing leads was associated with visible distortion at the endocardial tissue–lead interface in at least 60% of swine and human hearts.

Many implanting physicians commonly use the coronary sinus in interventional cardiac procedures, however, complications can arise from certain anatomic structures, such as obstructing Thebesian valves, which are difficult to visualize under fluoroscopic and echocardiographic imaging. Our laboratory endoscopically visualized the coronary sinus ostia in 15 isolated human hearts and observed varying

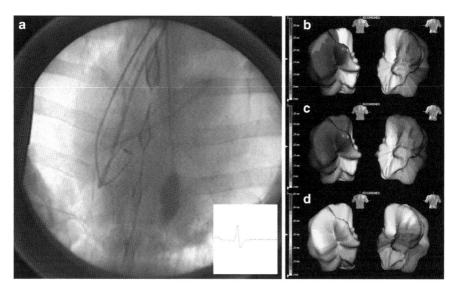

Fig. 12.3 (**a**) Fluoroscopic image of a typical study employing high-resolution, noncontact mapping to assess pacing configurations. Endocardial electrical activation sequences observed during pacing from (**b**) the right atrial appendage (intrinsic rhythm), (**c**) the right ventricular outflow tract, and (**d**) the right ventricular apex. The reconstructed geometry of the left ventricle is shown in an anterior-to-posterior orientation on the left and a posterior-to-anterior on the right, with *white* representing the region of maximal depolarization and *purple* representing isoelectric regions of the endocardium. *Other colors* represent varying levels of depolarization

Thebesian valve morphologies in 12 of 15 hearts.[9] The study of the coronary sinus ostium and subsequent access has aided design engineers in the design of specialized catheters that can be used to deploy left heart pacing leads (i.e., transvenous leads are positioned into various branches of the cardiac veins).

Beyond catheter and lead placement, several investigators have utilized isolated heart models for the study of valvular motion and impact of different valve designs and surgical interventions.[23,36,37] In our laboratory, we have deployed several different surgical and transcatheter valve designs into in vitro animal and human hearts to characterize interactions with the implant locations.[38] Specifically, Quill et al. recently visualized the deployment of the Melody™ transcatheter valve into an isolated human heart.[8] In other studies, we have examined transcatheter valve placements with specific focus on sizing, paravalvular leak, and impact of placement on surrounding anatomy, such as transcatheter aortic valve interactions with the aortic leaflet of the mitral valve (Fig. 12.5).

12.3   Limitations

One of the major limitations of using an isolated heart model is that there is a subsequent decrease in performance over time; this is especially true if a nonblood perfusate is employed. In other words, following completion of the transplantation

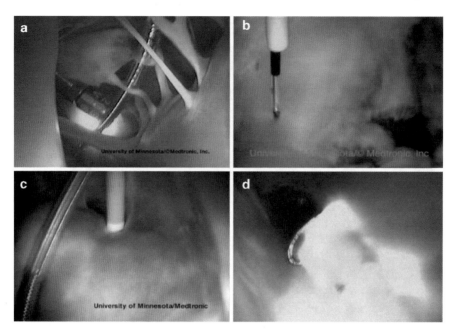

Fig. 12.4 Examples of device–heart interaction are shown. (**a**) Pacing lead (Medtronic, Inc., Minneapolis, MN) being viewed with a second endoscope (Olympus) implanted in the right ventricle. (**b**) 4.1 Fr pacing lead being delivered through a deflectable catheter (Medtronic, Inc.) and implanted into the triangle of Koch in the right atrium. (**c**) Catheter placed within the coronary sinus (Medtronic, Inc.). (**d**) Laser extraction of a lead within the right atrium (Spectronetics)[11]

procedure, suturing and cannulation of the vasculature, and reperfusion/stabilization of the heart in the apparatus, a constant deterioration process will occur after several hours with the induction of regional and eventual global ischemia. Furthermore, whether considered an investigational advantage or disadvantage, explicit effects due to various sympathetic and parasympathetic hormones in vitro are not able to be studied. However, this could be remedied with the addition of catecholamines, other neurotransmitters, and/or other performance enhancing agents (e.g., calcium) to the perfusate in a controlled manner. Administered anesthetics, which were not present in vitro, have also been shown to depress cardiac function. For instance, large decreases in ventricular relaxation were observed following explantation into the apparatus. Part of this difference may be due to the lack of compliance (and therefore vascular capacitance) of the filling tubing in vitro. The passive and constant filling nature of the in vitro filling pressure did not allow for elastance observed in systemic physiological systems.

The majority of isolated animal heart models lack pulmonary vasculature, and the geometry of these hearts is not 1:1 with that of humans. For example, if one wants to use an isolated heart model to study methodologies to isolate the pulmonary veins using ablation, the swine heart is a poor choice. Specifically, these hearts have only two main pulmonary vein ostia that subsequently branch within a short

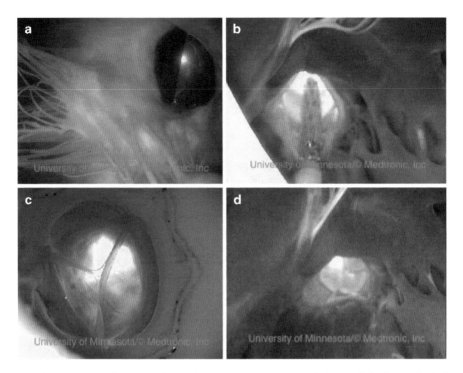

Fig. 12.5 Examples of valve–heart interaction are shown. (**a**) Videoscopic image of bileaflet mechanical valve (St. Jude Medical, St. Paul, MN, USA) within a reanimated donor human heart, viewed from the ascending aorta. (**b**) Transcatheter pulmonic valve (Melody™ Transcatheter Pulmonary Valve, Medtronic, Inc., Minneapolis, MN, USA) being delivered into a reanimated donor human heart via a balloon catheter, viewed from within the right ventricle looking up the outflow tract.[8] (**c**) In the same procedure as (**b**), the deployed valve is viewed via an endoscope placed within the trunk of the pulmonary artery (above). (**d**) Similar view as in (**b**) of the valve properly delivered

distance, and do not have myocyte projections into their ostia.[39] Therefore, choosing the best experimental model of a given human condition requires a number of decisions and compromises, especially relative to obtaining the optimal balance between the quantity and quality of the data produced versus the relevance of the data to the condition under investigation.[2]

12.4   Conclusion

This chapter summarizes some of the major methodologies used to support a large mammalian heart model. We provided examples of usage, and discussed several of the advantages and disadvantages of these experiments in comparison with other types of cardiovascular research.

In developing an in vitro apparatus to sustain a given heart ex vivo, considerations about the natural physiological conditions of the various species of heart to be used should be made. For example, numerous working small animal models have recently implemented biventricular modes[40–42] given right- and left-side function interdependence.[43] Additionally, perfusion apparatuses for isolating large animal hearts have been developed as investigational tools to assess hyperacute rejection,[44,45] blood flow characteristics for valve simulation and bioprosthesis evaluation,[8,46] cardiac ischemia,[47,48] and edema.[15,16,49]

In vitro human heart experiments have become relatively more frequent, using explanted human hearts from donor recipients.[8,12,14] Nevertheless, in many of these studies, the hearts are often fairly compromised, i.e., obtained from organ donors whose hearts are deemed not viable for transplantation and often with the RA damaged as the inferior vena cava is isolated for liver transplantation. Nevertheless, from such investigations, we have learned much about the functional ability to reanimate human hearts in vitro, knowledge that can then be applied to subsequent animal models. Furthermore, because all isolated heart studies eventually aim to approximate in vivo human heart function, it is essential to attribute hemodynamic differences to the various stages of explantation and the mode of reanimation. For example, it should be noted that, in the large mammalian heart, a significant change in ventricular performance (comparable to explantation to the apparatus) occurred with excision of the pericardium.[13]

As evidenced by the experiences in our laboratory, the clear perfusate allowed detailed imaging during ex vivo physiological working conditions. This visual ability aids in interactive device studies during cardiac movement in vitro, providing benefits in assessing orientation and interaction of implanted devices, chamber and valve movements to varying inputs, and reactions to other various physiological factors. The transient ex vivo model provides interactive cardiac electrophysiological function separated from systemic effects.

In summary, the isolated large mammalian heart model remains a unique experimental approach to gain insights on the electrophysiologic properties of the heart. Furthermore, it allows for the critical evaluation of clinical methodologies and/or application of devices to influence or treat abnormal cardiac electrical function, while simultaneously allowing one to monitor hemodynamic performance without influence of systemic parameters.

References

1. Langendorff O. Untersuchungen am uberlebenden Saugethierherzen (Investigations on the surviving mammalian heart). Arch Gesante Physiol 1895; 61:291–332.
2. Hearse DJ, Sutherland FJ. Experimental models for the study of cardiovascular function and disease. Pharmacol Res 2000; 41:597–603.
3. Neubauer S, Ingwall JS. The isolated, buffer-perfused ferret heart: a new model for the study of cardiac physiology and metabolism. Lab Anim 1991; 25:348–53.
4. Jacob AD, Elkins N, Reiss OK, et al. Effects of acetate on energy metabolism and function in the isolated perfused rat heart. Kidney Int 1997; 52:755–60.
5. Coetzee A, Kotze J, Louw J, et al. Effect of oxygenated crystalloid cardioplegia on the functional and metabolic recovery of the isolated perfused rat heart. J Thorac Cardiovasc Surg 1986; 91:259–69.

6. McCarthy PM, Fukamachi K, Fukumura F, et al. The Cleveland Clinic-Nimbus total artificial heart. In vivo hemodynamic performance in calves and preclinical studies. J Thorac Cardiovasc Surg 1994; 108:420–8.

7. Von Scheidt W, Neudert J, Erdmann E, et al. Contractility of the transplanted, denervated human heart. Am Heart J 1991; 121:1480–8.

8. Quill JL, Laske TG, Hill AJ, et al. Direct visualization of a transcatheter pulmonary valve implantation within the visible heart: a glimpse into the future. Circulation 2007; 116:e548.

9. Hill AJ, Ahlberg SE, Wilkoff BL, et al. Dynamic obstruction to coronary sinus access: the Thebesian valve. Heart Rhythm 2006; 3:1240–1.

10. Anderson SE, Skadsberg ND, Laske TG, et al. Variation in pacing impedance: impact of implant site and measurement method. Pacing Clin Electrophysiol 2007; 30:1076–82.

11. Love CJ, Ahlberg SE, Hiniduma-Lokuge P, et al. Novel visualization of intracardiac pacing lead extractions: methodologies performed within isolated canine hearts. J Interv Card Electrophysiol 2009; 24:27–31.

12. Laske TG, Skadsberg ND, Iaizzo PA. A novel ex vivo heart model for the assessment of cardiac pacing systems. J Biomech Eng 2005; 127:894–8.

13. Chinchoy E, Soule CL, Houlton AJ, et al. Isolated four-chamber working swine heart model. Ann Thorac Surg 2000; 70:1607–14.

14. Hill AJ, Laske TG, Coles JA Jr, et al. In vitro studies of human hearts. Ann Thorac Surg 2005; 79:168–77.

15. Sigg, DC, Coles JA Jr, Gallagher WJ, et al. Opioid preconditioning: myocardial function and energy metabolism. Ann Thorac Surg 2001; 72:1576–82.

16. Coles JA Jr, Sigg DC, Iaizzo PA. The potential benefits of 1.5% hetastarch as a cardioplegia additive. Biochem Pharmacol 2005; 69:1553–8.

17. Liu CT. Techniques for isolation and performance of the perfused guinea pig working heart. Am J Vet Res 1986; 47:1032–43.

18. Glower DD, Spratt JA, Snow ND, et al. Linearity of the Frank-Starling relationship in the intact heart: the concept of preload recruitable stroke work. Circulation 1985; 71:994–1009.

19. Neely JR, Libermeister H. Effect of pressure development on oxygen consumption by an isolated rat heart. Am J Physiol 1967; 212:804–14.

20. Fragata JI, Areias JC. Acute loads applied to the right ventricle: effect on left ventricular filling dynamics in the presence of an open pericardium. Pediatr Cardiol 1996; 17:77–81.

21. Schafer S, Schlack W, Kelm M, et al. Characterisation of left ventricular -dp/dt in the isolated guinea pig heart. Res Exp Med 1996; 196:261–73.

22. Hess OM, Bhargava V, Ross J Jr, et al. The role of the pericardium in interactions between the cardiac chambers. Am Heart J 1983; 106:1377–83.

23. Araki Y, Usui A, Kawaguchi O, et al. Pressure-volume relationship in isolated working heart with crystalloid perfusate in swine and imaging the valve motion. Eur J Cardiothorac Surg 2005; 28:435–42.

24. Hasegawa H, Araki Y, Usui A, et al. Mitral valve motion after performing an edge-to-edge repair in an isolated swine heart. J Thorac Cardiovasc Surg 2008; 136:590–6.

25. Bowditch HP. Über die Eigenthümlichkeiten der Reizbarkeit, welche die Muskelfasern des Herzens ziegen. Berichte über die Verhandlungen der Königlich Sächsischen Gesellschaft zu Leipzig. Mathematisch-Physische Classe 1871; 24:652–89.

26. Banville I, Chattipakorn N, Gray RA. Restitution dynamics during pacing and arrhythmias in isolated pig hearts. J Cardiovasc Electrophysiol 2004; 15:455–63.

27. Barold S, Lau C-P. Primary prevention of heart failure in cardiac pacing. Pacing Clin Electrophysiol 2006; 29:217–9.

28. Manolis A. The deleterious consequences of right ventricular apical pacing: time to seek alternate site pacing. Pacing Clin Electrophysiol 2006; 29:298–315.

29. Steinberg JS, Fischer A, Wang P, et al.; MADIT II Investigators. The clinical implications of cumulative right ventricular pacing in the multicenter automatic defibrillator trial II. J Cardiovasc Electrophysiol 2005; 16:359–65.

30. Schwaab B, Fröhlig G, Alexander C, et al. Influence of right ventricular stimulation site on left ventricular function in atrial synchronous ventricular pacing. J Am Coll Cardiol 1999; 33:317–23.
31. Lee MA, Dae MW, Langberg JJ, et al. Effects of long-term right ventricular apical pacing on left ventricular perfusion, innervation, function and histology. J Am Coll Cardiol 1994; 24:225–32.
32. Laske TG, Skadsberg ND, Hill AJ, et al. Excitation of the intrinsic conduction system through His and interventricular septal pacing. Pacing Clin Electrophysiol 2006; 29:397–405.
33. Rosenqvist M, Bergfeldt L, Haga Y, et al. The effect of ventricular activation sequence on cardiac performance during pacing. Pacing Clin Electrophysiol 1996; 19:1279–87.
34. De Cock CC, Giudici MC, Twisk JW. Comparison of the haemodynamic effects of right ventricular outflow-tract pacing with right ventricular apex pacing. Europace 2003; 5:275–8.
35. Skadsberg ND, Coles JA, Iaizzo PA. Electrophysiologic assessment of right ventricular cardiac pacing sites employing non-contact electrical mapping. IJBEM 2007; 7:325–8.
36. Hasegawa H, Araki Y, Usui A, et al. Mitral valve motion after performing and edge-to-edge repair in an isolated swine heart. J Thorac Cardiovasc Surg 2008; 136:590–6.
37. Mihaljevic T, Ootaki Y, Robertson JO, et al. Beating heart cardioscopy: a platform for real-time, intracardiac imaging. Ann Thorac Surg 2008; 85:1061–6.
38. Iaizzo PA, Hill AJ, Laske TG. Cardiac device testing enhanced by simultaneous imaging modalities: the Visible Heart®, fluoroscopy, and echocardiography. Expert Rev Med Devices 2008; 5:51–8.
39. Hill AJ, Iaizzo PA. Comparative cardiac anatomy. In: Iaizzo PA, editor. The Handbook of Cardiac Anatomy, Physiology and Devices, 2nd edition. New York: Humana Press, 2009 (Chapter 6).
40. Demmy TL, Magovern GJ, Kao RL. Isolated biventricular working rat heart preparation. Ann Thorac Surg 1992; 54:915–20.
41. Klima U, Guerrero JL, Levine RA, et al. A new, biventricular working heterotopic heart transplant model: anatomic and physiologic considerations. Transplantation 1997; 64:215–22.
42. Igic R. The isolated perfused "working" rat heart: a new method. J Pharmacol Toxicol Methods 1996; 35:63–7.
43. Bove AA, Santamore WP. Ventricular interdependence. Prog Cardiovasc Dis 1981; 23:365–88.
44. Forty J, White DG, Wallwork J. A technique for perfusion of an isolated working heart to investigate hyperacute discordant xenograft rejection. J Thorac Cardiovasc Surg 1993; 106:308–16.
45. Dunning J, Pierson RN, Braidley PC, et al. A comparison of the performance of pig hearts perfused with pig or human blood using an ex-vivo working heart model. Eur J Cardiothorac Surg 1994; 8:204–6.
46. Van Rijk-Zwikker GL, Schipperheyn JJ, Huysmans HA, et al. Influence of mitral valve prosthesis or rigid mitral ring on left ventricular pump function. Circulation 1989; 80:1–7.
47. Kimose H, Ravkilde J, Helligso P, et al. Influence of pre-existing ischemia on recovery from chemical cardioplegia. A study on pig hearts in an isolated blood-perfused model. Scand J sssssThorac Cardiovasc Surg 1992; 26:23–31.
48. Sandhu R, Diaz RJ, Wilson GJ. Comparison of ischaemic preconditioning in blood perfused and buffer perfused isolated heart models. Cardiovasc Res 1993; 27:602–7.
49. Weng ZC, Nicolosi AC, Detwiler PW, et al. Effects of crystalloid, blood, and University of Wisconsin perfusates on weight, water content, and left ventricular compliance in an edema-prone, isolated porcine heart model. J Thorac Cardiovasc Surg 1992; 103:504–13.

Chapter 13
Small Animal Models for Arrhythmia Studies

Jong-Kook Lee and Yukiomi Tsuji

Abstract Varieties of small animal models for arrhythmia study have been created using genetic and nongenetic techniques. However, data obtained from small animals must be interpreted carefully compared to larger animals such as dogs or pigs, because some electrophysiological properties of small animals such as constituents of action potentials are different from those of humans. This chapter briefly describes various small animal nongenetic models such as the myocardial infarction model and chronic atrioventricular block model as well as genetically engineered small animal models such as long QT syndrome and catecholaminergic polymorphic ventricular tachycardia.

Abbreviations

AF	atrial fibrillation
APD	action potential duration
ARVD/C	arrhythmogenic right ventricular dysplasia/cardiomyopathy
AV	atrioventricular
CPVT	catecholaminergic polymorphic ventricular tachycardia
ESCM	embryonic stem cell-derived cardiac myocytes
HF	heart failure
LQT	long QT
LV	left ventricular
MI	myocardial infarction
PV	pulmonary veins
RF	radiofrequency
TdP	Torsades de Pointes

J.-K. Lee (✉)
Department of Cardiovascular Research, Research Institute of Environmental Medicine, Nagoya University, Nagoya, Japan
e-mail: jlee@riem.nagoya-u.ac.jp

D.C. Sigg et al. (eds.), *Cardiac Electrophysiology Methods and Models*,
DOI 10.1007/978-1-4419-6658-2_13, © Springer Science + Business Media, LLC 2010

13.1   Introduction

For arrhythmia studies, wide varieties of experimental models have been created with small mammals including mice, rats, guinea pigs, hamsters, and rabbits. Compared to large animals such as dogs and pigs, small animals show various differences from humans. For example, mice and rats lack the plateau phase in action potentials of ventricular myocytes that is observed in large animals (similar to humans). In addition, ion channels as constituents for action potentials play different roles between rodents and dogs. In rodents, for instance, the transient outward potassium current (I_{to}) is one of the major determinants for repolarization of action potentials, while rapid and slow voltage-gated K channels (I_{Kr} and I_{Ks}) play critical roles in repolarization of large animals. These differences could pose problems in applying obtained results to clinical situations. Technically, the tiny anatomical structures of small animals, especially in mice, make surgical intervention difficult.

Nevertheless, there are increasing demands for small animal models using mice and rats. The mouse is a mammalian species in which substantial genomic information has been analyzed (second to the human). In addition, the Human Genome Project has revealed that most of the genes are conserved among mammalian species from mice to humans. Thus, once novel genes are cloned from inherited diseases or syndromes in humans, it is often required to confirm that the phenotype can be reproduced in genetically engineered animals. In stem cell research, regenerated myocardium can be differentiated or obtained from stem cells or other cell sources. To investigate the feasibility of cell transplantation as a potential therapeutic strategy, in vivo cell transplant studies are often conducted. Because most of these stem cell-derived cardiomyocytes are obtained from mice and humans, murine models have an advantage when homologous transplantation is feasible (i.e., transplantation of murine-derived cells to mice). In this chapter, commonly used experimental animal models with genetic engineering or nongenetic surgical techniques are introduced.

13.2   Nongenetic Small Animal Models for Arrhythmia Studies

A variety of small animal models have been created for studying cardiac arrhythmias. Genetically altered mice are the largest contributor to the recent advancement in cellular and molecular aspects of arrhythmia mechanism. On the other hand, traditional animal models by conventional techniques are still utilized. Here, we describe nongenetic small animal models that have provided insights into arrhythmia mechanisms (Table 13.1).

13.2.1   Myocardial Infarction Model

Coronary artery ligation to induce myocardial infarction (MI) has been long used in several species (dogs, pigs, cats, rabbits, and rats).[27] Based on findings from

Table 13.1 Small animal models of arrhythmia in the presence of diseases

Models	Methods	Species	References
Myocardial infarction	Coronary ligation	Rat	Ytrehus et al.[1]; Takamatsu[2]
		Mouse	Gehrmann et al.[3]
Hypertrophy and heart failure (HF)	Aortic constriction (ascending, transverse, abdominal)	Rat	Volk et al.[4]; Gomez et al.[5]; Tomita et al.[6]
	Transverse aortic constriction	Mouse	Marionneau et al.[7]
	Spontaneous hypertensive	Rat	Cerbai et al.[8]
	Daily injection of isoproterenol	Rat	Meszaros et al.[9]
	Monocrotaline injection (RVH)	Rat	Lee et al.[10]
	Pulmonary artery constriction (RVH)	Ferret	Potreau et al.[11]
	Tachypacing	Rabbit	Tsuji et al.[12]
	Aortic regurgitation/banding	Rabbit	Pogwizd et al.[13]; Vermeulen et al.[14]
Complete AV block	Chemical/RF ablation	Mouse	Lee et al.[15]; Piron et al.[16]
		Rabbit	Tsuji et al.[17]; Suto et al.[18]
Cardiac dyssynchrony	Overdrive RV pacing	Mouse	Bilchick et al.[19]
Atrial fibrillation	RA tachypacing	Rat	Yamashita et al.[20,21]
	Spontaneous hypertensive	Rat	Choisy et al.[22]
	HF after coronary-ligated infarction	Rat	Boixel et al.[23]
	Diabetes	GK Rat	Kato et al.[24]
	RA tachypacing	Rabbit	Bosch et al.[25]
	RV tachypacing-induced HF	Rabbit	Shimano et al.[26]

AV atrioventricular; *GK* Goto–Kakizaki; *RA* right atrial; *RF* radiofrequency; *RV* right ventricular; *RVH* right ventricular hypertrophy

these animal models, mechanisms of ventricular tachyarrhythmia associated with MI are well characterized.[2,28,29] Metabolic differences between the ischemic and nonischemic tissues in early phase acute MI, and remodeling of ion channels and transporters in the infarction border zone over days and weeks following acute MI, cause important changes in cellular electrical activity and impulse propagation; these changes promote enhanced automaticity, reentry, and triggered activity due to early and delayed after-depolarization. Increased tissue anisotropy, slowed conduction, and refractoriness heterogeneity favor unidirectional block with resultant reentry in the border zone, which is an important arrhythmia mechanism in healed MI. Gap junction changes (Connexin43, or Cx43, downregulation and redistribution) as well as alternations of K^+, Na^+, and L-type Ca^{2+} currents, and Ca^{2+} handling in the border zone cells have been demonstrated extensively in the dog[29] and also in the rat model.[2,29]

In recent years, the application of coronary artery ligation in the mouse model has allowed researchers to explore novel therapeutic approaches such as cell-based genetic therapies to prevent left ventricular (LV) remodeling and heart failure (HF) secondary to MI. Although there are many studies assessing their effects on global myocardial performance, information on how the electrophysiological substrate is modulated in the mouse is limited. Roell et al. demonstrated in mice, 11–14 days after MI, that transplantation of Cx43-expressing cells (either embryonic cardio-myocytes or genetically engineered skeletal myoblasts) suppressed conduction block and wave break in infarct border zone and decreased the incidence of ventricular tachycardia induced by pacing.[30] Kuhlmann et al. showed that treatment with granulocyte colony-stimulating factor and stem cell factor reduced inducible ventricular tachyarrhythmias via increased Cx43 expression in mice 5 weeks after MI.[31] Regarding mice in the control groups in these studies, the arrhythmogenic substrate seems comparable to that in other species. However, cellular and molecular electrophysiological changes associated with MI have been less investigated in the mouse. In addition, the mouse has high mortality (about 35–50%) because of ventricular fibrillation, acute HF, or LV rupture occurring within 1 h after MI, and develops HF if it survives over 2 weeks, which is similar to other species.[3,32]

13.2.2   Hypertrophy and Heart Failure Model

Experimental cardiac hypertrophy and HF have been induced in mice, rats, and rabbits using a variety of techniques. Transverse/ascending aortic banding,[4–7] daily injection of isoproterenol,[9] renal artery banding,[33] monocrotaline injection,[10] and pulmonary artery banding[11] produce left/right ventricular hypertrophy and/or HF, although the development of HF varies depending on the procedure. Spontaneous hypertensive rats have LV hypertrophy[8]; coronary artery-legated mice and rats develop HF following MI.[27] Ventricular tachypacing and aortic regurgitation/banding-induced HF models have been established in rabbits.[12–14]

Electrical remodeling associated with cardiac hypertrophy and HF predisposes to lethal ventricular tachyarrhythmias. Action potential duration (APD) prolongation is consistently observed. Downregulation of K^+ currents including transient outward and inward rectifier K^+ currents and alterations in Ca^{2+} handling have been demonstrated by many investigators (see review articles by Nattel et al.,[29] Furukawa et al.,[34] and Tomaselli et al.[35]). Studies in small animal models have shown that APD prolongation and alternation of membrane currents and Ca^{2+} handling protein expression (ryanodine receptor, sarcoplasmic reticulum Ca^{2+}-ATPase, and phospholamban) are normalized by pretreatment with ACE inhibitors,[36,37] angiotensin II type 1 receptor blockers,[38–40] mineral corticoid receptor antagonists,[41] and endothelin receptor-A antagonists,[42–44] suggesting antiarrhythmic effects. These results might be quite conceivable, along with our current understanding that Ca^{2+}-activated signals including calcineruin/NFAT and Ca^{2+}/calmodulin-dependent protein kinase II (CaMKII) pathways are major contributors to the arrhythmogenic remodeling in cardiac hypertrophy and HF,[45,46] because angiotensin II, aldosterone, and endothelin-1 increase intracellular Ca^{2+} concentration by activating L-type Ca^{2+} channels which, in turn, increase calcineurin and CaMKII activities.[34] However, molecular basis of ion channel remodeling remains largely unknown.

The arrhythmic phenotype may vary in the model even when the same species is used. It has been reported that rabbits subjected to ventricular tachypacing at 350–370 bpm for 3–4 weeks developed HF and some died prematurely.[12,47] But continuous 24-h telemetry ECG recording of seven tachypaced rabbits showed a single seven-complex run in only one animal. Pogwizd et al. have produced a rabbit HF model by aortic regurgitation and, 2–4 weeks later, by thoracic aortic constriction.[13] Nine of ten HF rabbits had nonsustained ventricular arrhythmias during serial Holter monitoring. The differences are likely due to the various methods of HF induction. Differences in etiology, duration, and severity of HF might influence the resulting ion channel remodeling and arrhythmic phenotype of HF.

13.2.3 Chronic Complete Atrioventricular Block Model

Bradycardia due to complete atrioventricular (AV) block is a well-known precipitator of Torsades de Pointes (TdP) arrhythmia in humans. Chronic AV block (CAVB) produces susceptibility to TdP in animals. Vos and coworkers described a dog model with CAVB as an animal model of acquired QT prolongation and TdP.[48] The ventricular remodeling seen after ablation of the AV node enhances the susceptibility for TdP arrhythmias. The cellular and molecular basis of ventricular remodeling has been well characterized.[49] CAVB cardiomyocytes show APD prolongation and increases in cell-shortening, systolic $[Ca^{2+}]_i$ transients and SR Ca^{2+} contents. Downregulation of subunits responsible for rapid and slow components of the delayed-rectifier K^+-current underlie APD prolongation, and CaMKII-activation and Ca^{2+}-handling alterations contribute to enhanced contractile function but at the same time promote arrhythmogenic after-depolarizations.[49,49-b]

Complete AV block has been created in rabbits, rats, and mice by chemical or radiofrequency (RF) ablation of the AV node. Following thoracotomy, 20 μl of 10–20% formaldehyde in rabbits,[17,47] 5–10 μl of 70% ethanol in rats,[50] or 5 μl of 10% glycerol in mice[15,51] was injected into the myocardium (the AV nodal area) below the epicardial surface between the aortic root and the right atrial medial wall to ablate AV node chemically (Fig. 13.1a, b; see Lee et al.[50] for details on the technique). Transvenous catheter ablation was performed in rabbits[18] and mice.[16] It has been reported that both the rabbit (Fig. 13.1c) and mouse develop sudden cardiac death with prominent QT prolongation and spontaneous TdP. The incidence of sudden cardiac death and TdP was 75% for rabbits[47] and 49% for mice,[15] respectively, which is clearly high compared with those in the dog model.[49] Transcriptional downregulation of KvLQT1 and minK responsible for I_{Ks} and ERG for I_{Kr} were documented in the rabbit model.[17,47] DNA microarray

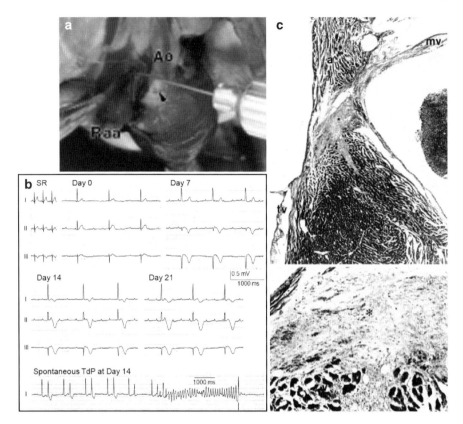

Fig. 13.1 Complete AV block model. (**a**) Surgical view for AV block creation. Right atrial appendage (Raa) was reflected laterally with forceps to expose the area between the aortic root (Ao) and medial wall of right atrium. The tip of needle, prepared by making a 90° bend in the shaft, penetrated the epicardial surface with the direction parallel to aorta. The epicardial fat pad (see *arrow*) located at this area was used as a marker for the insertion site in rats. Image from Lee et al.[50] (**b**) ECGs in a rabbit model. QT prolongation with abnormal QTU complex was observed at day 14 and 21. Spontaneous TdP was recorded during day 14 of ECG recording. *SR* sinus rhythm. Image from Tsuji et al.[17] (**c**) Histological section of AV conduction system from a rat 7 days after ethanol injection. Granulation tissue (*asterisks*) replaced the specialized muscle. Damage in working myocardium of either atrium (a) or ventricle (v) seemed very limited. Image from Lee et al.[50]

analysis showed downregulation of $Kv^\beta 1.5$, $Kv4.2$, $Kir2.1$, $Kir6.2$, and $Cav1.3$ and upregulation of $Kir2.2$ and $Cav^\beta 1$ in the mouse model.[15] It is believed that the animal models of sudden cardiac death might be a great tool to study the molecular basis of acquired modifications of ion channels and open up new strategies for arrhythmia therapy.

The novel biological therapy for bradyarrhythmias has been attempted in the mouse AV block model.[16,51] It was found that transplantation of embryonic stem cell-derived cardiac myocytes (ESCMs), which expressed the gene of transcriptional factor Nkx2.5, restored the AV conduction in the mouse model. In the nontransplanted mice, marked fibrosis and discontinuity of Cx43/Cx40 expression were observed in the AV nodal region, whereas in the mice injected with ESCMs, substantial amounts of Cx43/Cx40 were recognized between ESCMs and the host cardiac myocytes.[51] Piron et al. performed a gene transfer of hyperpolarization-activated HCN2 channel combined with β_2-adrenergic receptor into the LV free wall of the AV block mouse.[16] The biological pacemaker appeared to be functional but did not suppress TdP, perhaps because the biological pacemaker rhythm rate was not fast enough.

13.2.4 Cardiac Dyssynchrony Model

Left ventricular dyssynchrony due to intraventricular conduction delay induces regional heterogeneity of mechanical load and is a predictor of mortality and sudden death in patients with HF. In order to study the pathophysiological basis of dyssynchrony, dogs subjected to left bundle branch ablation and/or pacing have been commonly used.[52] Recently, a mouse model of dyssynchrony has been developed, using a custom-designed miniature implantable pacemaker (3 V lithium battery, programmable rate: 450–1,050 bpm, weight: 1.5 g, diameter: 1.2 cm, bipolar lead).[19] One-week overdrive right ventricular pacing (720 bpm, baseline heart rate 520–620 bpm) resulted in differential expression between the LV septal and lateral wall >1.5 times in only 18 of the 22,000 genes surveyed. Seven of these genes, which showed prominent disparities, encoded for proteins involved with stretch responses, matrix remodeling, stem cell differentiation to myocyte lineage, and Purkinje fiber differentiation.[19]

13.2.5 Atrial Fibrillation Model

Atrial fibrillation (AF) is the most common arrhythmia and is associated with cardiovascular morbidity and mortality. The management of AF has advanced in recent years due to a better understanding of the arrhythmia mechanisms. Studies in human and large animal models with AF have identified three important paradigms: (1) atrial remodeling referring to changes in atrial function or structure that promote atrial arrhythmogenesis; (2) genesis of macro- and micro-reentrant circuits in the atria; and (3) arrhythmogenic activity in pulmonary veins (PVs).[29,53] Conventional antiarrhythmic drugs and catheter ablation are therapies targeting the reentrant circuits and pulmonary vein isolation, respectively, which have been termed *downstream* approaches. Pharmacological approaches targeting remodeling have been highlighted as potential *upstream* therapy for AF.

Traditional small animal models have been used to investigate atrial structural remodeling in the setting of diseases. Kato et al. showed increased atrial arrhythmogenicity in association with diffuse interstitial fibrosis in a diabetic rat model (Goto–Kakizaki rat) with the defects in glucose-stimulated insulin secretion, peripheral insulin resistance, hyperinsulinemia, and hyperglycemia, a model relevant to human type II diabetes.[24] One study in a rabbit model with ventricular tachypacing-induced HF showed similarities to the dog HF model, including significant atrial fibrosis, conduction slowing, and susceptibility to AF.[26,53] In this study, pioglitazone, an antidiabetic drug of the class thiazolidinedione, attenuated HF-induced atrial structural remodeling and AF promotion, with effects similar to those in an angiotensin II type 1 receptor blocker, candesartan.[26] Based on the fact that diabetic patients have increased risk of both AF development and thromboembolic complications from AF, these two studies in small animals may provide important clinical findings and implications.[54] In addition, atrial arrhythmogenic fibrotic remodeling has also been reported in spontaneous hypertensive rats[22] and in rats with HF after MI.[23]

The paroxysmal AF model has been created by rapid atrial pacing in small animals. Bosch et al. described a rabbit model of rapid atrial pacing.[25] Two bipolar custom-made electrode leads inserted via right and left cervical veins were positioned at the lateral wall of the right atrium for pacing and at the coronary sinus for recording. They evaluated, in this model, pacing duration between 6 and 96 h molecular mechanism of early ion channel remodeling. Reduction in L-type calcium and transient outward currents, which began 12–24 h after pacing onset, was closely paralleled to transcriptional downregulation of underlying channel subunits.[25] Yamashita et al. performed 1,200 bpm right atrial pacing for 8 h through an electrode catheter via the cervical vein of anesthetized rats.[20,21] They demonstrated the short-term high-rate pacing to differentially alter mRNA levels of Kv1.5, Kv4.2, and Kv4.3 in a rate-dependent manner,[20] and the ability to acutely downregulate gene expression of intrinsic anticoagulant factors, thrombomodulin, and tissue factor pathway inhibitor in the atrial endocardium.[21] It is noteworthy that the ventricular rate was not controlled in these small animal models. Rapid ventricular rates can produce ventricular dysfunction that may alter the atrial remodeling response to atrial tachypacing.

The myocardial sleeves of PVs are an important source of ectopic foci that initiate and maintain AF in humans. The PV myocardial sleeves have been demonstrated to possess arrhythmic electrical properties including pacemaker activity and early/delayed after-depolarization diathesis in isolated tissues and Langendorff perfused hearts of rabbits,[55–58] guinea pigs,[59,60] and rats.[61] Aging,[57,61] stretch,[56] glycolytic inhibition,[61] and pharmacological interventions inducing abnormal Ca^{2+} regulation[55,57,58] enhanced the arrhythmogenic PV activities. However, in vivo small animal models relevant to human AF originating from PVs have not yet been developed.

13.3 Genetically Engineered Small Animal Models for Arrhythmia Studies

A number of genetically engineered animal models have been created mostly in mice used for arrhythmia studies. These genetic models can be classified into the following categories: (1) models with the *structurally normal heart*; and (2) models with the *structurally abnormal heart*. The former group includes channelopathies such as LQT syndromes or Brugada syndromes, and the latter includes so-called cardiomyopathy, such as arrhythmogenic right ventricular dysplasia/cardiomyopathy (ARVD/C). In both groups, there are animal models to "reproduce" known inherited arrhythmogenic diseases or syndromes in humans, while there are other models in which genes encoding ion channels/pumps or other structural proteins were modified regardless of disease entities, which have turned out to show arrhythmogenicity.

In most cases, these mouse models have been created by (1) transgenic overexpression (dominant negative suppression); (2) knock-in; (3) knock-out; and (4) targeted mutagenesis. Transgenic overexpression (random insertion of mutated genes), however, may sometimes lead to unexpected outcomes such as abnormal expression of other ion channels (i.e., electrical remodeling).[62] Thus, careful attention must be paid in the interpretation of "transgenic" mouse models.

13.3.1   Long QT Syndromes

Experimental animal studies of the LQT syndromes have been conducted extensively. In human LQT syndromes, ten culprit genes have been found in:

- *K⁺channels* (LQT1: KCNQ1 encoding KvLQT1, α-subunit of I_{Ks} channels; LQT2: KCNH2 encoding HERG1, α-subunit of I_{Ks} channels; LQT5: KCNE1 encoding MinK/IsK, β-subunit of I_{Ks} channels; LQT6: KCNE2 encoding MiRP1, β-subunit of I_{Kr} channels; LQT7: KCNJ2 encoding Kir2.1, α-subunit of I_{K1} channels, also called Andersen syndrome).
- *Na⁺channels* (LQT3: SCN5A encoding $Na_v1.5$, α-subunit of fast Na channels; LQT10: SCN4B encoding $Na_v1.5β4$: β-subunit of fast Na channels; in LQT3, Na channels show gain-of-function abnormalities).
- *Ca²⁺channels* (LQT8: CACNA1 encoding $Ca_v1.2$, α1C subunit of L-type Ca channels, also called Timothy syndrome).
- *Ankyrin-B* (LQT4: ANK-B encoding ankyrin-B, anchoring ion channels in the cell membrane).
- *Caveolin-3* (LQT9: CAV3 encoding caveolin-3).

Genetically engineered LQT animal models have been created in each loci and phenotypes were analyzed (Table 13.2). Figure 13.2 shows one of the LQT models (LQT3) with mutated SCN5A channels (Na channels). Although half of these mouse models showed prolonged APD and QTc, the incidence of spontaneous arrhythmias or the inducibility of arrhythmias was not necessarily high.

Because contribution of ion channels as constituents of action potentials are different between mice and humans, various mutants has been studied. For example, mutants with Shaker-type voltage-gated K channels were created. Those mutant mice resultantly show prolonged APD and QTc, and some of these mutants demonstrate marked arrhythmogenicity.

Table 13.2 Animal models of the LQT syndromes found in humans

	Gene mutations	Affected protein/subunit	Ion channel	Species	References
LQT1	KCNQ1	KVLQT1	I_{Ks}	Mouse	Casimiro et al.[63]
				Mouse	Demolombe et al.[64]
				Mouse	Brunner et al.[65]
LQT2	KCNH2	HERG	I_{Kr}	Mouse	London et al.[66]
					Lees-Miller et al.[67]
				Mouse	Babij et al.[68]
				Mouse	Brunner et al.[65]
LQT3	SCN5A	Nav1.5α	I_{Na}	Mouse	Nuyens et al.[69]
LQT4	Ank2	Ankyrin-B	–	Mouse	Chauhan et al.[70]
LQT5	KCNE1	MinK	I_{Ks}	Mouse	Drici et al.[71]
					Kupershmidt et al.[72]
				Mouse	Marks et al.[73]
LQT6	KCNE2	MiRP1β	I_{Kr}	Human, dog, rat	Jiang et al.[74]
LQT7 (Andersen syndrome)	KCNJ2	Kir2.1	I_{K1}	Mouse	Zaritsky et al.[75]
LQT8 (Timothy syndrome)	CACNA1 c	Cav1.2α1c	$I_{Ca,L}$	Rat	Thiel et al.[76] Sicouri et al.[77]
LQT9	CAV3	Caveolin-3	–		
LQT10	SCN4B	Nav1.5β4	I_{Na}	Mouse	Remme et al.[78]

13.3.2 Brugada Syndrome

Brugada syndrome is a genetic disease characterized by right bundle branch block, ST elevation in the right precordial leads (V1, V2, V3), and susceptibility to ventricular tachyarrhythmias. Mutation in the SCN5A (Na$_v$1.5) accounts for a certain proportion of the syndromes (<25%). It has been reported that the syndrome is sometimes related to progressive cardiac conduction defects (also called Lev–Lenegre disease). Mutated Nav1.5 channels in Brugada syndrome show loss of function as phenotype, while mutated Nav1.5 channels show gain of function in long QT syndrome (LQT3). Papadatos et al. reported that SCN5A(+/−) mice show phenotype with slowed conduction in the atrium and AV node, and increased inducibility of ventricular tachyarrhythmias (Fig. 13.3).[79] In the following several studies, the model provided useful information regarding underlying mechanisms of the arrhythmogenesis of Brugada syndrome and the relationship with other conduction defects such as sick sinus syndrome.[80–82]

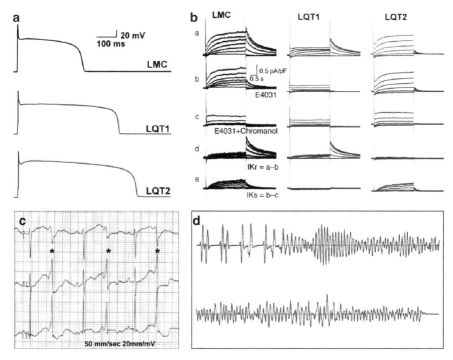

Fig. 13.2 Rabbit models for LQT1 and LQT2. (**a**) Action potentials of rabbit ventricular myocytes from LMC (littermate control), LQT1, and LQT2 rabbits. (**b**) Representative tracing of I_{Kr} and I_{Ks} from control (LMC), LQT1, LQT2 rabbits. The cells were perfused with 5 μM E-4031 (I_{Kr} blocker) (*line b*) and 30 μM chromanol 293B (I_{Ks} blocker), then the E4031-sensitive current (I_{Kr}) (*line d*) and chromanol-sensitive current (I_{Ks}) (*line e*) were calculated. The downregulation of I_{Kr} (in LQT1) (*line e*) and I_{Ks} (in LQT2) (*line d*) were demonstrated, respectively. (**c**) Sample ECGs (lead II) of the founders and a control (LMC) rabbit with sedation (midazolam 2 mg/kg, i.m.). Note the markedly prolonged QT interval and the lack of an isoelectric T-P line in both transgenic rabbits. (**d**) Sample telemetric ECGs (lead II) of awake, free-moving male rabbits. Cited from Brunner et al.[65]

13.3.3   Catecholaminergic Polymorphic Ventricular Tachycardia

Catecholaminergic polymorphic ventricular tachycardia (CPVT) is a genetic disease characterized by ventricular tachyarrhythmias (typically) triggered by exercise or emotion. Typically, VTs show a bi-directional nature. Recent studies have shown that mutations in ryanodine receptor (RY2)[83] and calsequestrin (CASQ2)[73] have been related with CPVT. Both abnormalities cause serious disruption of intracellular Ca^{2+} homeostasis. Genetic mouse models related to these mutations have been created and analyzed in detail. Wehrens et al. reported that mutations at Protein kinase A-induced phosphorylation sites of RYR2 induced incomplete closing of RYR2 channels during the diastolic phase, which causes Ca^{2+} leak from sarcoplasmic reticulum.[84]

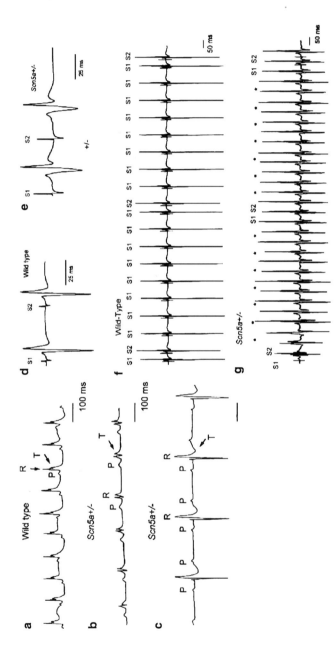

Fig. 13.3 Murine model for Brugada syndrome. (**a**) Representative ECG (lead I) from wild-type mouse. (**b**, **c**) Representative ECGs recorded from Scn5a+/− mouse. In trace (**b**), Scn5a+/− mouse shows 1:1 atrioventricular conduction with increased P-wave duration and prolonged PR interval. In trace (**c**), Scn5a+/− mouse shows second-degree atrioventricular block (2:1 AV conduction). The PR interval is prolonged (60 ms) with a rightward shift in the QRS axis. Panels (**d**–**g**) show conduction properties and ventricular tachycardia in Langendorff perfused mouse ventricular preparations. (**d**, **e**) Electrical recordings from the base of the left ventricle in response to stimuli applied to the right ventricular septum in wild-type and Scn5a+/− mouse. Note that latency and duration of QRS are greater in Scn5a+/− than in wild-type. (**f**, **g**) Representative continuous electrical recording from wild-type (**f**) and Scn5a+/− (**g**) ventricular preparation. In Scn5a+/−, S2 is followed by a delayed ventricular response that initiates ventricular tachycardia (*asterisks* represent points of S1 delivery with shock artifacts removed for clarity). Cited from Papadatos et al.[79]

Wehrens et al. also demonstrated that JTV519 (a derivative of 1,4-benzothiazepine) effectively prevented VTs by increasing the affinity of calstabin2 for RyR2, which decreases the Ca^{2+} leak.[85]

13.3.4   Arrhythmogenic Right Ventricular Dysplasia/ Cardiomyopathy (ARVD/C)

The ARVD/C is a genetic disease characterized by a progressive fatty degeneration of the right ventricle. Previous studies have reported that mutations in genes encoding desmosomal proteins (junctional plakoglobin, desmoplakin, plakophilin, and desmoglein) cause ARVD/C. On the other hand, in ARVD2, mutations in RyR2 that cause Ca leak from RyR channels show similar pathophysiological conditions with CPVT. Cardiac restricted transgenic mice with a mutation in desmoplakin have been created as an ARVD/C model.[86] A mouse model which has mutation in laminin receptor (lmmr1) has also demonstrated ARVD/C phenotype.[87]

13.3.5   Familial Atrial Fibrillation

Atrial fibrillation (AF) is the most frequently observed arrhythmia in clinical situations and often associated with structural heart diseases such as valvular heart disease, cardiomyopathy, and hypertensive heart disease. However, 2–16% cases have no obvious structural abnormalities, and those cases are called *lone AF*. Some portion of the lone AF population has familial history, suggesting genetic background. Recent studies have identified various culprit genes for familial atrial fibrillation,[88] and have attributed the disease to abnormalities of ion channels such as voltage-gated K channels and Na channels. In addition, several studies have reported that proteins related to intracellular Ca handling (Fig. 13.4), nuclear pore component, and transcription factors are involved in familial AF. Murine models corresponding to these abnormalities have been genetically engineered.[89-93]

13.4   Summary

Varieties of small animal models for arrhythmia study have been created using genetic and nongenetic techniques. Although small animals can be obtained relatively easily, data obtained from small animals must be interpreted carefully compared to data obtained from larger animals such as dogs or pigs, because electrophysiological properties of small animals such as constituents of action potentials are different from those of humans.

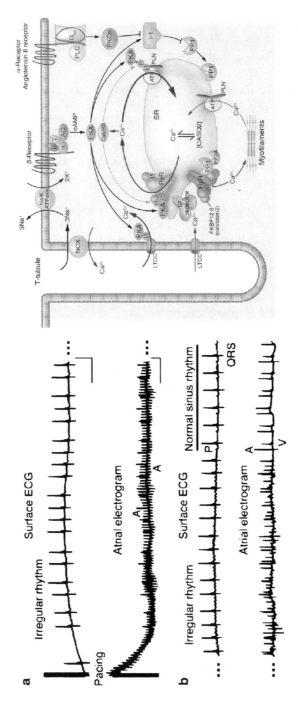

Fig. 13.4 Atrial fibrillation demonstrated in Ryr2[R176Q/+] knock-in mouse. *Left*: (**a**) Representative surface ECG (*upper*) and intracardiac atrial electrogram (*lower*). Lack of P-wave and irregular RR intervals were demonstrated in surface ECG. (**b**) Abrupt transition from AF to normal sinus rhythm. *P* P-wave; *QRS* QRS complex; *A* atrial wave; *V* ventricular wave. Modified from Chelu et al.[94] *Right*: Schematic illustration of intracellular Ca^{2+} handling in cardiomyocytes. *AC* adenylyl cyclase; α G protein subunit α; α-*receptor* α-adrenergic receptor; β G protein subunit β; β-*receptor* β-adrenergic receptor; γ G protein subunit γ; *LTCC* L-type Ca^{2+} channel; *CAMKII* Ca^{2+}-calmodulin kinase II; *I-1* inhibitor 1; *NCX* Na+/Ca^{2+} exchanger; *P* phosphate group; *PLC* phospholipase C; *PLN* phospholamban; *PP1* protein phosphatase 1; *PP2A* protein phosphatase 2A; *SERCA2a* SR Ca^{2+}-ATPase isoform 2a; *T-tubule* transverse tubule. *Image on right from Rubart and Zipes*[95]

According to recent progress in molecular biology and genetics, techniques of genetic manipulations have been widely applied to create genetically engineered animal models. The genetic models are useful for analyzing pathophysiological conditions that mimic human-inherited arrhythmic disease such as LQT syndromes or CPVT. However, data should be analyzed carefully, because persistent exposure to genetic abnormality from embryonic to adult stages may cause unexpected myocardial and electrical remodeling. On the other hand, nongenetic models induced with surgical techniques or drugs are helpful to regenerate heart diseases such as myocardial infarction or congestive heart failure. Although these nongenetic models are advantageous in light of the negligible effect caused by genetic manipulation, the variance between individual animals is relatively larger compared to genetic models which usually have stable phenotypic manifestations.

References

1. Ytrehus K, Liu Y, Tsuchida A, et al. Rat and rabbit heart infarction: effects of anesthesia, perfusate, risk zone, and method of infarct sizing. Am J Physiol 1994; 267:H2383–90.
2. Takamatsu T. Arrhythmogenic substrates in myocardial infarct. Pathol Int 2008; 58:533–43.
3. Gehrmann J, Frantz S, Maguire CT, et al. Electrophysiological characterization of murine myocardial ischemia and infarction. Basic Res Cardiol 2001; 96:237–50.
4. Volk T, Nguyen THD, Schultz JH, et al. Regional alterations of repolarizing K+ currents among the left ventricular free wall of rats with ascending aortic stenosis. J Physiol 2001; 530:443–55.
5. Gomez AM, Benitah JP, Henzel D, et al. Modulation of electrical heterogeneity by compensated hypertrophy in rat left ventricle. Am J Physiol 1997; 272:H1078–86.
6. Tomita F, Bassett AL, Myerburg RJ, et al. Diminished transient outward currents in rat hypertrophied ventricular myocytes. Circ Res 1994; 75:296–303.
7. Marionneau C, Brunet S, Flagg TP, et al. Distinct cellular and molecular mechanisms underlie functional remodeling of repolarizing K+ currents with left ventricular hypertrophy. Circ Res 2008; 102:1406–15.
8. Cerbai E, Barbieri M, Li Q, et al. Ionic basis of action potential prolongation of hypertrophied cardiac myocytes isolated from hypertensive rats of different ages. Cardiovasc Res 1994; 28:1180–7.
9. Mészáros J, Ryder KO, Hart G. Transient outward current in catecholamine-induced cardiac hypertrophy in the rat. Am J Physiol 1996; 271:H2360–7.
10. Lee JK, Kodama I, Honjo H, et al. Stage-dependent changes in membrane currents in rats with monocrotaline-induced right ventricular hypertrophy. Am J Physiol 1997; 272:H2833–42.
11. Potreau D, Gomez JP, Fares N. Depressed transient outward current in single hypertrophied cardiomyocytes isolated from the right ventricle of ferret heart. Cardiovasc Res 1995; 30:440–8.
12. Tsuji Y, Opthof T, Kamiya K, et al. Pacing-induced heart failure causes a reduction of delayed rectifier potassium currents along with decreases in calcium and transient outward currents in rabbit ventricle. Cardiovasc Res 2000; 48:300–9.
13. Pogwizd SM, Qi M, Yuan W, et al. Upregulation of Na+/Ca2+ exchanger expression and function in an arrhythmogenic rabbit model of heart failure. Circ Res 1999; 85:1009–19.
14. Vermeulen JT, Mcguire MA, Opthof T, et al. Triggered activity and automaticity in ventricular trabeculae of failing human and rabbit hearts. Cardiovasc Res 1994; 28:1547–54.
15. Lee JK, Yuasa D, Iwase M, et al. Gene profiling in a novel mouse model of sudden cardiac death with acquired QT prolongation and Torsades de Pointes secondary to complete AV block. Circulation 2004; 110:98.

16. Piron J, Le Quang K, Briec F, et al. Biological pacemaker engineered by nonviral gene transfer in a mouse model of complete atrioventricular block. Mol Ther 2008; 16:1937–43.
17. Tsuji Y, Opthof T, Yasui K, et al. Ionic mechanisms of acquired QT prolongation and torsades de pointes in rabbits with chronic complete atrioventricular block. Circulation 2002; 106:2012–8.
18. Suto F, Cahill SA, Wilson GJ, et al. A novel rabbit model of variably compensated complete heart block. J Appl Physiol 2002; 92:1199–204.
19. Bilchick KC, Saha SK, Mikolajczyk E, et al. Differential regional gene expression from cardiac dyssynchrony induced by chronic right ventricular free wall pacing in the mouse. Physiol Genomics 2006; 26:109–15.
20. Yamashita T, Murakawa Y, Hayami N, et al. Short-term effects of rapid pacing on mRNA level of voltage-dependent K+ channels in rat atrium – electrical remodeling in paroxysmal atrial tachycardia. Circulation 2000; 101:2007–14.
21. Yamashita T, Sekiguchi A, Iwasaki YK, et al. Thrombomodulin and tissue factor pathway inhibitor in endocardium of rapidly paced rat atria. Circulation 2003; 108:2450–2.
22. Choisy SCM, Arberry LA, Hancox JC, et al. Increased susceptibility to atrial tachyarrhythmia in spontaneously hypertensive rat hearts. Hypertension 2007; 49:498–505.
23. Boixel C, Fontaine V, Rüker-Martin C, et al. Fibrosis of the left atria during progression of heart failure is associated with increased matrix metalloproteinases in the rat. J Am Coll Cardiol 2003; 42:336–44.
24. Kato T, Yamashita T, Sekiguchi A, et al. What are arrhythmogenic substrates in diabetic rat atria? J Cardiovasc Electrophysiol 2006; 17:890–4.
25. Bosch RF, Scherer CR, Rub N, et al. Molecular mechanisms of early electrical remodeling: transcriptional downregulation of ion channel subunits reduces I-Ca, I-L and I-to in rapid atrial pacing in rabbits. J Am Coll Cardiol 2003; 41:858–69.
26. Shimano M, Tsuji Y, Inden Y, et al. Pioglitazone, a peroxisome proliferator-activated receptor-gamma activator, attenuates atrial fibrosis and atrial fibrillation promotion in rabbits with congestive heart failure. Heart Rhythm 2008; 5:451–9.
27. Halapas A, Papalois A, Stauropoulou A, et al. In vivo models for heart failure research. In Vivo 2008; 22:767–80.
28. Janse MJ, Wit AL. Electrophysiological mechanisms of ventricular arrhythmias resulting from myocardial ischemia and infarction. Physiol Rev 1989; 69:1049–169.
29. Nattel S, Maguy A, Le Bouter S, et al. Arrhythmogenic ion-channel remodeling in the heart: heart failure, myocardial infarction, and atrial fibrillation. Physiol Rev 2007; 87:425–56.
30. Roell W, Lewalter T, Sasse P, et al. Engraftment of connexin 43-expressing cells prevents post-infarct arrhythmia. Nature 2007; 450:819–24.
31. Kuhlmann MT, Kirchhof P, Klocke R, et al. G-CSF/SCF reduces inducible arrhythmias in the infarcted heart potentially via increased connexin43 expression and arteriogenesis. J Exp Med 2006; 203:87–98.
32. Wang QD. Murine models for the study of congestive heart failure: implications for understanding molecular mechanisms and for drug discovery. J Pharmacol Toxicol Methods 2004; 50:163–74.
33. Li Q, Keung EC. Effects of myocardial hypertrophy on transient outward current. Am J Physiol 1994; 266:H1738–45.
34. Furukawa T, Kurokawa J. Potassium channel remodeling in cardiac hypertrophy. J Mol Cell Cardiol 2006; 41:753–61.
35. Tomaselli GF, Marban E. Electrophysiological remodeling in hypertrophy and heart failure. Cardiovasc Res 1999; 42:270–83.
36. Yokoshiki H, Kohya T, Tomita F, et al. Restoration of action potential duration and transient outward current by regression of left ventricular hypertrophy. J Mol Cell Cardiol 1997; 29:1331–9.
37. Rials SJ, Xu XP, Wu Y, et al. Regression of LV hypertrophy with captopril normalizes membrane currents in rabbits. Am J Physiol Heart Circ Physiol 1998; 44:H1216–24.

38. Rials SJ, Xu XP, Wu Y, et al. Restoration of normal ventricular electrophysiology in reno-vascular hypertensive rabbits after treatment with losartan. J Cardiovas Pharmacol 2001; 37: 317–23.

39. Cerbai E, Crucitti A, Sartiani L, et al. Long-term treatment of spontaneously hypertensive rats with losartan and electrophysiological remodeling of cardiac myocytes. Cardiovasc Res 2000; 45:388–96.

40. Shao QM, Ren B, Saini HK, et al. Sarcoplasmic reticulum Ca^{2+} transport and gene expression in congestive heart failure are modified by imidapril treatment. Am J Physiol Heart Circ Physiol 2005; 288:H1674–82.

41. Perrier E, Kerfant BG, Lalevee N, et al. Mineralocorticoid receptor antagonism prevents the electrical remodeling that precedes cellular hypertrophy after myocardial infarction. Circulation 2004; 110:776–83.

42. Allan A, Fenning A, Levick S, et al. Reversal of cardiac dysfunction by selective ET-A receptor antagonism. Br J Pharmacol 2005; 146:846–53.

43. Matsumoto Y, Aihara H, Yamauchi-Kohno R, et al. Long-term endothelin a receptor blockade inhibits electrical remodeling in cardiomyopathic hamsters. Circulation 2002; 106:613–9.

44. Sakai S, Miyauchi T, Yamaguchi I. Long-term endothelin receptor antagonist administration improves alterations in expression of various cardiac genes in failing myocardium of rats with heart failure. Circulation 2000; 101:2849–53.

45. Bers DM, Guo T. Calcium signaling in cardiac ventricular myocytes. Commun Cardiac Cell 2005; 1047:86–98.

46. Anderson ME. Multiple downstream proarrhythmic targets for calmodulin kinase II: moving beyond an ion channel-centric focus. Cardiovasc Res 2007; 73:657–66.

47. Tsuji Y, Zicha S, Qi XY, et al. Potassium channel subunit remodeling in rabbits exposed to long-term bradycardia or tachycardia – discrete arrhythmogenic consequences related to differential delayed-rectifier changes. Circulation 2006; 113:345–55.

48. Vos MA, Verduyn SC, Gorgels APM, et al. Reproducible induction of early afterdepolarizations and torsade de pointes arrhythmias by d-sotalol and pacing in dogs with chronic atrio-ventricular block. Circulation 1995; 91:864–72.

49. Oros A, Beekman JDM, Vos MA. The canine model with chronic, complete atrio-ventricular block. Pharmacol Ther 2008; 119:168–78.

49b. Qi XY, Yeh YH, Chartier D, et al. The calcium/calmodulin/kinase system and arrhythmogenic after odepolarizations in bradycardia-related acquired long-QT syndrome. Circ Arrhythm Electrophysiol 2009; 2:295–304.

50. Lee RJ, Sievers RE, Gallinghouse GJ, et al. Development of a model of complete heart block in rats. J Appl Physiol 1998; 85:758–63.

51. Lee JK, Yuasa D, Iwase M, et al. A novel mouse model of sudden cardiac death with acquired long QT and Torsade de Pointes secondary to complete AV block. Biophys J 2005; 88:472A.

52. Kerckhoffs RC, Lumens J, Vernooy K, et al. Cardiac resynchronization: insight from experimental and computational models. Prog Biophys Mol Biol 2008; 97:543–61.

53. Nattel S, Shiroshita-Takeshita A, Brundel BJJM, et al. Mechanisms of atrial fibrillation: lessons from animal models. Prog Cardiovasc Dis 2005; 48:9–28.

54. Korantzopoulos P, Goudevenos JA, Liu T, et al. Role of pioglitazone treatment on atrial remodeling and atrial fibrillation(AF) promotion in an experimental model of congestive heart failure. Heart Rhythm 2008; 5:636.

55. Honjo H, Boyett MR, Niwa R, et al. Pacing-induced spontaneous activity in myocardial sleeves of pulmonary veins after treatment with ryanodine. Circulation 2003; 107:1937–43.

56. Chang SL, Chen YC, Chen YJ, et al. Mechanoelectrical feedback regulates the arrhythmogenic activity of pulmonary veins. Heart 2007; 93:82–8.

57. Wongcharoen W, Chen YC, Chen YJ, et al. Aging increases pulmonary veins arrhythmogenesis and susceptibility to calcium regulation agents. Heart Rhythm 2007; 4:1338–49.

58. Wongcharoen W, Chen YC, Chen YJ, et al. Effects of a Na⁺/Ca²⁺ exchanger inhibitor on pulmonary vein electrical activity and ouabain-induced arrhythmogenicity. Cardiovasc Res 2006; 70:497–508.

59. Cheung DW. Pulmonary vein as an ectopic focus in digitalis-induced arrhythmia. Nature 1981; 294:582–4.

60. Cheung DW. Electrical activity of the pulmonary vein and its interaction with the right atrium in the guinea-pig. J Physiol 1981; 314:445–56.

61. Ono N, Hayashi H, Kawase A, et al. Spontaneous atrial fibrillation initiated by triggered activity near the pulmonary veins in aged rats subjected to glycolytic inhibition. Am J Physiol Heart Circ Physiol 2007; 292:H639–48.

62. Salama G, London B. Mouse models of long QT syndrome. J Physiol 2007; 578:43–53.

63. Casimiro MC, Knollmann BC, Ebert SN, et al. Targeted disruption of the Kcnq1 gene produces a mouse model of Jervell and Lange-Nielsen Syndrome. Proc Natl Acad Sci U S A 2001; 98:2526–31.

64. Demolombe S, Lande G, Charpentier F, et al. Transgenic mice overexpressing human KvLQT1 dominant-negative isoform. Part I: phenotypic characterisation. Cardiovasc Res 2001; 50:314–27.

65. Brunner M, Peng XW, Liu GX, et al. Mechanisms of cardiac arrhythmias and sudden death in transgenic rabbits with long QT syndrome. J Clin Invest 2008; 118:2246–59.

66. London B, Pan XH, Lewarchik CM, et al. QT interval prolongation and arrhythmias in heterozygous Merg1-targeted mice. Circulation 1998; 98:56.

67. Lees-Miller JP, Guo JQ, Somers JR, et al. Selective knockout of mouse ERG1 B potassium channel eliminates I-Kr in adult ventricular myocytes and elicits episodes of abrupt sinus bradycardia. Mol Cell Biol 2003; 23:1856–62.

68. Babij P, Askew GR, Nieuwenhuijsen B, et al. Inhibition of cardiac delayed rectifier K⁺ current by overexpression of the long-QT syndrome HERG G628S mutation in transgenic mice. Circ Res 1998; 83:668–78.

69. Nuyens D, Stengl M, Dugarmaa S, et al. Abrupt rate accelerations or premature beats cause life-threatening arrhythmias in mice with long-QT3 syndrome. Nat Med 2001; 7:1021–7.

70. Chauhan VS, Tuvia S, Buhusi M, et al. Abnormal cardiac Na(+) channel properties and QT heart rate adaptation in neonatal Ankyrin(B) knockout mice. Circ Res 2000; 86:441–7.

71. Drici MD, Arrighi I, Chouabe C, et al. Involvement of IsK-associated K⁺ channel in heart rate control of repolarization in a murine engineered model of Jervell and Lange–Nielsen syndrome. Circ Res 1998; 83:95–102.

72. Kupershmidt S, Yang T, Anderson ME, et al. Replacement by homologous recombination of the minK gene with lacZ reveals restriction of minK expression to the mouse cardiac conduction system. Circ Res 1999; 84:146–52.

73. Marks AR, Priori S, Memmi M, et al. Involvement of the cardiac ryanodine receptor/calcium release channel in catecholaminergic polymorphic ventricular tachycardia. J Cell Physiol 2002; 190:1–6.

74. Jiang M, Zhang M, Tang DG, Clemo HF, Liu J, Holwitt D et al. KCNE2 protein is expressed in ventricles of different species, and changes in its expression contribute to electrical remodeling in diseased hearts. Circulation 2004; 109(14):1783–8.

75. Zaritsky J, Redell J, Tempel B, et al. The consequences of disrupting cardiac inwardly rectifying K(+) current (I(K1)) as revealed by the targeted deletion of the murine Kir2.1 and Kir2.2 genes. J Physiol 2001; 533:697–710.

76. Thiel WH, Chen BY, Hund TJ, et al. Proarrhythmic defects in Timothy syndrome require calmodulin kinase II. Circulation 2008; 118:2225–34.

77. Sicouri S, Timothy KW, Zygmunt AC, et al. Cellular basis for the electrocardiographic and arrhythmic manifestations of Timothy syndrome: effects of ranolazine. Heart Rhythm 2007; 4:638–47.

78. Remme CA, Scicluna BP, Verkerk AO, et al. Genetically determined differences in sodium current characteristics modulate conduction disease severity in mice with cardiac sodium channelopathy. Circ Res 2009; 104:1283–92.

79. Papadatos GA, Wallerstein PMR, Head CEG, et al. Slowed conduction and ventricular tachycardia after targeted disruption of the cardiac sodium channel gene Scn5a. Proc Natl Acad Sci U S A 2002; 99:6210–5.
80. van Veen TAB, Stein M, Royer A, et al. Impaired impulse propagation in Scn5a-knockout mice combined contribution of excitability, connexin expression, and tissue architecture in relation to aging. Circulation 2005; 112:1927–35.
81. Royer A, van Veen TAB, Le Bouter S, et al. Mouse model of SCN5A-linked hereditary Lenegre's disease – age-related conduction slowing and myocardial fibrosis. Circulation 2005; 111:1738–46.
82. Benson DW, Wang DW, Dyment M, et al. Congenital sick sinus syndrome caused by recessive mutations in the cardiac sodium channel gene (SCN5A). J Clin Invest 2003; 112:1019–28.
83. Mohamed U, Napolitano C, Priori SG. Molecular and electrophysiological bases of catecholaminergic polymorphic ventricular tachycardia. J Cardiovasc Electrophysiol 2007; 18:791–7.
84. Wehrens XHT, Lehnart SE, Huang F, et al. FKBP12.6 deficiency and defective calcium release channel (ryanodine receptor) function linked to exercise-induced sudden cardiac death. Cell 2003; 113:829–40.
85. Wehrens XHT, Lehnart SE, Reiken SR, et al. Protection from cardiac arrhythmia through ryanodine receptor-stabilizing protein calstabin2. Science 2004; 304:292–6.
86. Yang Z, Bowles NE, Scherer SE, et al. Desmosomal dysfunction due to mutations in desmoplakin causes arrhythmogenic right ventricular dysplasia/cardiomyopathy. Circ Res 2006; 99:646–55.
87. Asano Y, Takashima S, Asakura M, et al. Lamr1 functional retroposon causes right ventricular dysplasia in mice. Nat Genet 2004; 36:123–30.
88. Brugada R, Tapscott T, Czernuszewicz GZ, et al. Identification of a genetic locus for familial atrial fibrillation. N Engl J Med 1997; 336:905–11.
89. Temple J, Frias P, Rottman J, et al. Atrial fibrillation in KCNE-null mice. Circ Res 2005; 97:62–9.
90. Chelu MG, Sarma S, Sood S, et al. Calmodulin kinase II-mediated sarcoplasmic reticulum Ca2+ leak promotes atrial fibrillation in mice. J Clin Invest 2009; 119:1940–51.
91. Zhang XQ, Chen SH, Yoo S, et al. Mutation in nuclear pore component NUP155 leads to atrial fibrillation and early sudden cardiac death. Cell 2008; 135:1017–27.
92. Postma AV, van de Meerakker JBA, Mathijssen IB, et al. A gain-of-function TBX5 mutation is associated with atypical Holt-Oram syndrome and paroxysmal atrial fibrillation. Circ Res 2008; 102:1433–42.
93. Muller FU, Lewin G, Baba HA, et al. Heart-directed expression of a human cardiac isoform of cAMP-response element modulator in transgenic mice. J Biol Chem 2005; 280:6906–14.
94. Chelu MG, Sarma S, Sood S, et al. Calmodulin kinase II-mediated sarcoplasmic reticulum Ca^{2+} leak promotes atrial fibrillation in mice. J Clin Invest 2009; 119:1940–51.
95. Rubart M, Zipes DP. Mechanisms of sudden cardiac death. J Clin Invest 2005; 115:2305–15.

Chapter 14
Use of Large Animal Models for Cardiac Electrophysiology Studies

Jason L. Quill, Michael D. Eggen, and Eric S. Richardson

Abstract Large animal models can be utilized to recreate many cardiac electrophysiological disease states and procedures and to test new devices and imaging techniques. In this chapter, a brief summary of regulatory principles regarding animal models is presented. Factors for choosing an animal model, such as growth rate, ease of handling, and comparative cardiac anatomy, are detailed, with the cardiac anatomy presented in terms of common electrophysiologic procedures: lead placement, His pacing, and ablation studies. General anesthesia information is then provided, along with common methods of accessing the heart and invasive monitoring techniques. Finally, common electrophysiologic interventions are discussed such as different techniques for creating common pathologies including congestive heart failure models, acute and chronic atrial fibrillation models, ventricular fibrillation, and myocardial infarction (ischemia).

14.1 Introduction

Animal experimentation has resulted in numerous discoveries including the need for insulin, the creation of vaccines for polio and rabies, skin grafts for burn victims, and CT scanning technology. Furthermore, every drug and invasive medical device in use today has undergone some form of animal testing prior to human clinical studies and/or medical usage. Importantly, these advances in medical technology have benefited countless patients as well as veterinary science, in general. More specifically, it has been reported that dogs can now receive heart valves and hip replacements. And thanks to surgical research, vaccines and heart disease treatments for pets have resulted from medical research through animal experimentation.[1]

Currently, research on large animals primarily occurs at Universities in a regulatory environment described by the Animal Welfare Act of 1966 and the Health Research

J.L. Quill (✉)

Departments of Surgery and Biomedical Engineering, University of Minnesota, Minneapolis, MN, USA
e-mail: jason.l.quill@medtronic.com

D.C. Sigg et al. (eds.), *Cardiac Electrophysiology Methods and Models*,
DOI 10.1007/978-1-4419-6658-2_14, © Springer Science+Business Media, LLC 2010

Extension Act of 1985. The Public Health Service Policy on Humane Care and Use of Laboratory Animals, published through the Office of Laboratory Animal Welfare in 2002, supplements the Health Research Extension Act. In brief, the goals of these policies require:

- Procedures to be designed and performed with due consideration of their relevance to human or animal health, the advancement of knowledge, or the good of society.
- The selection of appropriate species and the minimum number of animals to be used to achieve valid results (including using alternate forms of testing, such as in vitro testing and computer simulations).
- The avoidance or minimization of animal discomfort, distress, and pain when consistent with sound scientific practices.
- The appropriate use of sedation, analgesia, or anesthesia during procedures that involve more than momentary or slight pain to the animal (acute studies should terminate with a painless ending of the animal's life).
- Appropriate living conditions and care for the animals and proper training for investigators.

Prior to animal experimentation, the study protocol must be approved by an independent regulatory body that ensures that investigators comply with the above goals. If the study is found to comply, all animals are kept in facilities overseen by a veterinarian and provided adequate food, housing, and medical care.

With these regulations in place, every effort is made to maximize health advancements while minimizing the number of animal experiments performed and the distress animals experience during the protocol. Since there are no computer simulations and/or adequate in vitro tests that are yet capable of mimicking the system responses of the human body, animal testing is not only necessary, but it is the best way to screen potential therapies and/or devices prior to human use.

14.2 Choosing the Right Animal Model

There are many factors that enter in to the careful decision of selecting the proper or correct animal model for pharmacological or device investigations, including: (1) the species (and breed); (2) size of the animal (or target organ of interest); and/ or (3) whether the study is acute or chronic. The three most common large animal models for cardiac investigations are the dog, pig, and sheep. Thus, this section will focus on and compare these three models to human anatomy, to aid in the choice of which species is appropriate for a proposed study. Nevertheless, the relative expertise and experience of the given investigator with the chosen animal model are important factors in the ultimate success of the planned experiments. In addition, an experienced investigator may be able to recall a previous study in which data from control animals could be used (i.e., historic data), thereby reducing the number of newly required experiments.

14.2.1   Rate of Growth

Pigs, dogs, and sheep can all be appropriate models for use in acute studies, but the study design for chronic studies must accommodate the natural growth of the animal when interpreting results. Dogs reach mature size by approximately 1 year of age. Sheep are also relatively slow growing and reach a standard mature weight with little growth beyond that age. An animal's final size is highly heritable and thus breed specific, but can also be nutrition dependent. The large growth rate of swine makes the results of chronic studies with these animals more difficult to interpret, e.g., the heart continues to enlarge with the size of the animal (within the age range of most swine during cardiac studies). There are mini-pigs available for chronic studies that have much lower adult weights or growth.[2]

In studies where a specific heart size is required, estimates have been established for each species comparing the excised heart weight to body weight. In general, the heart weight to body weight ratios for adult dogs, pigs, and sheep are 7, 2.5, and 3 g/kg, respectively.[3] For comparison, the heart weight to body weight ratio of humans is 5 g/kg. It should be noted that, for the pig model, a more realistic heart weight to body weight ratio may be obtained by using younger animals (25–30 kg, several months old).[4] However, these numbers are variable based upon breed of the animal or lifestyle of the population, so they should be used in the context of an animal experiment only, as a rule of thumb for ordering animals.

14.2.2   Arrhythmogenicity

There have not been any detailed studies comparing the relative onset of arrythmias in canine, swine, and sheep. Nevertheless, many investigators have noticed a qualitative order to the sensitivity with which the animals develop arrythmias. In general, dogs are thought to be relatively insensitive to arrythmias, followed by sheep and then pigs. Of interest, one highly experienced animal researcher (Dick Bianco, Experimental Surgical Services, University of Minnesota, USA) discussed the benefits of each animal model at the Bakken Surgical Device Symposium (University of Minnesota, December 2008), and stated that pigs would "fibrillate if you looked at them funny."

14.2.3   Comparative Anatomy

Detailed descriptions regarding comparative cardiac anatomy among canine, sheep, swine, and humans have become recently available.[5] In this section, we will describe the major differences in cardiac anatomy between animals and humans in the context of how those differences likely affect studies in cardiac electrophysiology such as lead placement and ablation studies.

It should be emphasized that all the animal models discussed in this chapter have cardiac anatomy that is generally similar to that of humans. All hearts contain four chambers, with two atrioventricular valves and two semilunar valves, and the same pathways of blood flow. The systemic blood enters the right atrium through the superior and inferior vena cavae, while the coronary venous system returns blood into the right atrium through the coronary sinus. The blood then flows through the tricuspid valve during diastole to the right ventricle, where it is pumped through the pulmonary valve during systole and into the pulmonary artery and the lungs. Upon oxygenation, the blood returns via the pulmonary veins to the left atrium. During diastole, the blood passes through the mitral valve and into the left ventricle. Finally, the left ventricle pumps the blood into the systemic arteries through the aortic valve. The coronary arteries are fed through backflow in the ascending aorta during diastole that enters the coronary system via the left and right coronary ostia, located within the sinus of Valsalva. The right and left heart pumps work in series in a coordinated fashion; in a healthy heart, the right and left atria contract in concert and, subsequently, so do the ventricles.

One of the most important things to recognize when choosing an animal model is that there are differences between animals, and the choice of an incorrect model can produce misleading results. An often stated example of incorrect model choice comes from pharmaceutical studies using an infarction model in dogs during the 1970s. These protocols were intended to create infarcts in sub-selected regions of the coronary arteries. However, canines have a high degree of collateralization within their coronary arteries compared with humans. Therefore, in these trials, the dog myocardium was still being fed in areas thought to be ischemic because of this collateralization, and it was reported that various drugs were effective at reducing damage caused by myocardial ischemia. Unfortunately, these drugs then failed in trials of human patients because the animal study data were not transferable.[6] It is considered that this could have been avoided if a different animal model was chosen (i.e., pigs or sheep), one that had a similar degree of collateralization as humans and produced consistent infarcts (not just myocardial stunning) as the protocol required.

The remainder of this section will describe some common devices and therapies that are used in animal models, and describe how the structural anatomy of the differing species can and will influence one's ultimate experimental design.

14.3 Lead Placement

The relative orientation of the heart within the thorax of quadrupeds differs from that of humans.[7] In humans, the right ventricle rests upon the diaphragm, with the long axis of the heart at approximately a 60° angle from the sternum, in such a manner that one third of the heart is in the right half of the thorax and two thirds of the heart is in the left half of the thorax. In contrast, the long axis of the heart in

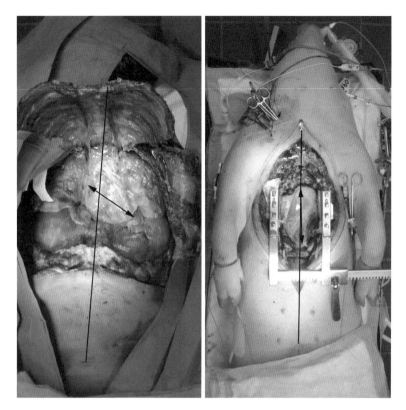

Fig. 14.1 The long axis of the heart in humans (*left*) is at approximately a 60° angle with the midline of the thorax, whereas quadrupeds, such as the pig (*right*), have a long axis of the heart more in line with the midline of the thorax

quadrupeds is much more in line with the sternum (Fig. 14.1). Thus, the relative orientation of a given heart within the thorax will ultimately affect the entrance angles of the superior vena cava into the right atrium. In humans, the superior and inferior vena cavae are essentially in line with each other, while in pigs, sheep, and dogs, they enter the atrium at nearly right angles. These differences become even more obvious and important when viewing a lead placement in a given heart location via fluoroscopy or any other imaging modality. For example, a physician or scientist may, at first, have difficulties in adjusting to these anatomical differences when placing leads in various animal models.

When a research protocol calls for left-sided lead implantation, anatomical variability of the Thebesian valve, coronary venous valves, and left azygous veins can all complicate such delivery. More specifically, the Thebesian valve covers the coronary sinus ostium and helps prevent backflow from the right atrium into the coronary sinus. In humans, this valve was found to be present in a variety of morphologies: remnant, nonobstructing valves, and prominent valves

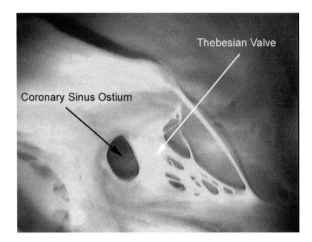

Fig. 14.2 A Thebesian valve covers the coronary sinus ostium within the right atrium of a human

covering more than 50% of the ostium.[8] In hearts with prominent Thebesian valves (Fig. 14.2), it has been shown, using an isolated heart apparatus, that coronary sinus access can be obstructed. While comparative anatomy studies of the Thebesian valve in animal models were not found, observation of swine hearts in isolated heart preparations in our laboratory has shown that prominent Thebesian valves are extremely rare and, in most cases, nonexistent. When testing devices requiring coronary sinus access in animal models, it should be noted that access may be more difficult in humans due to the Thebesian valve. The ostium of the dog is much smaller than that of the other animal models, hence the dog model would be most appropriate to use if one wants to increase the difficulty of assessing the coronary sinus by various means (e.g., studies to optimize catheter designs).

Although relative access to the coronary sinus in pigs and sheep is usually not impaired by the presence of Thebesian valves, the left azygous vein in each species drains into the coronary sinus near the ostium,[7] and this will often complicate left-sided lead implantations. Left-sided pacing is usually accomplished by positioning a lead within a venous branch which feeds into one of the larger main coronary veins: the posterior interventricular vein, the posterior vein of the left ventricle, the left marginal vein, or the anterior interventricular vein. It should be noted that the sub-selection process of implanting a lead can be helped or hindered by the presence of cardiac veins within the venous system. More specifically, intraluminal ridges and valves (Fig. 14.3) have been observed using fiberscopes (1.5 or 2.5 mm diameter) within the major cardiac veins of perfusion fixed human hearts.[9] Therefore, during a left-sided lead implantation, the location of these ridges and valves can angle a guidewire into a branch or hinder the sub-selection process by blocking access.[10] No published comparative anatomy studies have been found on

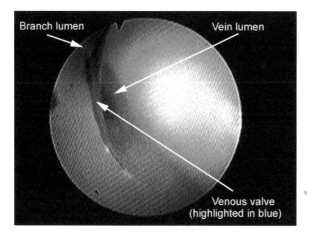

Fig. 14.3 A valve (*blue*) within the human coronary venous system is shown between the vein lumen (*right*) and the branch lumen (*left*)

cardiac venous valve anatomy, but qualitative observations of swine hearts by our group have indicated that these valves are less prevalent than in humans.

14.4   His Bundle Pacing

All the major large mammalian animal models have similar conductive pathways as humans, with the presence of an sinoatrial (SA) node, atrioventricular (AV) node, bundle of His, left and right bundle branches, and Purkinje cells. Yet, there are subtle differences between species in all portions of the conduction system, and we will discuss a few of the more notable ones here. For example, sheep have an os cordis, which is a bone at the base of the heart near the central fibrous body. This bone blocks the usual route of the His bundle to the crest of the ventricular septum, instead passing underneath the os cordis into the right ventricular septum before branching.[11] Pigs, dogs, and humans do not have an os cordis, with the His bundle located just beneath the membranous septum at the crest of the interventricular septum.[11]

In addition, the cells present in the His bundle and bundle branches of sheep differ from those of humans. In sheep, the Purkinje cells are most prevalent, whereas in human His bundles and bundle branches, they are composed of mainly transitional cells. In addition, human hearts elicit Purkinje cells throughout the pathways to the subendocardium. In contrast, sheep have comparatively more prominent cells that are present throughout the mural myocardium of the right and left ventricles.[12] As such, these differences in conduction pathways and cellular makeup should be noted by researchers attempting to pace from this site.

14.5   Ablation Studies

There are numerous published reports describing ablation studies in large mammalian models, hence this section is by no means comprehensive. Yet, listed here are some important anatomical differences between the various animal models and humans which should be kept in mind for any type of ablation study.

If a transseptal procedure is to be performed as part of the procedure, then the fossa ovalis is usually punctured via a catheter delivered from the inferior vena cava. As noted above, in quadripeds, the inferior and superior vena cavae enter the right atrium at right angles to each other, which differs from humans where the entrance of the vena cavae is in line, but with flows in opposite directions.[7] Yet, while the entrance angles of the vena cavae may differ slightly, the relative location of the fossa to the inferior vena cava in quadripeds is similar to human anatomy, and thus should have little effect on transseptal punctures.

It should also be noted that, in humans, there exists an interatrial groove for communication of electrical signals between the right and left atrium, named the Bachmann's bundle. The Bachmann's bundle has been claimed to be nonexistent in sheep,[11] but more recent studies have described pacing at the Bachmann's bundle as part of their methodology.[13] This apparent discrepancy between anatomical literature and electrophysiology studies is quite interesting, but is noted without further comment. Nevertheless, Bachmann's bundles have been reportedly found in both pig and canine hearts.[11]

Pulmonary vein isolation via ablation has been the focus of multiple papers as a site to eliminate atrial fibrillation. Humans typically have four pulmonary vein ostia, whereas pigs typically have two,[7] and dogs have five to six.[14] In addition, it has been noted that there is a more prominent myocyte border between the pulmonary veins and atria in the swine heart; in other words, there is no migration of myocytes into the lumen of the pulmonary veins in the swine heart.

Finally, an alternative ablation strategy is to use fractionation analysis and ablate at the site of dominant frequency. This technique is mentioned because it provides an excellent example of the value of animal models. These sites of dominant frequency were located and electrograms were simultaneously recorded with optical high-speed imaging within isolated sheep hearts; the clear perfusate employed allowed imaging within these hearts, and the electrical signals were correlated to regions with fast vortex-like reentry around miniscule cores.[15] This novel approach allowed the electrical signals to be compared with mechanical function of the atrial tissues through the use of a well-designed experiment in an animal model, helping to validate this technique's use on human patients.

14.6   Anesthetics and Monitoring

The choice of anesthetic(s) to be administered in a given study protocol depends on several factors, including: (1) the nature of the planned intervention, including the amount of pain or distress involved; (2) if the study is acute or chronic; (3) the known effect of the agents on suppressing hemodynamic function; and/or (4) if electrophysiology measurements will be taken during the intervention. It should be noted that general guidelines for the choice of anesthesia can be found on the Animal Welfare Information Center website (http://awic.nal.usda.gov). Nevertheless, the use of profound anesthesia will typically require intubation and ventilation of the animal, and therefore a proper ventilator will be needed. If the agent to be used is a volatile anesthetic, such as isoflurane, a vaporizer will also be required.

At the beginning of a typical acute animal study, the conscious animal is sedated with an induction agent (e.g., telazol and thiopental sodium), which then allows the investigator to gain intravenous access to provide supplemental agents if needed and to subsequently intubate the animal. Typically, at this point, the animal is moved to the operating table, where mechanical ventilation and anesthesia is initiated and levels are monitored. Nevertheless, all animals should be properly secured to the operating table (i.e., straps or ropes) to prevent movement or falls from the table, should anesthesia levels become too low. Care should be taken so that the restraints do not prevent proper limb circulation or alter respiration, especially if the animal will be recovering from the intervention.

During anesthesia, all animals should be closely monitored. At a minimum, a three-lead ECG should be continuously monitored and blood pressure should be assessed often (e.g., noninvasive cuff or direct arterial line). An excessively high heart rate, high blood pressure, and/or animal movement can be signs that the anesthesia is too low (the animal is *light*). Conversely, a low pressure and low heart rate may be indicators that the animal is receiving too much anesthesia. Typically, high-end anesthesia machines provide online inhaled and exhaled anesthetic levels, which can be assessed to ensure the animal is within an appropriate range of anesthesia. Given that many anesthetics can cause arrhythmias, the ECG should be monitored to detect dangerous arrhythmias. It should be noted that swine are particularly susceptible to rhythm abnormalities, yet this knowledge can be utilized to develop models to study various treatment regimes. Our laboratory always has a defibrillator available in case arrhythmias or fibrillation develop.

Under general anesthesia, both humans and animals have impaired ability to properly regulate their core temperatures, therefore, while under general anesthesia, it is important to constantly measure core temperatures and provide proper thermal management. In most large animal studies, core temperatures are monitored via a temperature probe placed in the rectum. However, in investigational studies employing a Swan–Ganz catheter, this system will provide continuous pulmonary artery temperatures (i.e., the *gold standard* measurement of core temperature). Nonetheless, active warming or cooling may be necessary to maintain the animal within an appropriate range for a given research protocol. For example, swine have a normal core temperature of 38°C, and our group attempts to control core temperature within 0.5°C. For a simple approach to therapy, blankets around the animal's abdomen and chest can help raise temperature, whereas wet cloths (water or rubbing alcohol), allowing for evaporative cooling, placed in the same locations can actively lower the temperature (the use of fans can also expedite convective losses). In addition, various heating (Fig. 14.4) and cooling systems are available commercially.

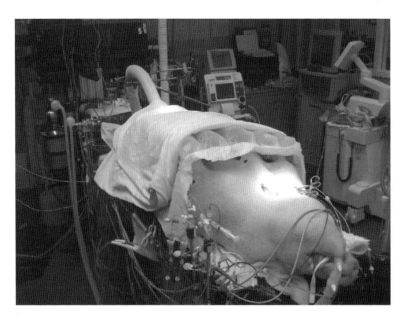

Fig. 14.4 A 90 kg swine that has been properly sedated and intubated. The animal is under general anesthesia (isoflurane) and is secured to the operating table using cords. A commercial warming system (Bair Hugger, Arizant Medical, Eden Prairie, MN, USA) is placed over the abdomen and covered with a cotton blanket

It has been our experience that electrophysiological parameters of the heart are extremely sensitive to temperature, particularly refractory periods and the induction of atrial fibrillation. Furthermore, mild hypothermia, even several degrees centigrade, is considered to confer some degree of cardioprotection against ischemic damage.

14.6.1 Invasive Monitoring

If more sophisticated hemodynamic monitoring is desired to accomplish the goals of a given study protocol, appropriate venous and arterial access will be necessary to introduce appropriate catheters into the heart for sensing. Access to large vessels such as the femoral arteries, carotid arteries, femoral veins, or jugular veins can be done: (1) with a blind stick; (2) under ultrasound guidance; or (3) after a direct surgical cut-down. In most acute investigational studies on large animal models, cut-downs or incisions of the skin and exposure of the vessel walls are commonly performed. Next, the vessels are accessed using the Seldinger technique with introducers; such sheaths typically have hemostasis valves which allow instruments to be passed in and out of the vessels without the loss of blood. In acute surgeries, where a given catheter will be placed in the vessel but will not be moved during the intervention, an introducer is not necessary. In such cases, a given vessel is isolated and then nicked and the catheter placed directly within; suture (ligatures) may then be used to cinch the vessel closed around the catheter (Fig. 14.5).

With venous and arterial access, various quantitative monitoring can be performed to obtain pressures, flows, and electrical information from each chamber of the heart. With a Swan-Ganz catheter, for example, the balloon-tipped catheter is advanced into the superior vena cava, and then continues through the right atrium, through the tricuspid valve into the right ventricle, and passes through the pulmonic valve into a small branch of the pulmonary artery (i.e., within the lungs). This catheter system can provide valuable real-time information on right atrial pressure, wedge pressure (an estimate of left atrial pressure), cardiac output, core temperature, and relative oxygen saturation. Also commonly employed in large animal cardiovascular research are Millar pressure catheters, which are small diameter catheters (5–7 Fr) that sense pressures at their tips via a diaphragm that covers a piezoelectric crystal sensor. For example, in our laboratory, we typically place Millar catheters within the right and left ventricles to obtain continuous pressure waveforms; e.g., from these, one can obtain parameters of cardiac contractility and relaxation. Pacing leads, defibrillation leads, and electrophysiology catheters can also be placed within these hearts using similar approaches (discussed later in this chapter).

14.6.2   *Accessing the Heart*

If epicardial access to the heart is needed, there are various approaches one may choose. Perhaps the least invasive of these is a *sub-xyphoid puncture*, which typically allows for access to the pericardial space at or near the apex of the heart. It should be noted that a number of commercially available tools and methods

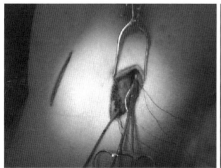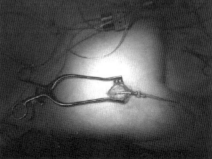

Fig. 14.5 On the left, catheters are placed into the right jugular vein of a swine without an introducer. Suture is used to cinch the vein around the catheter after it is placed. On the right, an arterial pressure line is shown after placement into a branch of the femoral artery. A cut-down was performed prior to placement, exposing the vessel for easier access

have been developed to facilitate a sub-xyphoid puncture. An added benefit of this procedure is that it can be done without perforating the pleural lining, thus preventing the need for intubation, general anesthesia, or postoperative chest tubes. However, it can be technically challenging because there are added risks of puncturing the myocardium or an epicardial vessel, which can result in cardiac tamponade. A *pericardial window* is a more invasive version of the sub-xyphoid approach. In this case, instead of a small puncture, the investigator makes a fairly large incision at the base of the rib cage and exposes the pericardium. Then a portion or the whole xyphoid process is removed, allowing for direct visualization of the pericardium and heart within.

A thoracotomy is generally described as a surgical window between two ribs, in which a spreader (i.e., a rib retractor holds the ribs apart) is placed to gain access to the heart. Such experimental procedures typically require intubation and also may necessitate collapsing one of the lungs to gain better visualization and/or access to the heart. The placement of the incision is important, because only a section of the heart is exposed during such a thoracotomy procedure.

A medial sternotomy is the most invasive method of accessing the heart, but gives the investigator complete access to almost all surfaces. In general, this experimental approach includes placing the animal under a deep surgical plane of general anesthesia, with a scalpel or electrocautery utilized to expose the sternum (cutting through skin, muscle, and other connective tissues). Next, the sternum is transected down its center using a bone saw. Note that extreme care must be taken when cutting the sternum because animals such as swine have ligaments that hold the heart close to the sternum (sternal-pericardial ligament). Then, a retractor is positioned to spread the opening of the rib cage, exposing the beating heart and lungs. The pericardium may be kept intact, excised, or sutured open to provide mechanical support (cradle). Hemodynamic parameters may change dramatically when the thoracic cavity is open, and also when the pericardium is removed.[16] Nevertheless, it is important to monitor all animals carefully during any of these procedures. Examples of parameters to be monitored include: end tidal CO_2 level, heart rate, blood pressure, cardiac output, anesthetic concentration, core temperature, arterial O_2 and pH values, renal output, hemoglobin level, and/or other parameters of specific interest (Fig. 14.6).

If the animal is to be recovered from a thoracic surgery, extreme care must be taken to use aseptic techniques, as any subsequent chest infections (mediastinitis) have a very high associated mortality rate for most large animal cardiovascular models. In general, the closure procedure can be complicated, including the placement of chest tubes, and the animal requires postoperative monitoring. Also, recovery from thoracic surgery may take anywhere from a few days to several weeks, and can be associated with considerable pain. Therefore, appropriate pain medication and antibiotics must be given to help ensure the comfort and survival of these animals. An excellent resource for more detailed information on these procedures can be found in David Gross' *Animal Models in Cardiovascular Research.*[17]

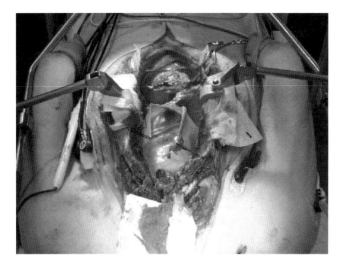

Fig. 14.6 A full medial sternotomy in an anesthetized 90 kg swine. A retractor is used to hold the ribs apart and a pericardial sling was created with suture

14.7   Common Cardiac Electrophysiology Interventions

Many common electrophysiology procedures and/or interventions performed by physicians in the hospital or clinic can be readily reproduced (or developed) in large animal models. For example, it is quite typical for our laboratory to perform the basic electrophysiology (EP) studies one would perform in a standard hospital catheter lab on large animal models employing the same equipment. In general, for such an EP study to be performed, animals are first administered an anesthetic that has minimal hemodynamic affects, such as pentobarbital. Venous access is commonly achieved via an introducer, and then EP catheters are placed in the right side of the heart under the guidance of fluoroscopy. Pacing leads may also be implanted at various sites to provide stimulation and sensing. Left-sided leads and EP catheters can be placed through arterial access, or a transseptal puncture may be performed to allow catheters to pass from the right atrium to the left atrium.[18]

After catheters are placed, various stimulation protocols are commonly employed to measure electrophysiological parameters. For example, a common protocol is to stimulate the right atrium eight times with a stimulus interval of 400–600 ms. After these eight stimuli (called S1 stimuli) have captured the rhythm of the heart, a ninth stimulus (the S2 stimulus) is given at a much smaller interval called the S1–S2 interval. This protocol is then repeated, each time shortening the S1–S2 interval. When the S1–S2 interval becomes so short that the S2 stimulus fails to propagate through the AV node, the S1–S2 interval is called the AV node effective refractory period. If the interval is shortened further, the S2 stimulus will eventually fail to evoke any response from the atria, and this S1–S2 interval is the atrial effective refractory period. The same stimulus protocol can be performed in the ventricle to measure the antegrade AV node refractory period and the ventricular effective refractory period.

It should also be noted that burst pacing, where a high-frequency train of stimuli are delivered to the heart, can be useful in testing fibrillation thresholds in both the atrium and ventricle. Thus, importantly, a defibrillator should always be nearby if sustained ventricular tachycardia or ventricular fibrillation might be induced. While atrial fibrillation is stable in most humans, some animals (particularly swine) may develop dangerous ventricular arrhythmias or become hemodynamically unstable if allowed to elicit atrial fibrillation for a long period of time.

Implantation of pacemaker and implantable cardioverter defibrillator (ICD) leads in various large animal models is also a common procedure. As such, leads can either have passive fixation, where the lead is lodged into trabeculae, or active fixation, where the lead tip has a helix and is screwed into the tissue. Yet, the relative degree of ventricular trabeculae greatly differs among the commonly employed animal models, e.g., swine can be considered to have minimal trabeculation relative to the dog. Nevertheless, after the lead is placed under fluoroscopy in the desired cardiac location, the introducer is removed and the lead is subsequently connected to the pacemaker or ICD. These devices are then implanted into a pocket formed under a skin or muscle flap. It is recommended that these devices be implanted where they will not be subjected to excessive external impact or motion (Fig. 14.7).

Ablation is another common EP procedure that has been incorporated into numerous animal study protocols. More specifically, an EP catheter can be used to

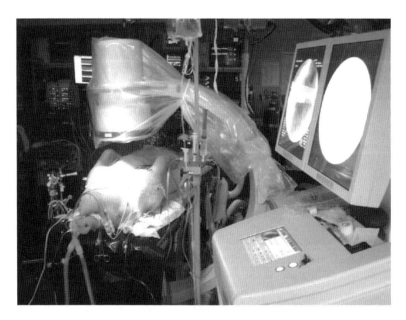

Fig. 14.7 Fluoroscopy is a commonly used imaging modality for placing leads and electrophysiology catheters

find the appropriate site of ablation, and typically the same catheter can be used to deliver therapy from an ablation system to the target tissue. Today, the therapy can be delivered either in the form of RF energy (which burns the tissue) or via cryotherapy (where the tissue fails due to freezing). The parameters, duration, energy, and temperature of the therapy will vary depending on the application, thickness of the tissue, and relative tissue viability, etc.

Large mammalian models have been extensively used to develop the technology of cardiac mapping which, in general, can measure relative activation patterns within the heart in order to study and/or subsequently treat arrhythmias. Typically, in such studies, a multielectrode EP catheter is placed on the right side of the heart; this can be considered as the most basic tool to map activation patterns. For example, properties of atrial, His, and ventricular activation and repolarization potential can be measured using this technique. To better understand the global activation patterns within a given heart chamber, mapping systems have been developed to measure 3D patterns. To date, St. Jude Medical's Ensite System, Medtronic Inc.'s Localisa system, and Biosense Webster's Carto system are all commercially available cardiac mapping systems that are used clinically. It should be noted that recent research from our lab has shown that body surface potential mapping may also be used to obtain similar 3D cardiac activation patterns and begin to provide transmural information; these emerging technologies and procedures may provide a cheaper alternative diagnostic tool, requiring only an array of ECG electrodes on the chest.[19]

Furthermore, a number of more advanced biological techniques have been introduced into large animal EP studies. More specifically, cell and gene therapies are emerging as a potential *cure* for heart rhythm disorders, e.g., cells, genes, and extracellular matrices can be injected with special needle catheters into various anatomical areas of the heart as specific means to treat arrhythmias.[20] In such cases, imaging beyond fluoroscopy (i.e., cardiac MRI and CT) can provide valuable anatomical information which is helpful in analyzing EP data.[19] As noted in Chap. 12, isolated heart models such as those developed in our Visible Heart® Lab (www.visibleheart.com) allow for direct endoscopic visualization of catheters, leads, and other devices while still maintaining the electrical and mechanical function of the heart.[21] Finally, postmortem histological analyses may also provide valuable insights into the structure of the cardiac conduction system.[22]

In summary, a number of techniques and methods are available for investigators to study the efficacy and feasibility of EP therapies, and large animal models enable the translation of cell- or tissue-level discoveries to become viable therapies that can be used in the clinic to benefit human lives.

14.8 Animal Models of Disease States

In any type of translational research, it is desirable to have an appropriate animal model which exhibits similar physiology and pathophysiology to the targeted disease state in humans. In the realm of heart failure, animal models have been developed by numerous laboratories to mimic a variety of myocardial disease states or conditions such as congestive heart failure, hypertrophic heart failure, myocardial infarction, atrial fibrillation, ventricular fibrillation, tachycardia, etc. Such models have been developed for use in either acute or chronic investigations. The following section briefly covers some of the more common disease states which can be created (modeled) in the large mammals commonly used for translational studies on associated cardiac EP.

14.8.1 Congestive Heart Failure Models

Dilated cardiomyopathy (DCM), a form of systolic heart failure, is characterized by ventricular dilation and functional impairment. Commonly, DCM is associated with conduction disturbances in the myocardium; for example, a left bundle branch block causes significant interventricular and intraventricular dyssynchrony in such patients. Furthermore, the current clinical practice in these cases is to provide cardiac resynchronization therapy (CRT), the implantation of a biventricular pacing system that is used to resynchronize the ventricles. Because there is no consensus regarding the optimal anatomical site for lead placement in CRT (or lead placement, in general, for pacing in a failing heart), numerous large animal models of DCM have been developed and employed to study the validation and optimization of such therapies.

Chronic high-rate pacing, or tachypacing, is considered the gold standard in creating animal models of DCM; it is highly reproducible and technically simple to produce.[1] Pacing the heart at 2–4 times the intrinsic rate from either the atria or ventricles will produce marked changes in both cardiac function and anatomy within a matter of weeks; the extent of remodeling can be controlled by both the pacing rate and duration (Fig. 14.8). Typically, a high-rate pacing model of DCM will cause the following functional and anatomical changes in the heart[23–25]:

- Increased filling pressures;
- Left and right ventricular systolic dysfunction (low cardiac output, contractility, and ejection fraction);
- Left ventricle, right ventricle, right atrium, and left atrium chamber dilatation, spherical left ventricular chamber geometry;
- Increased cardiac mass (not uniform across species);
- Mitral valve regurgitation.

In addition, high-rate pacing is associated with the following systemic effects:

- Neurohumoral activation;
- Increased systemic vascular resistance;
- Ascites (accumulation of fluid in the abdomen);
- Peripheral edema.

For example, Wilson et al. studied the effects of high-rate pacing in canines at endpoints of 3 and 8 weeks.[26] They demonstrated that high-rate pacing at a rate of

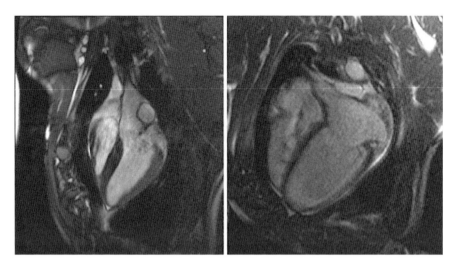

Fig. 14.8 A four-chamber MR image of a normal swine heart is shown in end-diastole (*left*), and after 3 weeks of high-rate pacing at 200 beats/min (*right*). The increase in chamber size and wall thinning after high-rate pacing can easily be discerned

240–260 beats/min in the canine model reduced cardiac output (control: 130 ± 20 ml/min/kg, 8-week pacing: 116 ± 14 ml/min/kg), elevated pulmonary wedge pressure (control: 10 ± 3 mmHg, 8-week pacing: 26 ± 8 mmHg), and increased right atrial pressure (control: 4 ± 1 mmHg, 8-week pacing: 9 ± 3 mmHg) (all $p < 0.01$ vs. control). They also noted that, after the study termination, the dogs in both pacing groups had left and right ventricular volumes which were approximately twice those of the controls. In addition, after 3 weeks of pacing, a functional assessment with echocardiography revealed a decreased percent of left ventricular shortening ($34 \pm 6\%$ to $17 \pm 7\%$, $p < 0.01$).

To date, the canine model has been the primary large mammalian model of pacing-induced DCM, with porcine and ovine models also utilized. It should be noted that the pacing time period necessary to reach the same hemodynamic endpoints varies by species, with pacing periods approximately twice as long in canines as in swine, partly due to the increased collateral coronary circulation in canines. Peripheral edema and ascites are common with this type of heart failure model, and the use of diuretics should be considered during the progression of the disease state for animal comfort and also to reduce mortality. In addition, for any procedure or measurement that cannot be made while the animal is awake, consideration should be given to the choice of anesthesia; a high dose of any administered anesthetic which may be a cardiovascular depressant (such as thiopental or isoflurane) could be fatal in such a heart failure model. Furthermore, there is general agreement that the cardiac and systemic effects of high-rate pacing are largely reversible after cessation of pacing, and the time period for recovery can be a matter of weeks.

It should also be noted that tachypacing-induced heart failure can also be fine tuned in order to more closely represent specific heart failure mechanisms in humans.

In one variation, for the study of ventricular timing and pacing site in CRT therapy, Helm et al. first created a left bundle branch block, followed by 3–4 weeks of tachypacing (210 beats/min) in canines to produce the combination of DCM and ventricular dyssynchrony.[27] In another example, Shen et al. sequentially clipped two regions of the left circumflex artery, followed by intermittent periods of chronic rapid pacing (220 beats/min).[28] Subsequently, in this canine model, severe left ventricular dysfunction resulted, and it was noted that left ventricular function and peripheral vasoconstriction did not recover after the cessation of pacing. In other words, the irreversibility of this later model indicates a different underlying mechanism for the induced heart failure than the tachypacing model alone, which is largely reversible.

14.8.2 Acute and Chronic Atrial Fibrillation Models

Atrial fibrillation (AF) is an uncoordinated tachyarrhythmia associated with a high level of morbidity and mortality as previously described (see Sect. 14.1 and Chap. 5). One necessary feature in a large animal model of AF is that the arrhythmia must be sustained for a period of time long enough to permit the electrical characterization of the rhythm and application of the therapy designed to correct the condition. To date, both acute and chronic large animal models have been developed for the study of AF.

There are various methods to generate AF in an animal model, which can be grouped into the following categories: (1) surgical; (2) pharmacological or chemical; and (3) electrical. Surgical methods used in the induction of AF involve creating an injury to the atrial tissue, such that there is a subsequent barrier for the propagating action potentials.[29] For example, this barrier can be created by clamping (traumatic injury), making an incision, or ablating the tissue. Once the anatomical block is formed, AF can typically be initiated by brief, rapid electrical stimulation and the presence of the created block allows the formation of a reentry loop. Yet, it should be noted that results can vary in this type of AF model, as they are sensitive to the location and size of the injuries, and also the relative placement of stimulating electrodes.

In general, pharmacological and chemical methods of inducing AF involve intravenous or local/targeted delivery of an agent which will increase the susceptibility of the heart to AF. Typically, pharmacological agents are chosen to alter specific ionic channels and their ionic currents in order to prolong the myocyte refractory periods, making it easier to electrically initiate AF. For example, in one study by Anadon et al., AF and atrial flutter were induced in swine with an intravenous delivery of ethanol followed by rapid stimulation of the right atrium to initiate an arrhythmia.[30] Furthermore, it was noted that as the intravenous concentration of alcohol was increased, the ability to generate sustained AF was also increased. However, this model was an acute model and AF was only sustained for a matter of minutes. In contrast, Kijtawornrat et al. have been successful in creating an acute animal model in canines, where AF was sustained for approximately 40 min.[31] In this study, AF was achieved through a combination of rapid atrial pacing and an infusion of phenylephrine. In general, rapid pacing decreased the atrial effective refractory period, slowed atrial conduction, and increased electrophysiologic heterogeneity, where the phenylephrine infusion increased the difference between left and right atrial and intra-atrial refractory periods. More specifically, AF in these canines was sustained for approximately 40 min following the infusion of phenylephrine and 20 min of tachypacing at 40 Hz.

Similar to animal models for DCM, high-rate pacing has been successfully utilized in developing chronic models of AF. For example, Bauer et al. used burst pacing at a frequency of 42 Hz in the right atrial appendage to cause AF-induced heart failure in swine.[32] In this case, the burst pacing resulted in very high ventricular rates, where an average ventricular rate of 270 ± 5 beats/min was reported during sustained AF. Furthermore, after 3 weeks of burst pacing, chronic heart failure was evident in these animals. In another experimental approach, Wijffels et al. created a chronic model of AF in goats through the use of an external fibrillator/pacemaker attached to epicardial electrodes on the atria.[33] Upon detection of a sinus rhythm, external stimulation of the atria was induced for 1 s at a rate of 50 Hz, which automatically maintained AF 24 h/day. It was reported that the repetitive induction of AF for a period of 1 week by this pacing method led to a progressive increase in the duration of AF, and subsequently AF became sustained for periods greater than 24 h without any maintenance pacing.

14.8.3   Animal Models of Ventricular Fibrillation

Common methods to induce ventricular fibrillation (VF) in large animals include electrical stimulation at high frequencies and/or the induction of acute ischemia. Since there are different mechanisms that cause VF, an appropriate animal for VF should be chosen based on the patient population for the therapy being studied (simulated). For instance, if targeting VF in children, which commonly occurs because of asphyxiation or circulatory shock, one would use a model in which the trachea is clamped in a anesthetized animal.[34] However, if the therapy is targeting VF due to an ischemic event, an acute or ischemic model would be more appropriate.[35] In addition, VF can be caused by an overdose of certain medications, and the appropriate animal model to mimic this type of mechanism can, in many cases, be achieved by treating an animal with the same medications. The methods and considerations involved in creating ischemic conditions in animal models is described in the next section, however, for a detailed description of other methods we refer the reader to the vast body of literature.

14.8.4   Animal Models of Myocardial Infarction, Ischemia

Myocardial infarction (more commonly known as a heart attack) refers to the focal or global damaging of myocardial tissue due to ischemia, a lack or stoppage of blood flow. Importantly, there are many electrical changes and resultant arrhythmias in the heart that arise from this condition that are of interest to the electrophysiologist (i.e., ventricular fibrillation, ventricular tachycardia, etc.) as previously described in Chap. 5.

Historically, there has been a wide variety of species employed and methods used to create large animal models of cardiac ischemia. Most common are acute experiments in which a targeted coronary artery is occluded in anesthetized animals. Typical methods of creating such an occlusion include opening the chest to gain access to the heart and the subsequent surgical ligation of the targeted branch of a coronary artery, or by placing a removable clip around the artery which gives the ability to study cyclic periods of ischemia (i.e., ischemia-reperfusion injury) (Fig. 14.9). As such, the size and location of the infarcted region will ultimately be dependent on the relative location of the artery occluded and the duration of the ischemic time.

If an investigational design requires a closed chest model, then a coronary occlusion can be induced via a balloon catheter placed into that given vessel (e.g., via access from the femoral artery). Although the potential for temperature variation is reduced in a closed chest model, there is a limitation regarding the type of physiological measurements that can be readily obtained. For example, in the open chest model, flow probes can be placed around the pulmonary artery and the aorta for online continuous measurement of cardiac output and total coronary artery flow; additionally, sonomicrometry crystals can be sutured to the epicardium for the assessment of focal wall motion and/or regional function.

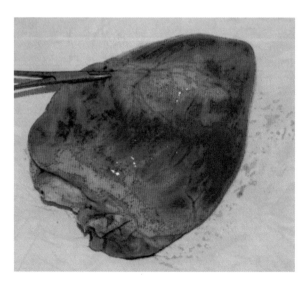

Fig. 14.9 An excised swine heart from an acute occlusion study after the injection of patent blue dye is shown. Regions stained *blue* indicate where perfusion occurred during the occlusion, and nondyed regions indicate the area at risk

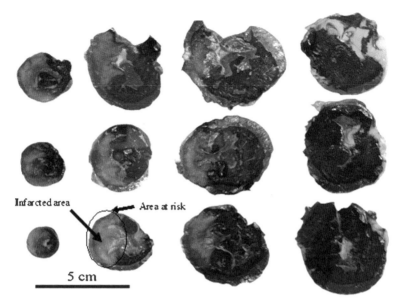

Fig. 14.10   Triphenyletrazolium chloride (TTC) staining after an acute infarct and the injection of patent blue dye in an acute model of myocardial infarction. In the nondyed regions, or area at risk, the infarcted regions are *pale in color*

There are multiple methods to quantify the size and location of an induced infarcted region. One common method used to identify the area at risk, or an area that is not perfused, is to inject microspheres or dyes while the vessels are still occluded. More specifically, the injected microspheres will then congregate in the capillaries of any tissues that are perfused. Therefore, following tissue digestion, any areas that contain microspheres can be identified as regions which were perfused, and visa versa. In contrast, if a dye injection is employed, the areas which were perfused will turn the color of the dye and areas which were not perfused will remain unaffected (Fig. 14.9). Triphenyletrazolium chloride (TTC) staining is a common histochemical method which is often used to delineate normal and infarcted myocardial tissue (postmortem), as the stain only adheres to infarcted (damaged) tissue (Fig. 14.10).[36] If an in vivo assessment of perfusion and myocardial infarction is desired, such as during a chronic study with progressive occlusion, a contrast enhanced cardiac MRI can be used.[37,38]

In an acute large animal infarct study, it is only possible to simulate where a myocardial infarction would likely be created. However, for scar formation (the replacement of dead myocardium), a chronic study would be necessary. An investigator's decision about designing an acute or chronic study is dependent on the relative pathophysiology and underlying mechanisms of the arrhythmia that is of primary interest. For example, in the case of a chronic study, where the animal recovers after the occlusion, careful consideration must be made about the location of the region occluded and the choice of the species used. Historically, dogs have been used in chronic ischemia models, as their increased collateral coronary circulation improves survivability, yet they also elicit fewer arrhythmias. However, as previously mentioned, the swine model has coronary anatomy more similar to that of a human heart; an induced large ischemic area would likely be more fatal in this species as compared to a dog.

14.9 Summary

Large animal models can be utilized to recreate many cardiac electrophysiologic diseases and procedures, in addition to being used to test new devices and imaging techniques. The three most common large animal models are dogs, sheep, and swine, but the choice of animal model is dependent upon many factors: anatomy of interest, skill and experience of the investigator, ease of handling, study design, and the ability to create specific pathological models. Used correctly, animal models are the best available method to predict systemic responses to therapies, while poorly designed experiments can lead to misleading and nontransferable results. Any animal studies conducted with government funding or at a major corporation or university are highly regulated, with the aim to maximize human benefit while minimizing animal use, pain, and suffering. Every invasive device used clinically today was once tested in a large animal model, and the continued use of animal models will make available the next generation of devices and therapies to patients in a safe and efficacious form.

Acknowledgment This work was partially funded by Grant Number T32AR007612 from the National Institute of Health.

References

1. NIH Publication Number 08-6436. Medical Research with Animals. http://science.education. nih.gov/AnimalResearchFS06.pdf. Accessed 14 January 2009.
2. Fox JG. Laboratory animal medicine, 2nd ed. San Diego: Academic Press/Elsevier; 2002.
3. Lee JC, Taylor FN, Downing SE. A comparison of ventricular weights and geometry in newborn, young, and adult mammals. J Appl Physiol 1975;38:147–50.
4. Hughes HC. Swine in cardiovascular research. Lab Anim Sci 1986;36:348–50.
5. Hill AJ, Iaizzo PA. Comparative cardiac anatomy. In: Iaizzo PA, editor. Handbook of Cardiac Anatomy, Physiology, and Devices, 2nd ed. New York: Humana Press; 2009.
6. Hearse DJ. Species variation in the coronary collateral circulation during regional myocardial ischaemia: a critical determinant of the rate of evolution and extent of myocardial infarction. Cardiovasc Res 2000;45:213–9.
7. Crick SJ, Sheppard MN, Ho SY, Gebstein L, Anderson RH. Anatomy of the pig heart: comparisons with normal human cardiac structure. J Anat 1998;193(Pt 1):105–19.
8. Hill AJ, Ahlberg SE, Wilkoff BL, Iaizzo PA. Dynamic obstruction to coronary sinus access: the Thebesian valve. Heart Rhythm 2006;3:1240–1.
9. Anderson SE, Quill JL, Iaizzo PA. Venous valves within left ventricular coronary veins. J Interv Card Electrophysiol 2008;23:95–9.

10. Anderson SE, Hill AJ, Iaizzo PA. Venous valves: unseen obstructions to coronary access. J Interv Card Electrophysiol 2007;19:165–6.
11. Frink RJ, Merrick B. The sheep heart: coronary and conduction system anatomy with special reference to the presence of an os cordis. Anat Rec 1974;179:189–200.
12. Ryu S, Yamamoto S, Andersen CR, Nakazawa K, Miyake F, James TN. Intramural Purkinje cell network of sheep ventricles as the terminal pathway of conduction system. Anat Rec (Hoboken) 2009;292:12–22.
13. Berenfeld O, Zaitsev AV. The muscular network of the sheep right atrium and frequency-dependent breakdown of wave propagation. Anat Rec A Discov Mol Cell Evol Biol 2004;280:1053–61.
14. Evans HE. The heart and arteries. In: Miller ME, Evans HE, editors. Miller's anatomy of the dog, 3rd ed. Philadelphia: Saunders; 1993, p. 586.
15. Kalifa J, Tanaka K, Zaitsev AV, et al. Mechanisms of wave fractionation at boundaries of high-frequency excitation in the posterior left atrium of the isolated sheep heart during atrial fibrillation. Circulation 2006;113:626–33.
16. Chinchoy E, Ujhelyi MR, Hill AJ, Skadsberg ND, Iaizzo PA. The pericardium. In: Iaizzo PA, editor. Handbook of Cardiac Anatomy, Physiology, and Devices. Totowa: Humana Press; 2005, p. 101.
17. Gross DR. Animal models in cardiovascular research. Boston: Nijhoff; 1985.
18. Naqvi TZ, Buchbinder M, Zarbatany D, et al. Beating-heart percutaneous mitral valve repair using a transcatheter endovascular suturing device in an animal model. Catheter Cardiovasc Interv 2007;69:525–31.
19. Liu C, Skadsberg ND, Ahlberg SE, Swingen CM, Iaizzo PA, He B. Estimation of global ventricular activation sequences by noninvasive three-dimensional electrical imaging: validation studies in a swine model during pacing. J Cardiovasc Electrophysiol 2008;19:535–40.
20. Qu J, Plotnikov AN, Danilo Jr P, et al. Expression and function of a biological pacemaker in canine heart. Circulation 2003;107:1106–9.
21. Chinchoy E, Soule CL, Houlton AJ, et al. Isolated four-chamber working swine heart model. Ann Thorac Surg 2000;70:1607–14.
22. Anderson RH, Yanni J, Boyett MR, Chandler NJ, Dobrzynski H. The anatomy of the cardiac conduction system. Clin Anat 2009;22:99–113.
23. Arnolda LF, Llewellyn-Smith IJ, Minson JB. Animal models of heart failure. Aust N Z J Med 1999;29:403–9.
24. Shinbane JS, Wood MA, Jensen DN, Ellenbogen KA, Fitzpatrick AP, Scheinman MM. Tachycardia-induced cardiomyopathy: a review of animal models and clinical studies. J Am Coll Cardiol 1997;29:709–15.
25. Recchia FA, Lionetti V. Animal models of dilated cardiomyopathy for translational research. Vet Res Commun 2007;31 Suppl 1:35–41.
26. Wilson JR, Douglas P, Hickey WF, et al. Experimental congestive heart failure produced by rapid ventricular pacing in the dog: cardiac effects. Circulation 1987;75:857–67.
27. Helm RH, Byrne M, Helm PA, et al. Three-dimensional mapping of optimal left ventricular pacing site for cardiac resynchronization. Circulation 2007;115:953–61.
28. Shen YT, Lynch JJ, Shannon RP, Wiedmann RT. A novel heart failure model induced by sequential coronary artery occlusions and tachycardiac stress in awake pigs. Am J Physiol 1999;277:H388–98.
29. Friedrichs GS. Experimental models of atrial fibrillation/flutter. J Pharmacol Toxicol Methods 2000;43:117–23.
30. Anadon MJ, Almendral J, Gonzalez P, Zaballos M, Delcan JL, De Guevara JL. Alcohol concentration determines the type of atrial arrhythmia induced in a porcine model of acute alcoholic intoxication. Pacing Clin Electrophysiol 1996;19:1962–7.
31. Kijtawornrat A, Roche BM, Hamlin RL. A canine model of sustained atrial fibrillation induced by rapid atrial pacing and phenylephrine. Comp Med 2008;58:490–3.
32. Bauer A, McDonald AD, Donahue JK. Pathophysiological findings in a model of persistent atrial fibrillation and severe congestive heart failure. Cardiovasc Res 2004;61:764–70.

33. Wijffels MC, Kirchhof CJ, Dorland R, Power J, Allessie MA. Electrical remodeling due to atrial fibrillation in chronically instrumented conscious goats: roles of neurohumoral changes, ischemia, atrial stretch, and high rate of electrical activation. Circulation 197;96:3710–20.

34. Adams JA, Bassuk JA, Arias J, et al. Periodic acceleration (pGz) CPR in a swine model of asphyxia induced cardiac arrest. Short-term hemodynamic comparisons. Resuscitation 2008;77:132–8.

35. Sridhar A, Nishijima Y, Terentyev D, et al. Repolarization abnormalities and afterdepolarizations in a canine model of sudden cardiac death. Am J Physiol 2008;295:R1463–72.

36. Lie JT, Holley KE, Kampa WR, Titus JL. New histochemical method for morphologic diagnosis of early stages of myocardial ischemia. Mayo Clin Proc 1971;46:319–27.

37. Manning WJ, Atkinson DJ, Grossman W, Paulin S, Edelman RR. First-pass nuclear magnetic resonance imaging studies using gadolinium-DTPA in patients with coronary artery disease. J Am Coll Cardiol 1991;18:959–65.

38. Judd RM, Lugo-Olivieri CH, Arai M, et al. Physiological basis of myocardial contrast enhancement in fast magnetic resonance images of 2-day-old reperfused canine infarcts. Circulation 1995;92:1902–10.

Chapter 15
Optical Mapping and Calcium Imaging

Rodolphe P. Katra

Abstract This chapter will cover basic theory, principles, and applications of optical mapping of transmembrane potentials, as well as of intracellular calcium imaging. Calcium plays a central role in both electrical and mechanical function of excitable tissue, and serves as an important player in many biochemical and biophysical cellular regulatory functions. Emphasis will be placed on practical applications, advantages, and limitations of both techniques.

15.1 Introduction

The fields of clinical and basic electrophysiology have benefited greatly from advances made in the techniques and technology of mapping electrical activity. A major technique widely used in preclinical research settings is optical mapping which relies on fluorescent dyes targeting specific biophysical phenomenon, specialized optics, and detectors to record the resulting fluorescence. Optical imaging, a noncontact mapping technique, allows for simultaneous multisite mapping of electrical activity across a certain area of tissue without the need for multiple electrodes in physical contact with the tissue, which arguably can disturb the physiologic condition being explored, alter the cellular milieu, and cause myocardial injury.

15.2 Brief Description of Optical Mapping Principles

Optical mapping is a basic research technique that is based on the principles of fluorescence where a fluorescent indicator – a compound that absorbs light photons at a certain wavelength and emits photons at a longer wavelength – is loaded into or

R.P. Katra (✉)

Department of Biomedical Engineering, College of Engineering, University of Alabama at Birmingham, Birmingham, AL, USA

e-mail: rkatra@uab.edu

D.C. Sigg et al. (eds.), *Cardiac Electrophysiology Methods and Models*,
DOI 10.1007/978-1-4419-6658-2_15, © Springer Science+Business Media, LLC 2010

onto a cell or tissue. The indicator is then excited by an external light source at a specific wavelength, which results in emission of fluorescent light from the dye at a characteristic wavelength. The emitted light is then processed through specialized hardware (optics and detectors) and software to yield a signal that correlates to the biophysical process being studied. These fluorescent indicators enable the investigation of cellular and sub-cellular processes without physical contact (e.g., suction electrodes) or damage of the cellular membrane caused by impalement (e.g., microelectrodes). For example, fluorescent dyes have been developed to respond to specific biophysical phenomena or reactions such as changes in transmembrane potential, changes in intracellular calcium, or changes in pH. A wide array of commercially available application-specific fluorescent dyes currently exists. These compounds vary greatly in number of excitation wavelengths and excitation spectral response, number of emission wavelengths and emission spectral response, quantum efficiency, linearity of response to biophysical phenomena, response dynamics, molecular weight, molecular stability, tissue permeability and affinity, and loading requirements. Table 15.1 describes some commonly used fast response potentiometric dyes and calcium-sensitive dyes as well as their properties.

The experimental setup of optical mapping can be tailored for observing a single biophysical process with a single fluorescent dye or, provided certain methodological considerations are managed carefully, multiple fluorescent dyes can be used to study multiple biophysical processes and their interactions simultaneously. This experimental flexibility marks one of many strengths of optical mapping. Practically, and of relevance to the field of basic cardiac electrophysiology and contractile function, this unique advantage permits the simultaneous study of electrical and mechanical activity of myocardial tissue in a relatively undisturbed and native environment. This chapter focuses on transmembrane potential and intracellular calcium imaging applications in optical mapping, but the principles covered in this chapter apply equally to other experimental applications and research interests such as measurement of pH, other ionic concentrations, etc. Figures 15.1–15.4 are schematic illustrations of experimental setups for optical mapping of voltage alone and dual voltage and calcium optical mapping systems. Actual setups may vary slightly according to vendors or experimental requirements, but the fundamentals and major components are represented in these schematic illustrations. The details of individual components of optical mapping and their respective applications are addressed in a later section of this chapter.

15.3 Principles of Wavelength Ratiometry in Optical Mapping

The development of ratiometric fluorescent indicators represented a significant advance in enabling the broad application of optical mapping for biomedical researchers.[1,2] As described previously, optical mapping relies on exciting a fluorescent indicator with light at a specific wavelength and collecting the resulting emitted light at another. This technique is further improved by exciting or collecting fluorescent light at two wavelengths instead of one. The ratio of the two wavelengths produces a value that is related strictly to the biophysical process, and the artifactual contributions of

Table 15.1 Common optical mapping dyes for imaging transmembrane potential and intracellular calcium

Fluorescent dye	Molecular weight	Ex λ	Em λ	Description
Fast potentiometric probes				
Di-4-ANEPPS	480.7	497 nm	705 nm	Sub-millisecond response to changes in membrane potential (10% change in fluorescence per 100 mV); smaller and more soluble than Di-8-ANEPPS; commonly used for cardiac applications
Di-4-ANEPPS	592.9	498 nm	713 nm	Sub-millisecond response to changes in membrane potential (10% change in fluorescence per 100 mV); good for long-term experiments; commonly used for cardiac applications
RH237/RH421	496.7/498.7	528/515 nm	782/704 nm	Principally used for imaging neurons
Calcium sensitive probes				
Fura-2	1001.9 for AM form	340 and 380 nm	510 nm	UV excitable, ratiometric (dual excitation, single emission); exists in membrane-permeant AM form and cell-impermeant salt form; commonly used for applications where dual light sources are employed
Indo-1	1009.9 for AM form	350 nm	405 and 485 nm	UV excitable, ratiometric (single excitation, dual emission); exists in membrane-permeant AM form and cell-impermeant salt form; commonly used for applications where dual detectors are employed
Fluo-3, Fluo-4 and Rhod-2	1129.9, 1097.0, and 1123.96 for AM forms	464, 456, and 550 nm	488, 488, and 571 nm	Visible light excitable, non-ratioable; exists in membrane-permeant AM form and cell-impermeant salt form; commonly used with confocal microscopy and flow cytometry

intensity and pattern of excitation light, dye concentration, and other methodological limitations are reduced.[3,4] The ratiometric method, for example, has enabled investigators to image intracellular calcium from a range of preparations from single cell to the intact heart, in different physiologic and pathophysiologic conditions. When studying transmembrane potentials, however, only the temporal response of the indicator is particularly important. This is due to the nature of changes in transmembrane potentials in excitable tissue. Action potentials in myocytes undergo a very characteristic change in voltage, which is amenable to linear scaling and spatial normalization.[5] It is important to note, however, that this scaling correction cannot be used when sub-threshold, nonsteady state electrical changes are being studied.

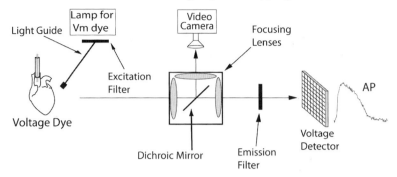

Fig. 15.1 Schematic illustration of a single dye optical mapping setup. The preparation is loaded with the fluorescent dye and then illuminated using a wavelength-filtered light source and light guide. The emitted light is then collected by the focusing lens assembly and emission-filtered before being directed at the detector array. A dichroic mirror is used to interrupt the light path and direct the image of the preparation to a video camera for image registration and localization. This example uses a voltage-sensitive dye and measures hundreds of action potentials simultaneously from a multicellular preparation like the Langendorff-perfused isolated heart or ventricular wedge preparation. The setup can easily be adapted to any other biophysical process by choosing the appropriate dye, excitation and emission filters, and dichroic mirror

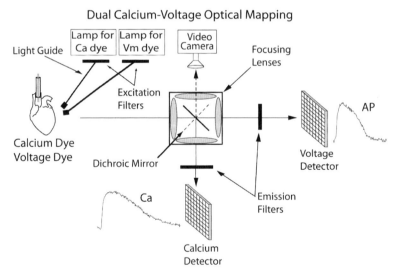

Fig. 15.2 Schematic illustration of a dual dye optical mapping setup. The preparation is loaded with two fluorescent dyes and illuminated using two different wavelength-filtered light sources and light guides, specifically chosen to match the dyes' requirements. The emitted light is collected by the focusing lens assembly. A dichroic mirror separates the light to direct wavelengths with the calcium content to a calcium-specific emission-filtered detector array and the voltage content to a voltage-specific emission-filtered detector array. The two detector arrays are in perfect register. The dichroic mirror is temporarily rotated by 90° to direct light to the camera to acquire an image of the preparation for registration and localization purposes. This example uses a voltage-sensitive dye and a calcium-sensitive dye loaded simultaneously to measure hundreds of co-localized action potentials and calcium transients from the same multicellular preparation

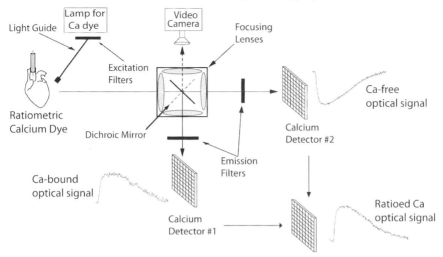

Fig. 15.3 Schematic illustration of a ratiometric optical mapping setup. The preparation is loaded with a ratiometric calcium-sensitive fluorescent dye and illuminated using a wavelength-filtered light source and light guide. The emitted light is collected by the focusing lens assembly. A dichroic mirror separates the light to direct light containing the calcium-bound wavelengths to an emission-filtered detector array and the calcium-free wavelengths to another emission-filtered detector array. The two detector arrays are in perfect register. The dichroic mirror is temporarily rotated by 90° to direct light to the camera to acquire an image of the preparation for registration and localization purposes. The signal from both detector arrays is then background-corrected and ratioed using custom software to yield ratiometric intracellular calcium transients from hundreds of sites of a multicellular preparation. This schematic uses the calcium-sensitive dye, Indo-1AM, and the respective light source, excitation filters, and emission filters

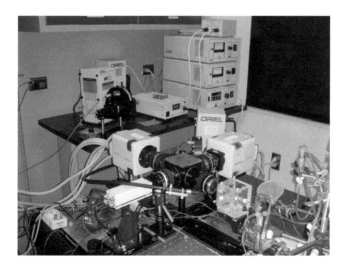

Fig. 15.4 Picture of a dual-detector optical mapping system. By incorporating multiple light sources and detectors, this custom-made optical mapping setup is capable of single-wavelength imaging, simultaneous voltage and calcium imaging, and ratiometric calcium imaging

15.4   Detailed Principles of Ratiometric Calcium Imaging

Calcium-sensitive dyes fall into two different functional classes: single-wavelength dyes and dual-wavelength ratiometric dyes. Single-wavelength dyes have a single peak emission wavelength in response to excitation. Dual-wavelengths dyes, on the other hand, have two peak emission or excitation wavelengths. These dual-wavelength ratiometric dyes are capable of emitting (e.g., Indo-1) or absorbing (e.g., Fura 2) two distinct wavelengths that are characteristic of that dye in response to two separate states – calcium-bound or calcium-unbound – and are classified as single-excitation dual-emission dyes or dual-excitation single-emission dyes, respectively.

Fluorescence from single-wavelength dyes can be calibrated to yield true intracellular calcium concentrations using equation:

$$[Ca]_i = K_d \frac{(F - F_{min})}{(F_{max} - F)} \tag{15.1}$$

where K_d is the effective dissociation constant of the dye expressed in moles/liter. The K_d of an indicator is defined as the concentration at which it reaches the half-saturation point; this value changes with ionic strength, pH, and temperature as well as the composition of the tissue. Fluorescence intensity (F) is measured at a particular wavelength, F_{min} and F_{max}, corresponding to the fluorescence at the same wavelength when the intracellular medium is calcium free and calcium saturated, respectively. Single-wavelength fluorescence imaging is sensitive to many artifacts like light intensity changes, dye loading, and dye degradation washout. Because of this, single-wavelength fluorescence needs to be calibrated at every site in multisite imaging and at every point in time during the course of an experiment.

Dual-wavelength ratiometric imaging, in contrast, is not sensitive to the mentioned artifacts of the single-wavelength technique. First, ratio signals are obtained from fluorescence at two peak wavelengths of emission or excitation using equation:

$$R = \frac{(F_{\lambda 1} - F_{back \lambda 1})}{(F_{\lambda 2} - F_{back \lambda 2})} \tag{15.2}$$

where F is the fluorescence signal, and F_{back} is the background or baseline signal before the dye is loaded. Therefore, the numerator is a background-corrected fluorescence measured at wavelength λ_1, and the denominator is a background-corrected fluorescence measured at wavelength λ_2. This ratio minimizes the effect of many artifacts that are unrelated to changes in [Ca], such as light intensity changes, dye concentration heterogeneities, dye washout, and motion artifact. The ratio of fluorescence accounts for these limitations but, without proper calibration, yields a nonlinear index of intracellular calcium. The ratio R can be calibrated to yield intracellular calcium levels using equation:

$$[Ca]_i = K_d \times \frac{F_{min \lambda 2}}{F_{max \lambda 2}} \times \frac{(R - R_{min})}{(R_{max} - R)} \tag{15.3}$$

where K_d is the dissociation constant of the dye used, and $F_{min\ \lambda2}$ and $F_{max\ \lambda2}$ are fluorescence signals obtained when the intracellular medium is calcium-free and calcium-saturated, respectively, measured at the longer of the two wavelengths. The ratio of $F_{min\ \lambda2}$ and $F_{max\ \lambda2}$ denotes absolute fluorescence levels obtained from the indicator, and is unnecessary if the chosen λ_2 wavelength corresponds to a non-variant wavelength on the fluorescence spectra, known as the *isosbestic point*. R is the ratio signal (15.2), and R_{min} and R_{max} correspond to the fluorescence ratio obtained when the intracellular medium is calcium-free and calcium-saturated, respectively. Although R_{min} and R_{max} vary between species and cell types, they only need to be measured once and applied in all subsequent calibrations, unless optical hardware in the setup is changed.

Calibration of the ratiometric values minimizes limitations of the single fluorescence technique and accounts for the nonlinearity of the dual-wavelength ratio technique without calibration. Practically however, the calibration process is very intensive and difficult to perform in intact multicellular preparations compared to isolated single cell preparations. The complexity stems, in part, from the difficulty in ensuring homogenous and fast transitions to the calcium-saturated and calcium-free conditions. A complexity that is significantly attenuated in single myocyte calibration, since calcium concentrations could easily be altered using pipette injections or other direct administration techniques. As a workaround, some researchers have resorted to mathematical calibration techniques that approximate the R_{max} and R_{min} parameters, whereas most others have resorted to in vitro calibration. Another complicating factor in intact tissue is the dissociation constant (K_d), which is mostly measured in vitro under room temperature using controlled buffer solutions. It is reported that the K_d value in vivo is significantly different from in vitro values, mainly due to differences in the measurement medium. In light of these complications, while recognizing the advantages over single-wavelength methods and the shortcomings compared to calibrated ratio values, the use of uncalibrated ratio measurements as an index of intracellular calcium has increased. Additional recommended readings and references that cover the principles and theory of ratiometry and calcium imaging in greater detail are listed at the end of this chapter.

15.5 Application and Practical Implementation

Fluorescence-based optical imaging of large multicellular preparations, like intact Langendorff-perfused hearts or ventricular wedge preparations, has been done almost exclusively using epi-illumination techniques, where the light source and the detector array are on the same side of the preparation, facing the surface to be studied. This mode of illumination has proven superior to trans-illumination, where the light source and detector array are on opposite sides of the preparation, since trans-illumination lacks the desired spatial resolution due to light scattering, a dominant light attenuation process in tissue. Therefore, the discussion in this chapter will focus mostly on practical implementation of optical mapping on anisotropic cardiac tissue, in epi-illumination mode. Specifically, the discussion focuses on the artifactual contribution of different optical components. This will promote a practical understanding of the implementation of optical mapping, of factors to account for, and of sources of artifact that need to be minimized in order to optimize optical signal acquisition and interpretation. Table 15.2 provides a brief summary of the application advantages and implementation limitations of non-ratiometric vs. ratiometric and trans-illumination vs. epi-illumination imaging techniques.

Theoretically, fluorescence imaging starts with excitation light generated by a light source, directed to and penetrating into tissue to various depths according to the properties of the tissue being studied and the incident light wavelength. After undergoing some reflection/refraction at the tissue interface, the penetrating light is either absorbed by the dye/tissue or scattered within the tissue to eventually be absorbed or exit the tissue. Once the dye is energized by absorbing photons of excitation light, it eventually fluoresces as a point source and emits light spherically. The emitted light will undergo the same process of scatter and ultimately either exit the tissue or get absorbed. After going through a series of

Table 15.2 Advantages and limitations of different imaging techniques

Imaging technique	Advantages	Limitations
Single-wavelength technique	Simple to perform Ideal for studying temporal relationships and processes Can easily incorporate multiple dyes simultaneously in one preparation	Not ideal for physiological responses that rely on changes in magnitude-like calcium transients Sensitive to methodological artifact Requires intensive spatial calibration if studying graded responses and processes
Ratiometric technique	Ideal for studying graded responses and processes Collected signal is less sensitive to excitation light intensity, illumination pattern, dye concentration, and other methodological artifacts	Requires special ratiometric dyes Requires complicated hardware and software Requires complicated dye calibration procedures
Trans-illumination	Most suitable for use with single cell and cultured monolayer imaging Usually incorporated with off-the-shelf macro/microscope systems Higher light throughput supports the use of low sensitivity light detectors	Not suitable for large preparations More excitation light and fluoresced light contamination Lacks high spatial resolution due to light scatter Plagued by high dye photobleaching
Epi-illumination	Suitable for thick multicellular preparations Has high spatial resolution due to limited light scatter Excitation light directionality and pattern is more customizable	Requires complicated excitation and emission light setup Low fluoresced light requires the use of high sensitivity light detectors Excitation light path and pattern may cause artifact

filters and optical components, the exiting fluorescent light is collected by detectors that convert the optical signals to electrical signals which, in turn, are processed by hardware and software to complete the process. Practically, the hardware in optical mapping is designed to produce and collect optical signals based on biological activity. Unfortunately, these components have the potential to introduce undesirable artifacts. Figure 15.5 describes the light path from light source to detectors and lists the potential complications introduced by each component along its path. Each component will now be discussed in detail below and summarized in Table 15.3.

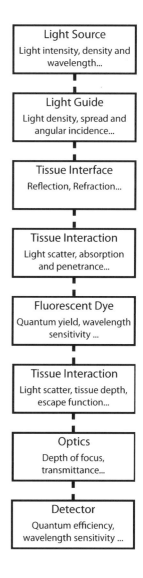

Fig. 15.5 Light path and basic components. Block diagram illustrating the light path through basic components for a fluorescence-based optical mapping setup. Each block also lists some of the artifacts introduced by each component

Table 15.3 Sources of artifact and suggested solutions

Source of artifact	Implementation pitfalls	Suggested solutions
Component artifact		
Light source	Mismatch light source specifications to dye characteristics	Use light source of the correct type with special consideration to wavelength, intensity, density, and bandwidth
	Excessive light intensity degrades dye	Use appropriate light intensity to ensure maximum dye excitation but not cause photobleaching
Light guide	Internal material may filter out certain wavelength	Use light guide that is appropriate for the light source's excitation wavelength
	Heterogeneous illumination pattern	Use multiple guides, collimators, or illumination rings to ensure homogeneous light delivery
Tissue interface and interaction	Varied illumination depth across the mapping field	Use homogeneous and perpendicular excitation to minimize reflection and scatter
	When using multiple light sources, the light penetration and interaction with tissue is different for each light source	Slightly reduce light intensity of longer wavelength relative to shorter wavelength in order to match light penetration
	Different tissue types have different spectral response	Use appropriate lighting conditions for the tissue type being studied
Fluorescent dye	Signal crosstalk when multiple dyes are used	Use the appropriate narrow excitation wavelength for each dye along with appropriate filters and dichroic mirrors to avoid spectral overlap
Optics	Wavelength sensitivity of lenses and filters	Use appropriate lenses and filters for excitation and emission light path in the setup
Detectors	Suitability of detector to experimental application	Match the detector's spectral quantum efficiency, spatial resolution, and temporal resolution to experimental needs

Experimental artifacts

Dye	Dye concentration heterogeneity across the preparation	Ratiometry minimizes dye heterogeneity, dye washout, and dye bleaching for calcium imaging; signal scaling eliminates these artifacts for voltage imaging
	Dye washout	Anionic transport blockers like probenecid and sulfinpyrazone reduce dye washout pharmacologically
		Running experiment at a slightly lower temperature reduces dye washout rate
	Dye bleaching	Reducing the excitation light intensity reduces dye bleaching
		Vitamin E reduces dye degradation
Light	Light intensity heterogeneity across the imaging surface	Ratiometry minimizes spatial heterogeneities and temporal variation in light intensity for calcium imaging; signal scaling eliminates these artifacts for voltage imaging
	Variations in light intensity over time	
Motion	Translational motion	Physical stabilization can reduce translational and rotational motion
	Changes in tissue density/focal plane	Reducing calcium content from the buffer solution reduces contractile strength of preparation
	Changes in surface curvature	Ratiometric imaging reduces motion artifact
		Electromechanical uncouplers like BDM and Cytochalasin-D minimize motion artifact
Multiple dye experiments	Tissue filtering effects	Balance dye selections to match fluorescence contribution across tissue depth and minimize spectral overlap
	Variability in depth contribution	Focal plane of optics reduces variability in depth contribution

15.5.1   Light Source

Numerous types of light sources have been used for exciting fluorescent dyes, each with advantages and disadvantages in terms of wavelength bandwidth capabilities, light intensity, and density. The ideal light source would be capable of delivering a consistent intensity with a uniform density at any wavelength for an indefinite amount of time. However, most sources fail to meet all these requirements simultaneously and, therefore, a compromise is necessary. For example, mercury arc lamps, a commonly used excitation source for fluorescent dyes, have unique discontinuous high intensity bands in the UV, near-UV, and deep blue ranges where irradiance intensity spikes orders of magnitude over neighboring wavelengths. This makes it difficult to tune the excitation intensity uniformly over different ranges of wavelength. The effect of such dramatic increases in intensity on the fluorescence from a dye and the resulting depth contribution of fluorescence in tissue (discussed in greater detail in later sections) are, therefore, difficult to gauge. This presents an even greater challenge when multiple excitation light wavelengths are needed to excite multiple dyes simultaneously, since the fluorescent light and depth contribution of tissue from each dye are proportional to the excitation light intensity and wavelength. It is easy to appreciate, then, the importance of delivering identical intensities of excitation light over a broad range of wavelengths.

15.5.2   Light Guide

In an epi-illumination setup, a light guide is needed whenever the excitation light is not incorporated into the optical light path (i.e., through the collecting lenses and filters). A variety of light guides are commercially available in a variety of lengths, diameters, transmittance, and internal materials to suit different applications. Simply though, a light guide is a flexible tube that serves as a means to move light from the source to the object, without relying on a fixed light path. This is achieved by the phenomenon of total internal reflection of light inside the guide. A light guide allows the investigator to selectively position light according to the specific tissue location being imaged without including the excitation light as part of the light path through the lenses and filters. Light exiting the light guide is not collimated and, therefore, not perfectly uniform in intensity, since the conical spread of light at the exit tip is governed by the acceptance angle of the input tip. Figure 15.6 (left panel) demonstrates the circular pattern that would manifest on the surface of the preparation due to the conical spread of light from the light guide, when the guide is perpendicular to the preparation. The intensity of light decays as the distance from the center increases. This illumination pattern can be altered by using certain components at the guide tip, like condensers and collimators. Figure 15.6 (right panel) illustrates how the circular pattern changes when the light guide is not perpendicular to the preparation. In this case, the illumination becomes a variable

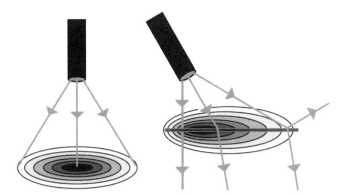

Fig. 15.6 Illumination patterns from light exiting a light guide. The *left panel* shows a circular illumination pattern of light when projected onto a 2D surface, if the guide is normal to the surface. The intensity of light decays monotonically as the distance from the center increases. The *right panel* shows an elliptical illumination pattern of light when projected onto the same 2D surface, but when the guide is not normal to the surface. This illumination configuration also introduces significant reflection. *Black zones* indicate largest illumination intensity

elliptical pattern with significant reflection occurring distal to the light guide, since incident light at very shallow angles reflects off the surface, while it refracts into the tissue at steeper angles. This angular dependence of light penetration is a complex artifact that is not easily quantified, especially when coupled with tissue curvature at the interface. A potential solution to this artifact involves using multiple light guides with reduced intensity to illuminate the preparation surface uniformly, from all directions. This is the motivation behind using illumination rings mounted at light guide tips. The illumination ring directs uniform excitation light around the entire area of interest on the preparation, minimizing this artifact.

15.5.3   Tissue Interface and Interaction

At the surface of the tissue, incident light will undergo reflection and/or refraction. Reflection involves light moving away from the medium, whereas refraction involves light moving toward the medium. In general, with a greater angle of incidence, light is reflected both as normal (specular) reflection and diffuse reflection, where light enters the tissue and re-exits upon scattering. Refraction depends on the angle of light incidence and the nature of the two media; this occurs anytime there is an index mismatch at the interface. Scattering is typically an elastic mechanism where a photon retains its energy but changes direction. For biological tissue, Rayleigh and Mie scattering are the dominant forms of scattering. *Rayleigh scattering* happens when light interacts with particles of a smaller size than the light wavelength (e.g., atoms and molecules). *Mie scattering* occurs when the light has a much smaller wavelength than the particle size (e.g., cell and tissue boundaries). In optical imaging of multicellular preparations, Mie scattering is the dominant light scatter artifact. Understanding light propagation within a medium requires detailed knowledge of the optical properties of the medium, as well as a model for how light behaves in that medium.[6] Light absorption in homogenous tissue can be simply described by exponential decay according to the Lambert–Beer theory. However, cardiac tissue is heterogeneous and behaves as a scattering medium. This presents a problem for studying excitation light propagation through tissue, but is extremely advantageous for fluorescence-based studies. Since excitation light is heavily scattered upon entering the tissue, the zigzag path within the tissue keeps the light in the medium for longer periods, thereby increasing the probability of reaching fluorescent dye molecules and getting absorbed by them. The scattering process, therefore, leads to an isotropic distribution of light in regions proximal to the surface and attenuates light exponentially with increasing depth. When fluorescent dyes return to their lower energy state, the emitted light is subject to the same exponential attenuation in heterogeneous tissue. The emitted light, however, has a longer wavelength, thereby ensuring higher penetration and a larger fraction of photons exiting the tissue, termed the *escape function*. Therefore, the spectral sensitivity of biological tissue provides a unique advantage in optical mapping. Every particular tissue type exhibits unique spectral characteristics that are commonly reported in a wavelength-sensitive absorption–emission spectrum, from which tissue excitation and emission decay constants can be calculated. This transmission spectrum is a result of the tissue's anisotropy, constituents (scatterers, absorbers), and other factors, giving the tissue a unique "fingerprint" in terms of light transmittance. Therefore, for fluorescence imaging, it is imperative that tissue transmittance properties be quantified in order to accurately obtain wavelength-dependent tissue excitation and emission decay constants, if an exact calculation of tissue depth contribution to light signals is desired.

15.5.4   Fluorescent Dye

A variety of commercially available fluorescent dyes exist with different quantum yields and spectral properties for a variety of applications. In cardiac tissue where electrical and mechanical functions are important, various combinations of commercially available voltage-sensitive and intracellular calcium-sensitive dyes may be used. In this chapter, we will specifically cover two commonly used dyes, di-4-ANEPPS for voltage and Indo-1 for intracellular calcium measurements, as examples to illustrate the theory and discuss implementation. The principles, however, can easily be extrapolated to apply to any other dye combinations. The membrane-binding, single-emission, voltage-sensitive dye, di-4-ANEPPS, exhibits a spectral excitation peak around 515 nm and emits light at around 640 nm, when bound to tissue. These values are slightly different from values measured in vitro instead of in situ, since the dye behavior is altered when tissue-bound. On the other hand, the cell-permeant, calcium-sensitive, ratiometric dye, Indo-1AM is excited at around 350 nm in situ (also slightly different from in vitro conditions, around 338 nm) and fluoresces at two different peak wavelengths simultaneously depending on its calcium-binding state (around 405 nm for calcium-bound and 485 nm for calcium-free). Experimentally, it is a complex process delivering two different wavelengths of excitation light and collecting emitted light selectively at three different wavelengths. This can be achieved, however, by judicious selection of excitation/emission filters and dichroic mirrors tailored to minimize spectral overlap.[7–11]

15.5.5   Tissue Interaction

As mentioned previously, the intensity of the excitation light in tissue is attenuated exponentially due to a combination of absorption and scatter, governed by wavelength of excitation light, tissue homogeneity, and transmission properties. Light absorption by the dye ultimately results in light emission at longer wavelengths. The emitted light intensity also undergoes an exponential decay due to a combination of absorption and scatter, governed mainly by wavelength of emitted light, the quantum yield of the dye, the tissue's homogeneity, and transmission properties. The light behavior in tissue, therefore, has strong depth dependence that can be modeled for each fluorescent dye (voltage and calcium) as a product of excitation and fluorescence intensity decaying exponentials, using the Lambert–Beer theory. This means that voltage and calcium signals would originate from slightly different tissue depth, with the longer wavelengths for voltage dye excitation penetrating deeper into the tissue and resulting emission escaping from deeper tissue layers compared to those used for the calcium dye. As an example, using the excitation and emission characteristics of di-4-ANEPPS and Indo-1, Fig. 15.7 illustrates the relative intensity contribution of voltage and ratiometric calcium signals along tissue depth, demonstrating that the voltage signal originates from a deeper region compared to the calcium signal. Furthermore, over the first 400 µm of tissue depth, 96% of the total calcium intensity is emitted vs. 90% from the voltage signal, which becomes about 96% relative intensity at about 600 µm of tissue depth.

15.5.6   Optics

Emitted fluorescence light needs to pass through an array of optical components that may alter the light based on their own optical properties. In some cases, the light and optical component interaction is intentional, for example, using beam splitters, dichroic mirrors, interference filters, and long pass filters. In other cases, the interaction is a side effect and may even be a source of artifacts. One such example is the wavelength sensitivity of lenses that serve to focus light on the detector. These lenses have varied wavelength-dependent transmittance efficiency, where shorter wavelengths are less transmitted. Newer generations of UV-grade filters and lenses have reduced that problem at the expense of total transmittance or

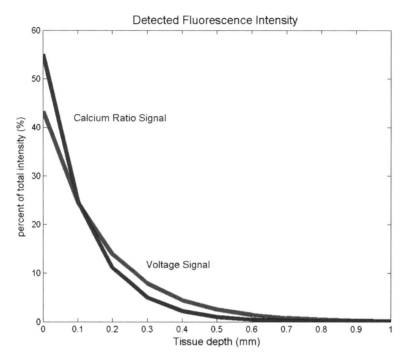

Fig. 15.7 Relative fluorescence intensity for voltage and ratiometric calcium signals. The calcium signal (*blue*) originates from shallower depth with a higher relative intensity compared to the voltage signal (*red*)

other compromises. In addition, the lenses, according to compound lens theory, have a depth of focus that relates to the light wavelength, the numerical aperture, and the optical magnification according to equation:

$$d = \left[\frac{1000}{7 \cdot NA \cdot M} \right] + \left[\frac{\lambda}{2 \cdot NA^2} \right] \tag{15.4}$$

where d is the depth of focus, NA is the numerical aperture of the objective, M is total magnification, and λ is the wavelength of light in μm. Continuing with the di-4-ANEPPS and Indo-1 example and assuming similar optics for both, this results in an effective depth of focus of about 323 μm for voltage signals and about 322 μm for calcium signals, indicating that the majority of the acquired light will originate from within that depth of focus. The light emanating from tissue outside the depth of focus will also contribute to the signal, but to a much lesser extent due to signal blurring. Furthermore, the depth of focus for the system is highly dependent on the magnification, such that as magnification is increased, the depth of focus will also be significantly decreased. Therefore, the artifact introduced by the compound lenses (i.e., limiting depth contribution of tissue to the total signal) seems to somewhat limit the artifact detailed in the previous section (i.e., depth of tissue contribution difference for different dye wavelengths).

Another integral part of the optical mapping system is optical filtering, which is needed for both the excitation and the emission light paths. Optical filters are commercially available for a wide variety of applications and to match the requirements of fluorescent dyes. They are mainly grouped into low-pass, high-pass, band-pass, dichroic, and neutral grade categories. Low-pass and high-pass filters selectively filter out high or low wavelengths, respectively. Band-pass filters have a selective transmission to a certain range of wavelengths. Dichroic mirrors transmit all light above a cutoff wavelength and reflect all light below the cutoff wavelength. Neutral grade density filters reduce total light intensity without altering wavelength transmittance. Optical filters can also be custom-made to fit specific applications, but most filter manufacturers have preconfigured sets of filters that can be used for common optical mapping applications. Note that the exact transmittance spectra need to be measured and the tradeoffs weighed for every optical filter since specifications can vary slightly from published theoretical specifications and can behave aberrantly at certain extended wavelengths. Additional readings are recommended to cover other relevant concepts in optics such as polarization, aberrations, and so on.

15.5.7 Detectors

A wide array of detectors varying by technology (e.g., photodiode array, photomultiplier tube, charge-coupled device, and complementary metal oxide semiconductor) are currently commercially available; each technology has its advantages and drawbacks. Some common issues of practical implementation and pitfalls are discussed here. Detectors have an inherent spectral sensitivity to certain wavelengths. Ideally, the detectors should have the same sensitivity and quantum efficiency to all wavelengths. In reality, however, they artifactually attenuate certain signal intensities depending on wavelengths, according to the detector's spectral quantum efficiency. Most detectors have a reduced efficiency at shorter wavelengths. This suggests that, all things being equal, the detector would not adequately detect light at shorter wavelengths (e.g., calcium signal) compared to longer ones (e.g., voltage signal). To remedy some of these shortcomings, photon amplifiers and multipliers have been introduced that can be coupled with detectors in order to boost their sensitivity. However, these intensifiers have their own set of limitations; therefore, a full understanding of the tradeoffs is warranted. Newer generations of detectors have improved spectral quantum efficiency, with some even specialized for certain applications in the UV and near UV ranges. An additional important factor to consider in detectors is their temporal resolution. The slower a detector responds to or processes collected light, the less suited it is for fast experimental and biological applications. Therefore, knowing technical specifications and features of the detector is essential to matching it to the right experimental application, typically requiring a compromise between spatial resolution, temporal resolution, and light collection efficiency.

15.6   Pitfalls, Limitations, and Artifacts

The tremendous advantages of fluorescence-based optical imaging over lower resolution, more invasive techniques have made this imaging modality an increasingly common tool used by basic researchers in studying excitable tissues, in particular in the disciplines of basic cardiac electrophysiology and neurophysiology. Fluorescence-based optical techniques, however, along with the recognized advantages, have their own set of drawbacks that need to be well understood in order to better tease out physiological phenomenon from experimental artifact. The major implementation pitfalls and some suggested solutions are listed in Table 15.3.

15.6.1   Artifacts of Dye and Excitation Light

Factors such as excitation light intensity, fluorescent dye concentration, dye degradation, and dye temporal washout and buffering need to be controlled in order to successfully record relevant reproducible physiological optical mapping signals. Over the last few decades, researchers have been able to minimize most of these limitations. Ratiometric imaging techniques have reduced: (1) the effects of spatial heterogeneity in light intensity; (2) spatial and temporal dye concentration differences; and (3) dye photobleaching. Creative approaches have been used to address other known limitations of optical mapping. The loss of dye over time can be drastically reduced by lowering the temperature of the preparation or by using pharmacological agents like probenecid or sulfinpyrazone[12,13] that target cellular anionic transporters. Artifacts related to dye degradation and bleaching[14] can be reduced by using Vitamin E in the solution. Though all of these measures have their own limitations, when used with caution, they can successfully limit artifacts in optical mapping and prove very useful experimentally.

15.6.2   Artifacts of Motion

A major complication associated with optical mapping is motion artifact, which occurs due to the noncontact nature of the imaging technique. There are three main kinds of motion artifact that may occur simultaneously with varying magnitudes: (1) the contracting heart or preparation moves relative to the optical setup (translational or rotational changes); (2) the preparation contracts while stationary (tissue density and focal plane changes); and (3) the preparation alters its planar imaging surface (surface curvature changes). Experimental and pharmacological solutions have been used to limit motion artifact including the following: (1) physical stabilization of the preparation with pistons and manipulator arms;

(2) reducing calcium concentration in the perfusion solution to reduce the contractile strength; (3) using ratiometric techniques to account for artifactual changes[15]; and (4) using electromechanical uncouplers such as Butanedione monoxine (BDM) or Cytochalasin-D to reduce motion artifact without significantly altering physiological processes.

15.6.3 Artifacts of Tissue Filtering and Interaction

Optical mapping is an indispensible tool for simultaneously studying basic cardiac electrophysiology and mechanics in large tissue preparations. Artifacts related to tissue filtering effects, however, arise from such an implementation. The wavelength-dependent tissue-filtering effect phenomenon occurs as a result of differential (i.e., nonuniform) light propagation and scatter in anisotropic tissue. The magnitude of this artifact, which frequently goes unaccounted for, varies greatly with wavelength of excitation/fluorescent light, angle of incident excitatory light, optical properties of tissue and in-tissue light scatter, and more. In some applications, tissue-filtering effect is significant and cannot be assumed negligible, since it would dramatically influence the experimental findings. To illustrate, when using a single dye to image action potentials in the heart, the recorded electrical activity would not exactly stem from the surface of the preparation, but would have a certain contribution from deeper layers of tissue. Some investigators have reported that action potentials recorded using di-4-ANEPPS originate from a depth of up to 700 μm, with the largest light intensity contribution originating from a shallower depth. This seems negligible, but to put things in perspective, an average cardiac myocyte has a diameter of about 10 μm. Therefore, optical mapping experiments using di-4-ANEPPS are measuring action potentials from an aggregate of cells with a depth of about 70 myocytes. Indo-1, on the other hand, due to its spectral characteristics, results in fluorescent light originating from much shallower depth, and hence less myocytes.

To study electromechanical function in intact preparations, di-4-ANEPPS and Indo-1 are used simultaneously to correlate electrical and mechanical activity. Unfortunately, these two dyes have different depth penetrations and target different tissue volumes. Since optical mapping is mainly a 2D representation of a 3D phenomenon, the depth contribution of each dye to the total signal is important to understand. Under steady-state conditions, the depth contribution is not as important and would not significantly alter any findings. Therefore, as a practical simplification, the recorded signals can be assumed to be mostly 2D and correlative under steady-state conditions. There are instances, however, where such assumptions might prove erroneous and invalid, such as when dyes with significantly different depth profiles are being used or during arrhythmia initiation. To illustrate, since the voltage dye can measure from deeper areas (about 600 μm) compared to the calcium dye (about 400 μm), an electrical event occurring at 500 μm would be detected whereas the calcium event, a marker for mechanical activity, would not. This would lead to the false interpretation that the electrical event was not accompanied by a mechanical event. Moreover, electrical events spread electrotonically, whereas calcium events do not, suggesting that electrical activity occurring at depth of about 1,500 μm can still theoretically spread passively to a depth of about 600 μm and influence membrane potential at that depth. In such an instance, electrical events would be detected but would have originated from a region outside the depth of view of the system. This emphasizes the need for matching depth contribution of different dyes when used together. Fortunately, the depth of focus from the optics can help limit the contribution of depth beyond about 300 μm, since they heavily weigh signals from shallower depths and blur signals from deeper regions.

15.6.4 Artifacts of Optical Signal Magnitude

Factors like intensity of excitation light, dye concentration, and physiologic phenomenon influence the magnitude of collected optical signals in optical mapping. However, when studying electrical activity only, the spatial differences in signal amplitude are not critical since action potentials exhibit all-or-none responses. This allows for normalization of action potential magnitude differences, both spatially and over the course of the experiment, to reflect physiological values, regardless of changes in excitation light differences or changes in dye concentration. In contrast, when studying intracellular calcium activity, the amplitude of the calcium transients cannot be normalized when using single wavelength dyes, since calcium-dependent events are graded (not all-or-none responses) and vary spatially and temporally. Dual-wavelength dyes are, thus, used to rectify this limitation through ratiometric techniques. Ratiometric techniques have also been used for certain single-wavelength dyes (voltage or calcium) that have an isosbestic wavelength, defined as the wavelength that does not change intensity in response to the physiologic response being studied.

15.7 New and Emerging Techniques/Models/Technologies

Over the last few decades, the uses of optical mapping have evolved from imaging isolated single myocytes to isolated multicellular preparations studied in an imaging chamber like Langendorff-perfused isolated hearts or arterially perfused wedge preparations (See Chaps. 11 and 12 for more information). More recently, however, technologies are being progressively adapted for use in intact hearts in vivo, in order to study cardiac tissue physiology and pathophysiology in its native environment, as well as noninvasively imaging whole small animals without even isolating tissue. These two approaches are still not very commonly used in mainstream basic research, but are indicative of the direction in which the field is headed.

15.8 Conclusion

In summary, optical mapping is a powerful technique for imaging cardiac function with high spatial and temporal resolution. Nonetheless, as with any methodology, the advantages and limitations of optical imaging need to be well understood in order to fully and accurately interpret information acquired by these means. This chapter covered some basic physical principles and fundamental knowledge of optical mapping in order to highlight its utility, limitations, and appropriate use in research. Please note that this chapter is not a comprehensive account of all optical mapping and calcium imaging applications. Rather, it is meant as a general introduction to be read and understood in the context of, and in concert with, other readings on this topic.

15.9 Additional References and Resources

This section contains a listing of recommended resources and references covering detailed aspects of optical mapping, in-depth discussion of the theory behind it, and its application-specific utilization. The partial listing of books constitutes important supplementary reading to better understand and implement optical mapping; select manuscripts are also meant to strengthen the reader's understanding of the field. Finally, a few websites are listed that can serve as a starting point for investigators interested in purchasing or building optical mapping systems. Note that these suggested readings and websites are only a partial listing and do not constitute an exhaustive reference list.

Books

- Bright GR. Fluorescence ratio imaging: issues and artifacts. In: Herman B, Lemasters JJ, editors. Optical microscopy: emerging methods and applications. San Diego: Academic Press; 1993.
  A thorough assessment of artifacts and errors related to fluorescence imaging of intracellular calcium using ratiometric techniques.
- Mason WT. Fluorescent and luminescent probes for biological activity: a practical guide to technology for quantitative real-time analysis. San Diego: Academic Press; 1999.
  An excellent reference discussing a variety of practical and implementation aspects of fluorescence imaging. This book addresses in-depth basics of fluorescence, fluorescent dyes, and practical applications in specific chapters covering fluorescence imaging in a variety of biological applications.
- Nuccitelli R. Methods in cell biology: a practical guide to the study of calcium in living cells. San Diego: Academic Press; 1994.
  A valuable reference covering various aspects of intracellular calcium measurements and techniques.

- Rosenbaum DS, Jalife J. Optical mapping of cardiac excitation and arrhythmias. Armonk: Futura Press; 2001.
  An excellent reference covering basic principles of optical mapping and its applications in cardiac electrophysiology.
- Slavik J. Fluorescent probes in cellular and molecular biology. Boca Raton: CRC Press; 1994.
  A good reference to learn more about fluorescent dyes, theory of fluorescence, instrumentation, and cellular applications.

Online References and Links

- http://www.Chroma.com A company that makes optical filters.
- http://www.newport.com A company that makes optics, light sources, and other essential equipment for a variety of optical and experimental applications. The website also is rich with educational references and covers fundamentals for applications.
- http://www.Invitrogen.com A company that sells fluorescent dyes for optical mapping applications. The website also includes educational references and covers fundamentals for applications.
- http://www.redshirtimaging.com A company that sells a complete optical mapping system with necessary hardware and software.
- http://www.scimedia.com A company that also sells a complete optical mapping system with necessary hardware and software.

References

1. Grynkiewicz G, Poenie M, Tsien RY. A new generation of Ca2+ indicators with greatly improved fluorescence properties. J Biolog Chem 1985;260:3440–50.
2. Sipido KR, Callewaert G. How to measure intracellular [Ca2+] in single cardiac cells with fura-2 or indo-1. Cardiovas Res 1995;29:717–26.
3. Brandes R, Figueredo VM, Camacho SA, et al. Investigation of factors affecting fluorometric quantitation of cytosolic [Ca2+] in perfused hearts. Biophys J 1993;65:1983–93.
4. Brandes R, Figueredo VM, Camacho SA, et al. Quantitation of cytosolic [Ca2+] in whole perfused rat hearts using Indo-1 fluorometry. Biophys J 1993;65:1973–82.
5. Girouard SD, Laurita KR, Rosenbaum DS. Unique properties of cardiac action potentials recorded with voltage-sensitive dyes. J Cardiovasc.Electrophysiol 1996;7:1024–38.
6. Wilson B, Jeeves W, Lowe D. In vivo and post mortem measurements of attenuation spectra of light in mammalian tissues. Photochem Photobiol 1985;42:153–62.
7. Choi BR, Salama G. Simultaneous maps of optical action potentials and calcium transients in guinea-pig hearts: mechanisms underlying concordant alternans. J Physiol(Lond) 2000;529:171–88.
8. Johnson PL, Smith W, Baynham TC, et al. Errors caused by combination of di-4 ANEPPS and fluo3/4 for simultaneous measurements of transmembrane potentials and intracellular calcium. Ann Biomed Eng 1999;27:563–71.
9. Katra RP, Laurita KR. Cellular mechanism of calcium-mediated triggered activity in the heart. Circ Res 2005;96:535–42.
10. Katra RP, Pruvot E, Laurita KR. Intracellular calcium handling heterogeneities in intact guinea pig hearts. Am J Physiol Heart Circ Physiol 2004;286:H648–56.

11. Laurita KR, Singal A. Mapping action potentials and calcium transients simultaneously from the intact heart. Am J Physiol 2001;280:H2053–60.
12. DiVirgilio F, Steinberg TH, Silverstein SC. Organic-anion transport inhibitors to facilitate measurement of cytosolic free Ca2+ with Fura-2. Meth Cell Biol 1989;31:453–62.
13. DiVirgilio F, Steinberg TH, Swanson JA, et al. Fura-2 secretion and sequestration in macrophages. A blocker of organic anion transport reveals that these processes occur via a membrane transport system for organic anions. J Immunol 1988;140:915–20.
14. Scheenen WJ, Makings LR, Gross LR, et al. Photodegradation of indo-1 and its effect on apparent Ca^{2+} concentrations. Chem Biol 1996;3:765–74.
15. Brandes R, Figueredo VM, Camacho SA, et al. Suppression of motion artifacts in fluorescence spectroscopy of perfused hearts. Am J Physiol 1992;263:H972–80.

Chapter 16
Electrophysiology of Single Cardiomyocytes: Patch Clamp and Other Recording Methods

Eric S. Richardson and Yong-Fu Xiao

Abstract The main function of the heart is to pump blood to the whole body. To accomplish this task, each individual myocyte in a normal heart needs to be electrically connected and mechanically coordinated with others during a cardiac cycle. The heart is composed of excitable myocytes and nonexcitable cells. The excitable cells are responsible for electrical initiation and conduction to activate the whole heart; they are also responsible for mechanical contraction to pump the blood. Therefore, methods and protocols used for studying cellular electrophysiology of single cardiomyocytes are crucial for understanding physiological functions of a normal heart or pathological mechanisms of a diseased heart. Electrophysiological activity of single cells can be investigated with different techniques either in situ in tissue or in isolated and cultured cells. The classical approach is intracellular recording of electrical activity via inserting a sharp electrode into a cardiomyocyte. However, with the patch clamp technique, scientists have learned more details about molecular structures and functions of ion channels, which are the basis of cardiac electrophysiology. Abnormalities of rhythmic initiation and/or wave conduction along the conductive pathway of a heart can lead to arrhythmias. The methods and techniques used in cellular electrophysiology in recent decades have greatly advanced the knowledge of cardiomyocyte function and arrhythmias at cellular and molecular levels. This chapter describes the patch clamp and other recording methods used for studying cardiac action potentials and ion channels.

16.1 Introduction

Cardiomyocytes can generate action potentials spontaneously. Cardiomyocytes can also be excited by action potentials propagated from adjacent exciting cells or by the stimulation of electrical pulses, chemical compounds, and mechanical stretches.

Y.-F. Xiao (✉)
Cardiac Rhythm Disease Management, Medtronic, Inc., Mounds View, MN, USA
e-mail: yong-fu.xiao@medtronic.com

D.C. Sigg et al. (eds.), *Cardiac Electrophysiology Methods and Models*,
DOI 10.1007/978-1-4419-6658-2_16, © Springer Science+Business Media, LLC 2010

Traditionally, cardiac action potentials can be recorded from the myocardium by inserting a sharp microelectrode into a single cardiomyocyte. This method has several advantages and disadvantages. In the 1970s, Neher and Sakmann invented the patch clamp recording technique for cellular electrophysiology.[1] Since then, this technique has been widely used in academic and industrial laboratories for studying cellular electrophysiology in excitable cells, such as cardiomyocytes, neurons, smooth muscle cells, skeletal muscles, and secretive cells.

16.1.1 Importance of Ion Channel Function in the Heart

The conduction system precisely controls the activation time of each cardiomyocyte to optimize mechanical pumping of the heart. The smooth operation of this system is imperative to the proper functioning of the heart; in settings of damage or disease, electrical chaos can lead to death within minutes. What separates excitable cells in the heart, brain, and elsewhere in the body from nonexcitable cells is the presence of specific ion channels that reside in the cell membrane. The type, population, activation, and/or inhibition of ion channels govern the whole-organ electrophysiology of the heart, as observed in the clinic. Heart rate, pacing and fibrillation thresholds, electrocardiogram (ECG) morphologies, and the presence of arrhythmias are all products of the function (or malfunction) of these ion channels. Many drugs that are prescribed to treat electrophysiological disorders are classified by which ion channels they target.[2] For example, procainamide, commonly used to treat ventricular arrhythmias, is classified as a class I anti-arrhythmic, because it inhibits Na^+ channels.

Almost all of what we have learned about these ion channels and the drugs that affect them are a result of decades of research using the techniques described in this chapter. Patch clamp and other single-cell electrophysiology techniques continue to be used not only to understand cardiac electrophysiology and mechanisms of arrhythmias but also to explore and screen treatments for heart disease.

16.1.2 Understanding Ion Channel Behavior Through Electrical Analogues

Before discussing the methods for studying ion channel behavior, it is helpful to understand the function of ion channels through electrical circuit models. This approach is convenient because we can also better understand the electrical equipment used in single-cell electrophysiology.

A basic knowledge of circuit elements and the physical laws that govern them can help the reader to better understand cellular electrophysiology. The following relationships are very important for a novice in electrophysiology to understand:

Ohm's Law
Voltage (V) = Current (I) × Resistance (R)
Definition of Capacitance
Current = Capacitance × Time Rate of Change of Voltage
Voltage Divider Law
Voltage Drop across Resistor (R1) = Total Voltage × R1/(R1 + R2 + …)

If required, more details of these relationships can be found in a basic physics text.

The simplest model of an ion channel is a resistor, as it offers resistance to the flow of ions across the cell membrane. The resistance of the lipid bilayer membrane itself is extremely large and in parallel with relation to the ion channel resistance; it may, therefore, be ignored. The membrane does play an important role, however, in providing capacitance to the system. This capacitance can be modeled as a capacitor in parallel with the resistance of the ion channels. The transmembrane potential serves as the voltage source of the system. Combining these elements, Figure 16.1 illustrates such a simplified model.

Should the transmembrane potential be changed in a step-wise manner (as in voltage clamping), we can record the resulting current that enters the cell (Fig. 16.2). The transient "spikes" that appear on the corners of the current waveform are due to the capacitive charge of the membrane (left) when the voltage pulse is applied and discharge of the membrane (right) when the pulse is turned off. Therefore, the membrane capacitance of a cell can be measured by the application of a small-step voltage pulse that does not activate any ion channels. The number of membrane capacitance reflects the size of a cell.

In practice, most ion channels of interest are not simply resistive. Rather, they have complex voltage-gating mechanisms, selectivities, and many kinetic properties that have been modeled by extremely complex electrical circuits. The development of these models helps us to understand the behavior of the channels to a greater degree, and the experimental results from techniques described in this chapter help us to develop and refine these models.

As the previous figure indicates, much can be learned about an ion channel if the transmembrane voltage or current can be measured; even more can be learned when either the voltage or current is controlled. This is the opportunity that single-cell

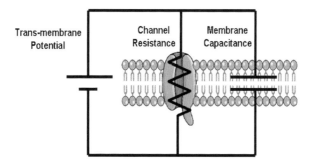

Fig. 16.1 A simplified electric circuit model of an ion channel and cell membrane

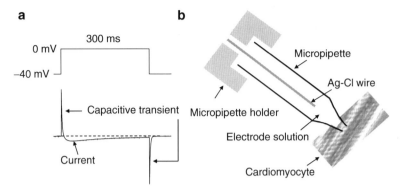

Fig. 16.2 Representative voltage-clamp experiment. (**a**) The whole-cell current trace (below) was elicited from a canine ventricular myocyte when a voltage step from −40 to 0 mV (above) was applied across the membrane. (**b**) Schematic assembly of a microelectrode holder used for patch clamp recording with the area of the cardiomyocyte patched (Cardiomyocyte)

electrophysiology techniques provide. In traditional extracellular recording, an electrode measures the changes in the electric field surrounding an active cell without any invasive disturbances. Intracellular recording allows us to passively measure the transmembrane voltage. With patch clamp methods, scientists can either control the transmembrane voltage and measure the current entering the cell (voltage-clamping), or control the current injected into the cell and measure the transmembrane voltage (current-clamping). In addition, the patch clamp technique allows scientists to control the components and concentrations of intra- and extra-cellular solutions. Under these conditions, a specific type of ion channel and its regulatory system can be carefully studied.

16.1.3 Terminology

Common terms are often used in cellular electrophysiology, and several of them are listed here:

Transmembrane potential: The potential difference caused by charged particles in the intra- and extra-cellular compartments. The extracellular side is often considered as ground potential (0 mV). The resting membrane potential of a human ventricular myocyte is around −90 mV.

Action potential: A time-elapsed change in membrane electrical potential due to channel activation and inactivation and flow of ions across the membrane.

Channel conductance: The ability of a channel to pass ion current.

Selectivity: The specificity of a channel preferably allows a certain type of ions through it. Selectivity is usually quantified experimentally as the ratio of the permeability of pairs of ions.

Gating: Conformational changes in an ion channel to open or close it in response to membrane voltage changes or to ligand stimulation.

Activation: Opening of a channel induced by a gating signal.

Deactivation: Closing of a channel after removing the gating signal.

Inactivation: Closing of a channel in the continued presence of the gating signal.

Tail current: A current that flows during the repolarizing phase of an action potential or voltage command.

Other terms used in cellular electrophysiology can be found in other textbooks and papers.[3–7]

16.2   Apparatus for Single-Cell Recordings

16.2.1   Microelectrodes

The ability to probe the electrical activity of a cell requires placement of an electrode near, on, or inside a cell that may only be a few microns wide or less. The function of a microelectrode is to transduce ion movement in an aqueous medium to electron movement in a wire. This is typically done by using a wire surrounded by an electrolyte solution and enclosed in a glass microelectrode, which is pulled by a micropipette puller (Fig. 16.3a). The micropipette allows only conduction to the interior solution

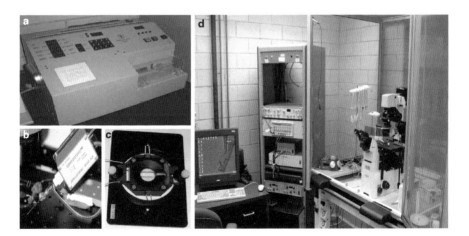

Fig. 16.3 A setup of apparatuses for cellular electrophysiology. (**a**) DMZ Universal Puller for fabricating micropipettes for intracellular or patch clamp recordings. (**b**) An assembled electrode holder and headstage. (**c**) Perfusion chamber used for patch clamp experiments. (**d**) A complete electrophysiology setup with the amplifier and acquisition system on the left, and the vibration isolation table, micromanipulator, faraday cage, perfusion bath, and microscope on the right

through a small opening at the tip (Fig. 16.2b and Fig. 16.3b). The conductive solution then transfers the electrical signal to the wire via an electro-chemical reaction.

Micropipette fabrication is often a tedious and iterative process. Micropipette pullers have made this process reproducible and much easier than when it was done by hand. Micropipette pullers heat and pull small glass tubes until they neck in the middle and eventually pull apart, producing two identical micropipettes at once. The force of the pull, the speed of the pull, and the intensity of the heat produce pipette tips of all varieties. Most pullers have the ability to store these parameters into a program that can be recalled when needed (Fig. 16.3a). Complex programs can include heat ramps, multistage pulls, and even small bursts of air on the newly formed tip to cool the glass. The composition and thickness of the glass wall, bevel angle, length of tip, and diameter of opening are all important characteristics of the finished micropipette, and puller parameters must be adjusted to satisfy the needs of each application.

The solution that couples the tip of the micropipette to the wire is a salt solution that varies in composition depending on the application. For traditional intracellular recording of cardiac action potentials, high concentrations of KCl (typically 2–4 M) are commonly used because there is little leakage of ions out of the tip and into the cytoplasm of the cell due to the much smaller tip. For patch clamp experiments, solutions that are more similar to the cytoplasm of the cell are used and can be modified according to the purpose of an experiment because there is more transfer of fluid through the tip. After a micropipette is pulled, it is filled with the aqueous solution using a long, flexible needle. It is important to ensure that no air bubbles are trapped in the micropipette, especially in the tip area, as this can interfere with the function of the microelectrode or affect patching.

The wire inside the micropipette is typically silver, with a silver chloride coating. This wire can be prepared by using fine sand paper to abrade the surface of clean silver wire, and then immersing the abraded and battery-connected (9 V) silver wire in a low HCl (0.01 N) solution for 1–2 min. The wire should then be rinsed with deionized water before placing it into the micropipette. The coating procedure may be repeated if the black silver chloride coating is scratched off after repeated insertions into micropipettes. The wire is typically mounted on a micropipette holder. The filled micropipette is placed over the wire and fastened to the holder. The assembly is then ready to be secured to the headstage for electrical recordings (Fig. 16.3b).

16.2.2   Headstage, Amplifier, and Data Acquisition System

The purpose of the headstage is to provide a high impedance input immediately next to the microelectrode (Fig. 16.3b). This protects the very small signal from noise as it travels through a shielded cable to the amplifier, which is typically a few feet away. Headstages and amplifiers typically are sold together and are available commercially through many companies (i.e., Axon Instruments from Molecular Devices, Sunnyvale, CA, USA or Dagan Corporation, Minneapolis, MN, USA). The type of headstage and amplifier is determined by the application. A simple bridge amplifier may be used for intracellular recording, but a more complex amplifier with current and voltage feedback mechanisms is needed for patch clamp experiments.[6] Further details about the amplifiers will be given in following sections; Figure 16.3d shows a complete patch clamp setup.

The role of an amplifier is to both amplify and condition the signal received from the headstage. Voltages measured from cells are typically in the millivolt to microvolt range, and in order to maximize the resolution of standard data acquisition systems, commercial amplifiers usually have gains from 0.1× to 100×. High-pass, low-pass, and notch filters may be employed to condition the signal. These filters may be adjustable, or they may be hardwired into the amplifier. Frequency responses of the filters must be taken into consideration when adjusting filter parameters. AC-coupling is almost always used in signal conditioning to prevent saturation of the downstream data acquisition system.

Additional features, such as blanking capabilities or audio monitors can also be incorporated into the amplifier. Blanking refers to the ability of the amplifier to ignore its input when given a logic-level pulse. During the pulse, the amplifier retains the output value just before the pulse. At the end of the pulse, the amplifier resumes function immediately. This feature is helpful in instances when a high voltage stimulus is used to evoke an electrophysiologic response. During the stimulus, the amplifier may easily saturate and take several milliseconds to recover, losing valuable data from the evoked response during the recovery period. If a blanking system is appropriately configured, a logic-level pulse is sent to the amplifier for the duration of the stimulus, avoiding the saturation and resuming recording as soon as the stimulus is complete. Audio monitoring converts the voltage or current measured at the electrode to an audible pitch. This provides real-time feedback to an investigator who is guiding a microelectrode under microscope guidance, preventing multiple glances back at the display on the amplifier.

Data acquisitions systems, commercially available for use with standard personal computers, convert the amplified, conditioned signal from the amplifier into a digital signal, which can be stored, manipulated, and analyzed by the investigator. The incoming analogue signal should be amplified to maximize the full range of the acquisition system (e.g., −15 to 15 V). Care should be taken, however, that the signal does not saturate the acquisition system. Many amplifiers and acquisition systems have overload detection circuitry that informs the user when the input is beyond an acceptable range.

Choosing an appropriate sampling rate is important to prevent aliasing. While the Nyquist theorem dictates that investigators choose a sampling rate at least twice the fastest component of the signal, a more practical guideline is to choose a rate 2.5 times the cutoff frequency of the highest low-pass filter (typically called an anti-aliasing filter). For electrophysiology systems, this rate can be as high as 25–250 kHz. After the signal has been acquired, various digital filters are available to further condition the signal. With the growing data storage capacities and higher maximum sampling rates that modern technology presents, it is easy to oversample to ensure that the signal is properly recorded. However, needless recording at extremely high sampling rates can lead to large data files that are hard to transfer and make post-process analysis difficult.[6]

Most data can be analyzed with commercially available software designed for electrophysiology applications (e.g., pCLAMP, Molecular Devices). For those who would like more flexibility and the ability to apply various digital filters, technical computing programs such as MATLAB (The Mathworks, Inc., Natick, MA, USA) have powerful signal processing capabilities.

16.2.3   Cell and Tissue Baths

For excitable cells and tissues to be studied, they must be kept in a physiologic environment to maintain their electrophysiological function during an experiment; this requires the use of a bath mounted on the stage of a microscope. The microscope is used for visualization and placement of the microelectrode in or near cells. Many patch clamp protocols call for single disassociated cells or cultured cells with a low density, usually attached to a coated glass cover slip. The cover slips can be taken directly from the incubator in which they were maintained and placed in a small bath (Fig. 16.3c) mounted on the microscope stage (Fig. 16.3d). Baths typically have an inflow port on one end, a glass-bottom well in the center, and an outflow on the other end. The inflow is attached to a reservoir of media that has a mechanically- or electrically controlled flow meter. In applications such as pharmacology studies, there may be several reservoirs with different media compositions and a system of valves so that the investigator can quickly switch the media in the bath. The outflow of the bath can be a passive wick that transfers excess fluid to a lower drainage container, or an active suction tube that removes liquid as it reaches a certain level. As many electrophysiology processes change dramatically with temperature, high-end baths often have integrated heating elements that warm the bath to a desired temperature.

The complexity of a bath increases slightly when using tissue. Although single cells have little problem extracting the oxygen they need from the surrounding medium, cells within tissue rely on the diffusion of oxygen from the surface of the tissue. To prevent hypoxia, therefore, the medium must be saturated with oxygen before entering the bath. This may be done in an adjacent reservoir where fluid is bubbled with oxygen using a sparger, and then continues on to the bath. Oxygenation of the bath solution may become particularly important for cardiac tissue because of its high metabolic rate and extreme sensitivity to hypoxia. Therefore, using small and thin tissue samples can reduce ischemic damage. Also, care must be taken that bubbling does not alter the pH of the medium. It is common to use a mixed gas of 95% oxygen and 5% carbon dioxide to maintain the solution pH unchanged after bubbling.

16.2.4   Microscope, Micromanipulator, and Vibration Isolation Table

Inverted microscopes are commonly used for patch clamp experiments, as space is needed above the bath to introduce the microelectrode. The microscope should be equipped with multiple lenses with various magnifications, and may have contrast enhancement. Electrophysiology microscopes will usually have fluorescence capabilities because cells of interest are often fluorescently labeled. In some extracellular and intracellular applications/recordings where tissue is used, upright dissection microscopes can be used, as high resolution is not necessary. Placement of the microelectrode near, on, or inside a micron-sized cell is perhaps the most challenging aspect of single-cell electrophysiology. A micromanipulator allows the investigator to move a microelectrode with sub-micron precision under the microscope. Micromanipulators can be mechanical, pneumatic, hydraulic, or servo-controlled. Most have three degrees of translation with both coarse and fine controls, and a mounting surface for the headstage.

Without a buffering system, small vibrations, even those of a person walking nearby, can lose a sealed patch. Therefore, vibration isolation is necessary and is usually achieved by setting up the microscope, bath, and micromanipulator on a very heavy slab of metal or stone. The slab is then supported by a mechanism that dampens vibrations; this can be as simple as the inner tube of a bicycle. Commercially available vibration isolation tables use pneumatic cylinders to achieve the same result. Additional vibrations can be avoided by mounting the micromanipulator as close to the bath as possible.

The location of the apparatus is important to minimize the ambient mechanical and electrical noise. Electrophysiologists often find that the basement or lower levels of tall buildings have less mechanical vibration than higher levels. Large equipment, such as heating and cooling systems, refrigerators, and elevators not only produce mechanical vibrations, but usually emit a large amount of electrical noise as well. Faraday cages can be used to limit the amount of electrical noise picked up by the microelectrode.

16.3 Recording Modes

Methodologies will vary greatly depending on the application and purpose of a study. The following are general guidelines for the major techniques in cardiac cellular electrophysiology. The investigator is encouraged to search the scientific literature for further details relating to their specific application.

16.3.1 Extracellular Recording

During extracellular recording, the microelectrode is placed in close proximity to one or more cells and measures the changes in the electrical field (or field potential) near the cell. This technique can provide valuable information without invasively disturbing the cell membrane. It can be used in both tissue and disassociated cell preparations. In this technique, a sharp microelectrode is advanced into the preparation until electrophysiological activity is detected. The microelectrode can be a liquid-filled glass micropipette like those described previously, or it can be made of metal with insulation up to the tip. Size of the electrode will vary with the application, specifically if the intention is to measure the field potential from a single cell compared to multiple cells.

Electrical signals measured by extracellular recording are very small compared to those measured in other techniques; they are typically less than 1 mV. In addition, the amplifier is typically AC-coupled so that only dynamic changes in the electrical field at the microelectrode are recorded. Such conditions make blanking features important when using an external stimulus. External stimuli are provided either by needle electrodes inserted into the tissue, or by paddle electrodes placed on either side of the preparations. Stimulus parameters should be tuned so that only the minimum duration, current, and voltage are used to evoke a response. This will prevent a large stimulus artifact. Typical stimulus parameters are 1–2 ms duration at 1–10 V. The parameters will vary with electrode surface area, composition, and placement. Hydrolysis, or bubbling on the surface of the stimulus electrodes due to molecular separation of water, is a sure sign that stimulus parameters are too high.

Arrays of extracellular electrodes can be patterned on the bottom of a culture dish using photolithography. The multielectrode array technique provides an investigator the ability to record electrical activity temporally and spatially from cardiac tissue slices or cultured cardiomyocytes. This technique is discussed further in Chapter 20: Multi-channel System for Analysis of Cardiac Rhythmicity and Conductivity *In Vitro*.

16.3.2 *Intracellular Recording*

To measure electrical activity within the cell, two types of microelectrodes can be used: sharp microelectrodes and patch electrodes. Sharp microelectrodes were the first to be developed and consist of a fluid-filled micropipette with the tip pulled to an opening less than one micron in diameter. They are typically filled with a high-molarity salt solution, such as 3 M KCl. The resistance of these electrodes is usually around 10 MΩ. These "sharp" electrodes are thus called because they can simply penetrate the cell membrane without significant damage to cell function and the membrane quickly seals itself around the microelectrode. Therefore, a transmembrane potential is measured around −90 mV for a ventricular myocyte and −70 mV for an atrial myocyte when the sharp electrode moves into a myocyte with a micromanipulator.

In the late 1970s, patch microelectrodes came into use.[1,4] Patch microelectrodes are pulled to have an opening usually greater than one micron. The pulls are performed in multiple stages, with a final heat polishing of the tip to remove ragged edges. The microelectrodes are filled with a solution that is similar to the extracellular or intracellular fluid of the cell because there is a considerable exchange of contents with the "patched" cell. These microelectrodes are not designed to penetrate into the cell, but are positioned such that they just touch

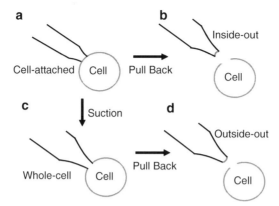

Fig. 16.4 Various patch clamp configurations frequently used in cellular electrophysiology. After forming a gigaohm seal and cell-attached configuration (**a**), additional suction or pull can create different configurations that can be used for single-channel (inside-out, **b**; outside-out, **d**) or whole-cell (**c**) recordings. The cell-attached configuration can also be used for single-channel recordings

the membrane. With small negative suction, these electrodes form a very tight seal with the membrane, often called a "giga-seal" because the seal resistance is typically several gigaohms.

Once the patch microelectrode is sealed to the membrane, the investigator can choose one of the several patch configurations (Fig. 16.4). The microelectrode can remain sealed to the intact membrane in the *cell-attached* configuration (Fig. 16.4a). If further suction is applied to the sealed microelectrode, the patch of membrane beneath the microelectrode will rupture, making the interior of the cell continuous with the interior of the microelectrode. This configuration is called the *whole-cell* patch (Fig. 16.4c). If one simply pulls the microelectrode away from a cell in the whole-cell configuration, a patch of membrane will separate from the cell and reform on the tip with the extracellular surface of the membrane facing away from the microelectrode. This is called the *outside-out* configuration (Fig. 16.4d). Finally, if a sealed microelectrode is pulled away from an intact membrane after forming cell-attached mode, a patch of membrane will form on the tip of the microelectrode with the extracellular surface towards the interior of the microelectrode and intracellular side facing the bath solution. This is called the *inside-out* patch (Fig. 16.4b). Figure 16.5 illustrates the changes of the currents during the operational process to form the whole-cell recording configuration.

16.3.3   Current Clamp

When using the current clamp, voltage is measured while the current passing through the microelectrode is controlled. Zero current clamp is often used for

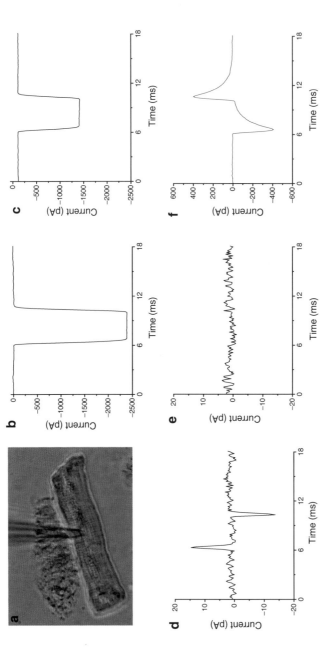

Fig. 16.5 A typical process for forming the whole-cell configuration. (**a**) One glass electrode and a human ventricular myocyte were selected for patch clamp recording. (**b**) The glass electrode was loaded with an internal solution and connected via an Ag-AgCl wire to an Axopatch 200A amplifier interfaced with a DigiData-1320 acquisition system (Axon Instruments). After the electrode was immersed in the bath solution, a current trace was evoked by a 5 mV pulse from 0 mV holding potential to −5 mV. Therefore, the resistance of the electrode was 2.08 MΩ. (**c**) When the electrode was touched and pushed to the cell membrane, the current amplitude was markedly decreased due to the increase in resistance (partially blocked the electrode tip). (**d**) A gigaohm seal was formed after a gentle suction of the electrode. (**e**) The electrode capacitance was compensated. (**f**) Additional burst suction ruptured the patched membrane and formed the whole-cell configuration. Cell membrane capacitance (C_m) could be measured with the pCLAMP program (version 9.2, Axon Instruments). After C_m measurement, the membrane capacitance and series resistance could be compensated and whole-cell currents or membrane potentials could be recorded

recording the resting membrane potential and spontaneous action potentials after inserting a sharp microelectrode into a myocyte or after forming the whole-cell configuration.[8] Also, a controllable current source can be connected to the electrode to simultaneously inject current into the cell and record voltage changes. In cardiac myocytes, intracellular injection of a negative current causes hyperpolarization of the resting membrane potential. On the contrary, intracellular injection of a positive current can depolarize the myocyte and induce an action potential.[8] Because of the injected current, compensation in the form of a *bridge* circuit (also know as a "voltage-follower") must be used to prevent distortion of the signal. Such circuitry requires a bridge balance to be performed with each new microelectrode. Instructions to perform the bridge balance are usually found in the amplifier's manual.

16.3.4 Voltage Clamp

The voltage clamp technique, which is one of the most commonly used techniques in electrophysiology, serves to measure the current passing through the microelectrode while a voltage pulse is applied. This technique is popular because most of the ion channels in excitable cells, including cardiomyocytes, are voltage-gated. There are several approaches to voltage clamping, the oldest of which uses two sharp electrodes placed into the same cell. In this approach, called *two-electrode voltage clamping*, one electrode serves as the recording electrode while the other injects current into the cell. A two-electrode voltage clamping amplifier has feedback circuitry that allows it to read the voltage from the recording electrode and then inject current into the cell to bring it to the user-defined voltage (or command voltage). The output of the amplifier is the real-time amount of current (represented as a voltage signal) needed to maintain a cell at a certain command voltage. Two-electrode voltage clamping is often used in recording electrical activities in oocytes after channel expression.

Because of the difficulty of penetrating small cells and large leakage currents with the two microelectrode methods, *single-electrode voltage clamp* was developed. In this approach, a patch electrode in one of the patch configurations described previously (Fig. 16.4) is used to control the membrane voltage and record the current passing through the membrane. This can either be done in a continuous fashion (continuous single-electrode voltage clamp) or in a discontinuous fashion (discontinuous single-electrode voltage clamp) where the electrode rapidly switches between only measuring voltage and only measuring current. To monitor the dynamic movements of ions in and out of the cell membrane during a cardiac cycle, a cardiomyocyte can be clamped by an action potential clamp protocol (voltage clamp). In addition, a single type of ion channels, such as the voltage-activated cardiac Na^+ or Ca^{2+} channel, can be investigated with different voltage clamp protocols.[9,10] More details about ion channel activation and recording can be found from other scientific papers and textbooks.[3–5]

16.4   Examples of Experimental Protocols

Single-cell cardiac electrophysiology is a very broad field with many tools and applications. Literature is the best resource for protocols to achieve a certain research goal. This section presents two representative protocols. The first is a standard intracellular recording protocol for measuring action potentials in human cardiac tissue, and the second is a more complex voltage clamp protocol for measuring human hyperpolarization-activated, cyclic-nucleotide-gated (hHCN) currents.

16.4.1   Protocol for Intracellular Recording of Human Cardiac Action Potentials

Antiarrhythmic medications are commonly prescribed for heart rhythm disorders. Most of these medications are classified by how they affect the morphology of the cardiac action potential. This protocol describes how human tissue samples can be used to gather this information using standard intracellular recording techniques, and is defined by the following steps:

1. Waste human cardiac tissue (usually right atrial appendage from a cardio-pulmonary bypass operation) is obtained from the operating room and immediately placed in a Tyrode's solution saturated with oxygen.
2. The tissue is pinned out on the bottom of a tissue bath to expose the endocardial surface. The tissue is constantly superperfused at 2 ml/min with Tyrode's solution supplemented with glucose and saturated with a mix of 5% carbon dioxide and 95% oxygen. The tissue bath is maintained at 37°C.
3. A sharp electrode (~10 MΩ) filled with 2 M KCl and connected to a headstage is advanced into the bath under the guidance of a dissection microscope. When the tip of the microelectrode is submersed in the bath, the DC offset is set to 0 mV.
4. The microelectrode is advanced very slowly into the tissue until the voltage sensed at the tip drops close to the membrane resting potential.
5. Plunge electrodes previously placed in the tissue then stimulate the preparation with a 2-ms square wave at 20 V and 1 Hz using a stimulator. The motion of contraction may cause the electrode tip to come out of the cell, a situation that can be prevented by overstretching the cardiac tissue when it is originally pinned out in the bath.
6. Action potentials measured by the microelectrode and amplifier are acquired by a data acquisition card and LABVIEW program that samples at a rate range from 10 to 25 kHz. Figure 16.6 shows a representative action potential obtained from a human cardiac myocyte using an intracellular recording protocol.
7. After baseline data have been recorded, pharmacologic agents may be added to the superperfusate to observe changes in action potential morphology. The preparation can be viable for several hours.

Fig. 16.6 Cardiac action potential recorded from a human cardiomyocyte. A sharp microelectrode loaded with 2 M KCl was used for the classical intracellular recording. The *y*-axis displays mV (~10 mV/unit) and the *x*-axis displays time (20 ms/unit). The initial spike of the upstroke is an artifact caused by the electrical stimulation

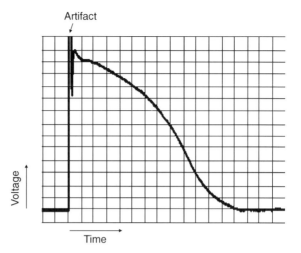

16.4.2   Protocol for Patch Clamp Recording of I_h in hHCN4-Transfected HEK293 Cells

An inward, nonselective cation current (I_f) through hyperpolarization-activated, cyclic-nucleotide-gated (HCN) channels plays a critical role in the generation of rhythmic action potentials in the sinoatrial node of the heart.[11,12] Four molecular isoforms (HCN1–4) of HCN channels have been identified in mammalian hearts,[13] but HCN4 is the dominant one in the human sinoatrial node.[14,15] The importance of HCNs in pacemaking stems from the association of HCN4 mutations and bradycardia in patients[16] and also from HCN transgenic mouse models.[17] We used HCN4-transfected human embryonic kidney (HEK293) cells (American Type Culture Collection, Manassas, VA, USA) for the assessment of human HCN4 current kinetics. Details of the protocol are described in the following steps:

1. Culture of HEK293 cells

   - Thaw frozen HEK293 cell aliquots quickly in 37°C water bath.
   - Dilute to 10 ml total volume in HEK293 culture medium and spin at 1,500 rpm for 4 min to pellet cells.
   - Remove supernatant and resuspend in 10 ml of fresh media.
   - Plate cells to 100 mm, 6-well, or 12-well culture dishes or 25-mm culture flasks.
   - Change medium every other day.
   - When cells reach 100% confluence or when needed for experiments, add 3–5 ml of 0.25% trypsin-EDTA and wait for 3–5 min to dissociate cells. Collect dissociated cells and add 10 ml medium to spin at 1,500 rpm for 4 min to pellet cells.
   - Cells can be replated at 1:5 or 1:7 subcultivation ratio, or store in liquid nitrogen for later use.

2. HCN4 transfer of HEK293 cells

- Generally, cells should be replated 24 h prior to transfection. Human HCN4 plasmid or adenovirus hHCN4construct is added to the HEK293 cells when the culture reaches a confluency of 40–60%.
- For hHCN4 plasmid transfection in 35 mm plate or 1 well of 6-well plate, add 6 μl of Fugene to 200 μl plain media (without serum or antibiotics) and allow to equilibrate for 5 min. Thaw plasmid DNA 2 μg to the Fugene/media mixed solution. Flick tube to mix and leave the tube for 15–30 min at room temperature. Add entire mixture to well/plate. Change media after 24 h exposure to plasmid.
- For Adv-HCN4 gene transfer in 35 mm plate or 1 well of 6-well plate, remove the media from the HEK293 cells and replace with 5×10^{10} PFU Adv-hHCN4 in 1 ml medium with low (0–2%) serum. Add 1 ml medium with 10% serum after 3 h. Change the media after 48 h exposure to virus.

3. Preparation for patch clamp

- Trypsinize and spin hHCN4-transferred cells as described above.
- Remove supernatant and plate cells at 1:20 to 1:25 dilution (or approximately 10,000 cells/cm^2) on 2–3 gelatin/laminin coated round cover slips placed in a 35-mm culture dish.
- Culture for another 24–48 h. The cells on the cover slips are ready for patch clamp experiments (Fig. 16.7).

4. Patch clamp recording of hHCN4 currents

- The electrode solution contains: 130 mM κ-glutamate; 15 mM KCl; 5 mM NaCl; 5 mM MgATP; 1 mM $MgCl_2$; 5 mM EGTA; 1 mM $CaCl_2$; 10 mM Hepes (pH adjusted to 7.2 with KOH). The bath solution contains: 140 mM NaCl; 25 mM KCl; 1.8 mM $CaCl_2$; 1 mM $MgCl_2$; 5 mM D-glucose; 10 mM Hepes (pH adjusted to 7.4 with NaOH).
- The whole-cell configuration is applied to obtain hHCN4 currents.[18] Briefly, glass electrodes (World Precision Instruments, Sarasota, FL, USA) with ~2 MΩ resistance are connected via an Ag-AgCl wire to an Axopatch 200A amplifier interfaced with a DigiData-1322 acquisition system (Fig. 16.3d). Green fluorescent protein positive cells are selected for patch clamps (Fig. 16.7). Data are sampled at 5 kHz and filtered at 2 kHz with the pCLAMP software (version 9.2). Experiments are conducted at room temperature (~22°C).
- The hHCN4 current (I_h) is activated by experimental voltage protocols similar to those in a previous study.[18] Specifically, I_h is elicited by 5–12 s test pulses from −140 to 0 mV in 10 mV increments every 30 s. The amplitudes of hHCN4 current at the end of the testing pulses are measured and plotted to obtain the current-voltage curves (Fig. 16.7). Other kinetics of hHCN4 can also be analyzed.[19,20]

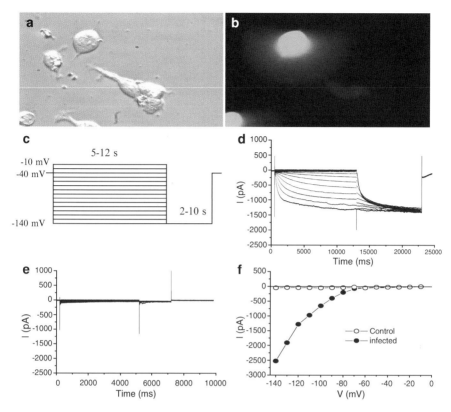

Fig. 16.7 Hyperpolarization-activated currents recorded from cultured HEK293 cells transferred with hHCN4 gene. HEK293 cells growing on a gelatin/laminin-coded cover slip were photographed under phase-contrast (**a**) and fluorescence (**b**) microscope. The green cells were hHCN4-infected cells after transferring with the hHCN4-eGFP (enhanced green fluorescent protein) gene construct. (**c**) The patch clamp protocol was used to elicit hHCN4 currents. (**d**) The superimposed current traces were elicited by the voltage pulse protocol (**c**) in a hHCN4-positive HEK293 cell. (**e**) No hHCN4 currents were elicited by the voltage pulse protocol (**c**) in a hHCN4-negative HEK293 cell. (**f**) Current-voltage relationships were plotted from the hHCN4 currents recorded from the control cell (*open circle*, Control) and hHCN4-transferred cell (*closed circle* Infected)

16.5   Pitfalls and Troubleshooting

Any investigators assembling an electrophysiology apparatus will inevitably have their patience tested. It is not uncommon to spend many hours chasing sources of noise, or managing to pull a desired microelectrode. Below are just some of the many common pitfalls that are likely to occur.

16.5.1   Tissue and Cell Viability

Good viability of myocardial tissue or isolated cardiomyocytes is a key factor for obtaining high quality results. As cardiac tissue and cells, in particular, are vulnerable to hypoxia and mechanical disruptions, an investigator needs to take extra precautions to handle the specimen. Myocardial tissue should be cared for properly before and during an experiment. Isolation and culture of cardiomyocytes need a great deal of practical experience and caution. More details on how to obtain high yield and high quality isolated single cardiomyocytes and how to culture them are described in Chapter 10: Cell Culture Models and Methods.

16.5.2   Microelectrodes

The shape of an electrode and the size and edge of the tip are crucial for successful high quality recording of action potentials or ion currents. Therefore, taking additional effort to work out how to get the desired electrodes may save considerable time during your late experiments and also increase your success rate. A microelectrode with inadequate size or a broken tip will prevent an investigator from properly penetrating or patching a cell. Check the electrode impedance to be sure that it is within an acceptable range. Most amplifiers with their software allow testing of the resistance of the microelectrode while it is submersed in the bath. Also, a small voltage-step (5 mV) protocol with zero holding potential can be continuously applied to measure the size of an electrode when its tip is in the bath solution (Fig. 16.5).

16.5.3   Electrical Noise

Noise is an extremely common problem in electrophysiology. If the noise is high, the first thing is to check whether the setup is grounded properly and whether the ground wire is coded and immersed in the bath solution. As mentioned before, a properly grounded faraday cage, an air floating table, and a properly positioned apparatus (setup away from large machinery) can lower the risk of noise. If these do not solve the noise problem, ground the microscope, micromanipulator, and any other equipment within the faraday cage using clips. Shielding the bath with aluminum foil may also prevent noisy measurements. In addition, cleaning the surface of microscope platform and solution chamber with alcohol and deionized water from time-to-time may reduce noise level because, during experiments, drops of the bath solution may be left behind in those areas and dry out; the salts can act as an antenna to cause noise. Sometimes, a solution drainage line can bring in noise to the recording system; grounding a suction system can thus significantly reduce the noise level. For good advice in troubleshooting such problems, the investigator is referred to Chap. 11 in the Axon Guide.[6]

16.6   Emerging Technologies for Cellular Electrophysiology

The techniques described in this chapter can provide valuable information not only about cellular electrophysiology but also about drug effects. Screening drugs is an important part of the pharmaceutical industry, and due to the long and tedious nature of conventional patch clamp techniques, automated patch clamp systems have been developed. Companies that sell automated systems include Molecular Devices, Nanion Technologies (Munich, Germany), Sophion Bioscience (North Brunswick, NJ, USA), and Flyion (Tübingen, Germany). These systems use complex microfluidic devices with suction capabilities to capture cells, seal onto the membrane, and form different patch configurations. Some systems are capable of patching 16 cells or more at the same time. These machines are costly, but they save greatly on the time that it takes to screen large libraries of potential pharmaceutical compounds.

In recent years, a novel technique for the high-resolution localization of single ion channels on a living cell surface has been developed and applied in patch clamp studies.[21,22] Compared with the conventional methods, this scanning patch clamp technique greatly facilitates single-channel recording from small cells or from submicron cellular structures. This technique combines scanning ion conductance microscopy and patch clamp recording to obtain a high-resolution topographic image via a single glass nanopipette probe, which also serves for patch clamp recording. This technique can be applied to various cell types, such as epithelial cells and neurons. Therefore, while the basic techniques and concepts of patch clamp have not changed much over the last two decades, technology is enhancing its reach by streamlining the process.

References

1. Neher E, Sakmann B. Single-channel currents recorded from membrane of denervated frog muscle fibres. Nature 1976; 260:799–802.
2. Gussak I, Antzelevitch C, Bjerregaard P, et al. The Brugada syndrome: clinical, electrophysiologic and genetic aspects. J Am Coll Cardiol 1999; 33:5–15.
3. Hille B. Ionic Channels of Excitable Membranes, third edition. Sunderland, MA: Sinauer Associates Inc., 2001.
4. Hamill OP, Marty A, Neher E, et al. Improved patch clamp techniques for high-resolution current recording from cells and cell-free membrane patches. Pflugers Arch 1981; 391:85–100.
5. Molnar P, Hickman JJ. Patch Clamp Methods and Protocols. Totowa, NJ: Human Press, 2007.
6. Sherman-Gold R. The Axon Guide for Electrophysiology & Biophysics Laboratory Techniques. Foster City, CA: Axon Instruments, 1993.
7. Walke MJA, Pugsley MK. Methods in Cardiac Electrophysiology. Boston, MA: CRC Press, 1997.
8. Kang JX, Xiao YF, Leaf A. Free, long-chain, polyunsaturated fatty acids reduce membrane electrical excitability in neonatal rat cardiac myocytes. Proc Natl Acad Sci USA 1995; 92:3997–4001.
9. Xiao YF, Kang JX, Morgan JP, et al. Blocking effects of polyunsaturated fatty acids on Na+ channels of neonatal rat ventricular myocytes. Proc Natl Acad Sci USA 1995; 92:11000–4.
10. Xiao YF, Gomez AM, Morgan JP, et al. Suppression of voltage-gated L-type Ca2+ currents by polyunsaturated fatty acids in adult and neonatal rat ventricular myocytes. Proc Natl Acad Sci USA 1997; 94:4182–7.

11. Baruscotti M, Bucchi A, Difrancesco D. Physiology and pharmacology of the cardiac pacemaker ("funny") current. Pharmacol Ther 2005; 107:59–79.

12. Brown H, Difrancesco D. Voltage-clamp investigations of membrane currents underlying pace-maker activity in rabbit sino-atrial node. J Physiol 1980; 308:331–51.

13. Stieber J, Hofmann F, Ludwig A. Pacemaker channels and sinus node arrhythmia. Trends Cardiovasc Med 2004; 14:23–8.

14. Dobrzynski H, Boyett MR, Anderson RH. New insights into pacemaker activity: promoting understanding of sick sinus syndrome. Circulation 2007; 115:1921–32.

15. Thollon C, Bedut S, Villeneuve N, et al. Use-dependent inhibition of hHCN4 by ivabradine and relationship with reduction in pacemaker activity. Br J Pharmacol 2007; 150:37–46.

16. Milanesi R, Baruscotti M, Gnecchi-Ruscone T, et al. Familial sinus bradycardia associated with a mutation in the cardiac pacemaker channel. N Engl J Med 2006; 354:151–7.

17. Stieber J, Herrmann S, Feil S, et al. The hyperpolarization-activated channel HCN4 is required for the generation of pacemaker action potentials in the embryonic heart. Proc Natl Acad Sci USA 2003; 100:15235–40.

18. Xiao YF, TenBroek EM, Wilhelm JJ, et al. Electrophysiological characterization of murine HL-5 atrial cardiomyocytes. Am J Physiol Cell Physiol 2006; 291:C407–16.

19. Azene EM, Xue T, Marban E, et al. Non-equilibrium behavior of HCN channels: insights into the role of HCN channels in native and engineered pacemakers. Cardiovasc Res 2005; 67:263–73.

20. Ludwig A, Zong X, Stieber J, et al. Two pacemaker channels from human heart with profoundly different activation kinetics. Embo J 1999; 18:2323–9.

21. Gu Y, Gorelik J, Spohr HA, et al. High-resolution scanning patch clamp: new insights into cell function. Faseb J 2002; 16:748–50.

22. Gorelik J, Gu Y, Spohr HA, et al. Ion channels in small cells and subcellular structures can be studied with a smart patch clamp system. Biophys J 2002; 83:3296–303.

Chapter 17
Invasive Electroanatomical Mapping and Navigation

Moussa Mansour and David Donaldson

Abstract An overview of electroanatomical mapping is described, including its history and current application in treating patients with atrial and ventricular arrhythmias. Using a roving catheter in 3D space relative to a fixed reference, electroanatomical mapping provides the electrophysiologist with important location and electrical data to carefully guide catheter ablation procedures. Both magnetic-based mapping and impedance-based mapping are briefly discussed.

17.1 Introduction

Catheter ablation has become one of the primary treatments for symptomatic drug-refractory cardiac arrhythmias. Initially, this procedure was performed under the guidance of X-ray fluoroscopy. This imaging modality however has significant limitations, most notably its inability to provide 3D views. In addition, X-ray fluoroscopy does not allow visualization of cardiac structures. Electroanatomical mapping was introduced in the mid 1990s and represented a major breakthrough in the way catheter ablations are performed. It allows the tracking of a roving catheter in 3D space relative to a fixed reference. By moving the roving catheter in the cardiac chamber of interest, data points that represent both location and electrical activity are collected. The integrated information is displayed in easily readable 3D maps. More recent advances, including image integration, allowed the visualization of cardiac structures such as the pulmonary veins and great cardiac vessels during the procedures. By allowing the display of electrical data in relation to anatomical data and by tagging ablation lesions and other areas of interest, these advances significantly facilitated catheter ablation. In this chapter, we present an overview of electroanatomical mapping and its applications in the treatment of various cardiac arrhythmias.

M. Mansour (✉)
Heart Center, Massachusetts, General Hospital, Boston, MA, USA
e-mail: mmansour@partners.org

D.C. Sigg et al. (eds.), *Cardiac Electrophysiology Methods and Models*,
DOI 10.1007/978-1-4419-6658-2_17, © Springer Science+Business Media, LLC 2010

17.2   The Use of Electroanatomical Mapping for the Treatment of Atrial Arrhythmias

Electroanatomical mapping is used extensively in the treatment of atrial arrhythmias, including atrial tachycardia, atrial flutter, and atrial fibrillation.

17.2.1   Atrial Tachycardia

Atrial tachycardia consists of an automatic focus or a micro-reentry circuit, located in the right atrium, left atrium, or the proximal portion of the thoracic vessels, including the pulmonary veins, the superior vena cava, the inferior vena cava, and the non-coronary cusp of the aorta. The ablation catheter is typically used to create a 3D reconstruction of the chamber of interest. By gating the acquisition of points in space to the cardiac electrical activity, points that represent both location and electrical activity at that location can be acquired and displayed on a computer screen. After acquiring a number of points, a 3D representation is constructed and may be displayed from any viewing projection. The point of earliest electrical activity can be easily recognized (Fig. 17.1a). Areas surrounding that point will have colors reflecting their activation times in relation to the earliest point and showing propagation in a centrifugal pattern. The ability to view the map in different projections helps to guide the ablation catheter to the location of earliest activation.

17.2.2   Atrial Flutter

Atrial flutter consists of a reentrant rhythm around an anatomical obstacle. The obstacle may be an area of scar from: (1) prior cardiac surgery, ablation, or fibrosis; (2) a valve such as the tricuspid or the mitral valve; or (3) the ostium of a cardiac structure such as a pulmonary vein or the left atrial appendage. As in the case of atrial tachycardia, the roving catheter is moved in the chamber of interest and electrical data are collected and superimposed on the anatomical information. The resulting map shows propagation of electrical impulse with the area of earliest activation, meeting the area of latest activation, as shown in Fig.17.1b. By having the anatomical data integrated with the electrical data, the narrowest isthmus along the path of the flutter circuit can be identified and ablated.

17.2.3   Atrial Fibrillation

Atrial fibrillation (AF) is divided into paroxysmal and persistent types. Paroxysmal AF is believed to be triggered and maintained by rapid electrical activity emanating

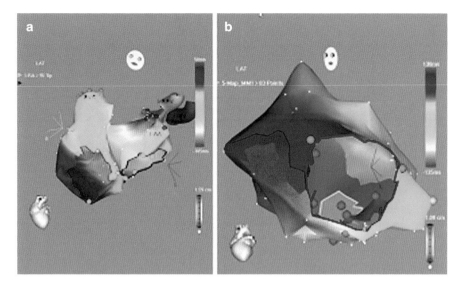

Fig. 17.1 Electroanatomical mapping of atrial arrhythmias. (**a**) Electroanatomical map of an atrial tachycardia originating from the left atrium, just outside of the left superior pulmonary vein. Timing of local electrical activity is color coded, with the earliest activation shown in *red*. *Red dots* represent ablation lesions. (**b**) Electroanatomical map of atrial flutter in the right atrium around the tricuspid valve annulus. The map demonstrates areas of earliest activation (*red*) adjacent to areas of latest activation (*blue*) indicating a reentrant rhythm. *LAA* left atrial appendage; *LIPV* left inferior pulmonary vein; *LSPV* left superior pulmonary vein; *SVC* superior vena cava

from foci in the pulmonary veins. As a result, the most common procedure for this type of AF is pulmonary vein isolation. During this procedure, ablations are performed in a circumferential fashion around the ostia of the pulmonary veins to achieve their electrical disconnection. It became evident soon after this procedure was introduced that X-ray fluoroscopy is not an adequate mode of imaging to guide this operation. In fact, the pulmonary veins exhibit a complex anatomy with significant inter- and intra-patient variability in size, shape, bifurcation, and branching pattern.[1,2] Application of ablation lesions in certain areas of the left atrium can be challenging. One area is the ridge between the left pulmonary veins and the left atrial appendage; another area is the ridge separating the right middle pulmonary vein from the right superior pulmonary vein or the right inferior pulmonary vein.[3]

The use of electroanatomical mapping represented a paradigm shift in the way that AF ablations are performed. Newly developed tools allow integration of real-time catheter-based electroanatomical mapping with imported MR or CT images.[4] This integration process allows precise anatomic detail provided by CT and MR images to be superimposed onto real-time electroanatomic maps, providing visualization of the ablation catheter in relation to relevant cardiac structures (Fig. 17.2a, b).

The use of electroanatomical mapping and image integration also facilitated ablation of persistent AF. In this AF subgroup, pulmonary vein isolation alone did not yield the success rate realized with paroxysmal AF. One promising adjunctive

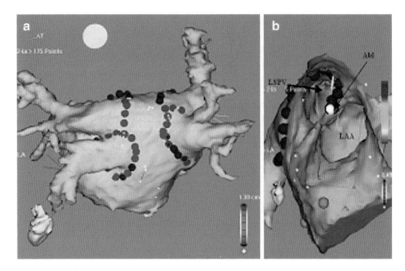

Fig. 17.2 Integration of 3D MRI with electroanatomical mapping. (**a**) External view of the posterior wall of the left atrium showing ablation lesions surrounding the pulmonary veins ostia. (**b**) Internal view of the left atrium showing placement of ablation lesions along the ridge between the left superior pulmonary vein and the left atrial appendage. *Abl* ablation lesion; *LAA* left atrial appendage; *LSPV* left superior pulmonary vein

approach involves the ablation of complex fractionated atrial electrograms (CFAE), which are areas of continuous electrical activity or short (<120 ms) cycle length. Ablation of these areas in addition to pulmonary vein isolation has been proposed to be effective in restoring and maintaining sinus rhythm in patients with persistent AF.[5] Mapping of CFAE areas can be challenging and time consuming; however, it can be facilitated by the use of high-density multi-electrode catheters, capable of covering a large area of the atrium, thus allowing the acquisition of CFAE maps in a rapid manner as well as the display of information in easily legible maps (Fig. 17.3).

17.3 The Use of Electroanatomical Mapping for the Treatment of Ventricular Tachycardias

Electroanatomical mapping is also an important tool for the treatment of ventricular tachycardia (VT), both automatic and reentrant.

17.3.1 Automatic Ventricular Tachycardia

Automatic VT can arise from any area in the left and right ventricles as well as the cusps of the aorta. As in the case of atrial tachycardia, electroanatomical maps containing

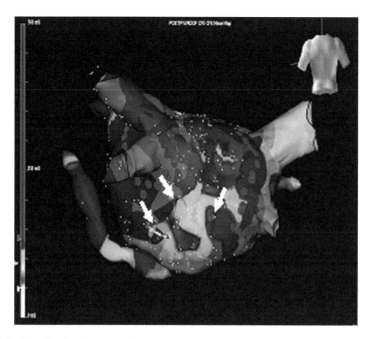

Fig. 17.3 Complex fractionated atrial electrograms map. Posterior view of an electroanatomical map of the left atrium. *Purple* colors represent slow cycle length, while other colors represent areas of faster conduction. *Red dots* indicate ablation lesions around the pulmonary vein ostia

electrical activation time and voltage amplitude superimposed on anatomical shells can be generated by moving the roving catheter in the chamber of interest. The point of earliest activation can then be identified and ablated.

17.3.2 Reentrant Ventricular Tachycardia

Reentrant VT occurs in various cardiomyopathies, including ischemic, dilated, and hypertrophic. It is also encountered in other less prevalent conditions such as sarcoidosis and arrhythmogenic right ventricular cardiomyopathy. The circuit of the reentrant rhythm typically involves a channel of preserved myocardium in the scar. Local electrograms in these channels are of low amplitude and fractionated, and occur after the QRS deflection on the surface ECG. If VT can be induced and tolerated, moving the catheter and recording electrograms relative to a fixed reference results in an activation map. The circuit of the VT can then be delineated on the map and targeted for ablation. The exit of the VT circuit is usually along one of the edges of the scar; as a result, scar localization and delineation is an important step in this procedure. This is even more important for hemodynamically unstable VT where ablations are often performed in normal sinus rhythm because of the inability to

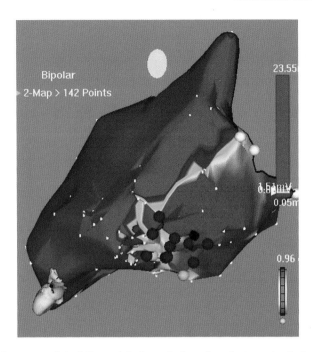

Fig. 17.4 Voltage map of the left ventricle. Lateral view of an electroanatomical map of the left ventricle showing the area of scar in the posterior wall. Areas of healthy myocardium are shown in *purple* and represent a local voltage greater than 1.5 mV. *Red dots* indicate ablation lesions at the scar border

perform entrainment and activation mapping. An anatomical shell of the ventricle is first obtained by moving the roving catheter during sinus rhythm. The maps are color coded (Fig. 17.4) with areas of scar typically indicating local voltage of less than 1.5 mV.[6] A transition zone between the scar and healthy myocardium can also be delineated. In addition, areas of fractionated and late potentials, representing channels inside the scar, are tagged. VT is then induced for a brief period to obtain an ECG; pace maps are then performed from the areas of late and fractionated potentials to match the ECG during VT and allow localization of the exit site. Electroanatomical mapping also allows tracking of ablation lesions; these can be tagged and revisited to localize gaps along the ablation lines if needed.

17.4   The Use of Electroanatomical Mapping for the Treatment of Arrhythmias in Patients with Congenital Heart Disease

Electroanatomical mapping proves highly useful in mapping and ablation of cardiac arrhythmias in patients with complex congenital heart disease.[7] Reentrant atrial and ventricular tachyarrhythmias are frequently encountered in these patients.

Catheter ablation in this patient population consists of localization of the surgical scars and identification of isthmus sites. This procedure can pose a great technical challenge and requires accurate identification of key anatomical locations and landmarks inside surgically modified structures. Electroanatomical mapping, especially when used with image integration, remarkably facilitates the ablation of these arrhythmias by enabling the operator to visualize the ablation catheter in relation to the complex cardiac anatomy with great accuracy and fine detail. Integration of CT images acquired prior to the procedure with real-time intra-procedural electroanatomical maps is performed by registering corresponding anatomical points inside the aorta.[8] The resulting image allows virtual navigation of the ablation catheter inside 3D accurate anatomical cardiac structures.

17.5   Types of Electroanatomical Mapping Systems

17.5.1   Magnetic-Based Mapping

Magnetic-based electroanatomical mapping was introduced first and allowed 3D mapping of the human heart. The system consists of three small magnets placed under the operating table and a location pad placed on the patient for standard orientation. The catheter tip contains a miniature location sensor, which is tracked by the magnets and displayed on a screen. This system has a series of monitors for visualization of electrograms and images and a processing unit. One of the disadvantages of this system is the inability, at the current time, to incorporate sensors on multiple catheters, limiting the visualization and localization to only one catheter.

17.5.2   Impedance-Based Mapping

This system is composed of several components, including the patient interface unit and a display workstation. This alternate system localizes catheter electrodes by considering the impedance between electrodes in the heart and electrode patches on the body surface. This system allows the visualization and localization of multiple electrodes and catheters. The accuracy of impedance-based mapping relative to magnetic-based mapping remains a controversial issue.

17.6   Pitfalls and Troubleshooting

Inaccurate catheter localization is sometimes encountered during electroanatomical mapping and results from numerous variables including movement of the patient. During the mapping process using the magnetic-based systems, any change in the position of the patient affects the localization of the catheter, rendering the map inaccurate. As a result, it is crucial to prevent movement of the patient, if possible. Similarly, using the impedance-based mapping systems, avoiding movement of the reference catheter is important for a successful procedure. In addition to patient's movement, other variables can affect image integration. As discussed above, the integration process is based on the fusion of CT and MRI acquired before the procedure with an intraprocedural 3D shell of the cardiac chamber of interest. As a result, changes in the respiration and volume status can affect the accuracy of the integration process. To minimize these potential errors, it is more beneficial to obtain the pre-procedure image during end expiration, rather than inspiration. Most points during map acquisition are also acquired during end expiration. Similarly, changes in volume status between the time of CT/MRI acquisition and the map creation can lead to discrepancies in location. This can be minimized by administering diuretics to the patient if excessive fluid has been given during the ablation procedure.

References

1. Schwartzman D, Lacomis J, Wigginton WG. Characterization of left atrium and distal pulmonary vein morphology using multidimensional computed tomography. J Am Coll Cardiol 2003; 41:1349–57.
2. Mansour M, Holmvang G, Sosnovik D, et al. Assessment of pulmonary vein anatomic variability by magnetic resonance imaging: implications for catheter ablation techniques for atrial fibrillation. J Cardiovasc Electrophysiol 2004; 15:387–93.
3. Mansour M, Refaat M, Heist K, et al. Three-dimensional anatomy of the left atrium by magnetic resonance angiography: implications for catheter ablation for atrial fibrillation. J Cardiovasc Electrophysiol 2006; 17:719–23.
4. Malchano ZJ, Neuzil P, Cury RC, et al. Integration of cardiac CT/MR imaging with three-dimensional electroanatomical mapping to guide catheter manipulation in the left atrium: implications for catheter ablation of atrial fibrillation. J Cardiovasc Electrophysiol 2006; 17:1221–9.
5. Elayi CS, Verma A, Di Biase L, et al. Ablation for longstanding permanent atrial fibrillation: results from a randomized study comparing three different strategies. Heart Rhythm 2008; 5:1658–64.
6 Marchlinski FE, Callans DJ, Gottlieb CD, et al. Linear ablation lesions for control of unmappable ventricular tachycardia in patients with ischemic and nonischemic cardiomyopathy. Circulation 2000; 101:1288–96.
7. Delacretaz E, Ganz LI, Soejima K, et al. Multi atrial macro-re-entry circuits in adults with repaired congenital heart disease: entrainment mapping combined with three-dimensional electroanatomic mapping. J Am Coll Cardiol 2001; 37:1665–76.
8. Aryana A, Liberthson RR, Heist EK, et al. Images in cardiovascular medicine. Ablation of atrial flutter in a patient with mustard procedure using integration of real-time electroanatomical mapping with 3-dimensional computed tomographic imaging. Circulation 2007; 116:e315–6.

Chapter 18
Cardiac Electrophysiological Imaging: Solving the Inverse Problem of Electrocardiography

Bin He and Chenguang Liu

Abstract In this chapter, we review the concepts, principles, and potential applications of cardiac electrophysiological imaging. First, the idea and history of the ECG inverse problem is introduced. Second, the following representative inverse methods are presented: (1) estimation of the cardiac electrical activity represented by equivalent moving dipole(s); (2) heart surface imaging approaches, including epicardial potential imaging and heart surface activation imaging; and (3) estimation of the distributed three-dimensional cardiac electrical activity. Finally, the potential applications and future trends of cardiac electrophysiological imaging are discussed.

18.1 Introduction

Electrocardiography is the noninvasive recording of electrical potentials varying over time on the body surface, originating from the heart. The standard 12-lead ECG is a popular recording method used widely in clinical settings for probing and characterizing cardiac electrical activities and diagnosing heart diseases. Due to the limited number of electrodes employed by the 12-lead ECG, it does not provide spatial details of the cardiac electrical activity. For example, it does not reveal information with regard to where arrhythmias originate.

In order to better characterize the cardiac electrical activities, invasive electrical mapping systems have been employed in electrophysiological (EP) labs. The CARTO® system (Biosense Webster Inc., Johnson & Johnson, Diamond Bar, CA, USA) conducts direct electro-anatomic mapping over the endocardial surface by sequential acquisition of electrograms and anatomical coordinates to construct spatial distributions of electrical activity over the endocardial surface.[1] On the other hand, the Ensite® system (St. Jude Medical, Inc., St. Paul, MN, USA) employs a multi-electrode array placed in the heart's intracavitary chamber to record instantaneous potentials at multiple sites.[2] Both of these systems have been widely used in clinical

B. He (✉)

Department of Biomedical Engineering, University of Minnesota, Minneapolis, MN, USA
e-mail: binhe@umn.edu

D.C. Sigg et al. (eds.), *Cardiac Electrophysiology Methods and Models*,
DOI 10.1007/978-1-4419-6658-2_18, © Springer Science+Business Media, LLC 2010

357

EP labs for treating cardiac arrhythmias, particularly for guiding catheter ablation. While these endocardial mapping systems have achieved reasonable success, they are still invasive procedures, and the lengthy mapping process might require patients to stay in the EP lab for quite a long duration.

Alternatively, the cardiac source can be estimated noninvasively from body surface potential maps (BSPMs). Body surface potential mapping[3] records the ECG signal from hundreds of electrodes over the patient's torso surface, and contains much more information than the 12-lead ECG recording, thus making it possible to estimate the characteristics of cardiac sources (location, magnitude, trend, etc.). For this purpose, the so-called inverse problem of electrocardiography has been studied to determine information about cardiac electrical sources from the measured body surface potentials. This problem is the counterpart of the forward problem. In the inverse problem, the thoracic ECG signals from a large number of leads are used to reconstruct cardiac electrical activity with the aid of a forward heart–torso volume conductor model. A schematic diagram of the forward/inverse problem is shown in Fig. 18.1a. Cardiac EP imaging, or the ECG inverse solution, is aimed at providing the same important information on cardiac electrical activity *noninvasively* that is currently obtained by invasive systems in clinical EP labs.

The reconstructed cardiac electrical sources, i.e., the results of cardiac EP imaging, can be either focal or distributed, as shown in Fig 18.1b. With the aim of extracting useful information regarding cardiac electrical activity, focal source models, such as equivalent moving dipole(s)[4] or an equivalent multipole,[5] are reasonable approximations of cardiac electrical sources in certain cases, especially for situations when there is a focal activity. On the other hand, distributed source models have gained much attention, because cardiac electrical activity is, in principle, distributed over the three-dimensional (3D) volume of the heart. Cardiac EP imaging shall refer to spatially characterizing and reconstructing the distributed (as well as focal) cardiac electrical activity. Heart surface imaging has been pursued in the past decades by various investigators, and has included imaging epicardial potentials[6-11] and the activation sequence on the heart surfaces (both epicardium and endocardium).[12-15] Imaging 3D distributed cardiac sources has been rigorously

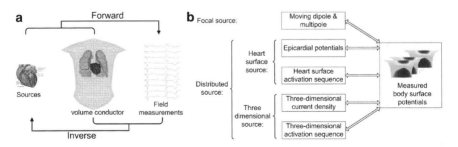

Fig. 18.1 (a) Schematic diagram of the forward/inverse problem. (b) Configurations of cardiac sources in the forward/inverse problem

studied recently; a detailed distributed 3D heart source model is used, allowing imaging of EP properties over the 3D volume of the heart.[16–24]

Solving the inverse problem requires tackling inherent mathematical difficulties. The ECG inverse problem is an under-determined problem as the number of measurements (surface leads) is generally smaller than the number of variables (say, the number of myocardial cells) involved. In order to obtain unique solutions, source models with implicit constraints have been introduced to represent cardiac electrical activity, such as equivalent moving dipoles, epicardial potentials, heart surface isochrones, and excitable heart models with embedded physiological knowledge. Such source modeling enables "constraint" imaging with *a priori* knowledge based on vast experimental observations of cardiac electrical activity.

Another difficulty is that the ECG inverse problem is ill-posed, due to the smoothing and attenuation effects of the torso volume. This is because body surface potentials are due to the flow of current within the passive torso volume conductor. As a result, cardiac electrical signals are smoothed and attenuated when traveling through the torso volume conductor. Little measurement noise could thus induce large perturbation on the ECG inverse solution. Fortunately a number of regularization techniques have been developed which can address the "ill-posedness" of the ECG inverse problem to obtain stable and meaningful inverse solutions.

In this chapter, we review the principles, methods, and potential applications of cardiac EP imaging (ECG inverse solutions). Some examples are provided with regard to the representative inverse methods.

18.2 Moving Dipole Source Imaging

Certain cardiac electrical activities, such as ectopic beats, can be represented reasonably by one or two equivalent moving dipoles. An electric dipole is a separation of positive and negative charge, which can be characterized by a vector. Electrical activity produced by excitable cardiac media may be modeled by a combination of current dipoles, where a current dipole is a separation of current source and sink, located in the vicinity of the current source. The location, direction, and magnitude of a current dipole(s) reflect the characteristics of cardiac electrical activity, in an equivalent sense that the dipole(s)-generated BSPM best represents the BSPM measured over a subject's torso surface. Notably, this representation is appropriate only when the cardiac electrical activity has one or two focal centers, so that the characteristics of the underlying sources can be tracked instant-by-instant by estimating the location, magnitude, and direction of one or two moving dipoles inside the volume. For instance, the accessory pathway of Wolff–Parkinson–White (WPW) syndrome can be tracked with the single-moving-dipole inverse solution.[4] In WPW syndrome, an accessory pathway exists between the atria and ventricles, which results in pre-excitation of the ventricles. The single-moving-dipole solution may contribute to localizing the pathway during the early pre-excitation period. In addition, the moving-dipole solutions are also useful for localizing and tracking the migration of excitation during ectopic beats.[25]

The mathematical principle of solving the moving-dipole inverse problem is to match measured body surface potentials with those generated by moving dipole(s) in the forward model. By adjusting the location, magnitude and orientation of the dipole(s), the dissimilarity between the measured and simulated body surface potentials is minimized. The dissimilarity can be quantified as follows:

$$R = \left\| \hat{V} - V \right\|^2 \tag{18.1}$$

$$V = AX \tag{18.2}$$

where $\hat{V}$ is the vector of the measured body surface potentials at one sampling instant, V is the vector of simulated body surface potentials from the dipole(s) within a given volume conductor, $\| \ \|^2$ denotes the square of the Euclidean norm of a vector referring to the difference between the measured and model-generated body surface potentials, X is the vector containing the unknown parameters of the moving-dipole inverse solution, and A is the transfer matrix relating the dipole sources to the body surface potentials. For a single-dipole model, the unknown parameters include three components of the dipole moment and three coordinates of the dipole location. For a two-moving-dipole model, the number of independent unknowns becomes 12. Notably, the relation between the simulated body surface potentials and the coordinates of a dipole is nonlinear. In an effort to minimize (18.1), iterative methods are employed to solve this nonlinear optimization problem, such as the Levenberg–Marquardt algorithm.[4] The number of assumed moving dipoles depends on the number of excitation centers that need to be represented, normally no more than two, due to the sensitivity to the measurement noise.[26]

18.3   Heart Surface Distributed Source Imaging

18.3.1   Epicardial Potential Imaging

Noninvasive imaging of the epicardial potentials from body surface potentials has been pursued since the 1970s. Intraoperative epicardial mapping was proved useful for diagnosing cardiac arrhythmias and guiding intervention procedures before the wide use of endocardial mapping systems.[27] Clearly, a noninvasive mapping method is desired to replace the invasive approach. Noninvasive imaging of epicardial potentials shares many of the benefits of distributed cardiac electrical source imaging. Providing the spatial details of cardiac electrical activity over the epicardial surface enhances our ability to image the EP characteristics of cardiac activities for clinical treatments and research. Epicardial potential imaging has been investigated in the past decades because it can be applied to general source configurations that are not limited to one or two focal activities.

In the late 1970s, it was demonstrated that epicardial potentials and body surface potentials can be related using a linear model with the aid of the boundary element method, which can be used to incorporate realistic geometry of a subject.[28] The mathematical equation can be represented as:

$$V_B = AV_H \tag{18.3}$$

where V_B is a vector of body surface potentials, V_H is a vector of epicardial potentials, and A is the transfer matrix from epicardial potentials to body surface potentials in a given torso volume conductor. The epicardial potential inverse problem is to reconstruct V_H from V_B. Such an inverse problem is usually ill-posed and regularization techniques need to be used.

A representative method is Tikhonov regularization which has been widely used in solving the inverse problem. In (18.1), the difference between the measured and model-generated body surface potentials is minimized to obtain the optimal estimate on the cardiac source. On the other hand, the Tikhonov regularization scheme minimizes the following equation:

$$\left\| \hat{V}_B - AV_H \right\|^2 + \left\| RV_H \right\|^2 \tag{18.4}$$

where the first part is the same as (18.1), and the second part is the regularized norm of the inversely estimated epicardial potentials. By minimizing the two parts simultaneously, an informative and stable solution can be obtained. The balance between the two parts is determined by the regularization parameter λ. In order to find the optimal value of λ, the *L-curve* method is widely used[29].

Noninvasive epicardial potential imaging techniques have been developed[6–10] and validated in animal studies,[9] in normal human subjects,[30] and in patients with heart diseases.[11] Figure 18.2 depicts an example of the imaged epicardial potentials during ventricular pacing in a human subject.[11] The epicardial potentials were estimated at each sampling time instant, and the electrogram at a certain location was plotted. As a result, the isochrone was estimated by picking up the activation time at the point of the maximum negative derivative of the electrogram ($-dV_H/dt$).

18.3.2 *Heart Surface Activation Imaging*

Since the 1980s, in parallel to epicardial potential imaging, heart surface activation imaging has been pursued,[12] where the spatial distribution of activation time over the entire heart surface is reconstructed from the BSPM. Here the heart surface includes both the epicardium and endocardium, and they form a closed heart volume in which the excitation occurs. While the principle applies to both the ventricles and atria,[14] most work has dealt with imaging activation times over the surfaces of ventricles, including the endocardium and epicardium of the ventricles. Heart surface activation imaging is a promising tool for evaluating heart function

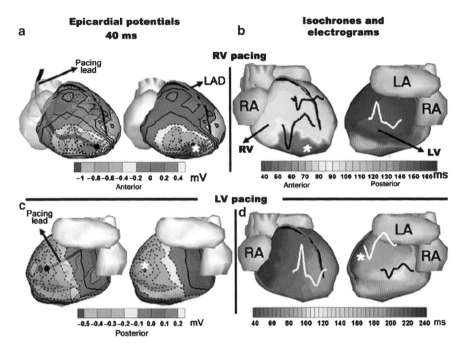

Fig. 18.2 Ventricular activation during RV (*top*) and LV (*bottom*) pacing in a human subject. (**a**) Anterior views of epicardial potential map during RV pacing. *Left*, translucent view showing pacing lead. *Right*, opaque view showing minimum at pacing site location (*asterisk*). Anterior view is tilted 10° to show pacing site location on inferior RV apex. (**b**) Anterior and posterior views of an epicardial isochrone map for RV pacing. Electrograms from three locations are shown at their respective spatial locations. (**c**) Posterior views of epicardial potential map during LV pacing (same format as in **a**). (**d**) Epicardial isochrone map with electrograms for LV pacing (same format as in **b**). *LA* left atrium, *LAD* left anterior descending coronary artery, *LV* left ventricle, *RA* right atrium, *RV* right ventricle. Reprinted by permission from Macmillan Publishers Ltd: Nature Medicine, Ramanathan C, Raja NG, Jia P, et al. Noninvasive electrocardiographic imaging for cardiac electrophysiology and arrhythmia, 2004[11]

in that it directly images EP properties of the heart (i.e., activation time), albeit on the surface of heart. Recent work has suggested its potential for clinical applications in assisting the diagnosis of cardiac abnormalities, such as Wolff–Parkinson–White syndrome,[15] bundle branch block,[31] and ventricular tachyarrhythmias.[15]

Regarding the inverse problem, the source model is again constrained on the heart surface. In order to find the activation time at critical locations on the heart surface, the so-called *critical points* theory[32] has been used. The "critical points" are defined as the extrema sites (minima, maxima, saddle points, etc.) on the heart surface activation map. The occurrence of the critical points will result in a changed slope in the temporal time course of an ECG, leading to a "jump" in the first derivative of the ECG time course corresponding to the activation time at critical points. By applying this principle, the critical points can be localized and the activation time at those critical points is determined by picking up the time instant when the "jump" happens.[13] The activation times at the detected critical points are then used to determine the activation time distribution over the heart surface.

More recently, another heart surface activation imaging algorithm has been proposed by Tilg et al.[14] In their method, building up the forward relation between the heart surface isochrone and body surface potentials includes two steps. First, based on the bidomain theory, a linear relation between heart surface transmembrane potentials and body surface potentials exists.[33] Second, the nonlinear relation between the transmembrane potential and activation time at each heart surface source point is modeled with *a priori* physiological knowledge. By combining those two steps, a nonlinear relation between the activation time τ and the body surface potentials can be obtained as follows:

$$V_B = F\tau \tag{18.5}$$

where F is a nonlinear operator, τ contains the activation time on the heart surface, and V_B is an $N \times N_t$ matrix containing the body surface potentials from N sensors at N_t time instants. To solve this nonlinear and ill-posed inverse problem, it is linearized by utilizing the derivative of F and then an iterative procedure is employed to update the value of τ in each step.[14] Notably, due to the nature of the linearization method, the initial estimation of τ should be close to the real value to ensure the convergence and accuracy of the final solution. For instance, the activation time obtained with the critical points theory could be used as the initial value in the current iterative approach.

This approach has been evaluated in patients with WPW syndrome. The imaged heart surface isochrone was used to localize the pre-excitation pathway. The pathway was localized with the inverse approach first, and then catheter ablation was performed during which the true location of the pathway was identified. The localization results were consistent with the outcome of catheter ablation (Fig. 18.3).

18.4   Three-dimensional Source Imaging

Heart excitation propagates throughout the 3D space. While heart surface imaging approaches have advanced the ECG inverse problem from point dipole solutions to distributed source imaging, there are limitations in their ability to characterize intramural activities, e.g., intramural delay.[34] On the other hand, 3D imaging of the intramural cardiac activation should provide important pathoanatomic information, for example, ventricular arrhythmias may arise from transmural regions within the myocardial tissue. Three-dimensional mapping of cardiac activities could not only be a powerful tool for research on the mechanisms of arrhythmias, but could also guide clinical management of cardiac arrhythmias in a more efficient way. This is like considering a number of "virtual" intramural sensors being placed in the heart from which detailed intramural information can be revealed, but in an intact heart.

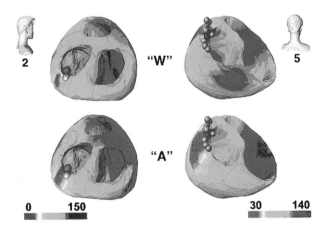

Fig. 18.3 Location of earliest ventricular activation as computed by noninvasive imaging of cardiac electrophysiology is indicated in red. Ablation points are denoted by grey markers, and the location of successful ablation is in purple, indicating the ventricular insertion site of the accessory pathway. A left posterolateral accessory pathway was identified in patient 2 (*left*), and a left ante-rolateral accessory pathway was noted in patient 5 (*right*). Upper panels show activation sequences during normal atrioventricular conduction ("W"), and lower panels show activation sequences during adenosine-induced atrioventricular block ("A"). Head icons indicate point of view. Isochrones are plotted in 20 ms intervals. Reprinted from the Journal of American College of Cardiology, Volume 48, Berger T, Fischer G, Pfeifer B, et al. Single-beat noninvasive imaging of cardiac electrophysiology of ventricular pre-excitation, pp. 2045–52, 2006, with permission from Elsevier[15]

18.4.1 Inverse Estimation of 3D Dipole Distribution

One of the 3D inverse source imaging approaches is to estimate a distribution of current dipoles within the 3D myocardium. Each of these dipoles represents, in an equivalent sense, the regional cardiac electrical source. The number of such dipoles is usually quite large in order to achieve the resolution of "imaging" of cardiac electrical activity. He and Wu reported a computer simulation study in which over 1,000 equivalent current dipoles were evenly distributed in the 3D ventricles.[16] The current density is approximated by the moment of current dipoles. The forward relation between the distributed dipoles and the body surface potentials can be represented by (18.2), and the unknowns are the dipole moments. Since the number of sensors is generally much smaller than the number of sources, such a problem is under-determined and ill-posed. Regularization techniques are thus needed in order to estimate the distribution of current dipoles. In their early work, He and Wu pro-posed to use the Laplacian weighted minimal norm (LWMN) algorithm to tackle this challenging problem.[16] In LWMN, the Laplacian of the source signal is mini-mized in order to obtain an estimate. It can be anticipated that such a 3D inverse solution is fairly smooth over space. He and Wu used an iterative approach further to enhance the sources with large energy concentration, and showed reasonable results in localizing and imaging of focal sources.[16]

18.4.2   Heart Model-Based 3D Activation Imaging

A major challenge in 3D dipole distribution imaging is the large number of unknowns, which makes the problem severely under-determined and ill-posed. He and co-workers have proposed a physiologically constrained 3D cardiac activation imaging approach in which a heart EP model is used.[17,18] A series of experimental studies have been conducted to validate this novel 3D activation imaging approach.[21,24] In this approach, a heart EP computer model with *a priori* knowledge about cardiac electrical activity can be deemed as explicit constraints on the inverse procedure so that the ill-posed nature of the inverse problem is circumvented. The heart–torso geometry of an individual subject is obtained from CT or MRI scans, and a heart EP computer model is then constructed based on the subject's anatomy and *a priori* physiological knowledge. Based on the bidomain theory, the spatial distribution of current dipoles is derived from activation patterns of the heart, and then are linearly related to the body surface potentials. The global 3D activation sequence is estimated after the parameters of the heart model are optimized by means of a nonlinear estimation procedure. In this technique, the heart model parameters are first initialized by using an artificial neural network. The model parameters are then iteratively adjusted in an attempt to minimize the dissimilarity between measured and heart model-generated body surface potentials. The 3D activation sequence is reconstructed by utilizing the adjusted heart model parameters when the simulated body surface potentials and the measured body surface potentials match well.

An important component of this approach is to use a cellular automaton heart computer model.[17–18,35] The heart model contains tens of thousands of cell units. The spatial resolution of the cell units determines the fineness of the heart model, usually between 0.5 and 1.5 mm in the reported work. In each cell unit, the parameters characterizing the waveform of the transmembrane action potential, conductivity, fiber orientation (in an anisotropic heart model), conduction velocity and others are individually defined based on *a priori* physiological knowledge. Based on the cellular automation principle, the excitation procedure of the whole heart is simulated. The anisotropy of the heart can be incorporated into the heart model.[35] The fiber orientation at the location of each cell unit is assigned. In practice, the fiber orientation of a realistic heart can be obtained by either histological study or diffusion tensor magnetic resonance imaging.[36] In simulation, a generalized principle of fiber orientation can be utilized. For each cell unit, the associated fiber orientation is approximately parallel to the epicardial surface and determined by its fiber angle. The myocardial fiber orientations rotate counterclockwise over 120° from the outermost layer (epicardium, –60°) to the innermost layer (endocardium, +60°) with identical increments between the consecutive layers. All units on the same myocardial layer of the ventricles have identical fiber angles. The excitation conduction velocity along the fibers is faster than that transverse to the fibers, and the conductivity along the fibers is higher than that transverse to the fibers. After simulating heart excitation, body surface potentials are calculated from the equivalent sources inside the heart. Based on the bidomain theory, the field potential Φ (body surface potential V_B is the subset of Φ) is simulated from the equivalent current sources and the V_B is numerically solved from the heart-excitation model by applying the boundary element method[35] or the finite element method.[37]

This 3D heart electrophysiological model-based activation imaging has been validated on a rabbit model[21] and swine model.[24] In the rabbit study, simultaneous intracardiac mapping and body surface potential mapping were conducted during pacing. The estimated ventricular activation sequence and site of activation initiation were quantitatively compared with the measured activation sequence and site of pacing. The experimental results indicate a ~5 mm localization error of initiation site and 0.32 in relative error between the measured and estimated activation sequence throughout the ventricles. In the swine study, simultaneous intracavitary recording and body surface potential mapping were conducted during pacing. The endocardial activation sequence as a subset of the 3D activation sequence was extracted and compared with the output of the Ensite® mapping system. An example is shown in Fig. 18.4. In pacing studies, the averaged error of localizing the initiation site of activation was ~7 mm. The inversely estimated endocardial activation sequence was consistent with the output of the Ensite® system in both healthy pigs and pigs with induced heart failure. These promising experimental results suggest that the 3D heart model-based activation imaging approach can image activation sequence and localize initiation sites of activation, which may become a useful tool for aiding clinical management of arrhythmias.

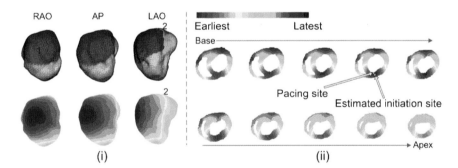

Fig. 18.4 Evaluation of inverse results when a control animal is paced from the endocardial left ventricular anterior. (**a**) Activation sequence (AS) on the left ventricular endocardial surface. The AS reconstructed by the Ensite® system is shown in the upper row in three views: RAO, AP, and LAO. RED represents the earliest activated area and BLUE represents the latest activated area. The earliest activated site is indicated by the number "1" and the latest activated site is indicated by "2" on the figure. The corresponding AS estimated by inverse approach is shown in the lower row. The earliest activated site and the latest activated site are also indicated by "1" and "2," respectively. (**b**) Location of the initiation site and the 3D AS. The geometry of the heart is shown by 10 horizontal sections, arranged from base to apex. The actual initiation site and estimated location of the initiation site are indicated. The 3D AS is shown on the 10 sections. Reproduced from Liu C, Skadsberg ND, Ahlberg SE, et al. Estimation of global ventricular activation sequences by noninvasive three-dimensional electrical imaging: validation studies in a Swine model during pacing. J Cardiovasc Electrophysiol 2008;19:535–40[24]

18.4.3 *Physical Model-Based 3D Activation Imaging*

The above 3D activation imaging method explicitly utilizes prior electrophysiological assumptions as embedded in the heart EP computer model. Most recently, a novel approach which images the 3D ventricular activation sequence without an explicit physiological heart model has been proposed,[22] an approach which is based on the fundamental biophysics relations of cardiac activation. This method is based on the physical modeling of the heart–torso volume conductor and distributed equivalent current sources arising from the transmembrane potential gradient throughout the ventricular myocardium. The equivalent current source distribution is first reconstructed from body surface potentials at every time instant during the period of ventricular activation. The activation time at any given location within the 3D myocardium can be estimated as the time instant corresponding to the occurrence of the maximum value of the estimated current density at this location.

As mentioned in Sect. 18.4.1, a linear relationship exists between the distributed current dipoles and body surface potentials at each time instant. This forward relation can be written as:

$$V_B(t) = Aj(t) \tag{18.6}$$

where $j(t)$ is a $3M \times 1$ matrix containing M current dipoles' moments at t. If one only considers the process of ventricular depolarization (e.g., during the QRS interval), the spatial distribution of $j(t)$ is dominated by its values at the interface between the depolarized and nondepolarized myocardium (known as the excitation wavefront), where the myocardial cells are undergoing rapid depolarization. Owing to the steepness of depolarization, these myocardial cells can only stay in the depolarization phase shortly; therefore, the excitation wavefront is expected to propagate by a given myocardial site only at its activation time. As a result, when one looks at the time-varying equivalent current dipole $j(r,t)$ at a fixed location r, its amplitude $|j(r,t)|$ reaches the maximum value at its activation time $\tau(r)$ for the entire duration T of the ventricular depolarization. Figure 18.5 illustrates this phenomenon and the principle of the algorithm. This concept can be mathematically expressed as:

$$\arg\left[\max_{t \in T}(|j(r,t)|) \right] = \tau(r) \tag{18.7}$$

The above equation implies that the activation sequence throughout the 3D ventricular volume can be determined by evaluating the time course of local equivalent current dipole at every myocardial site. Therefore, noninvasive estimation of the activation sequence from the body surface potential measurements consists of two steps: (1) imaging 3D equivalent current sources; and (2) detecting the temporal "marker" at which the inversely calculated source magnitude arrives at its maximum.

The first step can be solved by applying the Tikhonov regularization approach introduced in Sect. 18.3.1. The regularization matrix is chosen to be a weighting matrix.

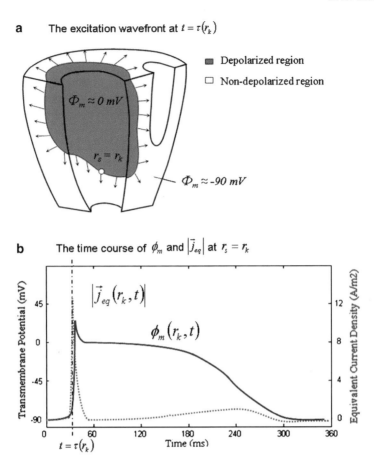

a   The excitation wavefront at $t = \tau(r_k)$

Depolarized region
Non-depolarized region

$\Phi_m \approx 0\ mV$

$r_s = r_k$

$\Phi_m \approx -90\ mV$

b   The time course of ϕ_m and $\left|\vec{j}_{eq}\right|$ at $r_s = r_k$

$\left|\vec{j}_{eq}(r_k, t)\right|$

$\phi_m(r_k, t)$

$t = \tau(r_k)$ Time (ms)

Fig. 18.5 (**a**) Ventricles are shown at the instant $t = \tau(r_k)$ ($\tau(r_k)$ is the activation time at r_k) when the excitation wavefront is propagating by a given location r_k (marked by a *circle*). Over each point along this wavefront, the local equivalent current density field (appearing as a current dipole) arises from the sharp spatial variation of the transmembrane potential across the wavefront, which is much larger than any other non-wavefront location. Therefore, these dipoles dominate the instantaneous cardiac electrical activity that accounts for the measurable torso electrical potentials. (**b**) Time courses of the transmembrane potential $\Phi(r_k)$ and the amplitude of the associated equivalent current density $|j_{eq}(r_k)|$. "Spike" of $|j_{eq}(r_k)|$ occurs exactly at $t = \tau(r_k)$, coinciding with the instant when the myocardial cells at r_k are undergoing steep depolarization. This relationship suggests that the activation time at a given myocardial site can be estimated by detecting the temporal peak of the magnitude of its local equivalent current density. Reproduced from Liu Z, Liu C, He B. Noninvasive reconstruction of three-dimensional ventricular activation sequence from the inverse solution of distributed equivalent current density. IEEE Trans Med Imaging 2006;25:1307–18[22]

Once the first step is completed, the next step is picking up activation time by simply detecting the time instant with the occurrence of the maximum current source estimate for each 3D source point.

Measured activation sequence   **Imaged activation sequence**

a Rabbit#1 LV pacing

b Rabbit#2 RV pacing

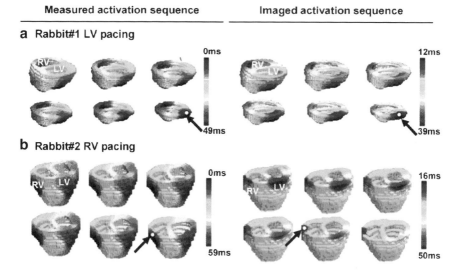

Fig. 18.6 Comparison between the 3D activation sequence measured via 3D intracardiac mapping (*left column*) and the inversely imaged 3D activation sequence (*right column*). The activation sequence is color coded from blue to red, corresponding to earliest and latest activation, respectively. The pacing site and estimated initial site of activation are marked by a red circle and purple arrow, respectively. (**a**) Activation was paced at the left posterior wall of the ventricle in rabbit 1. A realistic geometry of the ventricle for rabbit 1 is displayed (*top left view*). (**b**) Activation was induced by pacing at the right lateral wall of the ventricle in rabbit 2 (*top anterior view*). Reproduced from Han C, Liu Z, Zhang X, et al. Noninvasive three-dimensional cardiac activation imaging from body surface potential maps: a computational and experimental study on a rabbit model. IEEE Trans Med Imaging 2008;27:1622–30[23]

Validation study of this approach has been conducted on rabbits.[23] The precise 3D activation sequence was measured by intracardiac needle electrodes, and was used as a gold standard to evaluate the imaged activation sequence. Good consistency was observed between the imaged and measured 3D activation sequences, as shown in Fig. 18.6. The validation results indicate good performance of this algorithm in reconstructing the overall activation sequence and localizing the site of origin of activation. These experimental results are encouraging and suggest that the physical model-based technique may have potential to become a useful imaging means for mapping cardiac electrical activity noninvasively throughout the 3D myocardium.

18.5   Imaging Cardiac Sources from Intracavitary Recordings

Besides BSPM-based inverse approaches, intracavitary potential maps (ICPMs) have also been used to map cardiac electrical activity and are widely used in clinical EP labs. Compared to the BSPM-based source imaging techniques, ICPM-based inverse imaging has the following unique features. First, the recording electrodes are relatively close to the sources being imaged (compared to the distance between the body surface and the heart), thus more details revealing cardiac activities can be obtained. Second, the volume between the electrodes and the heart is composed only of blood (as opposed to multiple types of tissue or material between the body surface and heart), so less modeling error may exist in the transfer matrix.

Endocardial potential imaging from intracavitary recordings has been attempted by solving an endocardial inverse problem, that is, to estimate endocardial potentials from ICPMs in animals[38–39] and in humans.[2,40] The Ensite® system can image endocardial potentials from the ICPM recorded using a balloon catheter. Another endocardial mapping system is the widely used CARTO® system, in which electrical and anatomical information of the endocardium is recorded by using sequential placement of a catheter tip. The CARTO® system provides direct recording of endocardial electrical information, but requires sequential recording. On the other hand, the Ensite® system can map endocardial electrical potentials from instantaneous ICPM recordings, but needs one to solve an inverse problem. Nonetheless, both systems have been widely used in clinical EP labs to assist the management of arrhythmias, e.g., guiding radiofrequency catheter ablation.

Most recently, the idea of estimating 3D cardiac activation from intracavitary recordings has been proposed,[41] and the method has been evaluated in computer simulations.[42] He et al. used the heart model-based algorithm to estimate 3D activation sequence from ICPMs.[42] The finite element method was employed to build up the relationship between the 3D cardiac sources and intracavitary recordings. Similarly, by optimizing the parameters of the heart model in an iterative attempt to minimize the dissimilarity between the measured and modeled ICPMs, the algorithm can estimate the global activation sequence in 3D myocardium. Furthermore, intramural extracellular potentials can also be estimated with the aid of the finite element method. The detection of extracellular potentials/electrograms can increase our understanding of the mechanisms of arrhythmic events and aid clinical management of arrhythmias. Such estimated intramural electrograms can be considered as an approximation of extracellular potentials, which would be recorded if one placed a large number of electrodes within the ventricular volume. The ICPM-based 3D imaging approach provides a powerful tool to reveal the detailed EP activity of the heart in a minimally invasive way.

18.6   Discussion

We have reviewed the development of noninvasive cardiac electrical source imaging techniques. The ECG inverse problem has progressed from focal moving dipole solutions to heart surface imaging, and recently to 3D cardiac source imaging. This progress is due, in part, to our better understanding of the principles and development of new powerful computation imaging techniques, as well as the ever-increasing computational power we enjoy today. One important advancement in solving the ECG inverse problem was to move from point equivalent sources (such as moving dipoles) to distributed sources such as epicardial potentials and heart surface activation sequences. Another important development was to progress from two-dimensional heart surface imaging to 3D cardiac tomographic imaging. Three-dimensional cardiac EP imaging promises to become a useful electrophysiological imaging modality, providing a broad perspective of applications for clinical diagnosis and management of a variety of cardiac diseases. In clinical settings, the minimally invasive catheter-based endocardial mapping approaches are currently widely used in aiding catheter ablation of arrhythmias. The recently available 3D cardiac EP imaging from intracavitary recordings promises to greatly enhance our ability to image cardiac electrical activity, not only over the endocardium but also throughout the entire 3D volume of the heart.

Acknowledgement   This work was supported in part by NIH R01HL080093 and NSF CBET-0756331.

References

1. Gepstein L, Hayam G, Ben-Haim SA. A novel method for nonfluoroscopic catheter-based electroanatomical mapping of the heart: in vitro and in vivo accuracy results. Circulation 1997; 95:1611–22.
2. Gornick CC, Adler SW, Pederson B, et al. Validation of a new noncontact catheter system for electroanatomic mapping of left ventricular endocardium. Circulation 1999; 99:829–35.
3. Taccardi B. Distribution of heart potentials on the thoracic surface of normal human subjects. Circ Res 1963; 12:341–52.
4. Gulrajani RM, Roberge FA, Savard P. Moving dipole inverse ECG and EEG solutions. IEEE Trans Biomed Eng 1984; 31:903–10.
5. Geselowitz DB. Multipole representation for an equivalent cardiac generator. Proc IRE 1960; 48:75–9.
6. Barr RC, Spach MS. Inverse calculation of QRS-T epicardial potentials from normal and ectopic beats in the dog. Circ Res 1978; 42:661–75.
7. Shahidi AV, Savard P, Nadeau R. Forward and inverse problems of electrocardiography: modeling and recovery of epicardial potentials in humans. IEEE Trans Biomed Eng 1994; 41:249–56.
8. He B, Wu D. A bioelectric inverse imaging technique based on surface Laplacians. IEEE Trans Biomed Eng 1997; 44: 529–38.
9. Oster HS, Taccardi B, Lux RL, et al. Noninvasive electrocardiographic imaging: reconstruction of epicardial potentials, electrograms, and isochrones and localization of single and multiple electrocardiac events. Circulation 1997; 96:1012–24.
10. Greensite F, Huiskamp G. An improved method for estimating epicardial potentials from the body surface. IEEE Trans Biomed Eng 1998; 45:98–104.
11. Ramanathan C, Raja NG, Jia P, et al. Noninvasive electrocardiographic imaging for cardiac electrophysiology and arrhythmia. Nat Med 2004; 10:422–8.
12. Cuppen JJM, Van Oosterom A. Model studies with inversely calculated isochrones of ventricular depolarization. IEEE Trans Biomed Eng 1984; 31:652–59.
13. Huiskamp G, Greensite F. A new method for myocardial activation imaging. IEEE Trans Biomed Eng 1997; 44:433–46.
14. Tilg B, Fischer G, Modre R, et al. Model-based imaging of cardiac electrical excitation in humans. IEEE Trans Med Imaging 2002; 21:1031–9.
15. Berger T, Fischer G, Pfeifer B, et al. Single-beat noninvasive imaging of cardiac electrophysiology of ventricular pre-excitation. J Am Coll Cardiol 2006; 48:2045–52.

16. He B, Wu D. Imaging and visualization of 3-D cardiac electric activity. IEEE Trans Inf Technol Biomed 2001; 5:181–6.

17. Li G, He B. Localization of the site of origin of cardiac activation by means of a heart-model-based electrocardiographic imaging approach. IEEE Trans Biomed Eng 2001; 48:660–9.

18. He B, Li G, Zhang X. Noninvasive three-dimensional activation time imaging of ventricular excitation by means of a heart-excitation model. Phys Med Bio 2002; 47:4063–78.

19. Ohyu S, Okamoto Y, Kuriki S. Use of the ventricular propagated excitation model in the magnetocardiographic inverse problem for reconstruction of electrophysiological properties. IEEE Trans Biomed Eng 2002; 49:509–19.

20. Skipa O, Sachse NF, Werner C, et al. Transmembrane potential reconstruction in anisotropic heart model. Int J of Bioelectromagnetism 2002; 4:17–8.

21. Zhang X, Ramachandra I, Liu Z, et al. Noninvasive three-dimensional electrocardiographic imaging of ventricular activation sequence. Am J Physiol Heart Circ Physiol 2005; 289: H2724–32.

22. Liu Z, Liu C, He B. Noninvasive reconstruction of three-dimensional ventricular activation sequence from the inverse solution of distributed equivalent current density. IEEE Trans Med Imaging 2006; 25:1307–18.

23. Han C, Liu Z, Zhang X, et al. Noninvasive three-dimensional cardiac activation imaging from body surface potential maps: a computational and experimental study on a rabbit model. IEEE Trans Med Imaging 2008; 27:1622–30.

24. Liu C, Skadsberg ND, Ahlberg SE, et al. Estimation of global ventricular activation sequences by noninvasive three-dimensional electrical imaging: validation studies in a Swine model during pacing. J Cardiovasc Electrophysiol 2008; 19:535–40.

25. Ideker RE, Bandura JP, Cox JW Jr, et al. Path and significance of heart vector migration during QRS and ST-T complexes of ectopic beats in isolated perfused rabbit hearts. Circ Res 1977; 41:558–64.

26. Okamoto Y, Teramachi Y, Musha T. Limitation of the inverse problem in body surface potential mapping. IEEE Trans Biomed Eng 1983; 30:749–54.

27. Parson I, Downar E. Clinical instrumentation for the intra-operative mapping of ventricular arrhythmias. Pacing Clin Electrophysiol 1984; 7:683–92.

28. Barr RC, Ramsey M 3rd, Spach MS. Relating epicardial to body surface potential distributions by means of transfer coefficients based on geometry measurements. IEEE Trans Biomed Eng 1977; 24:1–11.

29. Hansen PC. Analysis of discrete ill-posed problems by means of the L-curve. SIAM Rev 1992; 34:561–80.

30. Ramanathan C, Jia P, Ghanem RN, et al. Activation and repolarization of the normal human heart under complete physiological conditions. Proc Nat Acad Sci U S A 2006; 103:6309–14.

31. Fischer A. Optimization techniques in cardiac resynchronization therapy. Future Cardiol 2009; 5:355–65.

32. Greensite F. Remote reconstruction of confined wavefront propagation. Inv Prob 1995; 11:361–70.

33. Geselowitz DB, Miller WT. A bidomain model for anisotropic cardiac muscle. Ann Biomed Eng 1983; 11:191–206.

34. Avari JN, Rhee EK. Cardiac resynchronization therapy for pediatric heart failure. Heart Rhythm 2008; 5:1476–8.

35. He B, Li G, Zhang X. Noninvasive imaging of ventricular transmembrane potentials within three-dimensional myocardium by means of a realistic geometry anisotropic heart model. IEEE Trans Biomed Eng 2003; 50:1190–202.

36. Helm P, Beg MF, Miller MI, et al. Measuring and mapping cardiac fiber and laminar architecture using diffusion tensor MR imaging. Ann N Y Acad Sci 2005; 1047:296–307.

37. Zhang Y, Zhu S, He B. A high-order finite element algorithm for solving the three-dimensional EEG forward problem. Phys Med Biol 2004; 49:2975–87.

38. Khoury DS, Taccardi B, Lux RL, et al. Reconstruction of endocardial potentials and activation sequences from intracavitary probe measurements. Localization of pacing sites and effects of myocardial structure. Circulation 1995; 91:845–63.
39. Khoury DS, Berrier KL, Badruddin SM, et al. Three-dimensional electrophysiological imaging of the intact canine left ventricle using a noncontact multielectrode cavitary probe: study of sinus, paced, and spontaneous premature beats. Circulation 1998; 97:399–409.
40. Schilling RJ, Peters NS, Davies DW. Simultaneous endocardial mapping in the human left ventricle using a noncontact catheter: comparison of contact and reconstructed electrograms during sinus rhythm. Circulation 1998; 98: 887–98.
41. He B. Imaging 3-dimensional cardiac electrical activity from intra-cavity potentials. Proceedings of the 28th Annual International Conference IEEE Engineering in Medicine and Biology Society 2006; 4519.
42. He B, Liu C, Zhang Y. Three-dimensional cardiac electrical imaging from intracavity recordings. IEEE Trans Biomed Eng 2007; 54:1454–60.

Chapter 19
Traditional Electrophysiological Mapping

Tushar V. Salukhe, Louisa Malcolme-Lawes, Pipin Kojodjojo, and Nicholas S. Peters

Abstract Technological advances over the last two decades have assisted the electrophysiologist in identifying tachycardia mechanisms and guiding ablation therapy. However, accurate analysis and interpretation of the surface electrocardiogram (ECG) and intracardiac signals remain fundamental to conventional mapping. This chapter details the three maneuvers most commonly employed, usually in combination, including activation sequence mapping, pace mapping, and entrainment. These techniques are essential in any standard electrophysiological study and apply to both focal and reentrant forms of tachycardia. Critical to the effective use of these maneuvers is a clear appreciation of the mechanism of tachycardia which is briefly outlined in this chapter.

19.1 Introduction

Enormous technological advances over the last two decades have assisted the electrophysiologist in identifying tachycardia mechanisms and guiding ablation therapy. Of late, these advances, however sophisticated, have done little more than convert data from conventional mapping maneuvers into a more a esthetic three-dimensional picture, a picture which most traditional electrophysiologists construct mentally. Accurate analysis and interpretation of the surface electrocardiogram (ECG) and intracardiac signals remain fundamental to conventional mapping. Three maneuvers most commonly employed, usually in combination, are activation sequence mapping, pace mapping, and entrainment. These techniques constitute the essentials of arrhythmia interrogation in any standard electrophysiological study and are applicable to both focal and reentrant forms of tachycardia. Critical to the effective use of these maneuvers is a clear appreciation of the mechanism of tachycardia. These will only be outlined here, as they are beyond the scope of this chapter.

T.V. Salukhe (✉)
Department of Cardiology, St. Mary's Hospital and Imperial College Healthcare NHS Trust, London, UK
e-mail: salukhe@aol.com

D.C. Sigg et al. (eds.), *Cardiac Electrophysiology Methods and Models*,
DOI 10.1007/978-1-4419-6658-2_19, © Springer Science+Business Media, LLC 2010

19.2   Description of Apparatus

19.2.1   Electrode Catheters

Diagnostic electrode catheter sizes 5–7 French (Fr) are most commonly used in adult electrophysiological studies. Each catheter has two or more electrode pairs to allow simultaneous pacing (via the distal pair in contact with endocardium) and recording (via the proximal pair). A selection of interelectrode spacing is available; 2 mm spacing provides very localized signals useful for understanding multicomponent electrograms, while greater electrode separation (5–10 mm) records signals reflecting a greater proportion of the cardiac chamber (Fig. 19.1).

19.2.2   Recording Apparatus

The physiological signals acquired via surface and intracardiac electrodes are typically <10 mV in amplitude. Considerable amplification is therefore required

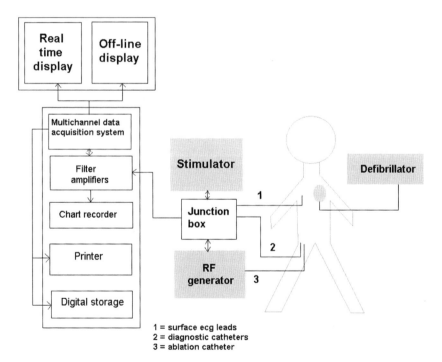

1 = surface ecg leads
2 = diagnostic catheters
3 = ablation catheter

Fig. 19.1 A standard digital electrophysiological monitoring setup is shown with patient stimulator and radiofrequency (RF) ablation generator. The diagnostic and ablation catheters are inserted via a sheath into the femoral vein and/or artery. The surface electrodes and defibrillator patch are attached via adhesive pads to the patient's skin

before the signals can be digitized, displayed, and stored. In addition, amplifiers require filters to eliminate any unwanted components of a signal. High-pass filters remove components below a certain frequency (typically 0.05 Hz to eliminate baseline drift), whereas low-pass filters remove components above a certain frequency (typically, filters of 500 Hz will eliminate any noise interference from nearby electrical equipment). A computerized data acquisition system will provide a real-time display from multiple selected recording channels, while providing a review screen for offline analysis and accurate measurement of intervals. Notch filters eliminate signals at a specific frequency (most commonly to eliminate main interference).

19.2.3   Stimulation Apparatus

A programmable stimulator is necessary to obtain data beyond the basic intracardiac conduction intervals and activation times. The stimulator is capable of delivering constant current pacing impulses, with expected thresholds of 3 mA and 2 mA in the atria and ventricles, respectively, with a 2-ms pulse width. Diseased myocardium may require higher current outputs. The stimulator is conventionally set at twice the measured diastolic threshold, and is capable of delivering simple pacing (inhibited or fixed), rapid pacing (rates of 300 bmp and over), single and multiple timed extra-stimuli following sensed beats, or a paced drive train.

19.3   Basic Mechanisms of Common Tachycardia

19.3.1   Reentry

Reentry is the most common mechanism for tachyarrhythmias. It is the first mechanism to consider for most arrhythmias interrogated at electrophysiological study and lends itself well to traditional mapping. Reentry is a perpetuating wavefront of activation rotating in circular fashion and requires three fundamental tissue properties to occur. These properties include two conduction conduits separated by non-excitable tissue, connected proximally and distally thus forming a circuit. Second, one conduit should have a refractory period significantly longer than the other. Third, the conduction velocity of the conduit with a shorter refractory period should be significantly slower than the other. At first, this complex arrangement may seem implausible. However, congenital (e.g., accessory atrioventricular or AV pathways) and acquired lesions (e.g., fibrotic scars of myocardial infarction) commonly harbor the properties required for reentry.

The final requirement for reentry is an appropriately timed premature extra-stimulus. When the premature stimulus arrives at the electrical conduit with fast conduction and long refractoriness (for example, conduit A), it will block as the conduit is still refractory from the previous stimulus. Instead, the premature impulse will conduct slowly via conduit B (slow conduction and short refractoriness). By the

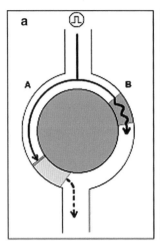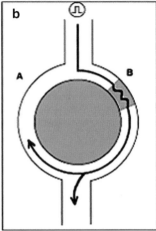

Fig. 19.2 (**a**) Premature beat propagating around the circuit. In conduit A, the wave of activation meets the refractory myocardium from the previous impulse and is blocked. In conduit B, the wave of activation slows as it passes through a zone of slow conduction. (**b**) The wave of activation in conduit B is able to continue propagating both onwards (anterogradely) from the circuit and back up (retrogradely) conduit A which is no longer refractory, and so the reentry circuit forms

time the premature stimulus has propagated via the slow conduit B, conduit A will have had time to recover from refractoriness and allow propagation in the opposite direction. If this impulse is again allowed to conduct down conduit B (as is likely, given its short refractory period), a perpetuating circuit is established (Fig. 19.2). As such, a premature impulse can also break the circus wavefront if it is timed to arrive and block in conduit B when it is refractory, and also block in conduit A as it collides with the wavefront advancing in the opposite direction.

19.3.2 Automaticity

All areas of myocardium have some degree of automaticity, most obviously in the sinoatrial node. This is due to (normal) acceleration of phase 4 of the action potential until threshold potential is reached, producing another action potential. Abnormally accelerated phase 4 depolarization results in abnormal automaticity and can occur in the atria, the AV junction, or ventricles. This mechanism accounts for 10% of tachycardia mechanisms (true focal tachycardias). Like the physiological properties of the sinus node, focal automatic tachycardias exhibit a warm and warm-down phenomenon at onset and offset, often due to physiological or metabolic stress such as ischemia, hypoxia, or electrolyte or acid–base imbalance. Such tachycardias are also amenable to mapping and ablation.

19.3.3   Triggered Activity

Late in phase 3 or early in phase 4 of the action potential, continued leakage of positive ions can cause smaller peaks of depolarization, called after-depolarizations. These can be of sufficient magnitude to reach threshold potential and generate another action potential, so-called triggered activity. Thus, triggered activity is similar to automaticity. However, triggered activity is not always spontaneous and can be provoked by an extra-stimulus much like reentry, and hence displays characteristics of both mechanisms. Early after-depolarizations, occurring in phase 3, are related to conditions which prolong the action potential such as hypokalemia, hypomagnesaemia, and class Ia and II antiarrhythmics. Prolongation of the action potential and early after-depolarization are exacerbated by increased cycle length of the previous beat, and this form of triggered activity is often called *pause-dependent*. Ischemia, congenital abnormalities, and digitalis can also lead to delayed after-depolarization in phase 4. These are generally not pause-dependant, but are exacerbated by sympathetic tone or so-called *catecholamine-dependent* triggered activity. Both pause-dependent and catecholamine-dependent triggered activity can manifest as QT interval prolongation and can result in significant ventricular arrhythmia. Arrhythmias with triggered mechanisms are generally amenable to ablation.

19.4   Activation Sequence Mapping

Activation sequence mapping is performed during tachycardia in an effort to describe a temporal sequence of myocardial activation. During activation mapping, the intracardiac signal is recorded at the tip of a roving mapping catheter and timed in as many chambers of the heart to which the arrhythmia mechanism is confined. Critically, the timing of the electrogram recorded at the tip of a roving catheter is compared with that of a constant and reliable reference, either a surface ECG or stable intracardiac signal, for example, a coronary sinus catheter electrogram. As the roving catheter is moved, the timing of the electrogram is continuously compared with the reference signal. In reentry tachycardias, this temporal relationship can be used to define the activation sequence during tachycardia around a well-defined circuit. Alternatively, the "earliest" endocardial signal can aide mapping focal or micro-reentrant tachycardias; this is done under fluoroscopic control and, as such, the temporal activation is given spatial connotation.

Focal arrhythmias are typically characterized by activation occurring less than 50 ms prior to systole timed from the surface ECG. Conversely, macro-reentrant arrhythmias demonstrate diastolic activity earlier (more) than 50 ms prior to systole. Intuitively, in macro-reentrant arrhythmias, intracardiac activity should be present at some location throughout the tachycardia cycle. For example, in typical anticlockwise atrial flutter, the macro-reentrant circuit is bound by two anatomic barriers: the tricuspid annulus anteriorly and the crista terminalis posteriorly. This circular activation route can be mapped throughout the cycle length of the tachycardia (Fig. 19.3).

In scar-related arrhythmias (e.g., ventricular tachycardia), the meandering, slow conducting route within scar provides the diastolic limb of the reentrant circuit. As the wavefront propagates out of this zone and into the healthy myocardium of the ventricle, the QRS complex of the ventricular tachycardia is generated. Thus during activation mapping any pre-systolic (pre-QRS) activation can be mapped at the exit site or in the diastolic conduit within the scar.

It is therefore essential to appreciate the mechanism involved when mapping, for what is early activation in focal tachycardia is not necessarily "early" in re-entrant tachycardia. The latter can be distinguished by activation throughout the tachycardia cycle length, earlier electrogram timing pre-systole, or mid-diastolic potentials. Mid-diastolic potentials are observed during tachycardia as discrete or complex signals within isoelectric signals which precede the systolic ECG deflection by more than 50 ms. These are thought to represent areas of slow conduction. Once recognized, it is important to establish their relevance to the tachycardia mechanism. If relevant, mid-diastolic potentials must be associated with every beat of tachycardia. This should be particularly evident at the onset of tachycardia. Importantly, these mid-diastolic potentials should be lost when tachycardia terminates and when pacing from the site in which they were recorded. If these criteria are satisfied, the potentials would be in keeping with a catheter position within the diastolic limb or critical isthmus of the reentrant tachycardia.[1] Mid-diastolic potentials which do not consistently precede every beat of tachycardia do not necessarily represent the critical isthmus of slow conduction to the tachycardia circuit, but rather a blind ally or bystander pathway within diseased myocardium or scar which is not integral to the tachycardia circuit.[2]

19.4.1 Local Electrogram Morphology

Electrogram timing is fundamental to the process of activation mapping, but valuable information can also be gained by assessment of the local electrogram morphology. Low amplitude (<0.5 mV in the atrium and <1.5 mV in the ventricle), high frequency signals are the hallmark of scar with duration and amplitude showing some correlation with zones of slow conduction.[3] In addition to myocardial health, local morphology can also give insight to tachycardia mechanism. Split potentials are high frequency potentials separated by an isoelectric interval of 50 ms and represent two local wavefronts colliding on either side of a zone of block or slow conduction (Fig. 19.4). Continuous, low-amplitude electrical activity (fractionated electrograms <70 ms duration) signifies local zones of slow conduction. Often, when recorded on bipoles of a single catheter, continuous fractionated signals can be seen to span the entire cycle length of tachycardia and represent a local micro-reentrant mechanism in a seemingly focal tachycardia.

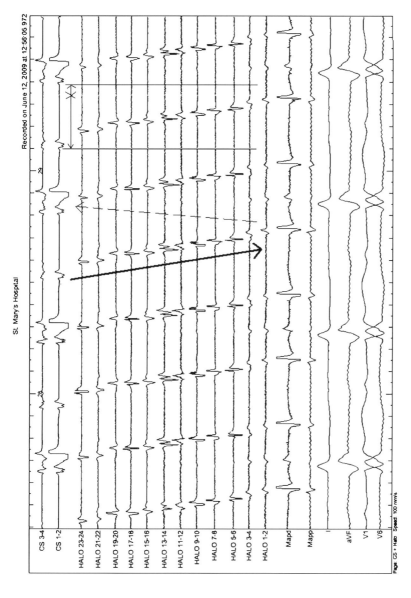

Fig. 19.3 Intracardiac electrograms from the top are quadripolar (4 pole) coronary sinus catheter, 20 pole catheter placed in the right atrium around the tricuspid annulus, proximal, and distal bipoles of the mapping catheter placed at the cavotricuspid isthmus and surface ECG leads. This demonstrates activation sequence from distal to proximal poles of the duodecapolar catheter; hence, in an anticlockwise direction around the tricuspid annulus during typical atrial flutter

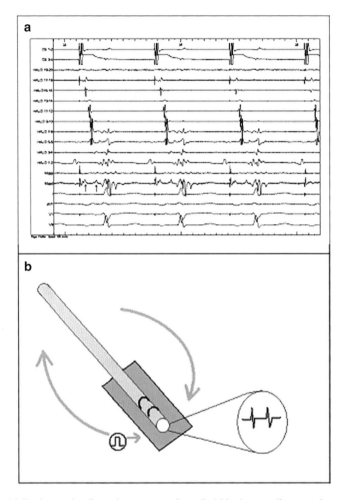

Fig. 19.4 (**a**) During pacing from the coronary sinus, 3–4 bipole recordings are demonstrated on the halo bipoles 1–20. A line of block has been produced by ablation at the cavotricuspid isthmus. Two discreet or "split" potentials can be seen on the distal bipole of the mapping catheter which is placed across the line of block. (**b**) The origin of these potentials is represented schematically as the first potential is caused by the activation front moving from the pacing site toward one side of the line of block, and the second potential is caused by the activation front traveling the long way round the circuit from the pacing site and toward the opposite side of the line of block

Activation mapping with unipolar potentials provides another useful dimension, particularly when mapping focal tachycardias. The unipolar "QS" morphology seen when mapping at the origin of a focal tachycardia has a sharp negative initial deflection because, at this point, the wavefront will always propagate away from the origin of the focal tachycardia. This unipolar "QS" potential configuration is associated with successful ablation of both focal atrial and ventricular tachycardias.[4]

19.4.2 Sinus Rhythm Mapping

In circumstances when tachycardia is poorly tolerated hemodynamically and activation mapping cannot therefore be performed, sinus rhythm mapping may be of value, specifically in scar-related reentrant arrhythmias. The areas of interest are those with abnormally late electrograms in sinus rhythm. These arise due to activation of slow conducting conduits within scar tissue, which is delayed after activation of the surrounding healthy myocardium.

Mapping studies have shown that up to 85% of ventricular tachycardias arise from areas of late potential activity in sinus rhythm. However, such potentials are widespread in diseased, infarcted myocardium and are not specific to the critical isthmus for the tachycardia.[5,6] Furthermore, 15% of ventricular tachycardias demonstrate normal electrogram morphology during sinus rhythm mapping at the point of successful ablation.

While new technologies which enable single beat maps may have helped the mapping of hemodynamically intolerant arrhythmias, sinus rhythm mapping of late potential provides a useful adjunct to conventional activation mapping and can be used to guide ablation, particularly to bisect or encircle culprit zones.[7] Further evaluation of the predictive value of late potential ablation is clearly needed.

19.5 Pace Mapping

Pace mapping is based on the principle that pacing at the site of tachycardia origin or exit site, at a cycle length similar to the tachycardia, will result in the same myocardial activation sequence, thus generating P-waves or QRS complexes identical to those of clinical tachycardia. As the site of pacing gets closer to the tachycardia focus or exit, the degree of concordance of paced and tachycardia ECG across the 12 leads improves. The distinct advantage of this technique is that it can be performed in sinus rhythm and does not necessarily require tachycardia to be present. Like sinus rhythm mapping, it is particularly useful when tachycardia is hemodynamically compromising because only short bursts of pacing are required to verify ECG concordance. Pace mapping should be performed at the clinical tachycardia cycle length to reduce rate-dependent aberrancy in P-wave or QRS morphology caused by incomplete repolarization and fusion with preceding P- or T-waves on the surface ECG.[8]

Using the surface ECG to predict the origin or exit site of tachycardia has significant limitations, particularly in diseased myocardium. The presence of scar, fibrosis, or ischemia, as well as changes in cardiac chamber size, shape and myocardial mass all impact on the predictive power or P-wave or QRS morphology to localize tachycardia origin. It is therefore not surprising that pace mapping suffers the same limitations. Although it is common to achieve a pace map with perfect or near-perfect concordance across all 12 surface ECG leads, performing this without knowledge of the general area of tachycardia origin from other mapping techniques can be very difficult. ECG concordance is critical to success, and most investigators will report high levels of success only when ablating areas with a perfect 12-lead ECG match.[9,10] Often, movements within a few millimeters will result in significant changes in axis or even bundle branch morphology.[11]

The size of the tip of the mapping catheter, its angulation, polarity, and pacing output all influence the area to which the current is delivered, the sequence of myocardial activation, and resulting ECG morphology. QRS morphology is particularly susceptible to this effect. In reentrant ventricular tachycardia, the tachycardia QRS morphology results from ventricular activation in a circus movement, while during pace mapping in sinus rhythm, the QRS morphology results from centrifugal activation of the ventricle. This is partly because the activation wavefront will follow the path of least resistance activating normal myocardium first and partly because the functional nature of the critical isthmus exhibits different properties in sinus rhythm and tachycardia. For tachycardias with focal mechanisms, pace mapping in sinus rhythm is applied very well as both result from centrifugal ventricular activation, but this has limitations for localizing the entrance or exit sites of recurrent arrhythmias.

Pace mapping can be somewhat refined by demonstrating that the timing of other intracardiac references (e.g., the right ventricular or RV electrogram) is the same during pace mapping and clinical tachycardia. Alternatively, by pace mapping during a reentrant tachycardia (entrainment), the paced wavefront is no longer centrifugal, but rather forced around the circuit of reentry by the ensuing tachycardia. Thus, during entrainment of reentrant tachycardia, the degree of surface ECG concordance with the clinical tachycardia is a much more reliable predictor of proximity of the pacing site to the entrance or exit site of the critical isthmus than pace maps in sinus rhythm. Furthermore, when exact ECG concordance is achieved, the interval from the pacing artifact to onset of QRS is indicative of the position of pacing site along the critical isthmus; the longer the interval, the closer to the entrance site and the ideal location for ablation.[12] The principles and applications of entrainment are discussed further in the next section.

19.6   Entrainment

Entrainment is the most powerful diagnostic maneuver at the electrophysiologist's disposal, and is also used to guide ablation. Entrainment provides evidence of an excitable gap, supporting reentry as the mechanism. In reentry, the circus wavefront is bound in front by the leading depolarized myocardium and behind by the trailing refractory myocardium. The rest of the circuit remains "excitable" and therefore vulnerable to intrusion by other activation fronts. By pacing close to the reentry circuit at a rate slightly faster than the tachycardia cycle length, it is possible to invade the excitable gap, breach the reentry circuit, and thus entrain the tachycardia.[13–16] On the surface ECG, entrainment manifests as progressive fusion of P-waves (in atrial tachy-cardia) or QRS complexes (in ventricular tachycardia). Fusion of the surface ECG occurs as the activation front spreading centrifugally from the pacing invades the excitable gap and is physiologically forced around the reentry circuit; during entrainment, it does not complete the circuit, as it collides with the next paced beat which arrives at the next excitable gap as entrainment continues. With progressive fusion entrainment is said to be manifest. When pacing stops, the last paced beat to invade the excitable gap continues uninterrupted around the reentrant circuit before tachycardia continues. This last paced beat is therefore entrained but not fused.

Once entrainment is confirmed (i.e., manifest), it can be used to map the tachycardia. This is done qualitatively by assessing the concordance between the fused and tachycardia ECG (Fig. 19.5a), and quantitatively by examining the post pacing interval (Fig. 19.5b). As the site of pacing approaches the tachycardia circuit, the concordance between tachycardia and paced ECG improves. When concordance is exact and fusion cannot be demonstrated, entrainment is said to be concealed. Thus, fusion (manifest entrainment) confirms reentry as the mechanism and concealed entrainment suggests the site of pacing is at or very close to the critical isthmus of the reentry circuit.

19.6.1 End-Entrainment Data

The post pacing interval (PPI) is the time taken for the activation front of the last entrained beat to reach the site of pacing after pacing has stopped. If the site of pacing is within the reentry circuit, then the PPI will equate to the tachycardia cycle length. If distant from the circuit, the PPI will be longer than the tachycardia cycle length because it will include the time taken for the last entrained beat to traverse the reentry

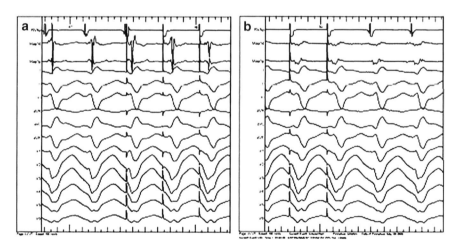

Fig. 19.5 (**a**) Pacing at the mapping catheter produces an identical ventricular morphology at a marginally faster cycle length compared with initial ventricular tachycardia. (**b**) With termination of pacing, the cycle length returns to its previous duration with a short post pacing interval, confirming concealed entrainment of ventricular tachycardia

circuit (the tachycardia cycle length), plus the time taken to reach the circuit from the pacing site and back again. Hence, the PPI provides a measure of proximity of the pacing catheter to the circuit, with a PPI of within 20–30 ms of the tachycardia cycle length considered to be within a critical part of the reentry circuit.

End-entrainment data can also provide critical diagnostic information. This is particularly helpful in the diagnosis of narrow complex tachycardia (NCT), where the three broad diagnostic groups include atrial tachycardia (AT), AV nodal reentry tachycardia (AVNRT), and accessory pathway-mediated AV reentry tachycardia (AVRT). The anatomy and physiology of these arrhythmias will be briefly outlined to support the relevant discussion. Atrial tachycardias, whether focal or reentrant, have an origin confined to the atria. When conducted to the ventricles (via the AV node) in a 1:1 ratio, ATs are often indistinguishable from AVNRT or AVRT on surface ECG and intracardiac signals. In AVNRT, the mechanism is always reentry with the circuit largely confined to the AV node. The atria and ventricles are not critical to the circuit and are most commonly activated simultaneously in a 1:1 ratio. In AVRT, the atria, AV node, ventricles, and an accessory pathway all constitute the reentry circuit. Very often, these tachycardias have very similar surface ECG morphologies and intracardiac signals, particularly if the accessory pathways of AVRT are central or close to the AV node. All three are amenable to ablation but require completely different techniques, therefore accurate diagnosis is critical. For this purpose, entrainment from the ventricles is a reliable and reproducible maneuver. The end-entrainment activation sequence and PPI are pertinent to diagnosis.

It is possible to entrain an AT via retrograde conduction through the AV node by pacing the ventricle (usually the RV apex) at a rate slightly faster than the tachycardia rate. Upon termination of pacing, the last paced beat in the ventricle (V) conducts retrograde to entrain the last atrial beat (A). The next recorded activation, as AT ensues, will occur again in the atrium (A) and subsequently conduct via the AV node down to the ventricle (V). This V–A–A–V response to the end of entrainment from the ventricle helps distinguish AT from AVNRT and AVRT (Fig. 19.6).[17] If the NCT terminates during ventricular pacing without any preceding change in atrial cycle length, then AT can be excluded as a possible diagnosis.

Entrainment of AVNRT and AVRT is also possible from the ventricle. Here the activation sequence and the end of entrainment is typically V–A–V as tachycardia continues. When a V–A–V sequence is observed, the PPI and the stimulation-to-A time (during entrainment) and V-to-A time (during tachycardia) can distinguish AVNRT from AVRT (Fig. 19.7). In AVNRT, the RV pacing site is distant from the reentry circuit within the AV node, whereas in AVRT, because the ventricle is part of the circuit, the RV pacing site is much closer to the circuit. Therefore, the PPI when entraining from the RV apex is typically longer in AVNRT (>115 ms) than AVRT (<115 ms).[17–19] For similar reasons, the difference between the RV stimulation-to-A time and the V-to-A time is longer in AVNRT (>85 ms) than AVRT (<85 ms). These boundaries of 115 ms for PPI and 85 ms for stimulation-to-A time/V-to-A time difference are generally reliable. Occasionally, measurements are very close to these cutoff times and it becomes

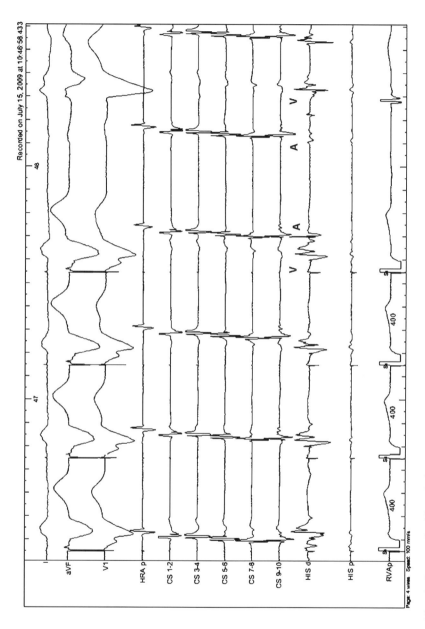

Fig. 19.6 After the last entrained beat during entrainment of tachycardia by ventricular pacing, a V–A–A–V response is seen, confirming atrial tachycardia as the mechanism of tachycardia

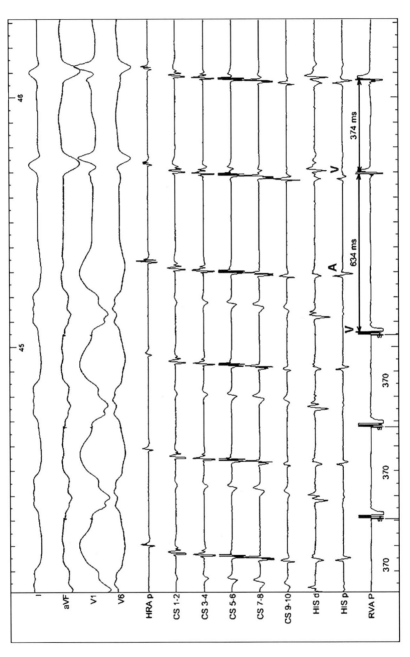

Fig. 19.7 After the last entrained beat during entrainment of tachycardia by ventricular pacing a V–A–V response is seen with resumption of the tachycardia. The post pacing interval is 364 ms, which is greater than 115 ms, demonstrating atrioventricular nodal reentry tachycardia (AVNRT) as the likely mechanism of tachycardia

more difficult to confidently distinguish the two arrhythmias. In this situation, alternative pacing maneuvers can be employed to support a diagnosis. These are discussed in the next section.

19.7   Additional Mapping Maneuvers

19.7.1   Node-Refractory Ventricular Pacing During NCT

Perhaps the most common maneuver used when a NCT is observed in the electrophysiology laboratory is the delivery of a single, premature ventricular paced beat (PVC) at the precise time the AV node is refractory, therefore not allowing retrograde nodal conduction to the atrium. To achieve this, a PVC is timed to synchronize with the His signal on the His catheter. A His-synchronous PVC is confirmed by a fused QRS complex. The His-synchronous PVC becomes of diagnostic utility if it advances or delays the next atrial beat or if it terminates tachycardia (Fig. 19.8). All three results indicate the presence of an accessory pathway. However, only if the subsequent atrial beat is delayed or if tachycardia consistently terminates does it imply that the accessory pathway is part of the circuit and the diagnosis is AVRT. If the atrial cycle length remains unaltered when a PVC is delivered greater than 30 ms prior to the next expected His bundle complex and close to the earliest A, it is considered diagnostic of absence of an accessory pathway.

19.7.2   Parahissian Pacing

When the existence of an accessory pathway (particularly a central accessory pathway) is in doubt, Parahissian pacing can be helpful. In this maneuver, the VA time is the relevant observation. The His bundle is paced directly at the His catheter position; this results in retrograde activation of the atrium via the AV node, normal activation of the ventricles via the His-Purkinje system, and a normal QRS complex. The pacing voltage is then reduced such that the His bundle captures longer and only the local myocardium is activated. The subsequent ventricular activation now spreads via direct activation of the local RV myocardium and manifests on the ECG as left bundle branch block. Retrograde atrial activation then takes much longer as it spreads through myocardium, into the Purkinje system, into the His bundle, and back up the AV node. Thus, in the absence of a centrally located accessory pathway and if VA conduction is exclusively nodal, Parahissian pacing results in a short VA time with direct His capture and long VA time without His capture (Fig. 19.9). In the presence of an accessory pathway, VA conduction occurs via the pathway and is therefore independent of His capture. Hence, the VA time will remain constant during this maneuver.[20]

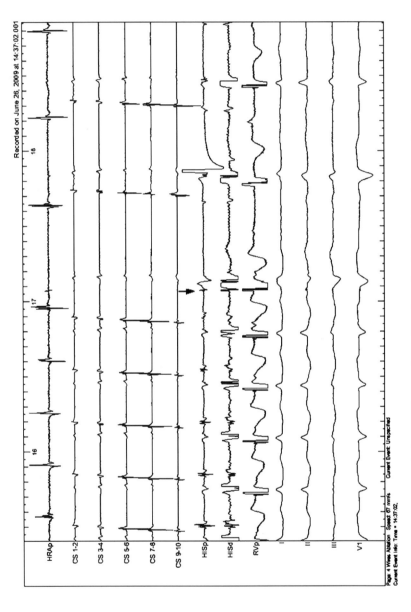

Fig. 19.8 A His-synchronous premature ventricular paced beat terminates the tachycardia without atrial capture, suggesting the presence of an accessory pathway

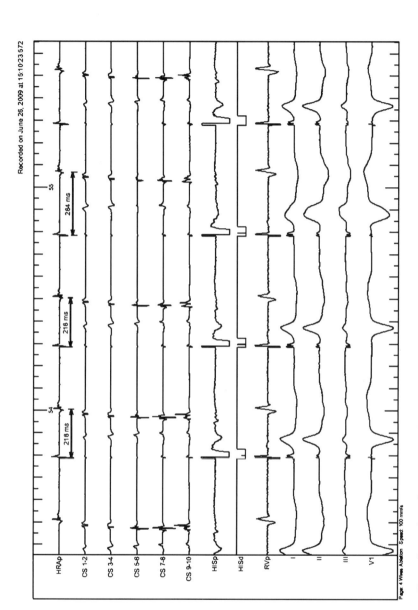

Fig. 19.9 Intracardiac catheters from the top are the high right atrial, coronary sinus, His, right ventricular and mapping catheters, then surface ECG leads. The first and second paced beats have a VA time of 218 ms, whereas the third beat has a VA time of 284 ms. This prolongation of conduction time (nodal response) with loss of His capture is suggestive that a retrogradely conducting accessory pathway is not present

19.8   Pitfalls and Troubleshooting

While it is important to use appropriate filters to provide clean intracardiac signals, it is also necessary to be aware of the effects of specific filters on physiological signals to avoid misinterpretation and the loss of clinically relevant signals. Close attention should be paid to elimination of the noise source rather than filtering in the first instance, and careful skin preparation should be carried out when placing surface electrodes to prevent poor contact. Arrhythmias are commonly, often intentionally, induced during electrophysiological studies. However, occasionally, if the arrhythmia is poorly tolerated, it may be necessary to terminate the arrhythmia; this can be done either by programmed stimulation or an external cardiac defibrillator.

Even the perfect electrophysiological study is not without risk to the patient. The access route for catheters is via the femoral vein or artery, and significant vascular damage and or hemorrhage may occur in a small percentage of cases. The risk of hemorrhage is increased by the requirement for routine anticoagulant use in order to prevent the formation of thrombus on the catheter surface. In spite of anticoagulant use, thromoembolism causing stroke or transient neurological deficit occurs in a small number of cases. Tamponade (perforation of the ventricle or atrium) is one of the most serious complications that can occur during catheter manipulation within the cardiac chambers. It is more likely, however, to occur during the application of radiofrequency energy required for ablation procedures. The overall occurrence of complications is approximately 2–4% of cases, however less than 0.1% of these are life-threatening.

19.9   Summary

There are various techniques at the electrophysiologist's disposal to confirm or refute diagnoses and, rarely in clinical electrophysiology, can a single pacing maneuver or mapping technique confirm a diagnosis or guide definitive treatment. The successful electrophysiologist will use a combination of observation of spontaneous phenomenon and forced maneuvers to reach the most likely diagnosis. Fundamental to the interpretation of these events is a clear appreciation of arrhythmia mechanism and normal physiology. Many complex electro-anatomical mapping systems have been developed to facilitate this process (as described in more detail in Chap. 17), but the basic data inputs for any and all of these systems are exactly those described above in tradition mapping techniques, namely the ECG, electrograms, their timing and morphology. Thus, in the midst of ongoing technological progress, traditional mapping remains the bread and butter of clinical electrophysiology.

References

1. Wen MS, Yeh SJ, Wang CC, et al. Successful radiofrequency ablation of idiopathic left ventricular tachycardia at a site away from the tachycardia exit. J Am Coll Cardiol 1997; 30:1024–31.
2. Stevenson WG, Weiss JN, Wiener I, et al. Fractionated endocardial electrograms are associated with slow conduction in humans: evidence from pace-mapping. J Am Coll Cardiol 1989; 13:369–76.
3. Cassidy DM, Vassallo JA, Miller JM, et al. Endocardial catheter mapping in patients in sinus rhythm: relationship to underlying heart disease and ventricular arrhythmias. Circulation 1986; 73:645–52.
4. Man KC, Daoud EG, Knight BP, et al. Accuracy of the unipolar electrogram for identification of the site of origin of ventricular activation. J Cardiovasc Electrophysiol 1997; 8:974–9.
5. Cassidy DM, Vassallo JA, Buxton AE, et al. The value of catheter mapping during sinus rhythm to localize site of origin of ventricular tachycardia. Circulation 1984; 69:1103–10.
6. Schilling RJ, Peters NS, Davies DW. Simultaneous endocardial mapping in the human left ventricle using a noncontact catheter: comparison of contact and reconstructed electrograms during sinus rhythm. Circulation 1998; 98:887–98.
7. Marchlinski FE, Callans DJ, Gottlieb CD, et al. Linear ablation lesions for control of unmappable ventricular tachycardia in patients with ischemic and nonischemic cardiomyopathy. Circulation 2000; 101:1288–96.
8. Goyal R, Harvey M, Daoud EG, et al. Effect of coupling interval and pacing cycle length on morphology of paced ventricular complexes. Implications for pace mapping. Circulation 1996; 94:2843–9.
9. Klein LS, Shih HT, Hackett FK, et al. Radiofrequency catheter ablation of ventricular tachycardia in patients without structural heart disease. Circulation 1992; 85:1666–74.
10. Calkins H, Kalbfleisch SJ, el-Atassi R, et al. Relation between efficacy of radiofrequency catheter ablation and site of origin of idiopathic ventricular tachycardia. Am J Cardiol 1993; 71:827–33.
11. Kadish AH, Childs K, Schmaltz S, Differences in QRS configuration during unipolar pacing from adjacent sites: implications for the spatial resolution of pace-mapping. J Am Coll Cardiol 1991; 17:143–51.
12. Brunckhorst CB, Stevenson WG, Soejima K, et al. Relationship of slow conduction detected by pace-mapping to ventricular tachycardia re-entry circuit sites after infarction. J Am Coll Cardiol 2003; 41:802–9.
13. Stevenson WG, Khan H, Sager P, et al. Identification of reentry circuit sites during catheter mapping and radiofrequency ablation of ventricular tachycardia late after myocardial infarction. Circulation 1993; 88:1647–70.
14. Waldo AL. Atrial flutter: entrainment characteristics. J Cardiovasc Electrophysiol 1997; 8:337–52.
15. Waldo AL, Henthorn RW. Use of transient entrainment during ventricular tachycardia to localize a critical area in the reentry circuit for ablation. Pacing Clin Electrophysiol 1989; 12:231–44.
16. Henthorn RW, Okumura K, Olshansky B, et al. A fourth criterion for transient entrainment: the electrogram equivalent of progressive fusion. Circulation 1988; 77:1003–12.
17. Knight BP, Ebinger M, Oral H, et al. Diagnostic value of tachycardia features and pacing maneuvers during paroxysmal supraventricular tachycardia. J Am Coll Cardiol 2000; 36:574–82.
18. Michaud GF, Tada H, Chough S, et al. Differentiation of atypical atrioventricular node re-entrant tachycardia from orthodromic reciprocating tachycardia using a septal accessory pathway by the response to ventricular pacing. J Am Coll Cardiol 2001; 38:1163–7.
19. Miller JM, Rosenthal ME, Gottlieb CD, et al. Usefulness of the delta HA interval to accurately distinguish atrioventricular nodal reentry from orthodromic septal bypass tract tachycardias. Am J Cardiol 1991; 68:1037–44.
20. Hirao K, Otomo K, Wang X, et al. Para-Hisian pacing. A new method for differentiating retrograde conduction over an accessory AV pathway from conduction over the AV node. Circulation 1996; 94:1027–35.

Chapter 20
Multi-channel System for Analysis of Cardiac Rhythmicity and Conductivity In Vitro

Yong-Fu Xiao

Abstract The microelectrode array (MEA) technology has been widely used in academic and industrial laboratories for revealing electrical activity of multiple electrogenic cells noninvasively. Scientists use this technology to study rhythmicity and conductivity of excitable cells and to assess the biological effect and safety of new drugs. This chapter describes how to use MEA technology to assess cellular electrophysiology of multiple cardiomyocytes in vitro. The MEA technique can monitor short- or long-term electrical activity of various types of cardiomyocytes or myocardial tissues under a relatively native environment. Compared with other approaches, the MEA method has several advantages, such as assessment of electrical interactions among cardiomyocytes at multiple sites, long-term monitoring of electrophysiological changes after chemical or biological treatment, and exceptional stability of signal recordings from contracting cardiomyocytes without damaging and interfering with the cells. However, compared to the patch clamp method, the MEA approach has little controllability of intracellular components. Generally speaking, the MEA technique is a fast, easy to handle, and efficient method to study the electrophysiological activity of excitable cells or tissues.

20.1 Introduction

Myocardium and other excitable tissues, such as neuronal and skeletal tissues, are electrically active. Continuous generation of action potentials in a heart is crucial for impulse conduction and excitation–contraction coupling. In a healthy human heart, the sinoatrial node generates rhythmic action potentials which propagate to the whole heart through a specific conduction system. Abnormalities of cellular excitability and/or wave conduction along the electrical pathway in a

Y.-F. Xiao (✉)
Cardiac Rhythm Disease Management, Medtronic, Inc., Mounds View, MN, USA
e-mail: yong-fu.xiao@medtronic.com

D.C. Sigg et al. (eds.), *Cardiac Electrophysiology Methods and Models*,
DOI 10.1007/978-1-4419-6658-2_20, © Springer Science+Business Media, LLC 2010

heart can lead to arrhythmias. In clinical cardiac electrophysiology, invasive or noninvasive methods are used to monitor cardiac electrical activity and determine the cause of rhythmic disturbances, as well as to provide the potentially best treatment. Cellular electrophysiology has been used to study electrical activity at cellular and molecular levels, which is invaluable for understanding the underlying mechanisms of cardiac rhythm and arrhythmia. Intracellular recordings, patch clamp methods for whole-cell or single channel recordings, or noninvasive extracellular recordings are widely used in experiments for studying action potentials, ion channels, and electrical conduction in single or multiple excitable cells.

Ion components (charges) of cardiomyocytes are different between the interstitial fluid and cytoplasm due to the separation of the lipid bilayer membrane inserting with numerous protein channels and transporters. The electrochemical gradients result in a resting membrane potential. Chemical or electrical stimulation opens ion channels and initiates an action potential due to the movement of ions along their electrochemical gradients. Extracellular signals of excitable or electrogenic cells and tissues, such as neurons and cardiomyocytes, can be recorded with multiple electrodes in vitro. In the 1970s, Jerry Pine, Guenter Gross, and Charles Thomas independently created planar microelectrode arrays for simultaneously recording electrical activity from hundreds of neurons to investigate the computational properties of small neural networks.[1,2] This approach has been used in different studies for noninvasive recordings of extracellular electrical activity in the last three decades. More sophisticated Multi-channel Systems (MCS GmbH, Reutlingen, Germany) have since been developed, and recording methods and software have been greatly improved. In myocardium or in cultured cardiomyocytes, action potentials can propagate from one myocyte to the next via gap junctions. Such electrical propagation can be recorded and analyzed by microelectrode array (MEA) technology; such technology can be used noninvasively with a relatively undisturbed intracellular and extracellular environment and is able to simultaneously record electrical activity of a large number of cells for long-term observation.[3,4] This chapter discusses how to use MEA technology to assess rhythmicity and conductivity of cultured cardiomyocytes from an atrial cell line (HL-5 cells)[5] or from isolated neonatal rat heart cells. In some experiments, cultured cardiomyocytes were transfected with the gene of human cardiac pacemaker channels (hHCN4),[6] and the effect of hHCN4 on the spontaneous rate was assessed.

Cardiac conduction damage was induced by mechanical abrasion of cultured myocyte monolayers in MEA arrays and conduction repair was investigated by adding myocytes or noncardiomyocyte cells. The effects of pharmacological compounds on myocyte rhythmicity and conductivity were also investigated. Furthermore, this chapter summarizes the progress in research with MEA technology on rhythmicity and conductivity of cardiomyocytes derived from embryonic stem cells (ESCs),[7-10] on myocardial slices,[11-13] and on cardiac conduction repair with mesenchymal stem cells[14-16] or with ESC-derived cardiomyocytes.[17]

20.2   Multi-channel System

The Multi-channel System (MCS GmbH, Reutlingen, Germany) has been used to noninvasively assess electrical activity of excitable cells or tissues and interactions between cells. Extracellular field potentials of cardiomyocytes obtained with the MEA technique are smaller than transmembrane potentials, and amplitudes decrease with increasing distances of the signal source to the electrode. Therefore, attachment (interface) of cells or tissue to the electrodes of an array is crucial for having better biological signals. The time course of an extracellular field potential represents the same one of the change of the transmembrane potential. One setup of the Multi-channel System includes the hardware, data acquisition software, vibration isolation table, and other accessories.

20.2.1   Hardware

Dependent on experimental needs, different system configurations can be obtained from the supplier (MCS GmbH). Hardware includes an amplifier (MEA 1060-1 or 1060-2), array (typically 60 electrodes), computer, MC_Card, temperature controller (TC01 or TC02), stimulator (1000 or 2000 series), perfusion system (PH01), and various accessories (Fig. 20.1). Detailed information on each item can be obtained from the website of the manufacturing company (http://www.multi-channelsystems.com).

20.2.2   Data Acquisition and Analysis

The standard MEA60 System (MCS GmbH) is a complete system and is primarily recommended for in vitro recordings and data analysis of electrical activity from cardiomyocytes (Fig. 20.1). An array with an electrode diameter of 30 µm and spacing of 200 µm from the next electrode is generally used for obtaining electrograms from cultured cardiomyocytes (Fig. 20.1c, d). Raw data from up to 60 MEA electrodes are amplified by 60 channels of filter amplifiers. A computer with preinstalled data acquisition software from the manufacturer can effectively record electrical signals from the cardiomyocytes cultured on the top of the electrodes of an array. The MC_Card acquires and digitizes analog input signals. The MC_Rack program can be easily used for recording and displaying data during or after an experiment. This program also can graph, analyze, review, and export recorded data. In parallel to MEA extracellular recording, additional signals (such as from patch clamp amplifiers or camera imaging) can be synchronized and recorded.[3,4,18]

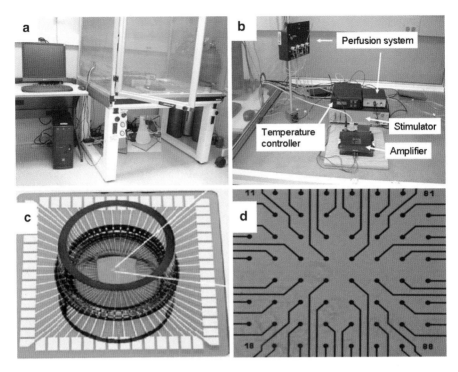

Fig. 20.1 Setup of a microelectrode array (MEA) obtained from Multi-channel Systems (MCS GmbH, Reutlingen, Germany). (**a**) Complete system for the MEA technology with a Faraday cage, isolating air-float table, amplifier, temperature controller, computer loaded with the data acquisition and analysis software, and solution perfusion system. (**b**) Enlarged photo of the amplifier, temperature controller, stimulator, and perfusion system. (**c**) Array of 60 electrodes (200 μm apart from the next electrode and 30 μm in diameter of each electrode) routinely used in many cardiomyocyte experiments for field potential recordings. (**d**) 60 electrodes arranged at the bottom of the left MEA chamber (see details at http://www.multichannelsystems.com)

20.2.3   Vibration Isolation and Noise Reduction

Due to significant amplification of biological signals, vibration of the MEA recording system can cause significant noise which may deflect interested signals during data collection. According to our own experience, an isolating air-float table is needed for a MEA amplifier setup (Fig. 20.1). The amplitude of interested biological signals and level of background noise (the ratio) are critical for obtaining useful biological signals and for late data analysis. A Faraday cage and good ground connection can be very helpful to reduce noise level (Fig. 20.1). The ratio between biological signal and noise is also very much determined by the interface between the electrodes and cells. Therefore, any effort to improve the interface will reduce noise. To get better attachment and cell growth for different types of cardiomyocytes, such as HL-5 or neonatal rat cardiomyocytes, MEA chambers need to be coated with different optimized compounds (Figs. 20.2 and 20.3).

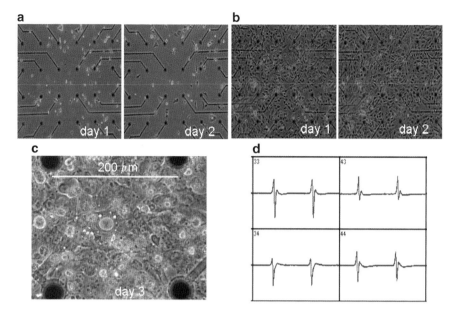

Fig. 20.2 Effects of microelectrode array (MEA) chamber coating on the growth of HL-5 cells. Phase-micrographs on day 1 and 2 of HL-5 cells plated to a MEA chamber coated with polyethyleneimine (0.1%) (**a**) and to a MEA chamber coated with gelatin (0.1%) plus fibronectin (0.02%) (**b**). Monolayer of HL-5 cells on day 3 after plating to the MEA chamber was formed (**c**) and spontaneous field potentials were recorded from electrodes 33, 34, 43, and 44 (**d**). The MEA chambers were coated overnight, washed three times with Dulbecco's phosphate-buffered saline (DPBS), and seeded with 1 to 1.25×10^6 HL-5 cells. Not many cells attached to the substrate by day 1 and 2, and little proliferation was observed in the chamber coated with polyethyleneimine [panel (**a**)]. However, many cells attached to the substrate on day 1 [panel (**b**)] and formed a monolayer on day 3 in the chamber coated with gelatin plus fibronectin [(panel **c**)]

20.3   Rhythmicity of Cultured Cardiomyocytes

Cardiac tissue in vitro or cultured cardiomyocytes can beat spontaneously under a physiological environment or can be stimulated by electrical pulses or chemical compounds. The Multi-channel System has made it possible to simultaneously and noninvasively record the rhythmicity and conductivity of large numbers of cardiomyocytes in vitro. Isolated cardiomyocytes or cardiac cells from a cell line or derived from ESCs can be plated and cultured in MEA chambers for days and weeks. Extracellular electrical signals from cardiomyocytes of multiple sites during excitation can be simultaneously assessed by MEA electrograms. In addition, cardiac tissue freshly sliced from a heart can be placed directly on the electrodes of an array. The electrical activity of the myocardial tissue on the electrodes can be studied. The effect and toxicity of pharmacological compounds or gene transfers on cardiomyocyte rhythm and rate can be assessed with the MEA technology.

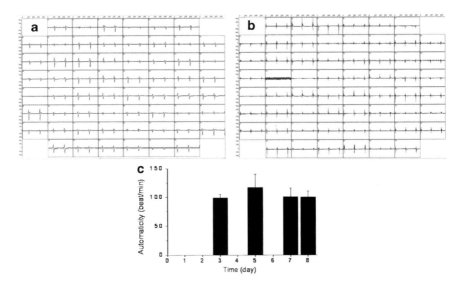

Fig. 20.3 Automaticity of mouse atrial HL-5 cells cultured in microelectrode array (MEA) chambers coated with gelatin/fibronectin. Electrograms show spontaneous beating activity of the HL-5 cells on day 3 after plating (**a**). The automaticity of the cultured HL-5 cells was very similar on day 8 (**b**), and was relatively stable during the culture for 8 days (**c**)

20.3.1 HL-5 Cells

HL-5 cells are cultured murine atrial cardiomyocytes. Both the HL-5 cell line and HL-1 cell line were derived from the AT-1 cell line by Claycomb and his coworkers.[5,19] HL-5 cells can be serially passaged after culture while maintaining a differentiated phenotype. An important feature is that both HL-1 and HL-5 cells can be recovered from frozen stocks or refrozen for later use. These cell lines have been used in studies to address cardiac cellular electrophysiology[20] and other important cellular and molecular questions.[21,22]

To study the rhythm and spontaneous beating rate, HL-5 cells were plated on standard planar MEAs containing 60 electrodes (inter-electrode distance, 200 μm; electrode diameter, 30 μm) and cultured at 37°C under an atmosphere of 5% CO_2 and 95% air with approximately 95% humidity. HL-5 cells attached and grew better in MEAs precoated with gelatin plus fibronectin (Fig. 20.2b) than in those coated with polyethyleneimine (Fig. 20.2a). Cells were maintained in Claycomb medium[19] (JRH Biosciences, Lenexa, KS, USA), supplemented with 10% fetal bovine serum (Life Technologies, Inc., Rockville, MD, USA), 4 mM L-glutamine (Life Technologies), and 10 μM norepinephrine (Sigma Aldrich, St. Louis, MO, USA). As each array had a limited volume (<2 ml) and as HL-5 cells proliferated quickly, nutrition in such a small volume to maintain a healthy culture was very limited. Therefore, the medium needed to be changed frequently (every 24 h) at early culture stage and every 12 h at late stage. However, if fewer numbers of HL-5 cells could be plated in a small surrounding area of the recording electrodes (Fig. 20.1d) of each array, the medium could be changed every 48 h without affecting cell growth and function. To do that, 30 µl of the medium containing HL-5 cells (1.25×10^6 cells) were plated into the central electrode area of each array. The arrays with plated cells were incubated in a culture incubator for 50 min to let cells attach to the bottom. Additional medium (1 ml/array) was carefully and gently added into each array for culture.

Fully confluent cultures of HL-5 cells were formed on day 3 after plating cells into an array (Fig. 20.2c) and beat spontaneously (Fig. 20.2d). Electrograms of synchronized field potentials were acquired from the 60 electrodes and recorded by a Multi-channel System which included the hardware and software (MCS GmbH). The recordings with a sampling rate of 5 kHz were conducted in 37°C controlled by a temperature control system (Fig. 20.1b). Spontaneous beating of cultured HL-5 cells lasted several days or weeks. Figure 20.3 shows that the rhythm and rate were relatively stable during an 8-day observation period, except for a minor increase on day 5. HL-5 cells proliferated quickly and the space of each array was very limited. Therefore, long-term observation (weeks or months) of electrical activity of HL-5 cells in the same array became difficult, because fast proliferation in a limited space and volume caused cell death and detachment from the electrodes.

20.3.2   Neonatal Rat Cardiomyocytes

Electrical properties of cultured newborn rat heart cells can be investigated by using microelectrophysiological methods. To assess the rhythm and spontaneous beating rate of cultured primary cardiomyocytes, atrial and ventricular myocytes were isolated from neonatal rats (Sprague–Dawley) according to a previous method.[23] Whole hearts were removed from newborn rats (1–3 days). The atria and ventricles were carefully dissected under a microscope and minced separately; minced heart tissue was incubated in an enzymatic solution. Isolated single cells were resuspended in a culture medium. Two 1.5 h preplating steps (incubation of cell suspension in 75 cm^2 flasks) were performed to separate slowly attaching cardiomyocytes from quickly attaching fibroblasts. After preplating, enriched cardiomyocytes were collected, resuspended, counted, and replated into pretreated MEAs with a density of 180,000 cells/cm^2. To improve the attachment of isolated cardiomyocytes, MEA chambers were pretreated with poly-L-lysine and coated with a complex of cell attachment factors containing collagen I, IV, fibronectin, and laminin on the day before cell isolation. Neonatal rat atrial and ventricular cardiomyocytes were cultured with norepinephrine (1 µM)/bromodeoxyuridine (BrDu, 100 µM) for 2 days, and then with BrDu alone for another 2 days. After forming a synchronized spontaneous beating monolayer, the culture was maintained in serum-free culture media which contained insulin, bovine serum albumin, and Vitamin B12. Electrograms of each array were recorded under 37°C. Figure 20.4 shows the monolayer of cultured neonatal rat ventricular myocytes in an array and electrograms recorded from the monolayer.

Spontaneous beating of the cultured monolayer of neonatal rat cardiomyocytes could be observed with a MEA system. Field potentials showed that neonatal rat ventricular

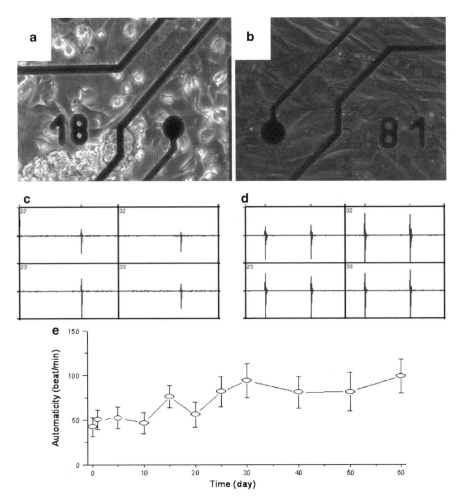

Fig. 20.4 Effects of microelectrode array (MEA) chamber treatment on the attachment and growth of neonatal rat ventricular myocytes. (**a**) Poor cell attachment and growth of neonatal rat ventricular myocytes were observed on day 5 after plating to a MEA chamber coated with collagen, fibronectin, and laminin. MEA recordings had unacceptably low amplitude of electrical signals. (**b**) Monolayer of neonatal rat ventricular myocytes was formed on day 5 after plating to a MEA chamber pretreated with poly-L-lysine and then coated with collagen, fibronectin, and laminin. Therefore, the bad attachment in panel (**a**) appeared related to the hydrophobic nature of MEA substrate. Cell attachment and growth, as well as quality of MEA recordings, were dramatically improved after pretreatment of MEA chambers with poly-L-lysine. Ventricular cells initially seeded with a density of 180,000 cells/cm^2 formed monolayer on day 5. Electrograms were recorded on day 0 (**c**) and day 60 (**d**) after forming a monolayer of neonatal rat ventricular myocytes. The average beating rates were gradually increased during the long-term culture (**e**)

myocytes beat at a relatively lower rate compared to atrial cells. Such rhythmic activity of cultured neonatal rat cardiomyocytes could last a few weeks or months if cells were cultured in an adequate medium and their medium was changed promptly every day (Fig. 20.4e). These data suggest that, as neonatal rat atrial or ventricular cardiomyocytes are primary cells with limited ability to proliferate, they can thus be very useful for studying long-term electrical activity of cardiomyocytes after treatment with biologics, such as antibodies, siRNAs, genes, or chemical compounds, such as drugs.

20.3.3   Cardiomyocytes Derived from Stem Cells

Embryonic stem cells derived from the inner cell mass of mammalian blastocysts can differentiate to cardiomyocytes which can be used for drug screen or toxicity testing; they can also potentially be used for cell transplantation. The MEA technology has been applied in in vitro studies of electrical properties of cardiac myocytes derived from mouse or human embryonic stem cells (mESCs or hESCs). During differentiation and cardiac maturation, molecular and functional changes associated with the development of electrical activity can be monitored when mESCs are cultured in MEA chambers.[7–10] Electrophysiological properties of multicellular cardiac clusters derived from ESCs can be examined during the ongoing differentiation process. The beating frequency of growing mESC preparations increased significantly concomitant to a decrease of the action potential duration and action potential rise time. A developmental increase in the expression of connexin-43 gap junction channels resulted in an increase in the conduction velocity of cardiomyocyte clusters derived from mESCs, similar to the development of a mouse embryonic heart.[18,24]

The Multi-channel System has also been used as a research tool in drug discovery and safety pharmacology with a combination of the use of hESC-derived cardiomyocytes.[25–27] ESC-derived cardiomyocytes can be cultured over an extended time in MEA chambers. Their electrophysiological properties can be continuously monitored under sterile conditions for acute or long-term drug testing. A major issue in cardiac safety pharmacology is QT prolongation by block of I_{Kr} currents (hERG channel), which can be monitored with a MEA system.[28] Another study has shown that functional cardiomyocytes can be differentiated from rhesus monkey rESCs.[29] MEA measurements revealed evidence of functionality, electrical coupling, and β-adrenergic signaling of the generated cardiomyocytes. These derived cardiomyocytes also can be used as a cell source for screening drugs for cardiac function and safety.[29] In addition, the spontaneous beating rates measured with the MEA technique are different among the cardiomyocytes derived from different sources or species. Specifically, HL-5 cells (120 ± 17 beats/min, $n = 17$) > neonatal rat atrial cells (100 ± 20 beats/min, $n = 24$) > cardiomyocytes derived from mESCs (72 beats/min varied with a range of 30–300 beats/min)[7,12] > neonatal rat ventricular cells (48 ± 15 beats/min, $n = 10$) > cardiomyocytes derived from hESCs (47 ± 5 beats/min, $n = 14$)[30] > cardiomyocytes derived from rESCs (42 ± 23 beats/min, $n = 6$).[29]

20.3.4   Myocardial Tissue Slices

In recent years, tissue slices from a heart have been used in studies for the evaluation of beating rate and signal propagation on standard planar MEAs.[11–13] The preparation and maintenance of slices from heart tissue of adult rats and guinea pigs for the evaluation of signal propagation on standard planar MEAs were described in a previous study.[31] The removed heart from an anesthetized animal was perfused with oxygenated physiological solution containing 10–15 mM 2,3-butanedione monoxime. Tissue blocks (4 mm × 6–8 mm) were prepared from the left ventricle. A block of tissue was glued to the cutting stage and sectioned by a precision vibratome to 300 μm thick transmural longitudinal, transverse slices. A slice was placed into an array chamber and an external stimulation electrode was implanted into the tissue. Extracellular field potentials and their propagation throughout the heart slice were assessed and combined with intracellular recordings simultaneously to verify tissue viability. Extracellular field potentials induced by electrical stimulation corresponded well to the first derivative of the intracellular action potentials and responded well to various chemical compounds for up to 30 h. These results demonstrated that acute heart slices prepared from adult rat or guinea pig heart could have normal physiological and pharmacological responses. Therefore, using heart slices for cardiac research can be highly valuable.

Another study evaluated extracellular field potentials of murine ventricular slices prepared from late-stage embryonic and neonatal murine hearts.[11] Field potentials of spontaneous beating or electrically stimulated tissue were recorded by a MEA system. The maximal negative deflection of the field potentials ($-dV/dt$) was assessed for the local activation time, creation of activation sequence maps, and estimation of conduction velocity. The results demonstrated that the combination of MEA with viable ventricular slice preparations provides a feasible and powerful technique to study cardiac anatomical structures and impulse propagation.

More recently, field potentials and activation sequences of Langendorff perfused guinea pig heart and rat cardiac tissue strips (5 mm × 5 mm) were studied by the MEA technique.[13] Field potentials recorded from the hearts showed a rate from 90 to 120 beats/min. The durations of the field potentials were 210 ± 78 ms for ventricular myocardium and 164 ± 58 ms for atrial myocardium. However, the durations of the field potentials were 115 ± 11 ms for ventricular strips and 83 ± 6 ms for atrial strips.[13] In addition, the MEA technique was used to assess whether mESC-derived cardiomyocytes served the pacemaker function after co-culture with mouse heart slices.[12] After 4 days in co-culture, beating rates were significantly higher in co-cultured slices (154 ± 22 beats/min, $p < 0.001$) than in control slices (49 ± 8 beats/min). These in vitro results suggest that mESC-derived cardiomyocytes can pace native heart tissue.

20.3.5 Biopacing Assessment

The sinoatrial node in the right atrium of a healthy human heart initiates rhythmic action potentials which propagate to the whole heart via the specific conductive system. A particular type of ion channel, the hyperpolarization-activated and cyclic nucleotide-gated (HCN) channel, plays a prominent role in the control of rhythmic electrical activity of the heart. HCN4 is the predominant isoform in the human sinoatrial node and thus plays a dominant role in cardiac rhythmicity.[32,33] Overexpression of hHCN4 could increase spontaneous beating rates of cardiomyocytes. We seeded mouse atrial HL-5 cells on the 60 electrodes of each array and measured electrograms to determine the effects of hHCN4 on beating rate. After 3 days in culture, HL-5 cells formed a monolayer (Fig. 20.5a) and showed synchronized spontaneous beating (Fig. 20.5c) with an average rate of 120 ± 17 beats/min ($n = 17$, Fig. 20.5e). Transfection of hHCN4-eGFP plasmid induced eGFP expression (Fig. 20.5b) and increased the beating rate by 65%, which reached 197 ± 16 beats/min ($n = 22$, $p< 0.01$, Fig. 20.5d, e). The effect of hHCN4 transfection on the automaticity of cultured HL-5 cells gradually increased over time and reached its peak on day 5 after transfection (Fig. 20.5f). After reaching its peak level, the rates

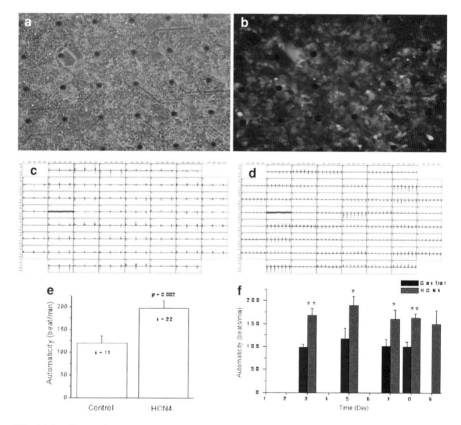

Fig. 20.5 Effects of hHCN4 transfection on automaticity of mouse atrial HL-5 cells. HL-5 cells were plated to gelatin/fibronectin-coded multielectrode arrays (MEAs) and transfected with hHCN4 gene. Monolayer was formed on day 3 (**a**, phase-contrast microscopy; **b**, fluorescence microscopy). Extracellular electrical activity (electrograms) was recorded from control (**c**) and hHCN4-transfected (**d**) HL-5 cells. (**e**) Averaged spontaneous firing rates of HL-5 cells with (HCN4) or without (control) hHCN4 plasmid transfection on day 5. (**f**) Time courses of spontaneous beating rates in control HL-5 cells (control, $n = 12$) and in cells with hHCN4 transfection ($n = 16$). *$p<0.05$; **$p<0.01$; versus control. n = number of arrays tested

began to decline, but still remained significantly higher than those of nontransfected cells (Fig. 20.5e). These results demonstrate that overexpression of hHCN4 increases myocyte automaticity for more than a week. Therefore, the MEA technology is a useful tool for the assessment of biological pacemaker activity in vitro.

20.3.6 Pharmacological Effects

The MEA approach is also very useful for assessing the pharmacological effect or toxicity of a compound on cardiac rhythmicity and conductivity.[4,34] Recently, we assessed the effects of the polyunsaturated fatty acid docosahexaenoic acid (C22:6n-3, DHA) on electrophysiology of multicellular preparations of cardiomyocytes. HL-5 murine atrial myocytes were cultured for 3 days to form a monolayer which showed spontaneous beating at a consistent rate. DHA inhibited the beating rate in a concentration-dependent manner (Fig. 20.6). Conduction velocity was slightly decreased by DHA. Washout of DHA with a solution containing 0.2% of bovine serum albumin was able to partially recover the rate.

It is well known that sympathetic stimulation increases heart rate. Therefore, we used the MEA technique to study the effect of cAMP on the spontaneous beating rate of cultured cardiomyocytes. To do that, cultured HL-5 cells in the arrays were perfused with a solution containing membrane permeable 8-Bromo-cAMP (200 μM) at 37°C. Figure 20.7 shows that cAMP stimulation caused an increase in the beating rate of HL-5 cells by 25.5 ± 8.5% for control ($n = 16$) and 39.5 ± 14.5% for hHCN4 transfection. These results demonstrate that HL-5 cells with or without hHCN4 transfection responded well to cAMP stimulation, and that the MEA technique can monitor these effects effectively.

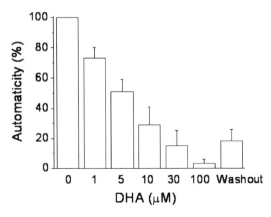

Fig. 20.6 The field potential frequency in the presence of various concentrations of docosahexaenoic acid (DHA). Note the decrease in frequency with an increase in DHA concentration; 100 μM DHA almost inhibited all activity. Washout (Washout) with the bath solution containing 0.2% bovine serum albumin partially recovered DHA-inhibited activity (mean ± SEM)

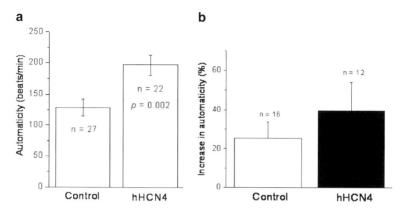

Fig. 20.7 Effects of cAMP on automaticity of HL-5 cells with or without hHCN4 transfection. (**a**) Averaged beating rates of HL-5 cells with (hHCN4) or without (control) gene transfection are shown. Rates were measured on day 3 after transfection and significantly increased after transfection. (**b**) Responsiveness to cAMP stimulation in HL-5 cells with (hHCN4) or without (control) gene transfection was measured on day 3 after transfection and normalized (%) to the beating rates in the absence of cAMP. Cyclic AMP significantly increased automaticity in the HL-5 cells with or without hHCN4 transfection, and had no significant difference between control and hHCN4-transfected groups. The p value is versus the control with the unpaired Student's t-test. n = number of arrays measured

Withdrawal or restrictions of a marketed drug can occur if it is found to cause a pro-arrhythmic side effect during clinical use. Therefore, a major concern in safety pharmacology is drug-induced QT interval prolongation. As the duration of action potentials of ventricular myocytes is closely related to the QT interval on an ECG, the ventricles of embryonic chickens have been used to partially reconstruct the shape and time course of the underlying action potential.[35] Field potentials recorded with the MEA technique can reflect the full range of mechanisms involved in cardiac action potential regulation. The MEA technology for screening compounds against QT interval prolongation in cardiomyocytes or heart tissue can avoid the problem of *false positives or negatives* by single cell assay.

Lack of an effective assay with human cardiac cells or tissue makes it difficult to detect side effects early during the development of a new medical drug. Recently, cardiomyocytes derived from hESCs were used for electrophysiological drug screening. Combination of single cell electrophysiology with MEA mapping in vitro detected the pro-arrhythmic property of a drug.[8] E-4031 and Sotalol (I_{Kr} blockers) significantly increased action potential duration and induced after-depolarizations. Multicellular aggregates of hESC-derived cardiomyocytes analyzed with the MEA technique showed that Class I (quinidine, procaineamide) and Class III (sotalol) antiarrhythmic agents, E4031, and cisapride (a noncardiogenic agent known to lengthen QT) resulted in dose-dependent prolongation of field potential duration. Conduction significantly slowed after adding the Na^+ channel blocker, quinidine or propafenone, and the gap junction blocker, 1-Heptanol.[8] In addition, the effects of a drug on QRS duration and amplitude, local activation time, T-wave amplitude, time of maximal slope of T-wave, QT interval duration, and activation refractory interval can be analyzed with the MEA technology.[35] Therefore, the MEA technique combined with hESC-derived cardiomyocytes can be very helpful for drug screening and cardiac toxicity analysis.

20.4 Cardiac Electrical Conductivity In Vitro

Signal propagation during excitation of cardiomyocytes in culture or in tissue slices can be captured by effective recordings of extracellular field potentials with a MEA system. Cellular electrophysiology of impulse conduction and propagation in cardiac tissue is extremely important for medical diagnosis, tissue repair, drug discovery, and toxicity analysis.

20.4.1 Conductivity Measurement

Conduction and propagation of cardiac impulses closely relate to electrical activity of the cardiomyocytes and the properties of their networks. Extracellular field potentials recorded from an electrode represent the assumption of electrical activity of a local cell population around the electrode. By analysis of a sequence in the occurrence of the spikes recorded from different electrodes, the direction of excitation spread can be determined (Fig. 20.8a). The origin of excitation and the direction of excitation spread in an array can be stable in the cardiomyocytes. The conduction velocity of field potential can be measured with a MEA system (Fig. 20.8). The delay of excitation spread from one electrode to another can be calculated against the respective distance between the electrodes. The conduction velocity was 2.96 ± 0.42 cm/s for cultured HL-5 mouse atrial cells and 1.24 ± 0.26 cm/s for neonatal rat atrial myocytes. Compared with neonatal rat atrial myocytes, the conduction velocity was faster for neonatal rat ventricular myocytes (2.76 ± 0.71 cm/s). Addition of the Ca^{2+} channel blocker nimodipine can cause failures of propagation.[36] Reduction of the voltage-gated Na^+ current by a channel blocker affects the negative spike amplitude and the maximal $-dV/dt$, which decrease conduction velocity of electrical impulse. Also, the duration of the spike plateau can be modulated by Ca^{2+} or K^+ channel blockers.[7] Therefore, the MEA technology can be helpful to determine the effects of a pharmacological compound on cardiac conductivity, which is a big concern related to drug safety.

20.4.2 Creation of Conduction Block

The MEA system can be very useful for assessment of cardiac conduction repair in vitro. Artificial conduction damage of cultured heart cells can be induced by a mechanical force. To do that, HL-5 mouse atrial cells were seeded on each standard planar MEA with 60 electrodes (inter-electrode distance, 200 µm; electrode diameter, 30 µm). A monolayer of cardiomyocytes was formed 3 days after seeding and beat

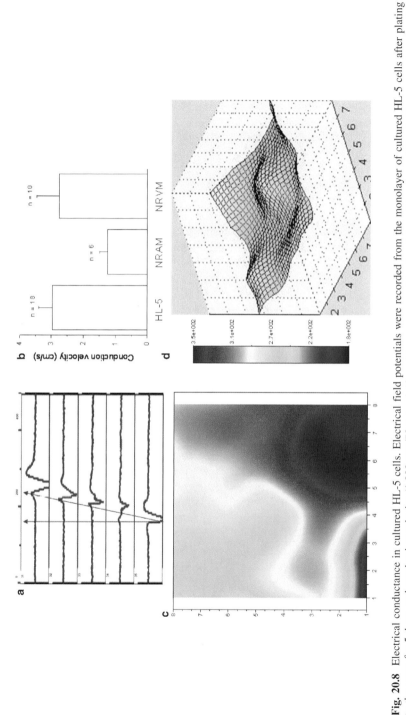

Fig. 20.8 Electrical conductance in cultured HL-5 cells. Electrical field potentials were recorded from the monolayer of cultured HL-5 cells after plating to the array for 5 days, and conduction velocity (1,000 mm/70 ms = 1.43 cm/s) was measured by the distance/time (**a**, *red lines*). The averaged conduction velocity of HL-5 cells, neonatal rat atrial myocytes (NRAM), and neonatal rat ventricular myocytes (NRVM) are shown in panel (**b**). Ventricular myocytes conducted impulses faster than the atrial cells. However, HL-5 cells also had high conduction velocity, which might result from their better attachment to the electrodes. Recorded electrograms could be reconstructed to 2D (**c**) and 3D (**d**) signal propagation waves

spontaneously and synchronously (Fig. 20.9). Conduction damage of a monolayer was created by carefully abrading a 600–700 μm channel in the middle of each array by using a 200 μl pipette tip (Fig. 20.9d). A thinner channel can be created if a smaller pipette tip (i.e., 50 μl) is used; however, a thinner channel may induce reconnection of originally separated cardiomyocytes, especially highly prolific HL-5 cells. Abrasion of the cardiomyocyte monolayer in each array should be done thoroughly to prevent any structure connection between the two sides. After abrasion, two fields of cardiomyocytes in each array were beating separately and asynchronously (Fig. 20.9e). After ensuring the presence of conduction block, cells targeted for conduction repair could be added to the abraded channel of each array for assessment of conduction repair. If electrical activity on one side crosses to the other side through the channel, conduction repair occurs. The two previously asynchronously beating cardiomyocyte fields should beat synchronously if electrical coupling forms.

In another study, electrograms of neonatal rat cardiomyocytes were recorded to confirm the presence of a synchronously beating monolayer.[37] The monolayer was divided into two fields of cardiomyocytes by an acellular channel from 250 to 350 μm wide, generated by two preprogrammed linear laser dissections. Removal of the strip of monolayer between the two laser dissection lines created an acellular channel that electrically separated the cardiomyocyte fields. After confirmation of conduction block, cells were added to the channel under a microscope with a pipette mounted in a micromanipulator to study conduction repair.[37]

20.4.3   Cardiac Fibrous Cells for Conduction Repair

As mature human myocardium has very limited ability to regenerate new myocardial tissue, cardiomyocyte death after myocardial infarction is replaced by scar tissue which contains electrically inert fibroblasts and an extracellular matrix. Areas with scar fibroblasts can cause slow conduction or conduction block. Also, fibroblasts modulate excitability and conduction properties of surrounding cardiomyocytes.[38] Previous studies have shown that cardiac fibroblasts have a limited capacity to conduct electrical current.[14,39,40] Electrical conduction among fibroblasts is slow and has a limitation in distance because of the nature of their nonexcitability and low levels of connexin expression. Therefore, scar tissue in the heart is potentially an arrhythmic substrate and prevention of its appearance can have an antiarrhythmic therapeutic value. Genetic modification of electrophysiology of scar tissue may provide potential therapy for scar-related arrhythmias or myocardial asynchrony.[41]

Fibroblasts are the predominant cell type of nonmyocardial cells in the heart. To assess how fibroblasts affect cardiac conduction, we cultured HL-5 cells in MEA chambers to form a monolayer and record their spontaneous beating signals. After control electrogram recordings, we abraded a channel (600–700 μm) of the monolayer in the middle of each array to create two asynchronously beating fields. We assessed the co-relation of the signals recorded from two electrodes located at the two sides of the abraded channel. We found that adding human cardiac fibroblasts did not repair the

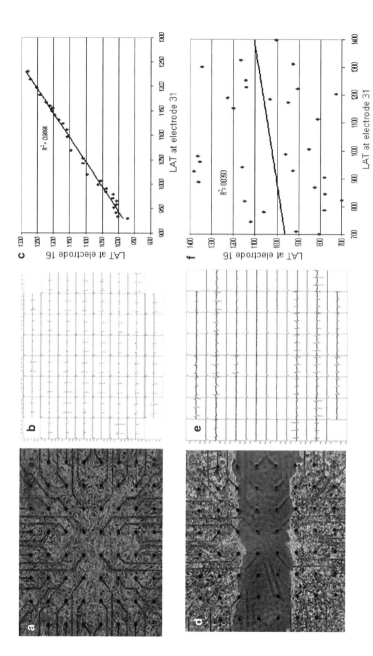

Fig. 20.9 Conductivity of cultured HL-5 cells. HL-5 cells formed a monolayer on day 3 after plating to a multi-electrode array (**a**). Spontaneous electrical field potentials were recorded on each electrode and the culture monolayer activated synchronously when the monolayer was intact (**b**). The local activation times (LATs) from two electrodes (16 and 31) correlated very well and fell on a straight line (**c**). Abrasion of the HL-5 cell monolayer in the center of the array with a 200-μl pipette tip formed a channel with a width of ~600 μm (**d**). After abrasion, the HL-5 cells on the two sides of the channel beat independently (**e**). Electrograms showed that two cardiomyocyte fields desynchronized. The correlation of the LATs obtained from the two electrodes (16 and 31) disappeared after abrasion (**f**)

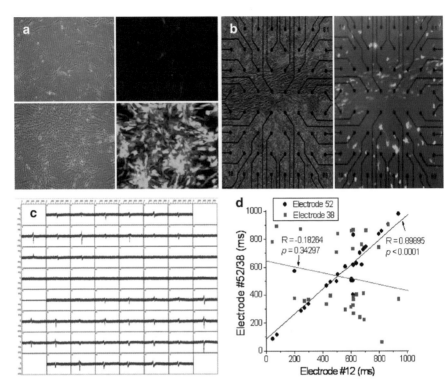

Fig. 20.10 Conduction repair with human cardiac fibrous cells (hCFCs). Human CFCs were transfected with eGFP gene (**a**, *upper panels* are control and *lower panels* are eGFP transfection, with phase-contrast on the left and fluorescence microscopy on the right). The myocyte monolayer was abraded in the middle of the array, and GFP-labeled hCFCs were carefully added to the channel under microscope (**b**, phase contrast on the left and fluorescence microscopy on the right). Electrograms show that cardiomyocytes on the two sides of the abraded channel beat independently and that no field potential was observed in the damaged area (**c**). (**d**) The electrical signals recorded from the electrodes (12 and 52) on the same side of the abraded channel correlated well (*black cycles and line*), but the field potentials recorded from the electrodes (12 and 38) on the different sides of the channel had no correlation at all (*red squares and line*)

conduction damage (Fig. 20.10). In addition, the amplitudes of field potentials from two beating areas along the abraded channel were significantly reduced after adding fibroblasts. These results suggest that cardiac fibroblasts are not only unable to repair the conduction damage, but they also sink electrical field potentials. Amplitude reduction of impulse can decrease conduction velocity and potentially cause arrhythmias.

The feasibility of resynchronization with genetically modified human ventricular scar fibroblasts was investigated with the MEA technique in a recent study.[37] A co-culture model of two rat cardiomyocyte fields separated by a strip of human ventricular scar fibroblasts (hVSFs) was used to study the effects of forced expression of the myocardin (*MyoC*) gene in hVSFs on resynchronization and the response of hVSFs to electrical pacing. Forced *MyoC* expression in hVSFs improved conduction of an electrical impulse at high velocity which resulted in resynchronization of two separated cardiomyocyte fields. Also, MyoC-hVSFs showed responsiveness to electrical stimulation. Intracellular recordings of MyoC-hVSFs coupled to surrounding cardiomyocytes displayed strong improvement of action potential conduction. Therefore, these electrophysiological alterations in hVSFs after forced *MyoC* expression were most likely mediated by MyoC-dependent activation of gene expression of various connexins and cardiac ion channels.

The results described above demonstrate that natural cardiac fibroblasts are unable to repair cardiac conduction damage in vitro and potentially induce arrhythmias by forming arrhythmic substrates which reduce impulse amplitude and slow or block electrical propagation. However, genetically modified cardiac fibroblasts can alter their electrophysiological properties and improve their ability to conduct impulse and respond to pacing.

20.4.4   Conduction Repair by Stem Cells

The ability of hESC-derived cardiomyocytes to integrate with primary cultures of neonatal rat ventricular myocytes was examined recently with a high-resolution MEA mapping technique.[42,43] Electrograms recorded simultaneously from 60 electrodes showed impulse initiation and conduction within the co-cultures. After adding hESC-derived cardiomyocytes, electrograms demonstrated that tight temporal coupling between the human and rat tissues occurred within 1 day and lasted continuously to the end of experiment, up to 21 days.[17]

Human mesenchymal stem cells (hMSCs) have been transplanted to myocardium in clinical trials in patients with ischemic heart disease.[44-46] The data have shown that transplantation of hMSCs derived from bone marrow is safe and feasible in patients with acute myocardial infarction or with old myocardial infarction. Implanted cells can contribute to regional regeneration of myocardial tissue and improve cardiac function, at least in the short term. One MEA study showed that adult hMSCs were able to conduct action potentials between two fields of cardiomyocytes induced by experimental conduction block and thereby to resynchronize these two fields.[14] Recently, the development of electrical transmission across hMSCs during 14 days of co-culture with cardiomyocytes was assessed in a model of experimental conduction block.[15] Neonatal rat cardiomyocytes were cultured in multi-electrode array dishes. A conduction block was induced by creating a channel, yielding two asynchronously beating cardiomyocyte fields. MSCs from ischemic heart disease patients were labeled with green fluorescent protein. Resynchronization of the two cardiomyocyte fields occurred after addition of hMSCs. Conduction velocity across hMSCs increased progressively after co-incubation with cardiomyocytes. This probably resulted from increases in Cx43 expression and functional gap junctional coupling between hMSCs and cardiomyocytes.[15]

More recently, the effects of forced alignment of neonatal rat MSCs with neonatal rat cardiomyocytes on their functional integration have been examined in a co-culture model.[16] Impulse transmission was measured with the MEA technique after MSCs were added to a laser-dissected channel in a monolayer of originally synchronized beating cardiomyocytes. Coatings in these channels were microabraded in a direction parallel or perpendicular to the channel or were left unabraded to establish different cell patterns. Cells cultured on microabraded coatings resulted in anisotropic cell alignment within the channel. The results showed that conduction velocity across MSCs was highest in the perpendicular, intermediate in the isotropic, and lowest in the parallel configuration. Immunostaining analysis showed alignment-dependent increases in connexin 43 expression. Therefore, forced alignment of MSCs affects the time course and degree of functional integration with surrounding cardiomyocytes.[16]

20.5 Summary

The microelectrode array technology has been greatly advanced in hardware and software since it was applied in scientific research more than 30 years ago. MEA measurements can reveal electrical activity of multiple electrogenic cells noninvasively and simultaneously. Therefore, this technology is increasingly attracting scientists who study rhythmicity and conductivity of excitable cells or who work on drug discovery and safety. This chapter provides an overview of MEA applications on cardiac cellular electrophysiology in vitro. The MEA technique can monitor long-term electrical activity of various cell types or tissues in a relatively native environment. Both acute and chronic effects of drugs or toxins on cardiomyocytes, neurons, or retinal cells can be assessed with MEAs under a physiological or induced pathophysiological condition that mimics in vivo damages. Several considerations on how to obtain better field potentials and how to analyze electrograms have been discussed in this chapter. Compared to the conventional methods for cellular electrophysiology, such as patch clamping or intracellular single electrode recording, the MEA approach has several advantages, such as: (1) being able to assess the electrical interactions among cells at different locations; (2) simultaneously recording electrophysiological activity of multiple cells or tissue sites to understand cell or tissue properties; (3) allowing long-term (weeks to months) monitoring of electrophysiological changes of cells or tissues with the same treatment of compounds or genes; and (4) the exceptional stability of the recordings from contracting cardiomyocytes without damaging and interfering with the cells. However, extracellular field potentials recorded by the MEA technique reflect the activity of the cells on and very near the electrode. Therefore, the morphology of MEA electrograms is not able to detect whether a field potential is from atrial or ventricular cells, as in the experiments with hESC-derived cardiomyocytes.[9] Compared to the patch clamp method, the MEA method has little controllability of the intracellular components. Also, although the cell–electrode interface can be optimized with coating, the coupling between the electrodes and the cells still presents a challenge. Generally speaking, the MEA technique is a fast, easy to handle, and efficient method for monitoring electrophysiological activity and drug or gene effects in excitable cells or tissue, such as cardiomyocytes or heart tissue.

Acknowledgements   I am very grateful to Alena Nikolskaya, PhD, Lepeng Zeng, PhD, Xiaohong Qin, MD, Daniel C. Sigg, MD, PhD, Eric S. Richardson, BS, and Paul A. Iaizzo, PhD for their collaboration and help.

References

1. Pine J. Recording action potentials from cultured neurons with extracellular microcircuit electrodes. J Neurosci Methods 1980; 2:19–31.
2. CA Jr, Springer PA, Loeb GE, et al. A miniature microelectrode array to monitor the bioelectric activity of cultured cells. Exp Cell Res 1972; 74:61–6.
3. Reppel M, Pillekamp F, Lu ZJ, et al. Microelectrode arrays: a new tool to measure embryonic heart activity. J Electrocardiol 2004; 37(Suppl):104–9.
4. Stett A, Egert U, Guenther E, et al. Biological application of microelectrode arrays in drug discovery and basic research. Anal Bioanal Chem 2003; 377:486–95.
5. White SM, Constantin PE, Claycomb WC. Cardiac physiology at the cellular level: use of cultured HL-1 cardiomyocytes for studies of cardiac muscle cell structure and function. Am J Physiol Heart Circ Physiol 2004; 286:H823–9.
6. Ludwig A, Zong X, Stieber J, et al. Two pacemaker channels from human heart with profoundly different activation kinetics. EMBO J 1999; 18:2323–9.
7. Reppel M, Igelmund P, Egert U, et al. Effect of cardioactive drugs on action potential generation and propagation in embryonic stem cell-derived cardiomyocytes. Cell Physiol Biochem 2007; 19:213–24.
8. Caspi O, Itzhaki I, Arbel G, et al. In vitro electrophysiological drug testing using human embryonic stem cell derived cardiomyocytes. Stem Cells Dev 2009; 18(1):161–72.
9. Hescheler J, Halbach M, Egert U, et al. Determination of electrical properties of ES cell-derived cardiomyocytes using MEAs. J Electrocardiol 2004; 37(Suppl):110–6.
10. Gepstein L. Experimental molecular and stem cell therapies in cardiac electrophysiology. Ann N Y Acad Sci 2008; 1123:224–31.
11. Pillekamp F, Reppel M, Brockmeier K, et al. Impulse propagation in late-stage embryonic and neonatal murine ventricular slices. J Electrocardiol 2006; 39:425.e1–4.
12. Hannes T, Halbach M, Nazzal R, et al. Biological pacemakers: characterization in an in vitro coculture model. J Electrocardiol 2008; 41:562–6.
13. Hou YM, Na JN, Rayile A. Cardiac field potentials and activation sequence in Langendorff perfused heart, cardiac tissue slices and cultured ventricular myocytes recorded by microelectrode arrays system. Zhonghua Xin Xue Guan Bing Za Zhi 2008; 36:944–6.
14. Beeres SL, Atsma DE, van der Laarse A, et al. Human adult bone marrow mesenchymal stem cells repair experimental conduction block in rat cardiomyocyte cultures. J Am Coll Cardiol 2005; 46:1943–52.
15. Pijnappels DA, Schalij MJ, van Tuyn J, et al. Progressive increase in conduction velocity across human mesenchymal stem cells is mediated by enhanced electrical coupling. Cardiovasc Res 2006; 72:282–91.
16. Pijnappels DA, Schalij MJ, Ramkisoensing AA, et al. Forced alignment of mesenchymal stem cells undergoing cardiomyogenic differentiation affects functional integration with cardiomyocyte cultures. Circ Res 2008; 103:167–76.
17. Kehat I, Khimovich L, Caspi O, et al. Electromechanical integration of cardiomyocytes derived from human embryonic stem cells. Nat Biotechnol 2004; 22:1282–9.
18. Halbach M, Egert U, Hescheler J, et al. Estimation of action potential changes from field potential recordings in multicellular mouse cardiac myocyte cultures. Cell Physiol Biochem 2003; 13:271–84.
19. Claycomb WC, Lanson NA Jr, Stallworth BS, et al. HL-1 cells: a cardiac muscle cell line that contracts and retains phenotypic characteristics of the adult cardiomyocyte. Proc Natl Acad Sci U S A 1998; 95:2979–84.

20. Xiao YF, TenBroek EM, Wilhelm JJ, et al. Electrophysiological characterization of murine HL-5 atrial cardiomyocytes. Am J Physiol Cell Physiol 2006; 291:C407–16.
21. Cicconi S, Ventura N, Pastore D, et al. Characterization of apoptosis signal transduction pathways in HL-5 cardiomyocytes exposed to ischemia/reperfusion oxidative stress model. J Cell Physiol 2003; 195:27–37.
22. Wu F, Yan W, Pan J, et al. Processing of pro-atrial natriuretic peptide by corin in cardiac myocytes. J Biol Chem 2002; 277:16900–5.
23. Nikolskaya AV, Nikolski VP, Efimov IR. Gene printer: laser-scanning targeted transfection of cultured cardiac neonatal rat cells. Cell Commun Adhes 2006; 13:217–22.
24. Banach K, Halbach MD, Hu P, et al. Development of electrical activity in cardiac myocyte aggregates derived from mouse embryonic stem cells. Am J Physiol Heart Circ Physiol 2003; 284:H2114–23.
25. Hescheler J, Wartenberg M, Fleischmann BK, et al. Embryonic stem cells as a model for the physiological analysis of the cardiovascular system. Methods Mol Biol 2002; 185:169–87.
26. Caspi O, Gepstein L. Potential applications of human embryonic stem cell-derived cardiomyocytes. Ann N Y Acad Sci 2004; 1015:285–98.
27. Harding SE, Ali NN, Brito-Martins M, et al. The human embryonic stem cell-derived cardiomyocyte as a pharmacological model. Pharmacol Ther 2007; 113:341–53.
28. Reppel M, Pillekamp F, Brockmeier K, et al. The electrocardiogram of human embryonic stem cell-derived cardiomyocytes. J Electrocardiol 2005; 38:166–70.
29. Schwanke K, Wunderlich S, Reppel M, et al. Generation and characterization of functional cardiomyocytes from rhesus monkey embryonic stem cells. Stem Cells 2006; 24:1423–32.
30. Xue T, Cho HC, Akar FG, et al. Functional integration of electrically active cardiac derivatives from genetically engineered human embryonic stem cells with quiescent recipient ventricular cardiomyocytes: insights into the development of cell-based pacemakers. Circulation 2005; 111:11–20.
31. Lohmann H, Bussek, A, Schmidt M, et al. Isolated living heart slices from adult rats and guinea pigs as a model for drug testing. Naunyn-Schmiedebergs Arch Pharmacol 2006; 372:90 (Abstract 332).
32. Dobrzynski H, Boyett MR, Anderson RH. New insights into pacemaker activity: promoting understanding of sick sinus syndrome. Circulation 2007; 115:1921–32.
33. Thollon C, Bedut S, Villeneuve N, et al. Use-dependent inhibition of hHCN4 by ivabradine and relationship with reduction in pacemaker activity. Br J Pharmacol 2007; 150:37–46.
34. Natarajan A, Molnar P, Sieverdes K, et al. Microelectrode array recordings of cardiac action potentials as a high throughput method to evaluate pesticide toxicity. Toxicol In Vitro 2006; 20:375–81.
35. Meyer T, Boven KH, Gunther E, et al. Micro-electrode arrays in cardiac safety pharmacology: a novel tool to study QT interval prolongation. Drug Saf 2004; 27:763–72.
36. Igelmund P, Zhao YQ, Heinemann U. Effects of T-type, L-type, N-type, P-type, and Q-type calcium channel blockers on stimulus-induced pre- and postsynaptic calcium fluxes in rat hippocampal slices. Exp Brain Res 1996; 109:22–32.
37. Pijnappels DA, van Tuyn J, de Vries AA, et al. Resynchronization of separated rat cardiomyocyte fields with genetically modified human ventricular scar fibroblasts. Circulation 2007; 116:2018–28.
38. Kizana E, Ginn SL, Smyth CM, et al. Fibroblasts modulate cardiomyocyte excitability: implications for cardiac gene therapy. Gene Ther 2006; 13:1611–5.
39 Gaudesius G, Miragoli M, Thomas SP, et al. Coupling of cardiac electrical activity over extended distances by fibroblasts of cardiac origin. Circ Res 2003; 93:421–8.
40. Miragoli M, Gaudesius G, Rohr S. Electrotonic modulation of cardiac impulse conduction by myofibroblasts. Circ Res 2006; 98:801–10.
41. Kizana E, Ginn SL, Allen DG, et al. Fibroblasts can be genetically modified to produce excitable cells capable of electrical coupling. Circulation 2005; 111:394–8.
42. Kehat I, Gepstein A, Spira A, et al. High-resolution electrophysiological assessment of human embryonic stem cell-derived cardiomyocytes: a novel in vitro model for the study of conduction. Circ Res 2002; 91:659–61.

43. Feld Y, Melamed-Frank M, Kehat I, et al. Electrophysiological modulation of cardiomyocytic tissue by transfected fibroblasts expressing potassium channels: a novel strategy to manipulate excitability. Circulation 2002; 105:522–9.
44. Katritsis DG, Sotiropoulou PA, Karvouni E, et al. Transcoronary transplantation of autologous mesenchymal stem cells and endothelial progenitors into infarcted human myocardium. Catheter Cardiovasc Interv 2005; 65:321–9.
45. Chen SL, Fang WW, Ye F, et al. Effect on left ventricular function of intracoronary transplantation of autologous bone marrow mesenchymal stem cell in patients with acute myocardial infarction. Am J Cardiol 2004; 94:92–5.
46. Katritsis DG, Sotiropoulou P, Giazitzoglou E, et al. Electrophysiological effects of intracoronary transplantation of autologous mesenchymal and endothelial progenitor cells. Europace 2007; 9:167–71.

Chapter 21
Cardiac CT/MRI Imaging for Electrophysiology

Mohammad Nurulqadr Jameel and Abdul Mansoor

Abstract Emergence of new management strategies in cardiac electrophysiology, including catheter ablation and device implantation, has lead to the development of better imaging modalities that provide accurate anatomic characterization. Standard fluoroscopy still remains the standard imaging modality during catheter ablation procedures and device implantation. However, fluoroscopy is insufficient for detailed imaging of important anatomical structures, and its desirability is also limited by the inherent patient and staff radiation exposure. Intracardiac echocardiography (ICE), computed tomography (CT), and magnetic resonance imaging (MRI) provide more detailed anatomic visualization. Currently, image integration with either CT or MRI is being used to enhance the acquisition of 3D electroanatomic mapping and to guide radiofrequency ablation. This involves imaging of the patient before the procedure and registration of the anatomy at the time of the procedure. In the future, real-time MRI would allow true real-time 3D imaging, displaying the exact catheter position in regard to the accurate cardiac anatomy without any ionizing radiation. Real-time MRI would allow direct monitoring of surrounding structures such as the esophagus and pericardial space, thus providing real-time feedback to reduce the chance of complications. Finally, fusion imaging with two different imaging modalities such as MRI and positron emission tomography (PET) may allow anatomic and metabolic characterization of a left ventricular scar that may provide improved guidance for ventricular tachycardia ablations. This chapter provides an overview of different imaging modalities in cardiac electrophysiology with an emphasis on CT and MRI.

21.1   Introduction

The field of cardiac electrophysiology has developed rapidly over the past decade with new exciting treatment strategies. Radiofrequency (RF) catheter ablation techniques have had a dramatic impact on the treatment of various forms of arrhythmias.

M.N. Jameel (✉)
Department of Medicine, University of Minnesota, Minneapolis, MN, USA
e-mail: jamee001@umn.edu

D.C. Sigg et al. (eds.), *Cardiac Electrophysiology Methods and Models*,
DOI 10.1007/978-1-4419-6658-2_21, © Springer Science+Business Media, LLC 2010

Similarly, transvenous device implantation has emerged as an important modality to prevent sudden cardiac death, and cardiac resynchronization therapy (CRT) has played a major role in management of heart failure patients.

Defining a patient's cardiac anatomy accurately has become essential for successful electrophysiologic procedures. Until recently, fluoroscopy provided the most important guidance while advancing and positioning catheters. However, fluoroscopy is often insufficient for the detailed imaging of important anatomical structures and its desirability is also limited by inherent patient and staff radiation exposure. Likewise, echocardiography also allows for real-time imaging of cardiac anatomy, e.g., intracardiac echocardiography (ICE) can be used for direct visualization of anatomic structures within the heart and real-time imaging during catheter placement. However, current systems for obtaining ICE windows may not be able to accurately delineate anatomic structures in the left atrium from the right atrium. Therefore, neither of these techniques employed alone allow for electrical mapping of the heart.

In the late 1990s, new nonfluoroscopic mapping techniques were developed in which the electrical and anatomic data were combined into 3D electroanatomic models. These systems continuously record the locations of roving mapping catheters and create maps of electrical activities in 3D space. However, these mapping systems are quite expensive and are also limited by the anatomic information collected by the roving catheters at certain points with a rough geometric approximation of the endocardial cavity. Of interest here, newer imaging modalities such as computed tomography (CT) and magnetic resonance imaging (MRI) have allowed detailed anatomical examination of the heart. Furthermore, this information can be integrated into electroanatomic maps. Currently, much research is being performed to assess the utility of real-time MRI for electrophysiologic procedures. In this chapter, we will briefly review the different imaging modalities used in cardiac electrophysiology. There will be a brief discussion of ICE followed by in-depth review of the roles of both CT and MRI in the evolving field of cardiac electrophysiology.

21.2 Intracardiac Echocardiography

Intracardiac echocardiography is currently a useful imaging modality in both the clinical and experimental electrophysiology laboratories. There are two types of ICE transducers – mechanical and phased array. Today, the only commercially available mechanical ICE catheter for clinical use is a 9 Fr and 4-cm radial imaging field.[1] Utilizing radial imaging, it only allows for views within the horizontal plane. Furthermore, this catheter does not have a deflectable tip or Doppler capabilities. On the other hand, phased array ICE catheters have Doppler capabilities, deflectable tips, and image capabilities in a longitudinal fashion with a 90° window that extends to 2–12 cm deep (8–10 Fr).[2,3] To date, ICE has several common clinical applications. It has been used to guide transseptal punctures for ultimate catheter access to the left atrium.[4,5] In other words, it can be employed to provide reasonable images of the fossa ovalis, and thus can be used for confirming needle placement prior to transseptal puncture to reduce the risk of atrial or aortic perforation. It can also aid in the identification of unusual anatomy in the atria that may ultimately impact ablation strategies.

Several strategies are being employed for 3D reconstruction from images obtained through ICE that can benefit the electrophysiologist during an ablation procedure. For example, the ICE images can be combined with an electroanatomic mapping system (CartoSOUND™). Other methods create reconstruction from standard phased array or single-element ICE catheters using special rotational or pull-back devices (Fig. 21.1).[7,8] Recently, it has been reported that 3D echocardiography may also be used for the precise assessment of cardiac dyssynchrony

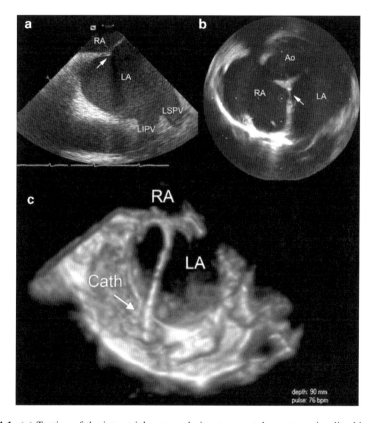

Fig. 21.1 (**a**) Tenting of the interatrial septum during transseptal puncture visualized by phase-array intracardiac echocardiography (ICE) (Acuson Siemens AG, Munich). (**b**) Fossa ovalis depicted by single-element ultrasound transducer-tipped catheter (Clearview, Boston Scientific, Natick, MA). Courtesy Dr. F. Lamberti, St. Filippo Neri, Rome, Italy. (**c**) 3D ICE sector (Acuson Siemens AG) image showing left atrium with mapping catheter. *Ao* aorta; *LA* left atrium; *LIPV* left inferior pulmonary vein; *LSPV* left superior pulmonary vein; *RA* right atrium. Reproduced from Kautzner et al.[6] with kind permission from Springer Science+Business Media, Fig. 3

before CRT in order to minimize the number of nonresponders to this treatment and optimize the left ventricular lead positioning for maximum hemodynamic benefits.[9]

21.3   Computed Tomography

In this section, we briefly summarize several key areas in clinical cardiac electrophysiology where cardiac CT has made an impact or is considered to have a strong future role. The ability of CT to image the cardiac structures with excellent temporal and spatial resolution has improved tremendously over the past two decades. Typically, cardiac CT utilizes either a moving electron beam or revolving X-ray source array to generate images of cardiac structures. The procedure is rapid and noninvasive with scanning times on the order of seconds and temporal resolution as low as 100 ms. Yet, quality image production of the functioning heart requires acquisition gating to ECG trigger points in order to overcome cardiac motion as well as time intravenous injection of iodinated contrast material. Common applications of CT relative to clinical cardiac electrophysiology include (1) atrial fibrillation ablation procedures; (2) atrial flutter ablation procedures; (3) biventricular lead insertions for CRT; and/or (4) evaluations of arrhythmogenic substrate. However, it should be realized that cardiac CT is not a zero-risk procedure. Radiation exposure is a necessary consequence of these procedures, and this exposure is actually increased with newer generation 64-slice scanners. The typical radiation dose for a cardiac structural evaluation is on the order of 10 mSv.[10] Nevertheless, this exposure can be reduced by as much as 50% by employing ECG-gated attenuation techniques that limit scanning during less informative parts of the cardiac cycle.[11] Yet, an increased heart rate is a known factor that can be associated with degraded image quality through motion artifact; this can often be minimized by the use of beta-blockers and optimal selection of reconstruction windows.[12,13] When employed, cardiac CT may also expose a patient to iodinated contrast materials that can be nephrotoxic.

21.3.1   Ablation of Atrial Fibrillation

It has been shown that pulmonary veins are an important source of ectopic beats initiating paroxysms of atrial fibrillation (AF) and that catheter ablation may successfully eliminate these triggers.[14] Ostial segmental isolation of the pulmonary vein and anatomically-based circumferential ablation are two commonly used ablation strategies.[14-17] Yet, it is the operator's understanding of intracardiac anatomy that is necessary for a successful and safe ablation procedure. More specifically, knowledge of the pulmonary vein anatomy and exact location of the junction of the pulmonary vein and left atrium, in particular, are required for ablation. Furthermore, only 70% of patients undergoing AF ablation have *traditional anatomy* with four pulmonary veins (each having an individual ostium), while the other 30% have various anatomic variants.[18–20] Nevertheless, multidimensional computed tomography (MDCT) can provide an accurate 3D reconstruction of the left atrium and associated pulmonary veins (Fig. 21.2).[22,23] Results of such imaging have also been compared to other modalities[24–26]; for instance, in a blinded head-to-head comparison, cardiac CT was considered superior to ICE, transesophageal echocardiography, and/or reflux venography in detecting the four typical pulmonary vein ostia.[26] In another study of 42 patients, MDCT was again reported as more sensitive than ICE in detecting variations in pulmonary vein anatomy.[24]

Most of the information regarding pulmonary vein location and ostia can be obtained from axial and multiplanar reformatted images. Yet, 3D and endoluminal views of the left atrium and pulmonary veins are also helpful in guiding electrophysiologists in procedure planning prior to AF ablation. At present, catheter ablation of AF is by far the most common electrophysiologic indication for cardiac multidetector CT. Knowledge of the location, length, and number of pulmonary vein ostia and branches, prior to an ablation procedure, help guide curative procedures. More specifically, MDCT can accurately define the pulmonary vein ostium at the junction with the left atrium, pulmonary venous branch points, and the saddle of left atrial tissue in between the ipsilateral pulmonary venous ostia.[20] It should be noted that the pulmonary venous trunk is typically defined as the distance from the

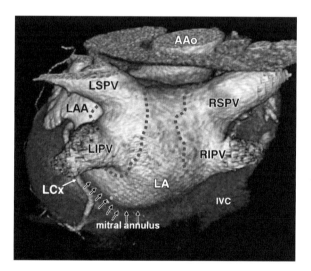

Fig. 21.2 Posterior 3D image of the left atrium and pulmonary veins demonstrates circumferential pulmonary vein ablation. Circumferential ablation lines (*red*) around two pulmonary vein lesions are connected by a roof ablation line (*green*). A mitral isthmus ablati on line (*blue*) was created between the left inferior pulmonary vein and the lateral mitral annulus (*arrows*). *AAo* ascending aorta; *IVC* inferior vena cava; *LA* left atrium; *LAA* left atrial appendage; *LCx* left circumflex artery; *LIPV* left inferior pulmonary vein; *LSPV* left superior pulmonary vein; *RIPV* right inferior pulmonary vein; *RSPV* right superior pulmonary vein. Reproduced from Saremi et al.[21]

ostium to the first-order branch. It is important to gain insight about the trunk length and ostial diameters of each vein which will, in turn, influence the selection of catheter diameters. It should also be recognized that the pulmonary veins and their ostia are usually oval. As such, with use of multiplanar reformations, two orthogonal pulmonary vein measurements can be obtained in a plane perpendicular to the long axis of a given vessel, to better define their shapes.

From a clinical imaging standpoint, the most common anomalies found include ipsilateral single pulmonary vein ostium, accessory pulmonary veins, and early branching (≤ 5 mm from the ostium of the main pulmonary vein). Additionally, single pulmonary vein drainage into the left atrium often occurs on the left side, and this is similar to that in the swine heart. Such common ostia are generally larger than the individual pulmonary venous ostia, and the myocardial sleeve around the common ostia is circumferential. As such, segmental PZ isolation is rarely feasible in these patients.[27] Accessory pulmonary veins in humans are more commonly found on the right side. Accessory veins usually drain a pulmonary lobe directly into the left atrium with the right middle and right lower lobes most commonly having accessory drainage. Thus, as would be expected, the ostia of these accessory veins are often smaller than those of the true pulmonary veins, thus they are at a higher risk for developing stenosis following an ablation procedure.[23] When an accessory vein is located between the upper and lower pulmonary veins, it may be difficult to deliver RF lesions between the upper and lower pulmonary veins due to the small amount of atrial tissue between the three ostia.[27] Unstable catheter position on a small isthmus of atrial tissue can lead to delivering lesions in the pulmonary vein, thus increasing the risk for pulmonary vein stenosis. Accessory veins may also drain into different locations in the left atrium. If this is not known prior to the ablation procedure, the accessory vein may be missed and not isolated with the lesions delivered. Early branching of the pulmonary vein may place the branch close to the left atrial wall. Ablation of the atrial wall at these sites can lead to damage to the pulmonary vein branch and stenosis or occlusion of the branch.[27]

In addition to the detailed pulmonary venous anatomy example above, MDCT can also be used to evaluate the presence of a left atrial thrombus prior to undergoing catheter ablation. To date, the transesophageal echocardiogram (TEE) is considered the gold standard for visualizing a thrombus, however, in a small study, MDCT reconstruction of the left atrium and left atrial appendage identified all patients with a left atrium and left atrial appendage thrombus as observed on TEE, with no false positive results.[28]

Multidetector CT is valuable for defining the relationship of the esophagus to the posterior left atrial wall prior to arrhythmia ablation.[29] Due to the proximity of the esophagus to the left atrium, RF lesions delivered in the left atrium over the esophagus can lead to atrioesophageal fistula formation.[30–32] However, the esophagus can migrate to different positions during ablation procedures and real-time imaging would be extremely useful to avoid creating lesions in high-risk areas.

Recently, image integration systems for catheter ablation procedures have been introduced.[33–35] With this new technology, 3D multidetector CT scans acquired prior to ablation can be fused with electroanatomic mapping data at the time of the procedure, with an accuracy of 2-mm distance between corresponding points on the two images.[35] This fusion approach allows for enhanced positioning of the catheter in the anatomic area of interest, thereby facilitating ablation procedures for AF.

The MDCT can also be useful in diagnosing the complications of ablation procedures such as pulmonary vein stenosis, dissection, and/or perforation. For example, when segmental pulmonary vein ostial ablations are performed, the ostial diameters can narrow by an average of 1.5 mm, and a 28–61% focal stenosis has been reported to occur within 7.6 mm from the ostium in 3% of cases.[36] In a recent prospective study using CT, it was shown that symptomatic pulmonary vein stenosis can even develop several months after a pulmonary vein isolation procedure, and this complication is more common when RF is applied inside the distal pulmonary veins.[37] Nevertheless, this delayed presentation of acquired pulmonary vein stenosis and the simplicity of outpatient cardiac CT make it a useful tool for potentially identifying this condition and for serial follow-ups.

It should be noted that the recurrence of atrial arrhythmias is not uncommon, particularly in the left atrial isthmus (the area between the orifice of the left inferior pulmonary vein and the posteroinferior mitral annulus).[38,39] For example, the length of the left atrial isthmus is highly variable, reported by Becker as ranging from 17 to 51 mm.[40] Of interest, it has been shown that the isthmus is longer in patients with AF.[41] Importantly, the use of multidetector CT can accurately demonstrate the boundaries of this area, including the exact location of the mitral valve ring, coronary sinus, and great cardiac veins (GCVs), as well as their anatomic variants.[41] It should be noted that a serious complication of left atrial isthmus ablation is potential injury to the adjacent vessels, including the LCx artery.[42] Again, the use of multidetector CT can demonstrate the relationships between the coronary sinus, LCx artery, and left atrial wall, thereby providing a safer approach in this type of ablation.

21.3.2   Atrial Flutter Ablation

The most common type of atrial flutter is isthmus-dependent atrial flutter, in which the reentrant circuit is confined to the tricuspid annulus with the wavefront progressing in either a counterclockwise or clockwise direction across the cavotricuspid isthmus between the inferior vena cava and the tricuspid annulus.[43] From an anatomical standpoint, this is a relatively narrow target but can easily be reached with ablation catheters introduced from the inferior vena cava. With new catheter techniques, the success rate for ablation of this form of atrial flutter is generally over 95%.[44] Most consider that cardiac CT is helpful in characterizing the cavotricuspid isthmus, including its size, depth, and anatomic relationship with the inferior vena cava, eustachian ridge, and coronary sinus ostium. Furthermore, cardiac CT imaging helps to depict the pouches and recesses that are commonly present along the cavotricuspid isthmus and that sometimes make it clinically difficult to create a complete ablation line of block in the isthmus.

21.3.3 Biventricular Lead Insertion for Cardiac Resynchronization Therapy

CRT with biventricular pacing can improve the synchrony of contractions of the two ventricles, leading to improved hemodynamics and left ventricular ejection fraction. Pacing of the left ventricle by placing transvenous leads is accomplished via access to the coronary sinus. However, the presence and identification of a suitable branch for placement from the coronary sinus is crucial for positioning the left ventricular lead with a transvenous approach. Recently, multidetector CT has been used to evaluate the coronary sinus and coronary veins prior to lead placement (Fig. 21.3).[45–48] This allows for visualization of the major components of the cardiac venous system, including the coronary sinus, GCV, and/or anterior and posterior interventricular veins. The GCV typically courses alongside the LCx artery and subsequently drains into the coronary sinus[48]; it receives two main branches, namely the left marginal vein (LMV) (which courses along the lateral border of the left ventricle) and the posterior vein or posterolateral vein (PLV). The LMV and PLV are often the target veins for left-sided pacemaker lead placement for CRT. Ideally, the anatomy of the cardiac venous system would be assessed

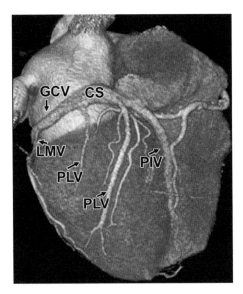

Fig. 21.3 Three-dimensional image depicts the cardiac venous anatomy. The great cardiac vein (GCV) receives two main branches: the left marginal vein (LMV), along the lateral border of the left ventricle, and the posterior vein or posterolateral vein (PLV). Implantation of the coronary sinus (CS) lead usually involves the lateral and posterior branches, which are quite variable in number, tortuosity, dimension, and angulation with the GCV. *PIV* posterior interventricular vein. Reproduced from Saremi et al.[21]

noninvasively on an outpatient basis, before referring the patient for CRT implantation. It should be noted that both electron-beam computed tomography and MDCT provide excellent images of the coronary venous system.[45,49–51] These structures are better identified during systole, but lead to greater motion artifact.[51] Furthermore, the 3D reconstruction of CT images has been instrumental in revealing the anatomic variability of the coronary venous system. Of course, such knowledge has implications for lead implantation because preprocedure identification of coronary venous anatomy would likely decrease overall procedure times. For example, common anatomic variants seen on CT include a small cardiac vein that drains into the right atrium by a separate ostium from the coronary sinus and a posterior interventricular vein that fails to connect to the coronary sinus.[45] Imaging with CT also shows variability in coronary vein branch angles and segment lengths.[47]

Several variations in coronary venous anatomy can, in some individuals, make the coronary sinus approach difficult and/or can lead to suboptimal resynchronization. Specific examples, all of which are well seen on cardiac CT, include (1) small or absent lateral branches; (2) veins with acute branch angles; (3) compression of the coronary sinus against the spine because of cardiomegaly; (4) prominent Thebesian valves blocking the coronary sinus ostium; (5) coronary sinus atresia; and (6) persistent left superior vena cava.[52–56] It should also be noted that left phrenic nerve stimulation after CRT is a well-recognized complication.[57] The left phrenic nerve passes at a distance of less than 3 mm from the LMV in 43% of cadaveric hearts.[58] Given the anatomic variability of the target coronary veins for CRT and the proximity of the left phrenic nerve to these structures, it is important to understand their relationship in order to avoid the phrenic nerve during left ventricular lead placement. As such, coronary multidetector CT angiography has the potential to help detect the left phrenic nerve in its neurovascular bundle as it passes over the left ventricular pericardium.[59] Finally, it should be noted that, to date, no controlled trial data exist to suggest that procedural success or complications are affected by the specific use of cardiac CT in CRT.

21.3.4 Evaluation of Arrhythmogenic Substrate

It has been recently reported that cardiac CT may be useful in identifying arrhythmogenic substrates within the myocardium. More specifically, it can be used to visualize the dysplastic changes of arrhythmogenic right ventricular dysplasia.[60] Similarly, in Brugada syndrome which is an inheritable cardiac membrane channel disorder, cardiac CT can be helpful to identify focal cardiac abnormalities.[61] Additionally, it should be mentioned that age-related fatty infiltration of the right ventricle can be seen on cardiac CT in asymptomatic patients, and it may lead to unnecessary workup if CT is used as the primary screening modality without adequate pretest suspicion.[62,63]

21.4   Magnetic Resonance Imaging

Magnetic resonance imaging is based upon the principles of nuclear magnetic resonance. The human body is primarily fat and water, both which contain hydrogen atoms. More specifically, the hydrogen nuclei have an inherent nuclear magnetic resonance signal which is imaged by MRI. Importantly, cardiac motion compensation is performed by synchronization of the image acquisition to the simultaneously recorded ECG signal. In addition to cardiac cycle motion, another potential source of image distortion is respiratory activity. Yet, due to the development of faster MR imaging techniques such as echo-planar imaging and turbo field echo imaging, it is possible to acquire images during short breath hold of around 15 s. To date, MRI has been commonly employed for the assessment of cardiac anatomy, congenital heart disease, blood flow, valvular pathology, myocardial infarction, and/or human heart viability. Both prospective and retrospective cardiac imaging studies can be performed.

One advantage of MRI over CT is that it has no associated radiation exposure and does not involve administration of a nephrotoxic contrast dye, although gadolinium exposure has been linked to development of nephrogenic systemic fibrosis in patients with renal insufficiency.[64] Recently, MRI has been increasingly used for electrophysiological applications and may have a very important role in the future. The relative role of MRI in specific fields in electrophysiology is discussed below.

21.4.1   Atrial Fibrillation Ablation

Imaging studies using MRI can be done prior to atrial fibrillation ablation to obtain the same important anatomic information as provided by CT. For example, abnormal pulmonary vein anatomy can be identified in up to 38% of patients by MRI[65–67]; this includes a common left or inferior truncus, additional right middle cardiac vein, or pulmonary roof veins. In many clinical electrophysiology centers, pre-ablation imaging of the left atrium has become part of the standard evaluation for atrial fibrillation ablation. In many cases, high-resolution MRI is able to visualize left atrial ganglionated plexi and could potentially be used to facilitate the newer ablation techniques targeting these plexi for atrial fibrillation treatment.[68] In addition, MRI along with CT also has a role in identifying procedural complications postablation. Specifically, MRI has been well validated in the diagnosis of symptomatic and asymptomatic pulmonary vein narrowing and long-term follow-up.[69–73] Furthermore, the use of MRI has the potential to delineate the course of the esophagus and potentially diagnose atrioesophageal fistulas which have a mortality of up to 50%.[31,32,74]

21.4.2   Ventricular Tachycardia Ablation

It is critical to identify that ventricular tachycardia ablation and other complex ablation procedures require detailed 3D information of the myocardial scar, its transmural extent, and border zones.[75-77] Specifically, contrast-enhanced MRI can be used to determine relative myocardial viability, and also allows for accurate localization and extent of nonviable scar tissue. The technique of delayed hyperenhancement is characterized by enhancement of myocardium more than 10 min after contrast injection, and the visualization is then suggestive of myocardial necrosis or scar tissue. Thus, in some cases, MRI can be useful to evaluate the myocardium for scar tissue that may be arrhythmogenic and act as a road map to guide ablation procedures. Yet, it should also be noted that channels of surviving myocardium within the scar can participate in the tachycardia circuit and may represent potential ablation targets. It is foreseen that newer mapping systems will utilize *volume imaging and integration* to display this information during the ablation procedure and provide additional anatomic guidance for ablations. Finally, MRI can also visualize the involved myocardial regions in diseases such as sarcoidosis and arrhythmogenic right ventricular dysplasia, and may provide new anatomically guided ablation approaches.[78,79]

21.4.3   Subsequent Imaging of Ablation Lesions with Magnetic Resonance Imaging

Myocardial scar tissue after myocardial infarction can be seen as delayed enhancement, and this same concept can be utilized to subsequently study formed ablation lesions. For example, in one recent study, RF ablation within the right ventricular apex could be visualized in six mongrel dogs after about 2 min, with an increase in signal intensity over the first 12 ± 2.1 min.[80] In another study, multiple RV lesions showed a characteristic enhancement pattern that differed significantly from the typical appearance seen in myocardial infarction.[81] In this study, four distinct phases of contrast enhancement were noted: (1) during the first phase, directly after injection of gadolinium contrast, RF lesions were clearly seen as contrast-free areas of low intensity; (2) a second phase demonstrated an increasing diffusion of the contrast material slowly diffusing from the lesion periphery to the lesion center; (3) complete delayed enhancement depended on the lesion size and was only reached after 98 ± 21 min; and (4) the lesions remained visible during a wash out period of >12 h, with slowly decreasing size, signal-to-noise ratio, and contrast-to-noise ratio. These different kinetics, compared to myocardial infarction, are likely due to a complete loss of the cellular architecture and total disruption of the vascular system. Thus, in the case of an ablation, enhancement relies mostly on a diffusion process starting from the lesion periphery. It should be noted that lesion size measured during the first three phases of contrast enhancement correlated well with the histopathological lesion size measured during necropsy.[81] Furthermore, knowledge about differential enhancement kinetics can be used to determine the relative age of an ablation lesion. Given the recent reports of nephrogenic systemic fibrosis associated with gadolinium, the noncontrast-enhanced visualization of ablation lesions is of increasing interest. Specifically, in a recent study, it was reported that noncontrast-enhanced MRI allowed for accurate assessment of RF ablation and its intralesional pathology during a 12-h follow-up.[82] It was shown that lesions were successfully visualized with T2- and T1-weighted images 30 min to 12 h after RF ablation. It was noted that T2 images were more consistent and displayed a characteristic elliptical, high-signal core with a surrounding 0.5-mm low-intensity rim that, on histopathology, corresponded to the central tissue necrosis and the transition zone, respectively; T1 images showed a less remarkable increase in signal intensity without a surrounding rim. Nevertheless, lesion sizes and appearances were well defined and unchanged during the 12-h follow-up, i.e., contrast-to-noise ratio was independent of applied RF energy and allowed accurate assessment of RF ablation at all time points. Importantly, transmural lesions, interlesional gaps, and intralesional pathology could be reliably predicted in >90% of cases.[82]

21.4.4 Real-Time Magnetic Resonance Imaging

Real-time MRI is an exciting tool that will likely have a tremendous impact on the field of electrophysiology. It is expected to allow true real-time 3D imaging that displays the exact catheter position in regard to accurate cardiac anatomy. Further, real-time MRI would allow direct monitoring of surrounding structures such as the esophagus and pericardial space, thus providing necessary feedback to reduce the chance of complications. It will also enable monitoring of the catheter–tissue contact and visualize ablation lesions and/or potential lesion gaps. Importantly, even lengthy electrophysiologic procedures would not require ionizing radiation. Finally, to date, while initial unit acquisition costs are high, they are in the same range as a current state-of-the-art biplane fluoroscopy system.

Despite the clinical potential for applying real-time MRI, to date, its use and assessment of utility has been limited to developmental work in only a few academic centers[83–85]; in its present form, real-time MRI has many technical challenges. For example, catheter guidance by real-time MRI may be limited by catheter heating,[86] yet this can be partially prevented by not allowing parts of the catheter to potentially function as a RF antenna, thus protecting the patient from hazardous heating effects.[87] Secondly, real-time MRI has the disadvantage of electromagnetic signal interference.[88] To avoid potentially hazardous magnetic forces, new electrophysiological equipment without ferro-magnetic properties or long fiberoptic connections is rapidly being developed. A third potential limitation is that image distortion may occur[89]; as such, new catheter designs have been developed to minimize any artifacts distorting the image quality. In a final example, during scanning protocols with high signal absorption rates, it is challenging to measure intracardiac signals in the millivolt range. Yet, faster imaging sequences continue to evolve to provide sufficient spatial and temporal resolution.

Recently, the first real-time MRI-guided electrophysiological studies in humans were performed at Johns Hopkins Hospital.[83] These investigators employed a real-time fast gradient-recalled-echo sequence to minimize metal susceptibility artifacts and specific absorption rate. In these studies, the imaging speed was approximately 5 frames/s and was considered adequate for catheter guidance. The investigators performed both passive (visualize catheter components based on magnetic properties) and active catheter tracking (utilize a signal received by the catheter to provide a local region of high signal through incorporation of RF coils). They noted that active catheters were easier to localize and also did not have any associated catheter trauma. Importantly, they noted that the catheters were successfully positioned at the right atrial, His bundle, and right ventricular target sites, and adequate target catheter localization was confirmed with recording of intracardiac electrograms.

Given the complication of gastroesophageal fistulas during ablation procedures, real-time MRI also offers the potential for thermometry, i.e., one could acquire temperature measurements in the adjacent esophagus. This is currently being performed during ablation of metastatic liver cancer[90] and could potentially be used to assess intracardiac energy delivery and prevent unnecessary complications.

In another recent study, an MRI-based electroanatomic system was designed to navigate catheters to the left ventricle, in vivo, in swine using MR tracking of microcoils incorporated into the catheters[91]; both retrograde aortic and transseptal approaches were used. More specifically, the catheters were manipulated to all desired endocardial locations to project electrophysiological electrogram information to the ventricular shell. Finally, to allow ventricular substrate mapping, these investigators were able to integrate this information with both 3D MR angiography and myocardial delayed enhancement images. Importantly, in all animals, the chronically infarcted myocardium was correctly identified. Thus, it appears that these findings support the potential to clinically use active MR tracking techniques to perform electrophysiology procedures completely in an MR imaging environment.

21.5   Fusion Imaging/Multimodal Imaging

In this investigative strategy, multiple imaging modalities are combined to allow supplemental and synergistic evaluation and guidance for ablation procedures. For example, MRI and positron emission tomography (PET) are simultaneously performed to allow the anatomic and metabolic characterization of a left ventricular scar to optimize guidance in ventricular tachycardia ablative procedures. In other words, this strategy can identify surviving myocardial channels or nontransmural infarcts that were not detected by the current gold standard of voltage mapping. Furthermore, in patients with structural heart disease, combined PET and CT has the potential to provide supplementary scar characterization by displaying additional metabolic (PET) and morphologic (CT) tissue-specific information.[92] Importantly, 3D scar maps can be created from the imaging datasets and uploaded into clinical mapping systems, and then employed to facilitate substrate-guided ablation procedures. This approach, although currently equipment heavy (i.e., a large facility investment), has the potential to shorten procedure times, decrease complications, and improve procedural success.

21.6   Conclusion

Enhanced cardiac imaging has become extremely important as a vital component of cardiac electrophysiology, as newer techniques provide for accurate anatomic characterization. To date, standard fluoroscopy remains the widespread standard imaging modality during catheter ablation procedures and device implantation. However, in centers of excellence, ICE, CT, and MRI techniques will have increasing roles in the future. Currently, image integration with either CT or MRI is being used to enhance the acquisition of 3D electroanatomic mapping and guide RF ablation; as such, this involves imaging of the patient before the procedure and registration of the anatomy at the time of the procedure. In the future, real-time MRI will likely allow for catheter navigation and enable the user to conduct procedures in an MR imaging environment.

References

1. Chu E, Fitzpatrick AP, Chin MC, et al. Radiofrequency catheter ablation guided by intracardiac echocardiography. Circulation 1994; 89:1301–5.
2. Bruce CJ, Nishimura RA, Rihal CS, et al. Intracardiac echocardiography in the interventional catheterization laboratory: preliminary experience with a novel, phased-array transducer. Am J Cardiol 2002; 89:635–40.
3. Bruce CJ, Packer DL, Seward JB. Intracardiac Doppler hemodynamics and flow: new vector, phased-array ultrasound-tipped catheter. Am J Cardiol 1999; 83:1509–12.
4. Daoud EG, Kalbfleisch SJ, Hummel JD. Intracardiac echocardiography to guide transseptal left heart catheterization for radiofrequency catheter ablation. J Cardiovasc Electrophysiol 1999; 10:358–63.
5. Epstein LM, Smith T, TenHoff H. Nonfluoroscopic transseptal catheterization: safety and efficacy of intracardiac echocardiographic guidance. J Cardiovasc Electrophysiol 1998; 9:625–30.
6. Kautzner J, Peichl P. 3D and 4D echo – applications in EP laboratory procedures. J Interv Card Electrophysiol 2008; 22:139–44.
7. Knackstedt C, Franke A, Mischke K, et al. Semi-automated 3-dimensional intracardiac echocardiography: development and initial clinical experience of a new system to guide ablation procedures. Heart Rhythm 2006; 3:1453–9.
8. Szili-Torok T, McFadden EP, Jordaens LJ, et al. Visualization of elusive structures using intracardiac echocardiography: insights from electrophysiology. Cardiovasc Ultrasound 2004; 2:6.

9. Kapetanakis S, Kearney MT, Siva A, et al. Real-time three-dimensional echocardiography: a novel technique to quantify global left ventricular mechanical dyssynchrony. Circulation 2005; 112:992–1000.

10. Morin RL, Gerber TC, McCollough CH. Radiation dose in computed tomography of the heart. Circulation 2003; 107:917–22.

11. Kuettner A, Beck T, Drosch T, et al. Diagnostic accuracy of noninvasive coronary imaging using 16-detector slice spiral computed tomography with 188 ms temporal resolution. J Am Coll Cardiol 2005; 45:123–7.

12. Choi HS, Choi BW, Choe KO, et al. Pitfalls, artifacts, and remedies in multi-detector row CT coronary angiography. Radiographics 2004; 24:787–800.

13. Leschka S, Scheffel H, Desbiolles L, et al. Image quality and reconstruction intervals of dual-source CT coronary angiography: recommendations for ECG-pulsing windowing. Invest Radiol 2007; 42:543–9.

14. Haissaguerre M, Jais P, Shah DC, et al. Spontaneous initiation of atrial fibrillation by ectopic beats originating in the pulmonary veins. N Engl J Med 1998; 339:659–66.

15. Morady F. Mechanisms and catheter ablation therapy of atrial fibrillation. Tex Heart Inst J 2005; 32:199–201.

16. Ouyang F, Bansch D, Ernst S, et al. Complete isolation of left atrium surrounding the pulmonary veins: new insights from the double-Lasso technique in paroxysmal atrial fibrillation. Circulation 2004; 110:2090–6.

17. Pappone C, Rosanio S, Oreto G, et al. Circumferential radiofrequency ablation of pulmonary vein ostia: a new anatomic approach for curing atrial fibrillation. Circulation 2000; 102:2619–28.

18. Cronin P, Sneider MB, Kazerooni EA, et al. MDCT of the left atrium and pulmonary veins in planning radiofrequency ablation for atrial fibrillation: a how-to guide. Am J Roentgenol 2004; 183:767–78.

19. Ghaye B, Szapiro D, Dacher JN, et al. Percutaneous ablation for atrial fibrillation: the role of cross-sectional imaging. Radiographics 2003; 23:S19–33; discussion S48–50.

20. Lacomis JM, Wigginton W, Fuhrman C, et al. Multi-detector row CT of the left atrium and pulmonary veins before radio-frequency catheter ablation for atrial fibrillation. Radiographics 2003; 23:S35–48; discussion S48–50.

21. Saremi F, Krishnan S. Cardiac conduction system: anatomic landmarks relevant to interventional electrophysiologic techniques demonstrated with 64-detector CT. Radiographics 2007; 27:1539–65; discussion 1566–7.

22. Jongbloed MR, Dirksen MS, Bax JJ, et al. Atrial fibrillation: multi-detector row CT of pulmonary vein anatomy prior to radiofrequency catheter ablation – initial experience. Radiology 2005; 234:702–9.

23. Stanford W, Breen JF. CT evaluation of left atrial pulmonary venous anatomy. Int J Cardiovasc Imaging 2005; 21:133–9.

24. Jongbloed MR, Bax JJ, Lamb HJ, et al. Multislice computed tomography versus intracardiac echocardiography to evaluate the pulmonary veins before radiofrequency catheter ablation of atrial fibrillation: a head-to-head comparison. J Am Coll Cardiol 2005; 45:343–50.

25. Schwartzman D, Lacomis J, Wigginton WG. Characterization of left atrium and distal pulmonary vein morphology using multidimensional computed tomography. J Am Coll Cardiol 2003; 41:1349–57.

26. Wood MA, Wittkamp M, Henry D, et al. A comparison of pulmonary vein ostial anatomy by computerized tomography, echocardiography, and venography in patients with atrial fibrillation having radiofrequency catheter ablation. Am J Cardiol 2004; 93:49–53.

27. Mansour M, Holmvang G, Ruskin J. Role of imaging techniques in preparation for catheter ablation of atrial fibrillation. J Cardiovasc Electrophysiol 2004; 15:1107–8.

28. Jaber WA, White RD, Kuzmiak SA, et al. Comparison of ability to identify left atrial thrombus by three-dimensional tomography versus transesophageal echocardiography in patients with atrial fibrillation. Am J Cardiol 2004; 93:486–9.

29. Lemola K, Sneider M, Desjardins B, et al. Computed tomographic analysis of the anatomy of the left atrium and the esophagus: implications for left atrial catheter ablation. Circulation 2004; 110:3655–60.
30. Cummings JE, Schweikert RA, Saliba WI, et al. Assessment of temperature, proximity, and course of the esophagus during radiofrequency ablation within the left atrium. Circulation 2005; 112:459–64.
31. Pappone C, Oral H, Santinelli V, et al. Atrio-esophageal fistula as a complication of percutaneous transcatheter ablation of atrial fibrillation. Circulation 2004; 109:2724–6.
32. Scanavacca MI, D'Avila A, Parga J, et al. Left atrial-esophageal fistula following radiofrequency catheter ablation of atrial fibrillation. J Cardiovasc Electrophysiol 2004; 15:960–2.
33. Dong J, Calkins H, Solomon SB, et al. Integrated electroanatomic mapping with three-dimensional computed tomographic images for real-time guided ablations. Circulation 2006; 113:186–94.
34. Sra J, Krum D, Hare J, et al. Feasibility and validation of registration of three-dimensional left atrial models derived from computed tomography with a noncontact cardiac mapping system. Heart Rhythm 2005; 2:55–63.
35. Tops LF, Bax JJ, Zeppenfeld K, et al. Fusion of multislice computed tomography imaging with three-dimensional electroanatomic mapping to guide radiofrequency catheter ablation procedures. Heart Rhythm 2005; 2:1076–81.
36. Scharf C, Sneider M, Case I, et al. Anatomy of the pulmonary veins in patients with atrial fibrillation and effects of segmental ostial ablation analyzed by computed tomography. J Cardiovasc Electrophysiol 2003; 14:150–5.
37. Saad EB, Rossillo A, Saad CP, et al. Pulmonary vein stenosis after radiofrequency ablation of atrial fibrillation: functional characterization, evolution, and influence of the ablation strategy. Circulation 2003; 108:3102–7.
38. Fassini G, Riva S, Chiodelli R, et al. Left mitral isthmus ablation associated with PV Isolation: long-term results of a prospective randomized study. J Cardiovasc Electrophysiol 2005; 16:1150–6.
39. Jais P, Hocini M, Hsu LF, et al. Technique and results of linear ablation at the mitral isthmus. Circulation 2004; 110:2996–3002.
40. Becker AE. Left atrial isthmus: anatomic aspects relevant for linear catheter ablation procedures in humans. J Cardiovasc Electrophysiol 2004; 15:809–12.
41. Chiang SJ, Tsao HM, Wu MH, et al. Anatomic characteristics of the left atrial isthmus in patients with atrial fibrillation: lessons from computed tomographic images. J Cardiovasc Electrophysiol 2006; 17:1274–8.
42. Takahashi Y, Jais P, Hocini M, et al. Acute occlusion of the left circumflex coronary artery during mitral isthmus linear ablation. J Cardiovasc Electrophysiol 2005; 16:1104–7.
43. Kalman JM, Olgin JE, Saxon LA, et al. Electrocardiographic and electrophysiologic characterization of atypical atrial flutter in man: use of activation and entrainment mapping and implications for catheter ablation. J Cardiovasc Electrophysiol 1997; 8:121–44.
44. Schreieck J, Zrenner B, Kumpmann J, et al. Prospective randomized comparison of closed cooled-tip versus 8-mm-tip catheters for radiofrequency ablation of typical atrial flutter. J Cardiovasc Electrophysiol 2002; 13:980–5.
45. Jongbloed MR, Lamb HJ, Bax JJ, et al. Noninvasive visualization of the cardiac venous system using multislice computed tomography. J Am Coll Cardiol 2005; 45:749–53.
46. Lemola K, Mueller G, Desjardins B, et al. Topographic analysis of the coronary sinus and major cardiac veins by computed tomography. Heart Rhythm 2005; 2:694–9.
47. Mao S, Shinbane JS, Girsky MJ, et al. Coronary venous imaging with electron beam computed tomographic angiography: three-dimensional mapping and relationship with coronary arteries. Am Heart J 2005; 150:315–22.
48. Meisel E, Pfeiffer D, Engelmann L, et al. Investigation of coronary venous anatomy by retrograde venography in patients with malignant ventricular tachycardia. Circulation 2001; 104:442–7.

49. Gerber TC, Sheedy PF, Bell MR, et al. Evaluation of the coronary venous system using electron beam computed tomography. Int J Cardiovasc Imaging 2001; 17:65–75.
50. Schaffler GJ, Groell R, Peichel KH, et al. Imaging the coronary venous drainage system using electron-beam CT. Surg Radiol Anat 2000; 22:35–9.
51. Tada H, Kurosaki K, Naito S, et al. Three-dimensional visualization of the coronary venous system using multidetector row computed tomography. Circ J 2005; 69:165–70.
52. Lane RE, Chow AW, Mayet J, et al. Biventricular pacing exclusively via a persistent left-sided superior vena cava: case report. Pacing Clin Electrophysiol 2003; 26:640–2.
53. Luik A, Deisenhofer I, Estner H, et al. Atresia of the coronary sinus in patients with supraventricular tachycardia. Pacing Clin Electrophysiol 2006; 29:171–4.
54. Shinbane JS, Girsky MJ, Mao S, et al. Thebesian valve imaging with electron beam CT angiography: implications for resynchronization therapy. Pacing Clin Electrophysiol 2004; 27:1331–2.
55. Singh JP, Houser S, Heist EK, et al. The coronary venous anatomy: a segmental approach to aid cardiac resynchronization therapy. J Am Coll Cardiol 2005; 46:68–74.
56. Yamada T, Plumb VJ, McElderry HT, et al. Left ventricular lead implantation in an unusual anatomy of the proximal coronary sinus. J Interv Card Electrophysiol 2007; 18:191–3.
57. Alonso C, Leclercq C, d'Allonnes FR, et al. Six year experience of transvenous left ventricular lead implantation for permanent biventricular pacing in patients with advanced heart failure: technical aspects. Heart 2001; 86:405–10.
58. Sanchez-Quintana D, Cabrera JA, Climent V, et al. How close are the phrenic nerves to cardiac structures? Implications for cardiac interventionalists. J Cardiovasc Electrophysiol 2005; 16:309–13.
59. Matsumoto Y, Krishnan S, Fowler SJ, et al. Detection of phrenic nerves and their relation to cardiac anatomy using 64-slice multidetector computed tomography. Am J Cardiol 2007; 100:133–7.
60. Wu YW, Tadamura E, Kanao S, et al. Structural and functional assessment of arrhythmogenic right ventricular dysplasia/cardiomyopathy by multi-slice computed tomography: comparison with cardiovascular magnetic resonance. Int J Cardiol 2007; 115:e118–21.
61. Takagi M, Aihara N, Kuribayashi S, et al. Localized right ventricular morphological abnormalities detected by electron-beam computed tomography represent arrhythmogenic substrates in patients with the Brugada syndrome. Eur Heart J 2001; 22:1032–41.
62. Jacobi AH, Gohari A, Zalta B, et al. Ventricular myocardial fat: CT findings and clinical correlates. J Thorac Imaging 2007; 22:130–5.
63. Kim E, Choe YH, Han BK, et al. Right ventricular fat infiltration in asymptomatic subjects: observations from ECG-gated 16-slice multidetector CT. J Comput Assist Tomogr 2007; 31:22–8.
64. Swaminathan S, Shah SV. New insights into nephrogenic systemic fibrosis. J Am Soc Nephrol 2007; 18:2636–43.
65. Kato R, Lickfett L, Meininger G, et al. Pulmonary vein anatomy in patients undergoing catheter ablation of atrial fibrillation: lessons learned by use of magnetic resonance imaging. Circulation 2003; 107:2004–10.
66. Lickfett L, Kato R, Tandri H, et al. Characterization of a new pulmonary vein variant using magnetic resonance angiography: incidence, imaging, and interventional implications of the "right top pulmonary vein." J Cardiovasc Electrophysiol 2004; 15:538–43.
67. Sra J, Malloy A, Shah H, et al. Common ostium of the inferior pulmonary veins in a patient undergoing left atrial ablation for atrial fibrillation. J Interv Card Electrophysiol 2006; 15:203.
68. Scherlag BJ, Nakagawa H, Jackman WM, et al. Electrical stimulation to identify neural elements on the heart: their role in atrial fibrillation. J Interv Card Electrophysiol 2005; 13(Suppl 1):37–42.
69. Arentz T, Jander N, von Rosenthal J, et al. Incidence of pulmonary vein stenosis 2 years after radiofrequency catheter ablation of refractory atrial fibrillation. Eur Heart J 2003; 24:963–9.

70. Dill T, Neumann T, Ekinci O, et al. Pulmonary vein diameter reduction after radiofrequency catheter ablation for paroxysmal atrial fibrillation evaluated by contrast-enhanced three-dimensional magnetic resonance imaging. Circulation 2003; 107:845–50.

71. Dong J, Vasamreddy CR, Jayam V, et al. Incidence and predictors of pulmonary vein stenosis following catheter ablation of atrial fibrillation using the anatomic pulmonary vein ablation approach: results from paired magnetic resonance imaging. J Cardiovasc Electrophysiol 2005; 16:845–52.

72. Kluge A, Dill T, Ekinci O, et al. Decreased pulmonary perfusion in pulmonary vein stenosis after radiofrequency ablation: assessment with dynamic magnetic resonance perfusion imaging. Chest 2004; 126:428–37.

73. Tsao HM, Chen SA. Evaluation of pulmonary vein stenosis after catheter ablation of atrial fibrillation. Card Electrophysiol Rev 2002; 6:397–400.

74. Kenigsberg DN, Lee BP, Grizzard JD, et al. Accuracy of intracardiac echocardiography for assessing the esophageal course along the posterior left atrium: a comparison to magnetic resonance imaging. J Cardiovasc Electrophysiol 2007; 18:169–73.

75. Marchlinski FE, Callans DJ, Gottlieb CD, et al. Linear ablation lesions for control of unmappable ventricular tachycardia in patients with ischemic and nonischemic cardiomyopathy. Circulation 2000; 101:1288–96.

76. Stevenson WG, Khan H, Sager P, et al. Identification of reentry circuit sites during catheter mapping and radiofrequency ablation of ventricular tachycardia late after myocardial infarction. Circulation 1993; 88:1647–70.

77. Verma A, Marrouche NF, Schweikert RA, et al. Relationship between successful ablation sites and the scar border zone defined by substrate mapping for ventricular tachycardia post-myocardial infarction. J Cardiovasc Electrophysiol 2005; 16:465–71.

78. Koplan BA, Soejima K, Baughman K, et al. Refractory ventricular tachycardia secondary to cardiac sarcoid: electrophysiologic characteristics, mapping, and ablation. Heart Rhythm 2006; 3:924–9.

79. Tandri H, Saranathan M, Rodriguez ER, et al. Noninvasive detection of myocardial fibrosis in arrhythmogenic right ventricular cardiomyopathy using delayed-enhancement magnetic resonance imaging. J Am Coll Cardiol 2005; 45:98–103.

80. Lardo AC, McVeigh ER, Jumrussirikul P, et al. Visualization and temporal/spatial characterization of cardiac radiofrequency ablation lesions using magnetic resonance imaging. Circulation 2000; 102:698–705.

81. Dickfeld T, Kato R, Zviman M, et al. Characterization of radiofrequency ablation lesions with gadolinium-enhanced cardiovascular magnetic resonance imaging. J Am Coll Cardiol 2006; 47:370–8.

82. Dickfeld T, Kato R, Zviman M, et al. Characterization of acute and subacute radiofrequency ablation lesions with nonenhanced magnetic resonance imaging. Heart Rhythm 2007; 4:208–14.

83. Nazarian S, Kolandaivelu A, Zviman MM, et al. Feasibility of real-time magnetic resonance imaging for catheter guidance in electrophysiology studies. Circulation 2008; 118:223–9.

84. Raval AN, Karmarkar PV, Guttman MA, et al. Real-time magnetic resonance imaging-guided endovascular recanalization of chronic total arterial occlusion in a swine model. Circulation 2006; 113:1101–7.

85. Razavi R, Hill DL, Keevil SF, et al. Cardiac catheterisation guided by MRI in children and adults with congenital heart disease. Lancet 2003; 362:1877–82.

86. Nitz WR, Oppelt A, Renz W, et al. On the heating of linear conductive structures as guide wires and catheters in interventional MRI. J Magn Reson Imaging 2001; 13:105–14.

87. Susil RC, Yeung CJ, Halperin HR, et al. Multifunctional interventional devices for MRI: a combined electrophysiology/MRI catheter. Magn Reson Med 2002; 47:594–600.

88. Laudon MK, Webster JG, Frayne R, et al. Minimizing interference from magnetic resonance imagers during electrocardiography. IEEE Trans Biomed Eng 1998; 45:160–4.

89. Wacker FK, Hillenbrand CM, Duerk JL, et al. MR-guided endovascular interventions: device visualization, tracking, navigation, clinical applications, and safety aspects. Magn Reson Imaging Clin N Am 2005; 13:431–9.

90. Melodelima D, Salomir R, Chapelon JY, et al. Intraluminal high intensity ultrasound treatment in the esophagus under fast MR temperature mapping: in vivo studies. Magn Reson Med 2005; 54:975–82.

91. Dukkipati SR, Mallozzi R, Schmidt EJ, et al. Electroanatomic mapping of the left ventricle in a porcine model of chronic myocardial infarction with magnetic resonance-based catheter tracking. Circulation 2008; 118:853–62.

92. Dickfeld T, Kocher C. The role of integrated PET-CT scar maps for guiding ventricular tachycardia ablations. Curr Cardiol Rep 2008; 10:149–57.

Part III
Putting It All Together

Chapter 22
Introduction to Translational Research

J. Kevin Donahue, Maria Strom, and Ian D. Greener

Abstract Translational research involves the process of validating ideas developed in nonclinical settings for use in patient care. It begins with the identification of a relevant and timely clinical problem (i.e., cardiac arrest, heart failure, atrial fibrillation), followed by investigation of the mechanisms responsible for disease pathogenesis, a step primarily performed at the scientific bench. Once the disease mechanisms are understood, potential therapy can then be rigorously tested in preclinical models (i.e., in silico, in vitro, in situ, in vivo). Efficacy and safety data in preclinical models can motivate early phase clinical testing. This chapter introduces the translational process and provides several examples.

22.1 Introduction

translate /tranz-lāt/ verb: to change from one place, state, form or appearance to another

The traditional goal of biomedical research is discovery of new knowledge (disease mechanisms, normal or diseased function of tissues, cells, organelles, proteins, genes, etc.). When the underlying research is patient based, application of the research findings to clinical practice is often straightforward (e.g., a clinical trial shows that a particular intervention improves survival in patients with certain characteristics, so use of that regimen is generalized to that specific population). When the new knowledge comes from research in test tube, cell culture, animal, or computer models, applicability to humans is less certain. The process of validating ideas developed in these nonclinical settings for use in patient care is the primary focus of the discipline called *translational research*.

Translational research has been called *mouse to man* or *bench to bedside* research to convey the notion that it applies knowledge gained in relatively

J.K. Donahue (✉)
Heart and Vascular Research Center, Case Western Reserve University School of Medicine, Cleveland, OH, USA
e-mail: kdonahue@metrohealth.org

D.C. Sigg et al. (eds.), *Cardiac Electrophysiology Methods and Models*, DOI 10.1007/978-1-4419-6658-2_22, © Springer Science+Business Media, LLC 2010

Fig. 22.1 Translational research design

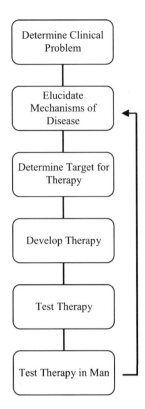

more controlled environments to the complex human situation. The translational process is really a feedback system (Fig.22.1). It begins with identification of a relevant and timely clinical problem, followed by investigation of the mechanisms responsible for disease pathogenesis – a step primarily performed at the scientific bench. Once an understanding of the disease mechanism is developed, certain elements of that mechanism can emerge as candidate targets for therapy. A method for manipulating these elements must then be conceived, and the potential therapy must be rigorously tested in preclinical models: in silico (theoretical predictions), in vitro (cell culture), in situ (tissue), and in vivo (small and large animal models of disease). Efficacy and safety data in these preclinical models can motivate *first in man* or early phase clinical testing. Clinical trials are designed in phases to determine a new therapy's effectiveness and ultimate acceptance. This process of going from mechanistic insights and proof-of-principle efficacy experiments to early phase clinical trials is the cornerstone of translational research.

In this chapter, we discuss these components of the translational process and provide a series of examples that are relevant to cardiovascular disease.

22.2   Determining the Clinical Problem

The decision to investigate a particular disease has both personal and societal implications. Very common diseases may have urgent public need, but the disease mechanism may not resonate with the individual researcher or the available technology may limit possibilities for mechanistic investigations. Very rare diseases may have individual appeal due to their unusual mechanisms or to personal experiences of the investigator, but they may not contribute greatly to improvement in public health. Common diseases with limited treatment options place the greatest financial burden on the healthcare system and, as such, should (and often do) receive the majority of research interest. Within the arena of cardiac electrophysiology, pervasive diseases include cardiac arrest (also known as sudden cardiac death), heart failure, and atrial fibrillation.

22.2.1   Cardiac Arrest

Cardiac arrest is defined as the cessation of cardiac mechanical activity and absence of signs of circulation. Approximately 315,000 deaths[1] occur each year as a result of cardiac arrest, making it the leading cause of death in the United States. By far, the most common cause of circulatory collapse is ventricular tachyarrhythmia, generally associated with acute ischemia or healed infarct scar. Cardiac arrest is sometimes referred to as *sudden cardiac death*, although this is not completely appropriate because death is not necessarily a part of this syndrome.

22.2.2   Heart Failure

Heart failure is a clinical syndrome that can result from any structural or functional cardiac disorder that impairs the ability of the ventricle to fill with or eject blood. The etiology of heart failure is related to the loss of a critical quantity of functioning myocardial cells after injury to the heart due to ischemic heart disease, hypertension, idiopathic cardiomyopathy, infections/inflammatory heart disease (e.g., viral myocarditis, Chagas disease), toxins (e.g., alcohol, cytotoxic drugs), valvular disease, and prolonged arrhythmias. However, the most common cause of heart failure is coronary artery disease with loss of functional myocardium due to prior infarction. The human heart is a highly vascularized organ and, if any one of the major vessels supplying blood to the myocardium is blocked (typically due to an acute rupture of an atherosclerotic plaque leading to acute thrombosis), invariable damage occurs to the tissue bed (i.e., a prolonged ischemic event leading to subsequent cell death). Clinically, this is termed myocardial infarction. The severity of tissue damage is dependent on the location and degree of vessel occlusion. If the occluding vessel is not immediately reopened, long-term tissue damage can ensue and chronic left ventricular dysfunction can develop. Coronary artery disease and myocardial infarction rates continue to rise in the developed world, predominately due to increases in obesity, diabetes mellitus, and median age of the population.[1]

Heart failure is associated with a significant reduction of quality of life, unacceptably high mortality (50% at five years), and enormous cost to the healthcare system. Hospitalizations for heart failure account for 6.8 million hospital days per year, and the annual costs amount to \$20–\$40 billion.[2] Alarmingly, heart failure rates are on the rise, with an estimated half a million new diagnosed cases per year in the United States alone.[3] The prevalence of heart failure in the United States is estimated at five million patients, while the worldwide prevalence is estimated at 22.5 million. However, the mechanisms responsible for structural and electrical remodeling during the development of heart failure are complex and poorly understood.

22.2.3   Atrial Fibrillation

Atrial fibrillation is the most common arrhythmia in the United States,[4] affecting 2–5 million people.[5] Furthermore, atrial fibrillation is responsible for 20% of all strokes,[6] being an independent factor for stroke severity[7] and stroke recurrence.[8] Atrial fibrillation can be lone (idiopathic) atrial fibrillation or associated with various disease states, for instance, hypertension, heart failure, mitral regurgitation, and aging. All cases produce sustained atrial fibrillation but different electrophysiological characteristics may be present.

22.3   Investigate Mechanisms of Disease

Since the etiology and nature of cardiac disease can be complex, it becomes important to focus our research on specific molecules, proteins, or pathways to understand the mechanism of disease. As with any therapy, the efficacy is dictated by a sound understanding of the disease mechanism. Therefore, it is imperative to explore and fully elucidate the electrophysiological substrates underlying arrhythmias.

22.3.1   Arrhythmias

Arrhythmia mechanisms include reentry, abnormal automaticity, and triggered activity (Fig. 22.2). Reentry is the most common mechanism of known arrhythmias. Reentry is the circulation of a cardiac impulse around an obstacle leading to repetitive stimulation of cardiac tissue. Two requirements must be met in order for reentry to occur: (1) the excitation wavefront must encounter unidirectional block; and (2) either the speed of the wavefront needs to be slow enough, or the path of the reentrant circuit must be long enough, in order for all cells along the circuit to regain excitability before the circulating

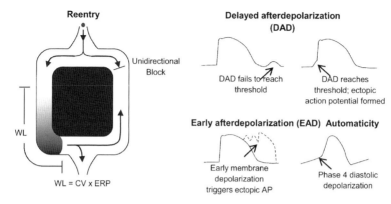

Fig. 22.2 Mechanisms of arrhythmias. *Reentry*: An anatomical barrier (black central zone) creates two pathways that a wavefront may propagate through. In the left pathway, the wavefront proceeds in a normal fashion. In the right pathway, the wavefront encounters refractory tissue and unidirectional block is formed. Since the bottom portion of the right pathway is not activated by the initial right-sided wavefront, the left-sided wavefront can wrap around and activate this tissue in a retrograde direction. If excitability recovers at the site of unidirectional block, the wavefront can continue uninterrupted around the circle. *Delayed after-depolarization (DAD)*: Small depolarizations in membrane potential may form after the cell has fully repolarized (for mechanism, see text). If the membrane depolarizations are of sufficient magnitude a full ectopic action potential is generated. *Early after-depolarization (EAD)*: Prolonged action potential (AP) durations predispose to early membrane depolarizations, i.e., before the action potential has fully repolarized. This may lead to the generation of ectopic action potentials. *Automaticity*: Abnormal automatic activity is produced by cells displaying a phase 4 diastolic depolarization

wave returns (i.e., the rotation time of the wavefront around the circuit must be longer than the recovery time of all segments of the circuit). Conduction speed can be influenced by the inherent excitability of the tissue (mediated by sodium channels) or the degree of cell-to-cell coupling (mediated by gap junctions). Additionally, the degree of heterogeneity of electrophysiological properties can create conditions of unidirectional block. Specifically, regions exhibiting the largest differences in action potential duration can have large gradients of repolarization where one area of tissue recovers excitability before another area, leading to conditions favoring conduction block.

Triggered arrhythmias fall into two groups: (1) early after-depolarizations (EADs); and (2) delayed after-depolarizations (DADs). EADs occur when a secondary electrical activation occurs during the later phases of an existing action potential. These events are commonly associated with delays in repolarization of the action potential allowing recovery of the depolarizing currents before completion of repolarization. This reactivation of the depolarizing currents drives the cell membrane potential toward depolarization rather than allowing repolarization to continue. If the depolarization has sufficient force, it can create a complete second action potential. Any process that results in prolongation of the action potential duration can predispose to the development of EADs. EADs have been implicated in the genesis of a number of arrhythmias in the heart including long-QT syndrome and heart failure.

On the other hand, DADs occur once the cell has fully repolarized. DAD occurrence is due, in part, to subcellular events. In particular, increases in cytosolic calcium levels, which lead to subsequent activation of inward I_{NCX}, thereby depolarize the membrane and reach threshold. Heart failure is the setting most associated with the presence of DADs. A number of cellular alterations in heart failure may increase the likelihood of a DAD occurring, especially a destabilized resting membrane potential and alterations in calcium handling.

Automatic arrhythmias arise from small focal discharges. Cells or tissues displaying automaticity contain a phase 4 diastolic depolarization which progressively takes the membrane potential to threshold. The mechanisms responsible for automatic arrhythmias are currently not well defined. However, components of the *calcium clock* and/or conventional ionic current mechanisms may underlie these arrhythmias.

22.3.2 Heart Failure

The underlying disease causing many patients to exhibit left ventricular dysfunction is dilated cardiomyopathy (DCM) in which the heart chamber is enlarged and the myocardial tissue is altered. The etiologies of DCM include ischemic cardiomyopathy, heredity, infections such as viral infections leading to myocarditis, alcohol, toxins such as cobalt, drugs such as cocaine/amphetamines/cytostatics, diabetes, and thyroid disease.[9]

After an ischemic insult, the left ventricular myocardium remodels electrically and mechanically.[10] While initial changes in the geometry, structure, and function of the left ventricle are adaptive, over time they prove to be maladaptive. Continuous activation of the neurohormonal axis overtaxing the remaining viable myocardium, unremitting loss of functioning myocytes, and maladaptive modifications to the extracellular matrix are a few of the factors leading to left ventricular dysfunction and eventual failure.[10]

Infectious cardiac disease occurs when bacterial or viral agents attack the cardiac muscle or heart valves, causing inflammation. Unfortunately, this common condition is often unrecognized, making its incidence unknown. Enteroviruses, adenoviruses, and cytomegaloviruses are implicated in the pathogenesis of inflammatory heart disease causing myocarditis. Irrespective of etiology, the structural and electrical remodeling of the myocardium in heart failure makes the heart vulnerable to perilous arrhythmias.

22.4 Define Target and Develop Therapy

One of the most difficult tasks of a researcher is finding a target with reasonable potential to modify the disease process. This is evident in the number of therapies failing to meet primary endpoints during key stages of clinical trials or even those drugs which have successfully met the most stringent criteria only to be proven less efficacious than competitor products in subsequent testing. Potential problems include identification of the wrong target, identification of a suitable target but with inappropriate tools to manipulate that target, or correct identification of the target and manipulation but uncontrollable toxicity from the manipulation. Therefore, this process often requires *out-of-the-box* or creative thinking, which is often discounted or rejected by the scientific establishment. In this section, we give examples of successful therapies that used this creative thinking approach.

Prior to publicizing a therapy, it is important to protect your intellectual property. The process of patent protection can be both time consuming and costly, and guidance is needed from external patent lawyers. However, academic institutions are beginning to recognize the financial potential of ideas borne out of academic research, therefore, universities are beginning to provide this service to researchers. These efforts have led to an explosion of *spin-out* or *start-up* companies in recent years. Increasingly, venture capitalists are being sourced for external funding in the initial phases.

22.4.1 Cardiac Arrest

Since cardiac arrest is primarily caused by disorganization of cardiac rhythm, it becomes important to target the processes responsible for organized electrical activity. The cardiac action potential, and subsequent electrical function of the heart, is mediated by the exquisite orchestration of ion channels. Hence, traditional approaches to restore electrical function have targeted ion channels. Unfortunately, many antiarrhythmic compounds actually cause arrhythmias at an unacceptable rate. The only currently reliable treatment for ventricular fibrillation is defibrillation, which shocks the heart to return back into normal rhythm but does nothing to prevent or alter the natural course of disease. With that said, there have been notable achievements in defibrillation therapy. Traditionally, patients in fibrillation were shocked with external paddles, the proof of principle first demonstrated in 1899 in animals and in humans in 1947. In the 1970s, Dr. Michel Mirowski miniaturized the defibrillating device sufficient to implant into patients.

Historically, pharmacologic approaches have dominated therapeutics, however, for the treatment of sudden cardiac death, these treatments were later proven ineffective, most likely due to their global effects. The 1990s was the advent of gene therapy, which offers curative potential by allowing specific modification of culprit genes and focal targeting – attributes that are attractive for the treatment of cardiac arrhythmias, especially cardiac arrest.[11,12] All of these examples required creativity and unconventional approaches to problem solving.

22.4.2 Heart Failure

Heart failure is the inability of the heart to pump adequate blood to meet the oxygen demands of the body. This is due to depressed contractile function of the failing myocardium. Research efforts aiming to decipher the cellular dysregulatory mechanisms have aided development of current therapies. Bioengineering advances have led to the development of several therapeutic options for people suffering from heart failure; ventricular assist devices and cardiac resynchronization therapy aid contractile function of the heart. These devices may offer the patient a certain degree of respite during this debilitating disease, but are far from ideal therapy.

More novel approaches to heart failure treatment are being sought, however. Stem cells are being exploited for their potential to differentiate into many cell types including cardiac myocytes.[13] These are particularly attractive, especially if they can restore contractile and electrical function. In addition, gene therapy is gradually beginning to live up to its potential. One particular molecule being targeted is SERCA2a which, when over expressed, is hoped to increase sarcoplasmic reticulum calcium loads, decrease cytosolic calcium, and improve contractile performance.[14]

22.4.3 Atrial Fibrillation

Therapy for atrial fibrillation has undergone two revolutionary advances in the last several years. The Cox–Maze procedure is a surgical dissection and reattachment of the atria based on the mechanistic understanding that chronic atrial fibrillation is a reentrant arrhythmia, so that carving the atria into sufficiently small sections will disrupt the reentrant circuits.[15] The full Maze procedure is reported to completely eliminate atrial fibrillation, but this is a difficult and complex procedure. Refinements to the surgery made it easier to implement, but at the cost of higher recurrence of atrial fibrillation.

In the vast majority of lone atrial fibrillation cases, rapid focal activity arises from the pulmonary veins, making them a suitable target. Radiofrequency ablation to isolate the pulmonary veins could terminate the arrhythmias, but prominent complications of this initial procedure included frequent recurrence of atrial fibrillation and stenosis of the pulmonary veins. Refinement of this procedure is an ongoing process. Improvements have reduced the complication rate, but cure rates remain in the 60–80% range.[16]

22.5 Test Therapy

It is imperative to study disease pathophysiology and the therapeutic strategies aimed to treat it in animal models that resemble the human disease. The selection of an appropriate, realistic, and relevant model is a crucial, yet delicate aspect of translational research because one must be able to draw inferences, extrapolate, and generalize results to human disease. While there does not exist an all-encompassing animal model of heart disease, a suitable model can be selected, instrumented, and proof of concept work can be achieved before translating therapies into human use.

22.5.1 Cardiac Arrest

A model of cardiac arrest should recapitulate the events leading up to sudden cardiac death in a human. Several have been developed, but the most extensively used model of cardiac arrest was developed by George Billman.[17] This model mimics the events seen in patients with a previous myocardial infarction, who then develop further acute ischemia culminating in ventricular fibrillation. To generate the model, an anterior infarction is created via ligation of the left anterior descending artery in the canine. Then acute ischemia is induced by positioning an arterial occluder over the left circumflex artery, and the animal's sympathetic tone is increased by a submaximal exercise test. This model has been used preclinically for the evaluation of numerous antiarrhythmic compounds including some currently being used in the clinic (i.e., amiodarone).

A similar approach has been used for investigation into the mechanisms of ventricular tachycardia. Ligation of the left anterior descending artery produces an anterior infarct, which provides the substrate for the formation of ventricular tachycardia, with the scar border being the site of origin of the lethal arrhythmia. Reimer et al. used the coronary occlusion model to investigate the time course of irreversible myocyte death with progressive ischemia, and described it as a wavefront that claimed subendocardial cells first and progressed transmurally to the epicardium.[18] This animal model was also used to show that reperfusing the coronaries early after ischemic injury can rescue myocardial tissue. This model has proven very useful for determining postmyocardial infarction changes in a number of major cardiac ionic currents and proteins underlying cardiac excitability and intercellular communication. Canine models of ischemia are not ideal, however, because the immense collateral circulation network makes it difficult to reproducibly create a necrotic lesion of the same size.[19]

Unlike canine hearts, the coronary anatomy of the porcine heart bears a striking resemblance to human hearts. Swine have scant coronary collaterals localized to the mid-myocardium and subendocardium unlike extensive epicardial collaterals in canines. Similar to the canine models, the left anterior descending artery is the target for infarct creation in the swine. More recently, our laboratory has developed a model whereby a balloon catheter is inflated in the left anterior descending artery just distal to the second diagonal for 150 min to create a large transmural infarction and reproducible ventricular tachycardia – key to the development of effective therapies. We eliminated the occurrence of ventricular tachycardia in this model using a gene therapy approach.[12]

22.5.2 Heart Failure

Chronic heart failure (CHF) is a debilitating manifestation of cardiac disease. Though many pathologic insults can contribute to the development of CHF, they all lead to the heart's inability to meet the metabolic demands of the body.

Relevant animal models of heart failure should best recapitulate human heart failure. The most commonly used instrumentation of heart failure is that of rapid ventricular pacing in the dog and myocardial infarctions in the rat. Alternative preparations include surgically-induced pressure and volume overload as well as delivery of cardiotoxic agents. While no ideal animal model exists, each offers advantages from which, with careful consideration of limitations, extrapolations from experimental to clinical heart failure can be made.

22.5.2.1   Chronic Myocardial Ischemia

Chronic myocardial ischemia leading to CHF in canines can be created by multiple sequential left-sided coronary artery microembolizations.[20] Titrating the number of repeated microembolization procedures can produce stable CHF. The disadvantage of the model, however, is that serial microembolization procedures are labor intensive, and may pose a threat to the survival of the animal under multiple anesthesia protocols. It is also noted that this model does not recapitulate CHF completely without exceedingly many embolic interventions.

Several other methods have been employed to induce ischemia/infarction such as ameroid constriction, hydraulic occlusion, and total acute coronary occlusion. The method of ameroid constriction is used to create coronary stenosis that is then followed by occlusion, which produces an ischemic bed of myocardium that is capable of meeting metabolic demands during rest but not exercise. Unlike ameroid occlusion, hydraulic occlusion has been used to deteriorate left ventricular wall motion at rest. Additionally, total acute coronary artery occlusion has been used as a model of ischemia/myocardial infarction, as it not only weakens left ventricular function but it also incites neurohormonal activation characteristic of human CHF.

22.5.2.2   Dilated Cardiomyopathy

Several large animal models of DCM have been developed. However, one that is predominately used is that of chronic tachypacing-induced heart failure first described in 1962.[21] Rapid pacing (either atrial or ventricular) has been used in ovine, canine, and swine models. The model provides several advantages, including straightforward implementation, similarity to human tachyarrhythmia-induced CHF, and predictability in CHF development; it remains a gold standard in heart failure research.[22] More precisely, to instrument this animal model, a pacing electrode must be implanted into the myocardium (atrial or, more often, ventricular) and connected to a pacemaker to pace at heart rates at a frequency three-to-fourfold higher than the spontaneous heart rate (between 210 and 240 beats/min). This pacing protocol generates severe left ventricular dysfunction evidenced by reduced cardiac output, neurohormonal activation, a rise in systemic vascular resistance, increased left ventricular systolic wall stress, electrical and metabolic alterations, and edematous failure.[22] Importantly, these changes closely mimic left ventricular dilation and dysfunction as seen in human DCM. Furthermore, the model creates reproducibly predictable CHF with severe left ventricular dysfunction, typically occurring as quickly as 3–4 weeks from the onset of rapid pacing. If a more stable, sustainable level of heart failure is desired, lower pacing rates can be used. The model's disadvantages include rapid onset, inability to produce similar left ventricular dysfunction as seen in patients with CHF due to ischemia, hypertension, or infection. Furthermore, unlike human CHF, the model is reversible, in that left ventricular function partially recovers once rapid pacing is halted.[23]

22.5.2.3 Other Models of Heart Failure

Cardiotoxic agents have been used to create models of CHF. For instance, serial exposure to doxorubicin has been shown to promote heart failure development (reduced ejection fractions, increased left ventricular end-diastolic diameters, elevated plasma norepinephrine and ANP levels).[24] The disadvantages of using cardiotoxic agents are the variability of heart failure that they produce and potential systemic toxicity.

Additionally, there exist several volume overload models of heart failure achieved by creating high pressure from aortic constriction, aortic regurgitation, renal artery constriction, pulmonary stenosis, or via mitral regurgitation.

22.5.3 Atrial Fibrillation

Due to the number of variables linked with the development of atrial fibrillation, creating a suitable animal model poses a significant challenge. In particular, studying the effects of aging in a large animal model is time and cost prohibitive. Nevertheless, other animal models of atrial fibrillation have provided invaluable insight into mechanisms of lone atrial fibrillation. By rapidly pacing the atria in goats, Allessie et al. were able to create a model of sustained atrial fibrillation.[25] Key properties of this model include (1) a shortening of the refractory period,[26] (2) disruption of atrial myocyte architecture and function, and (3) absence of atrial fibrosis.[27]

An alternative approach to model atrial fibrillation is one that incorporates heart failure. Nattel and colleagues rapidly paced canine ventricles, leading to the development of atrial fibrillation as a consequence of heart failure.[28] Prolonged atrial refractoriness and atrial fibrosis were evident in this model. Importantly, the Nattel model modifies the substrate and tests atrial fibrillation inducibility, but it is not a model of persistent atrial fibrillation. Alternatively, mitral regurgitation in canines has been shown to lead to atrial dilatation and consequent increased atrial fibrillation inducibility. This too was associated with a prolonged refractory period at all cycle lengths investigated.

We published a model that incorporated both atrial electrophysiological remodeling from burst atrial pacing and ventricular failure from uncontrolled heart rate in atrial fibrillation. Like the Allessie model, our pigs had sustained atrial fibrillation, but like the Nattel heart failure model, our pigs also had four-chamber dilation, extensive fibrosis, and apoptosis.[29]

22.6   Clinical Trials

Once a therapeutic target is identified and a specific therapy is developed, a clinical study can be started to determine the safety and efficacy of the new therapy in human volunteers. The notion of orderly experimentation of therapies on humans dates back to 1025 AD when Avicenna laid out, in *The Cannon of Medicine*, seven principles for proper experimentation of a new therapy, including that drugs need to be tested in man, because a drug's effect in a horse or in a lion might not be translatable to man.[30] Unfortunately, it took several hundred years before such principles were put into practice. Over the years, clinical trials have evolved into standardized procedures that focus on patient welfare to achieve medical progress.

22.6.1   Types of Clinical Trials

In a clinical trial, a potential therapy is tested in human volunteers to determine whether the therapy can be approved for use in the general population. Clinical trials can be categorized as interventional or observational. In interventional studies, the investigator assigns research subjects to an intervention and measures their outcomes compared to research subjects not receiving the intervention. In observational studies, on the other hand, research subjects are observed by the investigators. Irrespective of the type, clinical trials are organized in stages, such that information gathered at individual stages can be used to guide future studies.

22.6.2   Phases of Clinical Trials

In the United States, clinical trials for pharmacotherapy are organized into five phases to help guide potential therapies from concept to practical use. These phases are typically treated as separate clinical trials and may take several years to complete. Once a therapy adequately completes phases 0–III, it is submitted to a regulatory agency for approval to use in the general population. However, only 5–10% of all candidate therapies submitted for clinical trials are approved for marketing, owing in part to the stringent nature of the US drug approval process. Once approved, a therapy can enter phase IV (postmarketing) for further evaluation of less common adverse events.

It is important to note that clinical trials are only started after adequate demonstration of efficacy and safety in appropriate animal models. These first experiments are termed preclinical trials. The phases and their descriptions are outlined in Table 22.1.

Also noteworthy is that clinical trials are designed in phases for the development of pharmacotherapy. Devices, as well as stem cell and gene therapeutics, are paving their own clinical trial paths. Nevertheless, clinical trials conducted in humans are the ultimate step in translating scientific discoveries to practical applications.

Table 22.1 Clinical trial phases and descriptions

Phase 0	The candidate drug is administered in subtherapeutic doses to a small group of human volunteers ($n = 10$–15) to gather pharmacokinetic and pharmacodynamic data in the human body. The results of these *first in man* studies are used to decide whether to proceed with subsequent clinical trial phases
	Goal: Test whether the drug behaves in human subjects as would be expected from preclinical trial data
Phase I	The candidate drug is administered in small doses to a small group of healthy volunteers ($n = 15$–100) to test safety, tolerability, pharmacokinetic, and pharmacodynamic properties. If the pharmacokinetic data agrees reasonably with previously gathered data, the dosage is increased in a new set of volunteers until such time that relevant, predetermined pharmacokinetic endpoints are reached (single ascending dose). Alternatively, multiple doses are given to a group of volunteers to gather pharmacodynamic data (multiple ascending dose study)
	Goal: Test the safety of the drug
Phase II	The candidate drug is administered to a larger group of volunteers ($n = 300$), some of whom have the disease the drug is intended to treat, to determine the safety, efficacy, and potential toxicity of the drug. Typically, phase II trials are divided into phase IIA (determine proper safe dosing) and phase IIB (determine efficacy of the drug at the given doses)
	Goal: Test the efficacy of the drug
Phase III	The candidate drug is tested in a randomized, controlled, multicenter trial in a large population (several hundred to several thousand volunteers) designed to determine the efficacy of the drug in comparison to available treatments. These multicenter trials are expensive and time consuming. However, the results of these studies can be extrapolated to the general population and, as such, are key to gaining approval from regulatory agencies to make the therapy available for marketing
	Goal: Confirm safety, effectiveness, and proper dosage of the drug in large numbers of patients
Phase IV	*Post Marketing Surveillance Studies* are conducted after the therapy has been approved for general marketing and sale. Off label indications can also be explored and investigators can test the therapy for a purpose or in a manner other than what was described in the original indication. Additionally, long-term monitoring of the drug can reveal its effectiveness in large-scale use. During this phase, if the therapy proves to be ineffective or potentially harmful, the therapy can be pulled off the market
	Goal: Compare the therapy with others already on the market, determine the therapy's long-term effectiveness, and continue investigating associated risks

22.7   Conclusion

The processes underlying translational research are valuable and necessary if we are to provide novel efficacious therapies for the most devastating diseases. However, each translational step must be stringently met, which will require meticulous planning and creative thought. Nonetheless, if proven successful, clinical trials allow for new therapies to be used in the general population to improve quality of life and ameliorate disease. They also teach us that the assumptions made starting at the stage of investigating mechanisms of disease all the way to applying newly devised therapies in man need to be accurate, appropriate, and sound. What happens, though, when a new therapy fails to meet expectations in a clinical trial, or worse, turns out to be perilous? The truth is that lessons learned from failed clinical trials are just as valuable as those gleaned from successful trials because they provide invaluable insight into the molecular mechanisms of disease that drive the translational research process.

References

1. Lloyd-Jones D, Adams R, Carnethon M, et al. Heart disease and stroke statistics – 2009 update: a report from the American Heart Association Statistics Committee and Stroke Statistics Subcommittee. Circulation 2009; 119:e21–181.
2. Haldeman GA, Croft JB, Giles WH, et al. Hospitalization of patients with heart failure: National Hospital Discharge Survey, 1985 to 1995. Am Heart J 1999; 137:352–60.
3. DiBianco R. Update on therapy for heart failure. Am J Med 2003; 115:480–8.
4. Benjamin EJ, Wolf PA, D'Agostino RB, et al. Impact of atrial fibrillation on the risk of death. Circulation 1998; 98:946–52.
5. Go AS, Hylek EM, Phillips KA, et al. Prevalence of diagnosed atrial fibrillation in adults: national implications for rhythm management and stroke prevention: the AnTicoagulation and Risk Factors in Atrial Fibrillation (ATRIA) Study. JAMA 2001; 285:2370–5.
6. Rosamond W, Flegal K, Furie K, et al. Heart disease and stroke statistics – 2008 update: a report from the American Heart Association Statistics Committee and Stroke Statistics Subcommittee. Circulation 2008; 117:e25–146.
7. Penado S, Cano M, Acha O, et al. Atrial fibrillation as a risk factor for stroke recurrence. Am J Med 2003; 114:206–10.
8. Dulli DA, Stanko H, Levine RL. Atrial fibrillation is associated with severe acute ischemic stroke. Neuroepidemiology 2003; 22:118–23.
9. Braunwald, E. Braunwald's Heart Disease: A Textbook of Cardiovascular Medicine. Philadelphia: Elsevier Saunders, 1997.
10. Cohn JN, Ferrari R, Sharpe N. Cardiac remodeling – concepts and clinical implications: a consensus paper from an international forum on cardiac remodeling. Behalf of an International Forum on Cardiac Remodeling. J Am Coll Cardiol 2000; 35:569–82.
11. Donahue JK, Heldman AW, Fraser H, et al. Focal modification of electrical conduction in the heart by viral gene transfer. Nat Med 2000; 6:1395–98.
12. Sasano T, McDonald AD, Kikuchi K, et al. Molecular ablation of ventricular tachycardia after myocardial infarction. Nat Med 2006; 12:1256–8.
13. Smits AM, van Vliet P, Hassink RJ, et al. The role of stem cells in cardiac regeneration. J Cell Mol Med 2005; 9:25–36.
14. Hajjar RJ, Zsebo K, Deckelbaum L, et al. Design of a phase 1/2 trial of intracoronary administration of AAV1/SERCA2a in patients with heart failure. J Card Fail 2008; 14:355–67.
15. Cox JL. The surgical treatment of atrial fibrillation. IV. Surgical technique. J Thorac Cardiovasc Surg 1991; 101:584–92.
16. O'Neill MD, Jais P, Hocini M, et al. Catheter ablation for atrial fibrillation. Circulation 2007; 116:1515–23.
17. Billman GE. A comprehensive review and analysis of 25 years of data from an in vivo canine model of sudden cardiac death: implications for future anti-arrhythmic drug development. Pharmacol Ther 2006; 111:808–35.
18. Reimer KA, Jennings RB. The "wavefront phenomenon" of myocardial ischemic cell death. II. Transmural progression of necrosis within the framework of ischemic bed size (myocardium at risk) and collateral flow. Lab Invest 1979; 40:633–44.

19. Lowe JE, Reimer KA, Jennings RB. Experimental infarct size as a function of the amount of myocardium at risk. Am J Pathol 1978; 90:363–79.
20. Sabbah HN, Stein PD, Kono T, et al. A canine model of chronic heart failure produced by multiple sequential coronary microembolizations. Am J Physiol 1991; 260:H1379–84.
21. Whipple GH, Sheffield LT, Woodman EG, et al. Reversible congestive heart failure due to rapid stimulation of the normal heart. Proc New Engl Cardiovasc Soc 1962; 20:39–40.
22. Recchia FA, Lionetti V. Animal models of dilated cardiomyopathy for translational research. Vet Res Commun 2007; 31 Suppl 1:35–41.
23. Moe GW, Stopps TP, Angus C, et al. Alterations in serum sodium in relation to atrial natriuretic factor and other neuroendocrine variables in experimental pacing-induced heart failure. J Am Coll Cardiol 1989; 13:173–9.
24. Toyoda Y, Okada M, Kashem MA. A canine model of dilated cardiomyopathy induced by repetitive intracoronary doxorubicin administration. J Thorac Cardiovasc Surg 1998; 115:1367–73.
25. Allessie A, Bonke FI, Schopman FJG. Circus movement in rabbit atrial muscle as a mechanism of tachycardia: the role of nonuniform recovery of excitability in the occurrence of unidirectional block as studied with multiple microelectrodes. Circ Res 1977; 39:169–77.
26. Wijffels MCEF, Kirchhof CJHJ, Dorland R, et al. Electrical remodeling due to atrial fibrillation in chronically instrumented conscious goats – roles of neurohumoral changes, ischemia, atrial stretch, and high rate of electrical activation. Circulation 1997; 96:3710–20.
27. Ausma J, Wijffels M, Thoné F, et al. Structural changes of atrial myocardium due to sustained atrial fibrillation in the goat. Circulation 1997; 96:3157–63.
28. Li D, Melnyk P, Feng J, et al. Effects of experimental heart failure on atrial cellular and ionic electrophysiology. Circulation 2000; 101:2631–8.
29. Bauer A, McDonald AD, Donahue JK. Pathophysiological findings in a model of persistent atrial fibrillation and severe congestive heart failure. Cardiovasc Res 2004; 61:764–70.
30. Smith RD. Avicenna and the Canon of Medicine: a millennial tribute. West J Med 1980; 133:367–70.

Chapter 23
Clinical Perspective: Electrophysiology in the Young and Patients with Congenital Heart Disease

James C. Perry

Abstract Young patients and those with congenital heart disease (CHD) manifest all forms of cardiac arrhythmia, but the age of presentation varies considerably, and the indications for intervention differ from adults. Much remains to be discovered about the underlying mechanisms of pediatric and congenital heart arrhythmia and even more about the true indications and benefits of pacemaker, defibrillator, and resynchronization device management strategies. The purpose of this chapter is to review the age-dependent presentation of cardiac arrhythmias, their relation to structural congenital cardiac defects, and the growing implication of the needs of the adult population with CHD for improved heart failure and primary prevention guidelines.

Abbreviations

AAD	antiarrhythmic drug
AV	atrioventricular
ccTGA	congenitally corrected transposition of the great arteries
CHD	congenital heart disease
CRT	cardiac resynchronization therapy
d-TGA	d-transposition of the great arteries
EP	electrophysiologic
ICD	implantable cardioverter-defibrillator
RBBB	right bundle branch block
SNP	single nucleotide polymorphism
SVT	supraventricular tachycardia
TOF	tetralogy of Fallot
VSD	ventricular septal defect
VT	ventricular tachycardia
WPW	Wolff–Parkinson–White syndrome

J.C. Perry (✉)
Department of Pediatrics, Cardiology Division, University of California San Diego/
Rady Children's Hospital, San Diego, CA, USA
e-mail: jperry@rchsd.org

D.C. Sigg et al. (eds.), *Cardiac Electrophysiology Methods and Models*,
DOI 10.1007/978-1-4419-6658-2_23, © Springer Science+Business Media, LLC 2010

457

23.1   Introduction

In young patients, cardiac arrhythmias occur most commonly in the setting of a structurally normal heart, and the majority of cases are reentrant supraventricular tachycardia (SVT). Young individuals with and without structural heart disease manifest essentially all known forms of cardiac rhythm disturbances described in this book, with a frequency that varies by arrhythmia mechanism and also by the age of the patient. Additionally, patients with arrhythmia due to channelopathies have a mixed presentation based on age and sex as well as channelopathy mutation. Increasingly, both bradyarrhythmia and tachyarrhythmia are observed in those with structural congenital heart disease (CHD) of all ages. This has become an increasingly important issue because, with ongoing advances in the understanding of physiology and constant revisions of interventional and surgical techniques, more than 90% of infants born with CHD are expected to live well into adulthood. It has been estimated that there are now more survivors of CHD in the adult range (numbering close to one million over the age of 18 years) than are currently in the younger pediatric CHD age group in the USA.[1]

With the overarching theme of this book a focus on the basic science aspects of arrhythmogenesis, a simple iteration of each rhythm abnormality and its *pediatric* nuances would not give the reader the proper perspective of the aforementioned context. Older patients clearly tend to have arrhythmia more in the setting of the *structural* abnormalities of left-sided valve disease and heart failure due to ischemic cardiomyopathy, compared to the young population wherein numerically, normal heart arrhythmia mechanisms dominate, but proportionally more of those with CHD experience arrhythmia during their lives. If we are to gain new insights into potential electrophysiologic explanations and subsequent new therapeutic interventions for young patients with and without CHD, then we must be willing to attempt to look at the broad spectrum of cardiac rhythm abnormalities in different ways. Therefore, a chronologic approach to the *natural history* of pediatric and congenital heart tachyarrhythmia substrates will be described in this chapter, against the backdrop of three main influences on those rhythms: intrinsic anatomic and genetic factors, surgically-induced changes in the arrhythmia substrate for CHD patients, and the hemodynamic consequences of congenital heart defects that play a role (Fig. 23.1). In the course of this short chapter, the use of antiarrhythmic agents and cardiac rhythm device therapies will then be reviewed, followed by a short commentary on the near-future applications of emerging molecular electrophysiologic knowledge and invasive technologies.

23.2   "Natural History" Issues of Arrhythmias in Young Patients

23.2.1   Fetal and Newborn Arrhythmias

Prior to birth, both bradycardia and tachycardia can cause significant hemodynamic compromise in the fetus. In these cases, the intrinsic properties of anatomic and genetic cardiac development account for the arrhythmia. In many cases, arrhythmia

Fig. 23.1 Factors influencing pediatric and congenital heart arrhythmogenesis

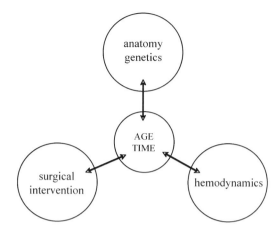

may be the initial manifestation of fetal cardiac structural abnormalities. The most common arrhythmias are those due to accessory atrioventricular (AV) pathways, resulting in orthodromic forms of SVT (~75%), atrial flutter (~25%), and rarely congenital complete AV block (~1%).[2] Accessory pathways occur most commonly as an isolated congenital abnormality, but can be associated often with Ebstein's malformation of the tricuspid valve and some ventricular septal defects (VSDs). In Ebstein's, there is a downward displacement of components of the tricuspid apparatus into the right ventricle. Accessory AV pathways in this setting essentially are universally on the tricuspid annulus, occurring in 5–25% of Ebstein's patients. Most often, these pathways conduct in both directions and Wolff–Parkinson–White (WPW) preexcitation is present during sinus rhythm. Approximately 10% of these pathways are *Mahaim* pathways, most often of the atrioventricular or atriofascicular type, inserting deeper into the body of the right ventricle.

The discussion of Ebstein's brings to the forefront a common finding in CHD arrhythmia care; the accessory pathway location tends to *follow the structural defect*. Therefore, essentially 100% of accessory pathways in Ebstein's are seen to be located in a right or septal position. Similarly, in tricuspid valve atresia 90% of accessory AV pathways are right or septal, in VSDs nearly all are septal, in aortic or mitral valve disease approximately 85% are left-sided, and in congenitally corrected transposition of the great arteries (ccTGA), where the systemic ventricle is a morphologic right ventricle and the systemic valve is a tricuspid valve, nearly all accessory pathways will be left or septal.[3] Accessory pathways are most often single, but in CHD patients they are multiple in 12% and when they occur in normal hearts are multiple in 6%.[4] The exact genetic determinants of these CHD types and their associated arrhythmia substrates are unknown.

Bradycardia in the fetus and newborn (not including perinatal fetal distress) is quite rare. Congenital complete AV block can be a result of maternal–fetal transmission of autoantibodies (anti-Ro and anti-La) that disrupt normal development of the AV node in utero. Fetal ventricular rates, if less than 50–70 beats/min, can result in in utero congestive heart failure and mortality. Structural CHD can also result in fetal complete

AV block due to ccTGA and, in some complex forms of CHD, is categorized as heterotaxy syndrome.

There are exceedingly rare anecdotal reports of in utero manifestations of channelopathy, restricted to long QT syndrome. Fetal and newborn cases of Brugada Syndrome, arrhythmogenic right ventricular dysplasia, and catecholaminergic polymorphic ventricular tachycardia have not been clearly recognized, perhaps due to either maturational changes in myocardial action potential characteristics necessary for arrhythmia or the required cumulative effects of rate and rhythm over many years for some of these syndromes to present clinically.

23.2.2   Arrhythmia Under One Year

Surgical interventions are now a matter of routine for most forms of CHD in the newborn or early postnatal stage. The predominant issue for these early surgical interventions, from an electrophysiologic standpoint, is the location of the AV node and bundle of His in relation to the planned procedure. Therefore, all operations in the region of the interventricular septum have some degree of associated risk of surgically-induced AV block. Surgical AV block has become a far less common adverse outcome of congenital heart surgery due to improved understanding of the location of the conducting tissues in each defect and improvements in overall surgical technique. However, surgical AV block still occurs. *Permanent* AV block can be expected in approximately 17% of operations involving the left ventricular outflow tract, as the His bundle lies directly beneath the plane of the aortic valve annulus. AV block is also seen in ~11% of operations for ccTGA with a VSD.[5] In this setting, the compact AV node and bundle arise from an anterior rather than posterior location and are in closer approximation to the area of suture placement for some defects. In general, tetralogy of Fallot (TOF), AV septal defects, and VSDs each have a risk of AV block on the order of ~2–4%.

Transient postoperative AV block occurs as well, likely due to the same localized trauma that results in permanent block. While a waiting period of ~8 days after surgery to assess return of AV conduction prior to implantation of a permanent pacing system is recommended,[5] it has been recognized that some patients who recovered AV conduction as early as 3–5 days after surgery can be at risk of later paroxysmal complete AV block and sudden cardiac death.[6] These patients likely require closer follow-up by ambulatory monitoring and exercise testing in the years after surgery and throughout life.

23.2.3   Recurrent and Onset of SVT

Natural history studies have shown that, of those patients who experience SVT in the newborn period, the rhythm disappears in 93% by the age of 8 months.[4] Rarer forms of persistent SVT, such as permanent junctional reciprocating tachycardia or some forms of atrial ectopic tachycardia, can continue beyond this and require earlier interventional therapies.

The factors that account for the waxing and waning course of some SVT substrates during the childhood years are unknown. Some data on maturational characteristics of AV node refractoriness and conduction properties[7] and on the observation of disappearance of overt preexcitation in patients with WPW lend credence to the notion that reentry circuits in young patients do not exist in a steady-state environment. Furthermore, there are reported observations of significant changes that are age-dependent in both the initiating mechanisms and the origin and frequency of extrasystoles (atrial, junctional, and ventricular).[8] Therefore, there are dynamic changes in both the underlying substrates and initiating factors necessary to establish reentry for most tachyarrhythmias in the young.

These natural history characteristics help guide plans for either interventional therapy or observation of the young patient with many forms of SVT.[9] One would not advocate an intervention such as catheter ablation for the patient with SVT as a newborn, as most will have their rhythm become quiescent early in life. For those who have recurrences in mid-childhood, the patient and cardiac sizes are such that risks of the procedure are then greatly reduced. Similarly, however, the very young patient with permanent junctional reciprocating tachycardia (under 5 years of age or so) is unlikely to have the rhythm resolve if it has persisted and intervention can be considered in selected cases.

23.2.4   Late Childhood and Early Adulthood: the Effects of Postoperative Anatomy and Physiology

Although patients in the early pediatric age range are subject to predominant intrinsic anatomic and genetic influences on arrhythmogenesis, patients in their late teen years and early to mid-20s become prone to rhythm abnormalities on the basis of the late effects of prior surgical interventions. Some of the earliest research into atrial reentry tachycardia or atrial flutter involved an epicardial application of an irritant (aconitine), resulting in nonuniform changes in action potential characteristics and the substrate for arrhythmia. Animal studies of atrial reentry utilizing a single and simple atrial incision (which approximated the surgeon's atriotomy incision approach for most CHD lesions) resulted in easily inducible atrial reentry around the surgical scar[10] or redirected conduction around other electroanatomic landmarks, such as the tricuspid valve annulus. It should not be surprising, therefore, that many patients with CHD suffer later complications of tachyarrhythmia following surgical procedures. The majority of CHD surgeries involve an atriotomy incision at a minimum, essentially reproducing the electrophysiologic substrate of the earlier animal studies. Similarly, incisions in the right ventricular outflow tract for muscle resections and/or placement of conduits to the pulmonary artery create a clear zone of conduction block and corridors for potential reentry circuits between the incision and the tricuspid valve annulus, crest of a VSD repair and, if it exists after surgery, the pulmonary valve annulus.[11]

Many of these patients have been led to believe that *repair* of their CHD lesion was equivalent to a *cure*. We have done these individuals a great disservice over the years, as many discovered in their teen and early adult years both electrophysiologic and residual hemodynamic consequences of surgery coming to clinical attention and requiring re-interventions. Table 23.1 shows an approximation of the overall frequencies of need for either pacing system implantation for bradycardia, defibrillator implantation for life-threatening ventricular tachyarrhythmia, or resynchronization therapies for heart failure in the wide spectrum of CHD types.

One of the notable growing populations for whom later onset rhythm abnormalities are a significant issue is that with *Fontan* surgical procedures for CHDs that have single ventricle physiology. There are a host of CHD lesions that result in the patient having one functional ventricular mass. Although variations on the Fontan approach have evolved over the prior decades, the essence of the procedure remains the same; one must design blood flow patterns that utilize the individual's single ventricle as the systemic pump for oxygenated blood returning from the lungs and have systemic venous return routed directly to the pulmonary circuit without the benefit of ventricular prograde force. The *best* Fontan patients therefore are those with good preservation of single ventricle contractility, minimal AV valve insufficiency, and unimpeded prograde systemic venous flow into a low resistance pulmonary vascular bed.

Table 23.1 Expected need for cardiac rhythm management (CRM) by device therapies by congenital heart defect type for pediatric and adult patients

Defect	CRM needs (pediatric) (%)	CRM needs (adult CHD) (%)
Patent ductus arteriosus	0.0	0.0
Pulmonary stenosis	0.0	0.0
Aortic coarctation	0.0	6.0
Ventricular septal defect	2.5	2.5
Atrial septal defect	6.0	25.0
Total anomalous pulmonary venous return	2.0	5.0
Atrioventricular canal	5.0	8.0
Aortic stenosis	5.5	38.0
Truncus arteriosus	34.0	26.0
Pulmonary atresia	8.0	29.0
Tetralogy of Fallot	28.0	42.0
Double outlet right ventricle	14.0	42.0
Hypoplastic left heart	14.5	49.0
Transposition of the great arteries	34.0	100.0
Other (single vent, ccTGA, heterotaxy, Ebstein's)	32.0	75.0

On the basis of the meta-analysis of literature. *ccTGA* congenitally corrected transposition of the great arteries; *CHD* congenital heart disease; *CRM* cardiac rhythm management

The initial hemodynamic consequences of the Fontan, most often via a three- or two-stage approach over the first 2–3 years of life, are beneficial and well tolerated. These frequently complex CHD anatomic substrates, however, combine all three of the factors involved in arrhythmogenesis in the young and the patients with CHD: anatomy/genetics and the sequelae of both surgical intervention and late hemodynamics. The anatomic factors dictate the surgical approach and nearly always require some component of atrial surgery, even if only an atriotomy or atrial septectomy. The surgical approach results in frequent atrial dilation on the systemic venous side of the Fontan, so atrial myocardial stretch and multiple electrophysiologic conduction barriers then coexist leading to a sustainable condition for reentry. AV valve insufficiency is a common contributor to atrial enlargement as well, leading to both reentry and abnormal automaticity. Many modifications of the Fontan have been utilized to reduce or avoid atrial surgery and later arrhythmia attempts to preserve function and reduce arrhythmogenesis. However, while there have been successful reductions in arrhythmia burden from the earlier reports of atrial reentry in 50–60% of patients by 8–10 years after surgery,[12] atrial tachycardias continue to be a significant problem in as many as 15–30% of patients even with so-called extracardiac Fontan procedures.[13]

In addition to tachycardia, sinus node dysfunction occurs very commonly in Fontan and other complex CHD anatomies in a nearly linear fashion with increasing age from the time of surgery. In many patients, the resulting chronotropic insufficiency leads to consideration of pacemaker therapy for as many as 50% or more of these patients by 20 years after surgery.[14]

Another fascinating group of patients with CHD who have survived childhood are those with d-transposition of the great arteries (d-TGA). At birth, these individuals have systemic venous blood returning to the right atrium, to the right ventricle, and out the rightward and anteriorly transposed aorta back to the body, while oxygenated blood from the pulmonary veins returns to the left atrium and left ventricle but returns back to the lungs out the posterior transposed pulmonary artery. A balloon atrial septostomy is generally required very soon after birth to tear the interatrial septum and provide atrial level mixing for these otherwise parallel circuits. Currently, the arterial switch procedure (which consists of relocating the great vessels and coronary arteries to their proper physiologic relationships) is performed in the newborn period with excellent early outcomes. However, in the past, the procedures utilized were the atrial level switch operations, Mustard and Senning, named after their respective surgical proponents. It has been surmised that arterial level switch operations were not possible in prior decades due to the inability to relocate the very small coronary vessels, possibly because of inadequate surgical suture material at the time. In any case, these atrial switch operations have not been performed as a matter of routine since ~1990 in most centers in the USA. The interesting Mustard/Senning population therefore represents a unique subset of patients moving through the growing adult population with CHD with a leading edge *head* at ~40 years of age and a *tail* end at ~18 years of age.

Mustard and Senning patients are prone to atrial reentry tachycardia, most often a form of atrial flutter around the tricuspid annulus on the systemic right ventricular side of the circulation. Interventional electrophysiologists need to be aware of the complexities of the atrial baffle anatomy, the location of the coronary sinus os, and the true isthmus of tissue that often serves as the target for catheter ablative therapies in this unique group of patients.[15] Atrial reentry clearly carries a risk of sudden death in the d-TGA Mustard patient,[16] possibly due to rapid 1:1 conduction and induction of ventricular arrhythmia, low cardiac output of a poorly functioning systemic right ventricle, or paroxysms of more advanced AV block during atrial tachycardia. Additionally, these patients develop sinus node dysfunction as a rule with increasing age. Transvenous approaches to pacemaker therapy must account for the fact that: (1) atrial leads need to be placed through to the native left atrial portion of the atrial baffle and avoid phrenic nerve stimulation; (2) ventricular leads will be placed through the atrial baffle to the left-sided, subpulmonary left ventricle; (3) resynchronization therapy by a pure transvenous route is not possible, as the coronary sinus is not only above the subpulmonary left ventricle, but accessible most often only from the pulmonary venous side of the baffle; and (4) intracardiac shunts are not an uncommon finding in this setting, leading to the risk of thromboembolism from intracardiac leads. Epicardial lead placement is a good solution to many if not all of these issues.

Finally, an important reentrant tachyarrhythmia in this age range of patients is ventricular tachycardia (VT) in the patient with repair of TOF.[17] The risk of sudden cardiac death in these patients has been appreciated since the early 1980s, as many TOF surgical survivors reached late adolescence and into their 20s. In fact, if one reviews the publications on sudden death since that time for TOF, one can see that the average age of death or significant, sustained VT has not changed in over 20 years and remains approximately 27 years of age. A surgical barrier creating a potentially critical isthmus of conducting tissue is again a factor. Many patients who undergo TOF repair require an incision in the infundibulum of the right ventricle. Even for those who have a *transatrial* surgical approach to this area of muscular stenosis or an approach through the pulmonary valve, a resection of ventricular myocardium is necessary and results in a transmural scar or subendocardial scar. There are created corridors of conduction then between that scar and the tricuspid annulus, the upper crest of the patch used to close the accompanying VSD, and, if it is still present, the pulmonary valve annulus. Reentry circuits can occur utilizing any or all of these created routes of conduction.[11]

There are many hemodynamic and other electrophysiologic factors that can contribute to VT in TOF.[18] Pulmonary valve regurgitation is a frequent finding in the postoperative TOF setting and results in dilation of the right ventricle (RV) and can cause RV failure. Ventricular arrhythmia correlates with RV size and may be reduced in many after reoperation to address the valvular insufficiency. Although still under some debate, the duration of the QRS complex may be associated with risk of VT. The QRS duration can be linked to RV enlargement, but may also reflect chronic effects of RV remodeling due to the late and slow activation of the ventricle in the face of right bundle branch block (RBBB). This is similar to the now well-appreciated association of left ventricular failure and left bundle branch block that spurred efforts at cardiac resynchronization therapy (CRT). From both surgical and catheter mapping and intervention studies, a strategy of arrhythmia therapy that targets these critical corridors of RV myocardium appears most likely to be beneficial.[11]

Before moving on to discuss CHD and arrhythmia in *middle aged* patients, one final comment could be enlightening going forward. Genetic factors can play a role in CHD arrhythmogenesis in the channelopathy patient. However, we have yet to appreciate the potentially wide implications of genetic factors in the CHD patient that play a role in arrhythmia. It has been shown that a small proportion of CHD patients with conotruncal defects (including TOF) can have single nucleotide polymorphisms (SNPs) in connexin 43 related to development of myocardial gap junctions.[19] Other connexin abnormalities have been associated with both atrial fibrillation and atrial bradycardia[20]; these have not been widely investigated in CHD. Therefore, there exists the possibility that arrhythmia may be inevitable in some patients with CHD on a purely genetic basis, regardless of the technique or timing of surgical interventions or of subsequent hemodynamic factors.

23.2.5 Arrhythmia and CHD in Middle Aged and Older Patients

As patients survive longer periods of time after CHD repairs, the effects of initially minor hemodynamic sequelae can become increasingly important in selected defects.[21] Heart failure then begins to play a major role in the appearance of potentially life-threatening arrhythmia.[22] A useful construct to begin to examine this issue is shown in Fig. 23.2. The underlying theme is that sudden death from arrhythmia and heart failure are intimately related.

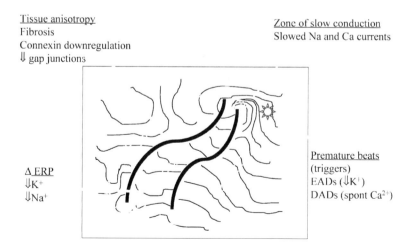

Fig. 23.2 Complexities of arrhythmia substrate in patients with congenital heart disease. The parallel dark lines represent a surgically created (incisional) corridor of myocardium

The long-term effects of CHD include those due to: (1) the volume load of left-to-right shunts and valvular insufficiency; (2) the inherent volume load from bradycardia in efforts to maintain cardiac output; (3) longstanding cyanosis and its effect on myocardial function and reserve; (4) macroscopic scar formation due to patches, incisions, conduits, and access for cardiopulmonary bypass; (5) chronic remodeling of both ventricles and atria due to stretch and dyssynchronous activation patterns and frequent tachycardia; and (6) the links between damage to either sarcolemma and sarcomere that can affect ion channel function and electrophysiologic properties.

Left ventricular (LV) failure can occur in patients with CHD, but often for different reasons than in the adult with ischemic disease. In patients with CHD and two ventricles, LV failure is often secondary to aortic valve insufficiency. This can present subsequent to interventions for congenital (not late-onset calcific) aortic valve stenosis, such as catheter valvuloplasty or surgical valvuloplasty. Another surgical intervention for severe cases of aortic stenosis, often coupled with aortic insufficiency, is the Ross operation. In this procedure, a dysfunctional stenotic or insufficient aortic valve is resected and the pulmonary valve and its support apparatus are surgically translocated posteriorly to the aortic position. This requires a reconstruction of the interventricular septum, a valved conduit placed from the RV to the pulmonary artery to take the place of the resected pulmonary valve, and a patch to augment the RV outflow tract. Mismatching between the aortic root and mobilized pulmonary segment, as well as intrinsic differences between the aortic and pulmonary valves' ability to tolerate systemic pressure, can lead to postoperative neo-aortic insufficiency in a not insignificant number of patients after the Ross operation. Aortic reconstructive surgery or replacement is needed in ~15%. Left ventricular stretch contributes to late VT and a risk of sudden death in ~30% of patients.[23]

An appreciation of RV and LV interactions has been found in patients with RV enlargement and RBBB.[24] The focus of attempts to prevent VT in patients with TOF history was concentrated on the RV and the factors that brought about VT circuits there. Lost in the analysis was the now recognized issue of LV failure in 10–15% of TOF patients, related to longer duration of a palliative aorto-pulmonary shunt (and its attendant LV volume load), RV enlargement, pulmonary insufficiency, and bundle branch block. Left ventricular ejection fractions are reduced in these patients and correlate with VT.

Systemic RV failure is seen often in patients with ccTGA where, even with otherwise normal physiologic relationships, the systemic ventricle is of right ventricular morphology.[22,25] The coronary circulation supplying the RV is unlikely to be adequate for systemic myocardial demands, and myocardial perfusion studies in ccTGA show both fixed and reversible perfusion defects essentially in all patients. In fact, myocardial perfusion in ccTGA may only be normal up to a point in very early childhood.[26] This makes RV failure in adult years inevitable, with the attendant risks of heart failure, VT, and sudden cardiac death. By the age of 45 years, two-thirds of ccTGA patients have systemic RV heart failure and more than one-fourth suffer early sudden death.[25]

For those with complex CHD anatomies and Fontan circulations, the insidious onset of heart failure in adult years would also appear a foregone conclusion.

For Fontan patients with systemic RVs, the intrinsic insufficiency of RV coronary arterial supply also applies. For those with Fontan, physiology of any ventricular morphology, or long-standing current or previous volume loads that alter myocardial function, may compromise systemic ventricular function. By mid-adulthood, up to 50–60% of patients have signs or symptoms of systemic ventricular failure and are at risk of sudden cardiac death from VT or ventricular fibrillation.[22]

23.2.6 Summary of "Natural History" Aspects

The influence of intrinsic CHD anatomy and genetic make-up on arrhythmogenesis are predominant in the youngest of patients. Orthodromic SVTs constitute the majority of rhythm abnormalities with a recognizable age-dependent disappearance, and recurrence pattern and accessory pathways tend to *follow the defect* as a general rule. Surgically induced arrhythmias are manifested: (1) initially at a very young age by surgical interruption of the AV node and His bundle for those with septal repairs; and (2) with late onset of reentrant tachyarrhythmia due to the electroanatomic surgical scar and barriers established in the atrium or ventricle at the time of surgery. Sinus node dysfunction is an important adverse event as well. The nature of the coronary arterial supply to the RV essentially dictates coronary insufficiency for those with systemic RV failure. Later in life, the hemodynamic effects of intrinsic CHD anatomy and residual valvular lesions and shunts result in ventricular stretch and failure, bringing about a significant risk of VT and sudden death.

23.3 Antiarrhythmic Drug Therapies in Young Patients

Rather than reviewing the electrophysiologic actions of all antiarrhythmic drugs (AADs) in this section of the chapter, we focus the attention on some of the pharmacokinetic findings and important clinical considerations in the use of AADs. For a complete review of AAD use in pediatrics, the reader is referred to any of the excellent textbooks on pediatric cardiology and pediatric cardiac intensive care.[27]

As a general rule, the *pharmacodynamics* of AADs in young patients is believed to have no significant differences from those in their adult counterparts. However, it is possible that it will be proved that there are age-dependent changes in cardiac membrane receptors to account for some differences in AAD responses. As in adult patients, the success or failure of an AAD trial is based on the general assumption that the AAD will target a predictable, known substrate (e.g., a sodium channel) and thereby control the arrhythmia. However, one must reexamine the results of previously published AAD efficacy studies in light of more recent findings showing that there are fairly common SNPs that have an effect on the expression of many cardiac ion channels and their response to AADs. An excellent example is SCN5A and the cardiac sodium channel, wherein a patient's response to Class I sodium channel blocking agents appears to be dictated by the presence of SNP-induced minor changes in sodium channel structure and function which otherwise would remain unimportant and undetected.[28] These minor alterations of channel function in the face of Class I drug action could result in either the successful, failed, or proarrhythmic response to the drug. It is unknown to what extent these common genetic polymorphisms have accounted for some portion of the findings of all AAD trial data and, for our review here, whether there are age-dependent expressions of these minor changes as well.

23.3.1 Pharmacokinetics of AADs in Pediatrics

In contrast to pharmacodynamic assumptions, the *pharmacokinetics* of AADs are known to be quite different in childhood versus adult years and have an effect on adverse drug reactions and proarrhythmia. A consideration of AAD use for pediatric arrhythmias begins with the occasional need to choose an appropriate agent for the treatment of fetal tachycardia. Therapy in this setting poses several challenges related to oral drug administration to the mother and drug transfer across the placenta to the fetus; placental transfer of drugs is related to drug size, polarity, protein binding, and the potential presence of fetal hydrops. The fetal metabolism of AADs is largely unknown; excretion of active drug or metabolites into the amniotic fluid can also result in continued absorption during fetal swallowing. Additionally, there is risk of proarrhythmia for both mother and fetus.

A relatively common finding and assumption of AAD pharmacokinetics in the fetus and newborn (based on umbilical cord sampling and drug levels immediately after delivery) is a prolonged elimination half life ($t_{1/2}$ β) in utero and in the first weeks and months of life. This has been shown for flecainide[29] and sotalol[30] and clearly has important implications for drug dosing, scheduling, and timing for sampling of *trough* levels. Calculations of volumes of distribution and clearance are similarly affected. Additionally, it is known in the infant that milk can block the absorption of flecainide from the GI tract, which can lead to increases in flecainide level in cases of gastroenteritis when milk and dairy products are removed from the diet, as is common during childhood. The $t_{1/2}$ for this drug is very prolonged in the fetus and in the first week of life, at ~20 h, decreases to approximately 12–14 h in early infancy, and drops in early childhood to 6–8 h from several months of age until the child reaches ~8 years of age. Thereafter, $t_{1/2}$ reverts to a more *adult* $t_{1/2}$ of 12 h.[29]

23.3.2 Important Clinical Considerations for AAD Administration in Pediatric and CHD Patients

One cannot simply take the adult dose of an AAD, divide by 70 kg, and establish a milligram per kilogram dosing schedule for younger patients. In light of the above comments on elimination half-lives, one must consider many other factors in dosing AADs in these patients. For some drugs, dosing body surface area (mg/m²) yields a better correlation to expected serum levels of AADs.

An excellent example of a disparity in use of AADs in children versus adults relates to the Class IC drugs (flecainide, propafenone, etc.). The Cardiac Arrhythmia Suppression Trial[31] showed a serious proarrhythmic risk of Class IC agents in attempting to suppress ventricular ectopy in adult patients after myocardial infarction. Appropriately, there was a rapid response in the adult cardiology community with subsequent withdrawal of these agents in most adult patients. In pediatric patients, the situation was quite different – the Class IC drugs were valuable tools for control of SVTs in many with normal cardiac anatomy.[32] In patients with CHD, however, there was a risk of arrest and death in those with atrial tachyarrhythmia, presumably due to the slowing of atrial reentry with IC drugs, allowing 1:1 AV conduction and either induction of ventricular tachyarrhythmia or low cardiac output.[33]

23.4 Clinical Use and Indications for Interventions in the Young

It is beyond the scope of this chapter to review adequately the place of arrhythmia interventions and device use in young patients and those with CHD. Brief comments related to catheter ablation, pacemaker implantation, defibrillator therapies, and CRTs are provided.

23.4.1 Catheter Ablation

An exceptional review of indications (or guidelines) related to catheter ablative techniques in the young and patients with CHD was provided first by the Pediatric EP Society in 2002.[9] In brief, catheter interventions in pediatric age patients must take into account:

- *Natural history features of each arrhythmia type.* Some rhythms, as discussed earlier in this chapter, have a waxing and waning course. AAD therapy as an interim measure would have benefits in the setting of, for example, the infant and very young child under the age of 5–6 years if one recognizes a high likelihood or disappearance of the (usually not life-threatening) arrhythmia and the wisdom of avoiding a potentially unnecessary interventional procedure.
- *Size of the patient.* This factor relates not only to the obvious size of catheters to be placed within smaller vessels and chambers, but also the increased risk of damage to the AV node,[34] a small risk of cardiac perforation, and the relationship of the size of an ablative lesion and the proximity of the coronary arteries to the endocardial ablation site.
- *Risk of AV block.* Although inadvertent AV block following catheter ablation in an adult patient may have minimal effect on that adult's healthcare consequences

and lifestyle over the ensuing decade or two, a pediatric patient who suffers AV block during a procedure (for what is most often not a life-threatening arrhythmia) looks toward multiple decades of risk inherent in pacemaker and lead revisions, explantations, device failures, infection, erosion, limitation of childhood and young adult activities, and the possible detrimental effects of long-term ventricular pacing on cardiac function.

- *Unknown long-term consequences of ablation lesions.* Data from nearly 20 years of ablation therapy suggest that the risk of lesion growth and long-term adverse effect is negligible. However, there are data from animal studies[35] showing potential *growth* of lesions, so the effect of a radiofrequency or cryoablative lesion placed at the age of 10 years when that patient reaches the age of 40 or 50 remains unknown. The Pediatric and Congenital EP Society has ongoing studies to address this concern.[36]

23.4.2 Pacemaker Implantation

Guidelines for pacemaker implantation in the young are published,[37] but typically the indications have very weak support from clinical studies. Considerations for pacemaker implantation include:

- *Epicardial or transvenous lead approach.* Most centers defer using a transvenous approach until patients are over 20 kg or, more likely, above age 8–10 years. While leads can be placed in the venous system of even the smallest patients from a technical perspective, the real concerns of venous obstruction, need for extraction, interference with valve leaflet function, fracture risk, and implantable cardiac defibrillator (ICD) coil size and location make an epicardial approach wise for most if not all of these patients. Additionally, the size of pulse generators, although much smaller than earlier models, remains a significant issue.
- *Effects of long-term ventricular pacing.* It is clear from adult patient data that excessive ventricular pacing, leading to asynchronous ventricular activation, not surprisingly mimics the negative hemodynamic effects of left bundle branch block that can result in heart failure. Optimization of single site pacing in young patients becomes more important considering the many decades of pacing the patient will need. Left ventricular apical epicardial sites appear best. Transvenous pacing shows the *standard* RV apex to be the worst location overall and other sites ranging from the mid-septum to RV outflow tract yield better hemodynamics. His bundle pacing cannot be achieved in a reliable and stable fashion in these patients and appears to offer no additional benefit over right ventricular outflow tract pacing sites. For most young paced patients, complete block is an indication for pacing, and pacing algorithms that minimize ventricular pacing are not appropriate.
- *Transvenous lead placement.* As young patients grow, transvenous leads can become quite taut and prop open the tricuspid valve leading to insufficiency, or become so tense that they dislodge and/or lose adequate capture and sensing

features. While some advocate that loops left within the heart and/or pacemaker pocket provide a reserve of lead length that will be drawn into the vascular system to accommodate growth of the patient, these techniques do not generally afford any such benefit other than curves left in the right atrium for atrial leads. In fact, loops of lead left within the heart have migrated out the pulmonary artery, causing insufficiency and ventricular ectopy. For leads in the RV, it has been shown that the RV outflow area does not grow in a downward direction with patient growth and likely yields an improved lead contour and stability.[38]

- *Heart rate.* Young patients have higher heart rates than adults at rest and with exertion. Programming of pacemakers must allow tracking of intrinsic atrial rates in those patients without sinus node dysfunction with AV delays and post-ventricular atrial refractory period programmed to allow 1:1 tracking up to at least 160/min.
- *Preserving battery life.* A patient who undergoes placement of a pacing system at a young age can expect a multitude of generator changes for battery depletion during their lifetime. Follow-up must be rigorous to reduce at least one or two procedures over that span of time, as well as the number of generator replacements needed by programming outputs as low as possible and minimizing unnecessary pacing. Use of the *sleep function* to allow lower heart rates at night is a useful tool.

23.4.3 Implantable Cardiac Defibrillators

Using conservative estimates of the distribution of CHD types, the effects of surgical interventions, and resulting need for primary or secondary prevention strategies for VT and/or sudden cardiac death, 2.6% of pediatric CHD patients and 5.2% of adult CHD patients are candidates for ICD therapies.[39] Factors that influence whether and how congenital cardiologists implement an ICD include:

- *Lack of clear clinical guidelines.* There are very few clinical studies that lead to CHD-specific guidelines for ICD implantation, and yet, sudden cardiac death remains the leading cause of demise in the adult with CHD. Extrapolation of adult ICD implant criteria to this group is problematic, as they apply generally to the ischemic and elderly heart disease substrate population.[40] Generating clinical studies with the requisite N in this population against the backdrop of already proven adult ICD therapies is difficult.
- *Device implantation can be problematic.* Transvenous approaches may be contraindicated in many CHD patients due to the presence of persistent intracardiac shunts and the risk of thromboembolism. Placement of a transvenous lead in a Fontan patient is likely to be associated with a much larger risk of thrombosis due to the sluggish flow characteristics of the Fontan circuit. In the single ventricle population, with rare exceptions where ventricular pacing can be carried out via a transvenous route and entry into a cardiac vein, a ventricular ICD coil-bearing lead must be epicardial, pericardial, in a vessel outside the myocardial

mass, or in the chest wall. Defibrillation vectors can then be problematic for these patients.[41] Additionally, there are a number of the complex CHD patients who have undergone so many previous catheter or surgical procedures that their venous system is thrombosed, preventing use of pacing or ICD therapy by a transvenous approach. Epicardial placement may resolve many of these issues, but epicardial scarring encountered by the surgeon can also be problematic.

- *Inappropriate shocks.* Young patients have higher sinus rates and patients with CHD have a very high risk of atrial tachyarrhythmia, leading to increased risks of inappropriate ICD discharges. These shocks occur in one-fourth to one-third of all young patients with ICD. The psychological effect of these shocks, in addition to the intrinsic psychological effect of ICD implantation, is significant.
- *Long-term risk of device-related failures.* In the past several years, there have been well-documented failures of cardiac rhythm device leads, batteries, and circuitry that have led to warnings and recalls. The majority of these serious issues have arisen within a relatively short period of time after market release. These failures have had a significant impact on the willingness not only of adult patients and their providers to recommend device implantation even when established criteria are met, but more so in the realm of the parent of a young patient or an adult CHD patient who may benefit from device implant. This is especially true for the large potential primary prevention in the population with CHD.

23.4.4 Cardiac Resynchronization Therapies

For young patients with a structurally normal heart but who have heart failure due to cardiomyopathy, carditis, or dysfunction from other causes, application of the adult-derived indications for CRT is relatively straightforward. As in the case of ICD implantation, however, the case for CRT in the CHD population likely has a myriad of applications but has not been clearly established. In addition to the examples below, Fig. 23.3 shows a template for consideration of CRT therapy in some patients with CHD:

- *CRT for the patient with CHD with left bundle branch block.* This setting bears some similarities to the adult, postischemic left bundle study group that has a clear benefit from CRT. Left bundle branch block occurs in any operation that involves the subaortic area, including aortic valve procedures, subaortic stenosis resections, Konno, and Kawashima procedures.
- *CRT for patients with RBBB.* RBBB is extremely common in the postoperative CHD population. There are identifiable patients with RBBB and two ventricle anatomies that develop right ventricular dysfunction in later years. In many, for example with TOF, the RBBB is accompanied by significant degrees of pulmonary insufficiency, adding a volume load onto the dyssynchronous activation of the RV. Restoration of pulmonary valve competency can improve many patients if the operation is performed before the RV becomes too large. An additional

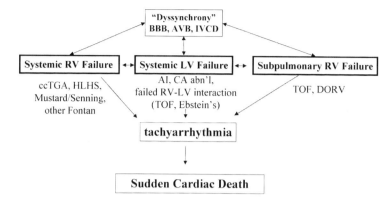

Fig. 23.3 Relationship of heart failure and sudden cardiac death in adult congenital heart disease. *AI* aortic insufficiency; *AVB* atrioventricular block; *BBB* bundle branch block; *CA* coarctation of the aorta; *ccTGA* congenitally corrected transposition of the great arteries; *DORV* double outlet right ventricle; *HLHS* hypoplastic left heart syndrome; *IVCD* intraventricular conduction delay; *LV* left ventricular; *RV* right ventricular; *TOF* tetralogy of Fallot

subgroup will likely show benefit of RV resynchronization, most often with the RV lead placed in a lateral location in the area of latest RV activation.

• *CRT for patients with single ventricle physiology.* This group of patients is perhaps the most difficult to investigate in any organized fashion to draw conclusions that would apply across the spectrum of CHD defects. Some patients in this group have relatively narrow QRS complexes but global dyssynchrony of the single myocardial mass. Electrophysiologic studies to test pacing sites may be necessary to prove potential benefit prior to attempting CRT. In some patients, a small outflow chamber remnant of the diminutive ventricle persists. In this setting, a *bundle branch block* pattern activation can result in this chamber behaving like a reservoir with the force of contraction spilling back and forth within the chambers rather than providing effective prograde cardiac output. This subgroup should benefit from CRT.

23.5 Looking Ahead: Cardiac Rhythm, Device Therapies, and Sudden Cardiac Death in the Adult Population with CHD

The adult population with CHD is increasing in overall complexity as those patients who began life with complex CHD lesions in the early 1990s are surviving in greater numbers into their adult years (Fig. 23.4). This group of patients is at high risk of sudden cardiac death, but receive ICD and CRT interventions in a small fraction of the candidate population based on published reports of device effectiveness in small numbers of patients. This dynamic of change in the adult CHD population clearly influences the scope of care for the adult CHD patient and

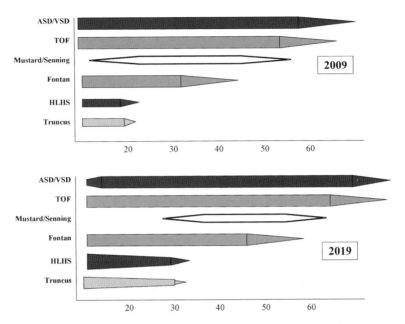

Fig. 23.4 A representation of the changing spectrum of adult congenital heart disease population. *ASD* atrial septal defect; *HLHS* hypoplastic left heart syndrome; *TOF* tetralogy of Fallot; *VSD* ventricular septal defect

should dictate a demand for both specialized training programs and regionalized adult CHD centers. Programs for quality adult CHD care in the USA will require collaboration of some of the best that the pediatric and adult cardiology communities have to offer. Given the politics of healthcare, the financial incentives in both academic and private physician settings, and the attitudes of many pediatric and adult providers that they are capable of taking care of these complex patients on their own, the development of an effective adult CHD care model in the USA will remain a daunting task. The solution that benefits the adult CHD patient will likely require eventual societal or institutional enforcement of some kind.

23.6 Putting It All Together

Those who care for arrhythmia issues in pediatric and CHD patients are constantly on the watch for research performed at the cellular level to lead to suggestions of new care paradigms for their patients. The pediatric and congenital heart electrophysiology world is one of constant adaptation and innovation for these special, often underserved, populations.

The arrhythmogenic framework for CHD of genetics and anatomy, surgical intervention, and hemodynamics can be used to examine areas of research that can advance the field and ultimately be integrated into the care of these patients.

From a *genetic* standpoint, one may well ask why, with the exception of some long QT patients, do we not see channelopathy patients presenting with arrhythmia and sudden death uniformly at a much younger age or even in utero? The effect of age-dependent changes in electrophysiologic (EP) parameters is paramount to the pediatric and CHD electrophysiologist, even to understand the background of *natural history* components of arrhythmia. Similarly, do SNPs found for cardiac ion channels have an age-dependent effect on arrhythmogenesis and the response to antiarrhythmic agents?

Anatomically, are there associations of ion channel dysfunction with specific CHD types that will dictate the presence and timing of arrhythmia? In the ccTGA population, why do we see some of these patients born with congenital complete AV block and not all? Are there EP manifestations of altered structural CHD that result in disparities of fiber orientation, refractoriness, functional block, and conduction velocities that make arrhythmia inevitable?

Surgically, what are the EP sequelae of the incision in the near-field that help maintain tachyarrhythmia? Are there protective EP mechanisms that prevent reentry or automaticity in this setting from being incessant and do they provide a basis for surgical revision, prevention, or therapy?

And lastly, when *hemodynamics* result in unfavorable effects on cellular remodeling, what specific factors in the sarcomere relate to associated and deleterious effects on ion channel function in the sarcolemma?

The descriptive phases of pediatric and congenital heart EP are almost complete, with the exception of the adult CHD population. The trend going forward must utilize a tighter link from the bench to the bedside in order to understand the intrinsic genetic and anatomic EP substrates present at birth, the EP effects of surgical intervention, and subsequent hemodynamic residua that will confront the patient throughout life.

References

1. Khairy P. EP challenges in adult congenital heart disease. Heart Rhythm 2008; 5:1464–72.
2. Ko JK, Deal BJ, Strasburger JF, et al. Supraventricular tachycardia mechanisms and their age distribution in pediatric patients. Am J Cardiol 1992; 69:1028–32.
3. Perry JC. Supraventricular tachycardia. In: Garson A Jr, Bricker JT, Fisher DJ, Neish SN, editors. The science and practice of pediatric cardiology, 2nd edition. Philadelphia: Lea & Febiger, 1997.
4. Perry JC, Garson A Jr. Supraventricular tachycardia due to Wolff-Parkinson-White in children: early disappearance and late recurrence. J Am Coll Cardiol 1990; 16:1215–20.
5. Weindling SN, Saul JP, Gamble WJ, et al. Duration of complete atrioventricular block after congenital heart disease surgery. Am J Cardiol 1998; 82:525–7.
6. Hokanson JS, Moller JH. Significance of early transient complete heart block as a predictor of sudden death after portative correction of tetralogy of Fallot. Am J Cardiol 2001; 87:1271–7.
7. Van Hare GF, Chiesa NA, Campbell RM, et al. Atrioventricular nodal reentry tachycardia in children: effect of slow pathway ablation on fast pathway conduction. J Cardiovasc Electrophys 2002; 13:203–9.

8. Dunnigan A, Benditt DG, Benson DW. Modes of onset ("initiating events") for paroxysmal atrial tachycardia in infants and children. Am J Cardiol 1986; 57:1280–7.

9. Friedman RA, Walsh EP, Silka MJ, et al. NASPE Expert Consensus Conference: Radiofrequency catheter ablation in children with and without congenital heart disease. Pacing Clin Electrophysiol 2002; 25:1000–17.

10. Frame LH, Page RL, Hoffman BF. Atrial reentry around an anatomic barrier with a partially refractory excitable gap. A canine model of atrial flutter. Circ Res 1986; 58:495–511.

11. Zeppenfeld K, Schalij MJ, Bartelings MM, et al. Catheter ablation of ventricular tachycardia after repair of congenital heart disease: electroanatomic identification of the critical right ventricular isthmus. Circulation 2007; 116:2241–52.

12. Cecchin F, Johnsrude CL, Perry JC, et al. Effect of age and surgical technique on symptomatic arrhythmias after the Fontan procedure. Am J Cardiol 1995; 76:386–91.

13. Giannico S, Hammad F, Amodeo A, et al. Clinical outcome of 193 extracardiac Fontan patients: the first 15 years. J Am Coll Cardiol 2006; 47:2065–73.

14. Villain E. Indications for pacing in patients with congenital heart disease. Pacing Clin Electrophysiol 2008; 31: S17–20.

15. Van Hare GF, Lesh MD, Ross BA, et al. Mapping and radiofrequency ablation of intra-atrial reentrant tachycardia after the Senning or Mustard procedure. Am J Cardiol 1996; 77:985–91.

16. Garson A, Gillette PC, McVey P, et al. Atrial flutter in the young: a collaborative study of 380 cases. J Am Coll Cardiol 1985; 6:871–8.

17. Khairy P, Landzberg MJ, Gatzoulis MA, et al. Value of programmed ventricular stimulation after tetralogy of Fallot repair: a multicenter study. Circulation 2004; 109:1994–2000.

18. Therrien J, Siu SC, Harris L, et al. Impact of pulmonary valve replacement on arrhythmia propensity late after repair of tetralogy of Fallot. Circulation 2001; 103:2489–94.

19. Chen P, Xie LJ, Huang GY, et al. Mutations of connexin43 in fetuses with congenital heart malformations. Chin Med J 2005; 118:971–6.

20. Juang JM, Chern YR, Tsai CT, et al. The association of human connexin 40 genetic polymorphisms with atrial fibrillation. Int J Cardiol 2007; 116:107–12.

21. Warnes CA, Williams RG, Bashore TM, et al. ACC/AHA 2008 Guidelines for the management of adults with congenital heart disease. J Am Coll Cardiol 2008; 52:e1–121.

22. Piran S, Veldtman G, Siu S, et al. Heart failure and dysfunction in patients with single or systemic right ventricle. Circulation 2002; 105:1189–94.

23. Pasquali SK, Marino BS, Kaltman JR, et al. Rhythm and conduction disturbances at midterm follow-up after the Ross procedure in infants, children and young adults. Ann Thorac Surg 2008; 85:2072–8.

24. Davlouros PA, Kilner PJ, Hornung TS, et al. Right ventricular function in adults with repaired tetralogy of Fallot assessed with cardiovascular magnetic resonance imaging: detrimental role of right ventricular outflow tract aneurysms or akinesia and adverse right-to-left ventricular interaction. J Am Coll Cardiol 2002; 40:204–52.

25. Graham TP, Bernard YD, Mellen BG, et al. Long-term outcome in congenitally corrected transposition of the great arteries: a multi-institutional study. J Am Coll Cardiol 2000; 36:255–61.

26. Hornung TS, Bernard EJ, Jaeggi ET, et al. Myocardial perfusion defects and associated systemic ventricular dysfunction in congenitally corrected transposition of the great arteries. Heart 1998; 80:322–6.

27. Perry JC. Pharmacologic therapy of arrhythmias. In: Wolff GS, Deal BJ, editors. Arrhythmias in the neonate, infant and child. Armonk, NY: Futura Pub. Co., 1998.

28. Ye B, Valdivia CR, Ackerman MA, et al. A common human SCN5A polymorphism modifies expression of an arrhythmia causing mutation. Physiol Genomics 2003; 12:187–93.

29. Perry JC, McQuinn R, Smith RT, et al. Flecainide acetate for resistant arrhythmias in the young: efficacy and pharmacokinetics. J Am Coll Cardiol 1989; 14:185–91.

30. Saul JP, Ross B, Schaffer MS, et al. Pharmacokinetics and pharmacodynamics of sotalol in a pediatric population with supraventricular and ventricular tachyarrhythmia. Clin Pharmacol Ther 2001; 69:145–57.

31. Epstein AE, Hallstrom AP, Rogers WJ, et al. Mortality following ventricular arrhythmia suppression by encainide, flecainide and moricizine after myocardial infarction. The original design concept of the Cardiac Arrhythmia Suppression Trial (CAST). JAMA 1993; 270:2451–5.
32. Perry JC, Garson A Jr. Flecainide acetate for pediatric tachyarrhythmias: review of world literature on efficacy, safety and dosing. Am Heart J 1992; 124:1614–21.
33. Fish FA, Gillette PC, Benson DW. Proarrhythmia, cardiac arrest and sudden death in young patients receiving encainide and flecainide. The Pediatric Electrophysiology Group. J Am Coll Cardiol 1991; 18:356–65.
34. Schaffer MS, Silka MJ, Ross BA, et al. Inadvertent atrioventricular block during radiofrequency catheter ablation. Results of the Pediatric Radiofrequency Catheter Ablation Registry. Circulation 1996; 94:3214–20.
35. Al-Ammouri I, Perry JC. Proximity of the coronary arteries to the atrioventricular valve annulus in young patients: implications for ablation procedures. Am J Cardiol 2006; 97:1752–5.
36. Van Hare GF, Javitz H, Carmelli D, et al. Prospective assessment after pediatric catheter ablation: demographics, medical profiles, and initial outcomes. J Cardiovasc Electrophys 2004; 15:759–70.
37. Epstein AE, DiMarco JP, Ellenbogen KA, et al. ACC/AHA/HRS 2008 Guidelines for device-based therapy of cardiac rhythm abnormalities. Heart Rhythm 2008; 5:e1–62.
38. Friedman RA, VanZandt H, Collins E, et al. Lead extraction in young patients with and without congenital heart disease. Pacing Clin Electrophysiol 1996; 19:778–83.
39. Boramanand NK, Perry JC. Expected prevalence of cardiac rhythm management device need in the adult congenital heart population: evidence of a large and under-treated population. Philadelphia Adult Congenital Heart Symposium, 2007.
40. Berul CI, Van Hare GF, Kertesz NJ, et al. Results of a multicenter retrospective implantable cardioverter-defibrillator registry of pediatric and congenital heart disease patients. J Am Col Cardiol 2008; 51:1685–91.
41. Jolley M, Stinstra J, Pieper S, et al. A computer modeling tool for comparing novel ICD electrode orientation in children and adults. Heart Rhythm 2008; 5:565–72.

Index

Printed by Printforce, the Netherlands